SPA

SCHÖNHEIT, GESUNDHEIT & DESIGN
BEAUTY, HEALTH & DESIGN
SPAS DE RÊVE
SCHOONHEID, GEZONDHEID & DESIGN

SPA

SCHÖNHEIT, GESUNDHEIT & DESIGN
BEAUTY, HEALTH & DESIGN
SPAS DE RÊVE
SCHOONHEID, GEZONDHEID & DESIGN

FKG

FKG

Editorial project:
2008 © **LOFT Publications**
Via Laietana, 32, 4.º, Of. 92
08003 Barcelona, Spain
Tel.: +34 932 688 088
Fax: +34 932 687 073
loft@loftpublications.com
www.loftpublications.com

Art director:
Mireia Casanovas Soley

Editorial coordination:
Simone Schleifer

Editor:
Daniela Santos Quartino

Texts:
LOFT Publications

Layout:
TRAMA, estudi gràfic
www.tramaestudi.com

Translations coordination:
Equipo de Edición, Barcelona
Translations: Heike Reissig (German), Éditions 360 (French),
Persklaar (Dutch)

ISBN 978-84-96936-80-5

Printed in China

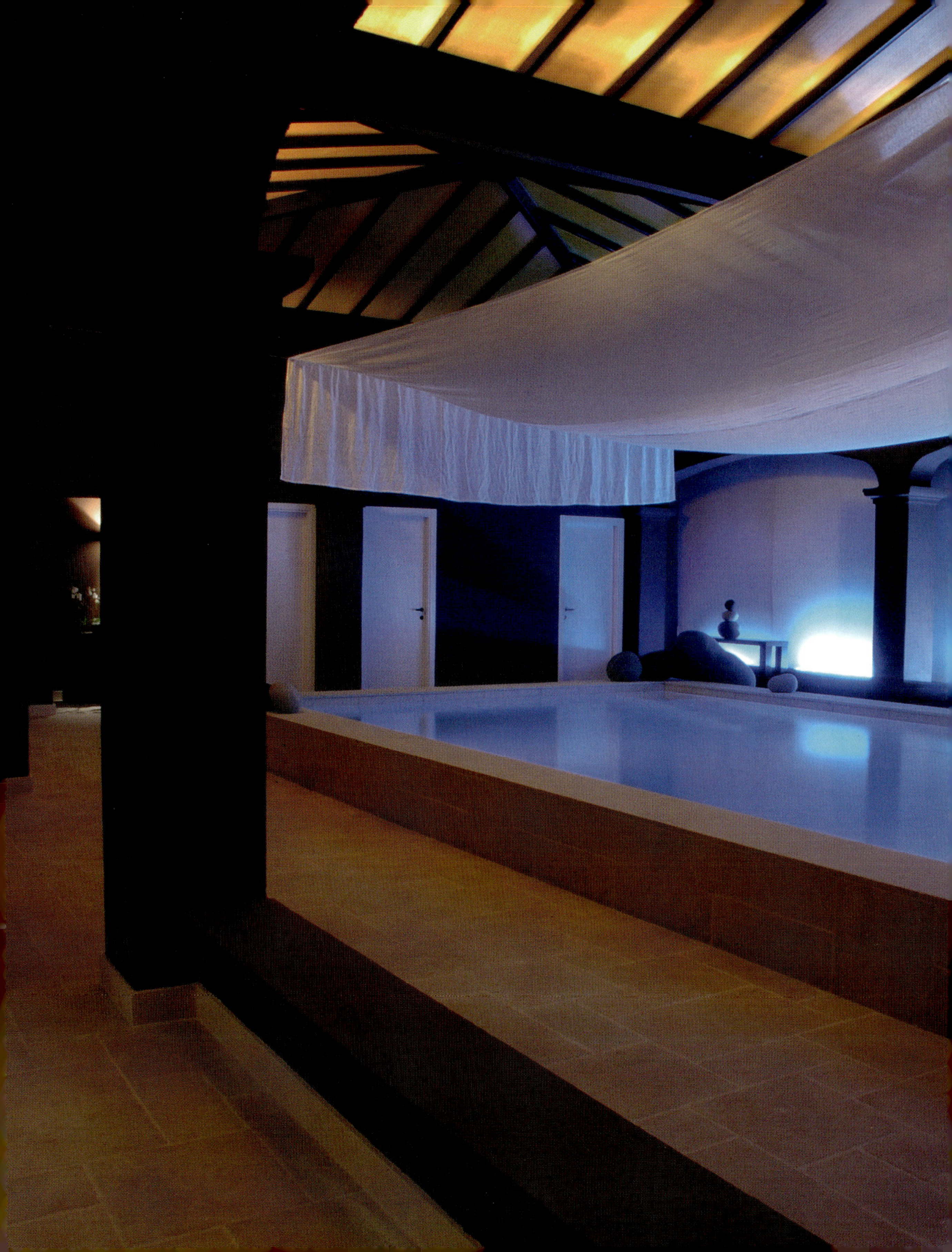

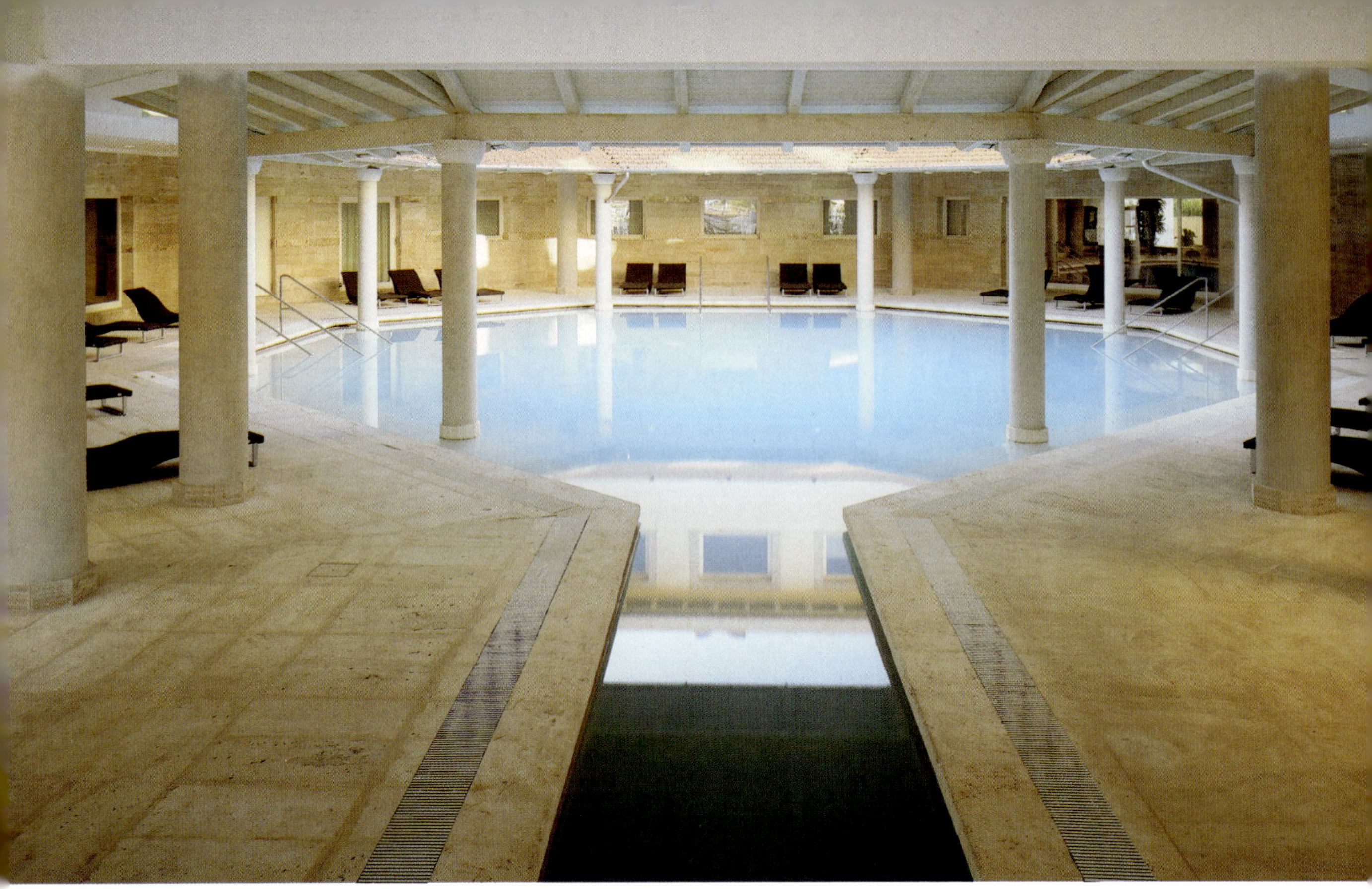

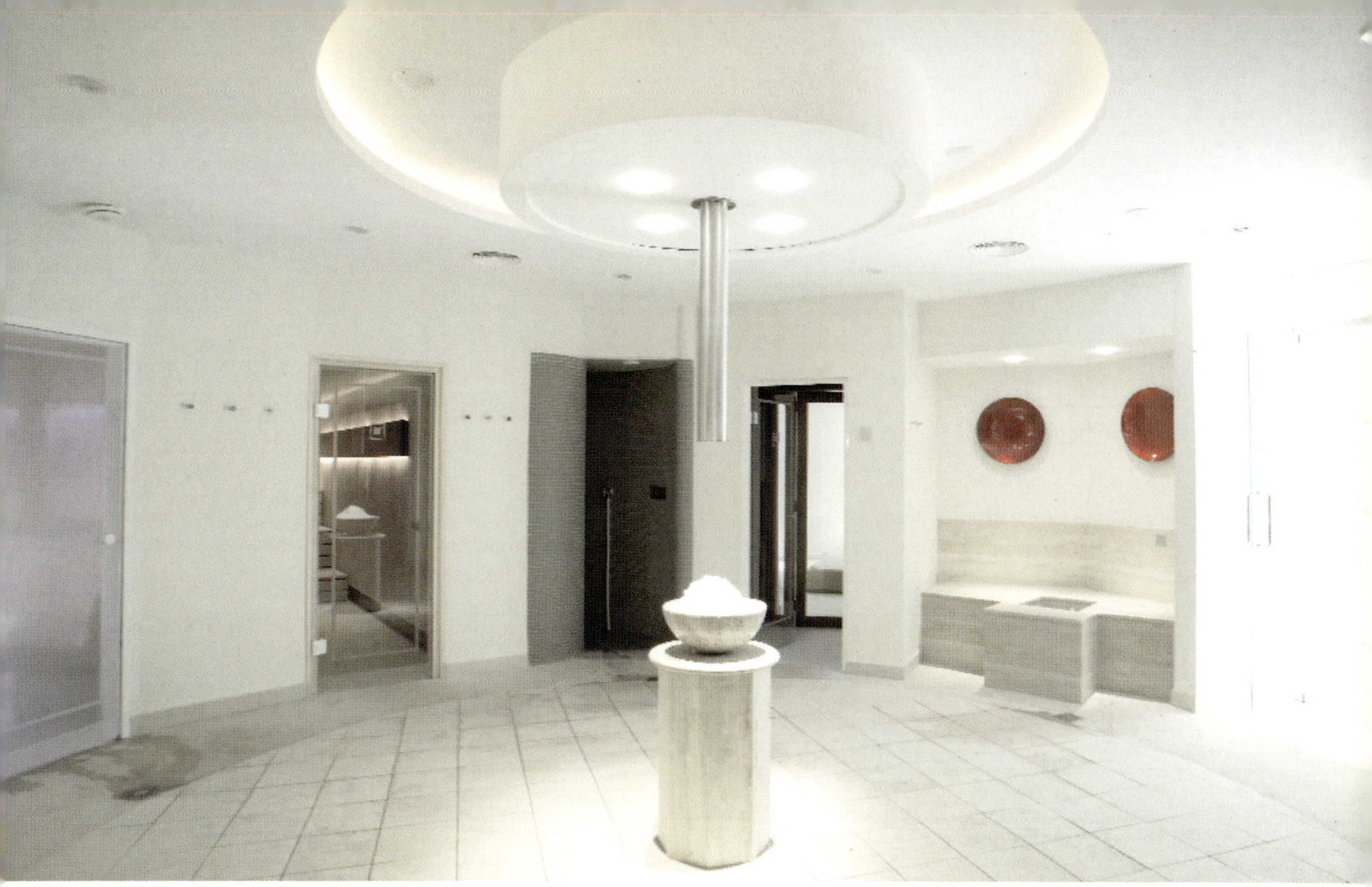

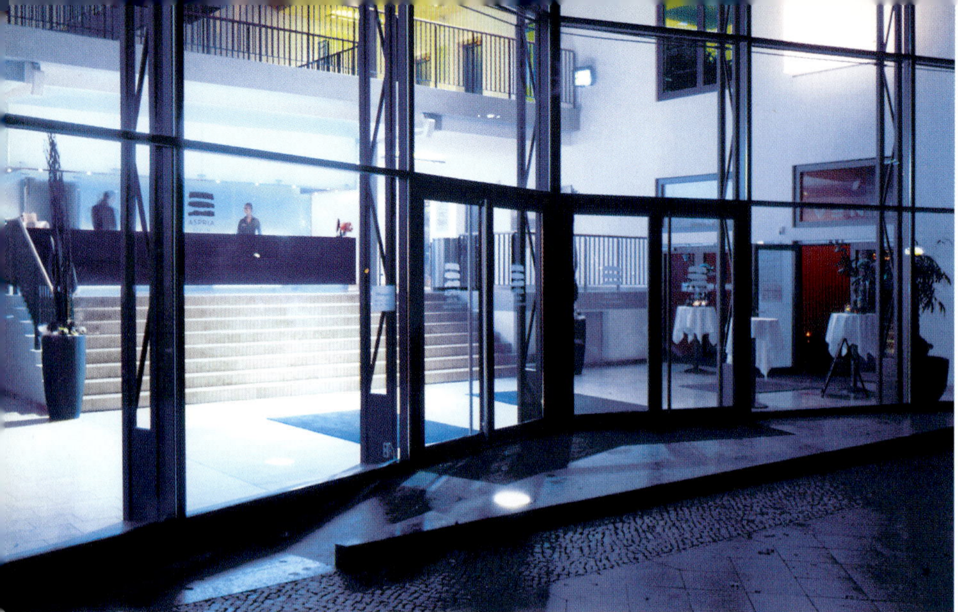

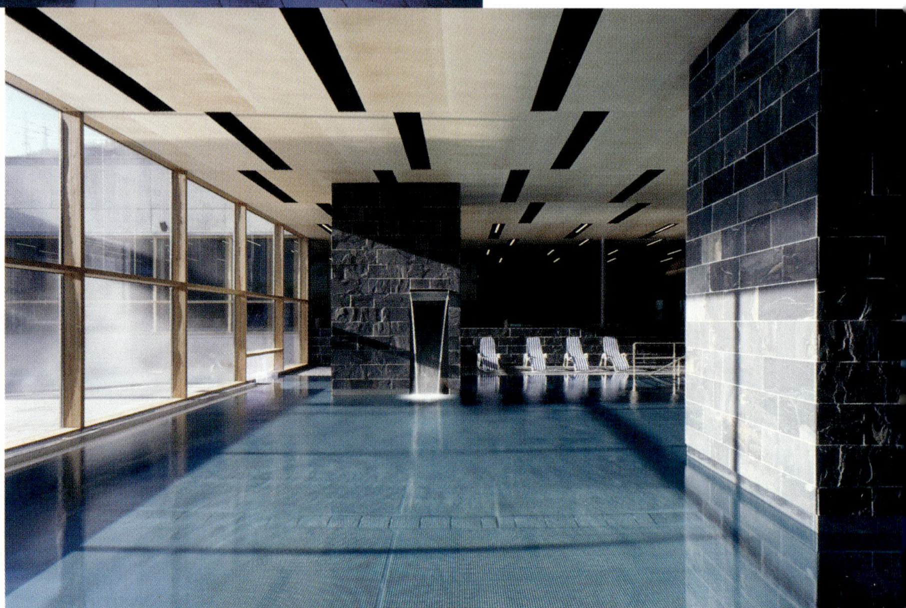

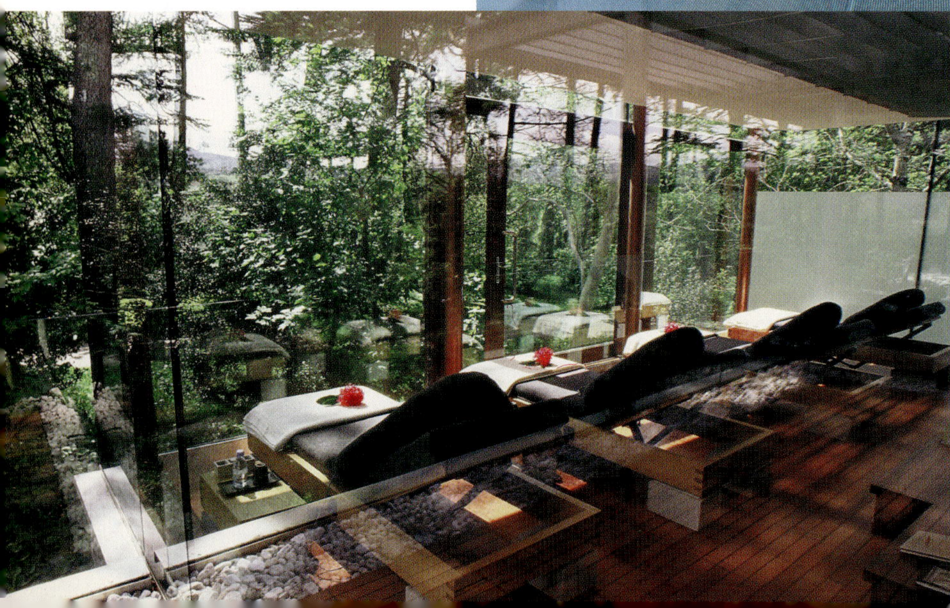

Europäische Spas sind in vielerlei Hinsicht einzigartig. Von türkischen Dampfbädern über Vinotherapie in Frankreich, Thalassotherapie in Griechenland bis hin zu alpinen Thermalbädern verfügt Europa über ein weitmaschiges Netzwerk renommierter Einrichtungen. Sie alle stützen sich auf eine seit vielen Jahrhunderten bewährte Tradition, deren jüngstes Element die Fitnessbewegung ist. Fitnessstudios sind heute nicht mehr wegzudenken, denn Wohlbefinden wird längst nicht mehr nur als Erfahrung des Ausruhens begriffen, sondern auch als das Ergebnis körperlicher Aktivität. Ein weiterer bedeutender Aspekt, der den Spas des alten Kontinents Sonderstatus verleiht, ist das Design: Hier entfaltet sich auf beeindruckende Weise die Kreativität vieler großer Architekten. Golf Spas, Ski Resorts, Thermalbäder und Health Clubs stellen nur einige der neuen Möglichkeiten für all jene dar, die sportliche Aktivität mit Entspannung und dem Vergessen des Alltags verbinden möchten.

Europe has more than one reason to believe its spas are special. From steam baths in the Turkish hammam, wine therapies in France, thalassotherapies in Greece and even Alpine thermal baths, the continent has a wide network of establishments that claim their identity based on a custom that has been followed for many centuries. The most recent addition to the European model is fitness. Nowadays, gyms are an essential part of the endeavors that conceive wellbeing not only as a pleasant and relaxing experience, but also as a product of physical activity. Design is another great element that makes the spas of the Old Continent stand apart. They awaken the interest of great architects and interior designers that do not hesitate to leave their imprint in these spaces. Golf spas, ski resorts, thermal resorts and health clubs are some of the new options available for a public that is eager to combine hobbies with relaxation and with the desire of escaping the daily routine.

L'Europe a plus d'une raison d'être persuadée que ses spas sont uniques. Hammam en Turquie, vinothérapie en France, thalassothérapies en Grèce, et même, bains thermaux dans les Alpes : le Vieux Continent possède un large réseau d'établissements qui revendiquent une identité basée sur des traditions transmises depuis des siècles. Des prestations nouvelles apparaissent toutefois, dont la dernière en date est le fitness. De nos jours, les salles de remise en forme sont un des éléments essentiels qui conçoivent le bien-être non seulement comme une expérience agréable et relaxante, mais aussi comme un produit d'activité physique. Le design est un autre des éléments essentiels faisant des spas européens des lieux à part. Ils éveillent l'intérêt de grands architectes et d'architectes d'intérieur qui n'hésitent pas à laisser leur empreinte dans ces espaces. Les spas de golfs, les stations de sports d'hiver, les stations thermales et les clubs de sports sont autant de nouvelles offres alléchantes pour un public qui désire conjuguer loisirs et relaxation afin d'échapper à la monotonie quotidienne.

Europeanen hebben alle reden om hun thermaalbaden bijzonder te vinden. Met stoombaden in de Turkse hammam, Franse wijntherapieën, Griekse thalassotherapieën en zelfs alpiene bronnenbaden kent het continent een uitgebreid netwerk aan gelegenheden die hun identiteit ontlenen aan een eeuwenoude gewoonte. Een recente toevoeging aan het Europese model is fitness. Fitnessruimten zijn een wezenlijk onderdeel gaan vormen van ondernemingen die 'wellness' niet alleen zien als een ontspannende ervaring, maar ook als een product van lichamelijke inspanning. Architectuur is een tweede element dat de baden in Europa iets bijzonders verleent. Deze etablissementen wekken de belangstelling van grote architecten en interieurontwerpers, die niet aarzelen er hun stempel op te drukken. Golfresorts, skioorden, bronnenbaden en fitnesscentra zijn nog maar een paar moderne mogelijkheden voor een publiek dat zijn liefhebberijen graag combineert met ontspanning om te ontsnappen aan het drukke dagelijkse bestaan.

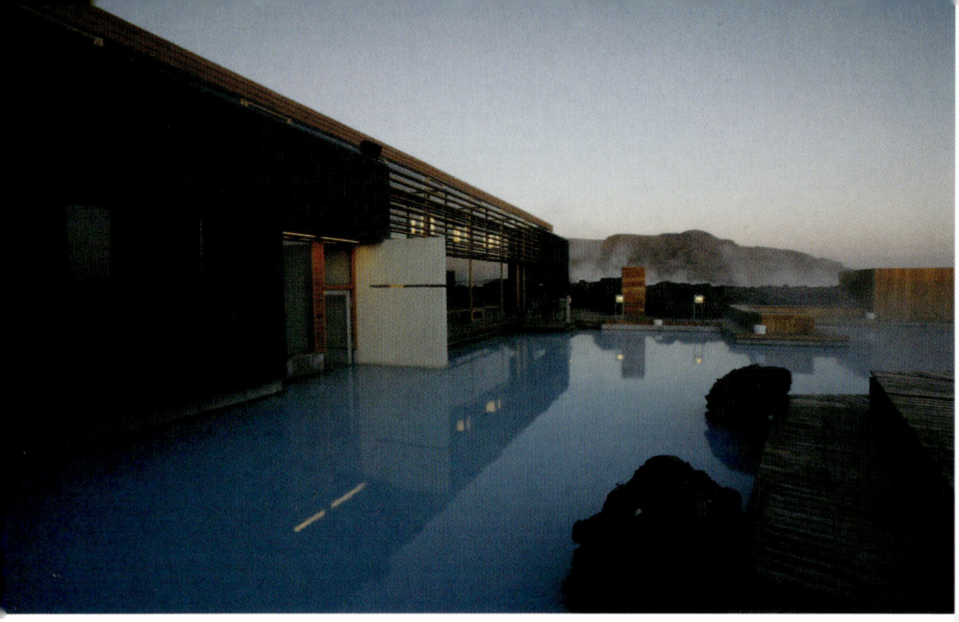
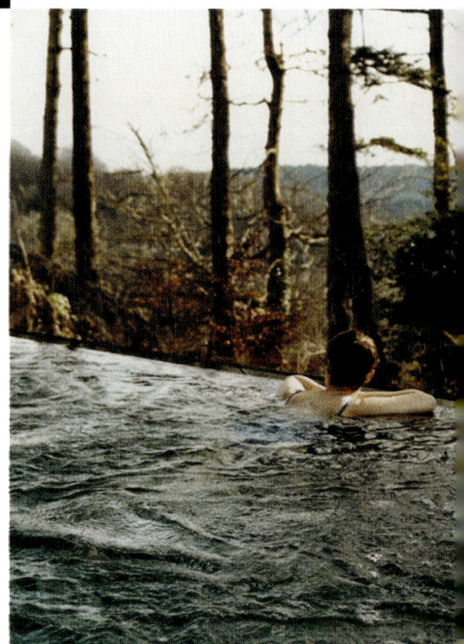
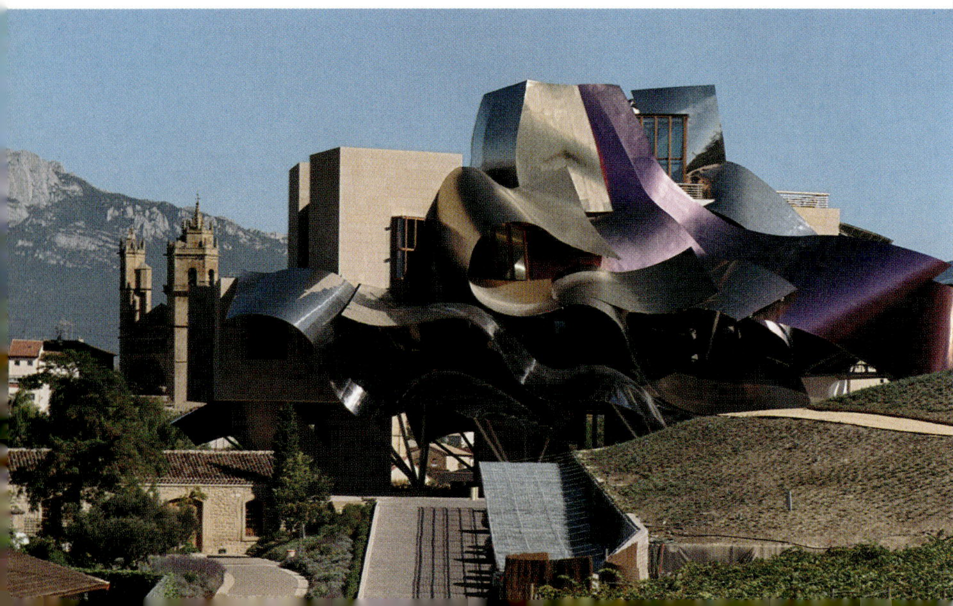

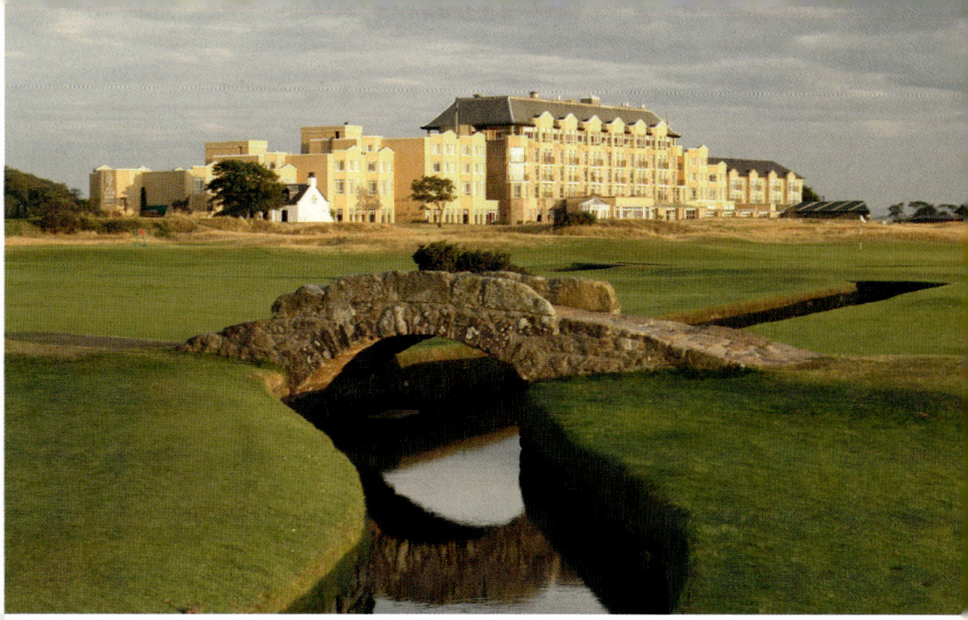

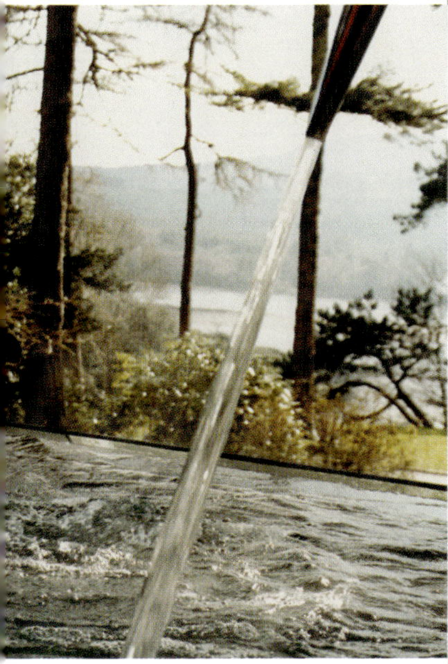

Country Spas

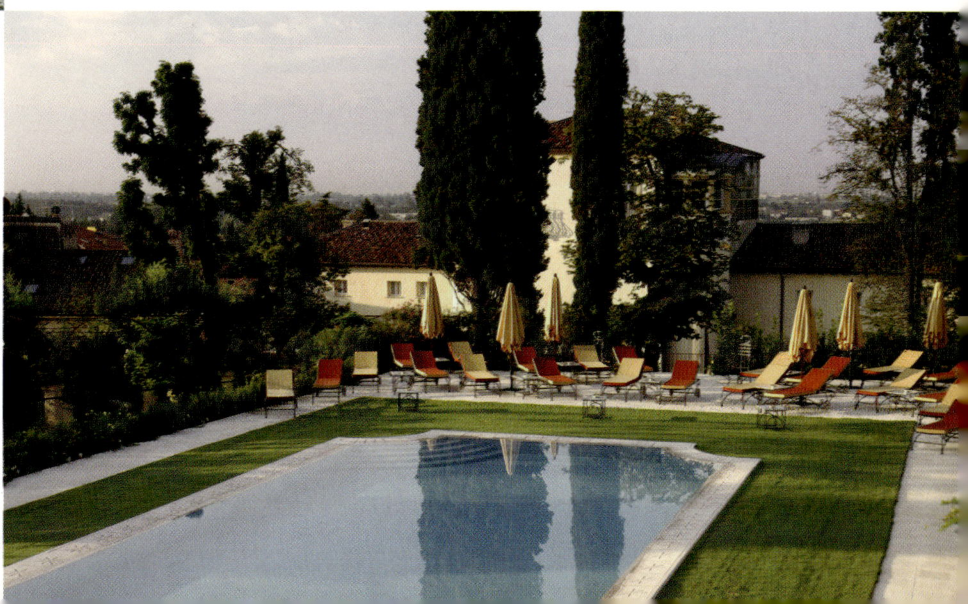

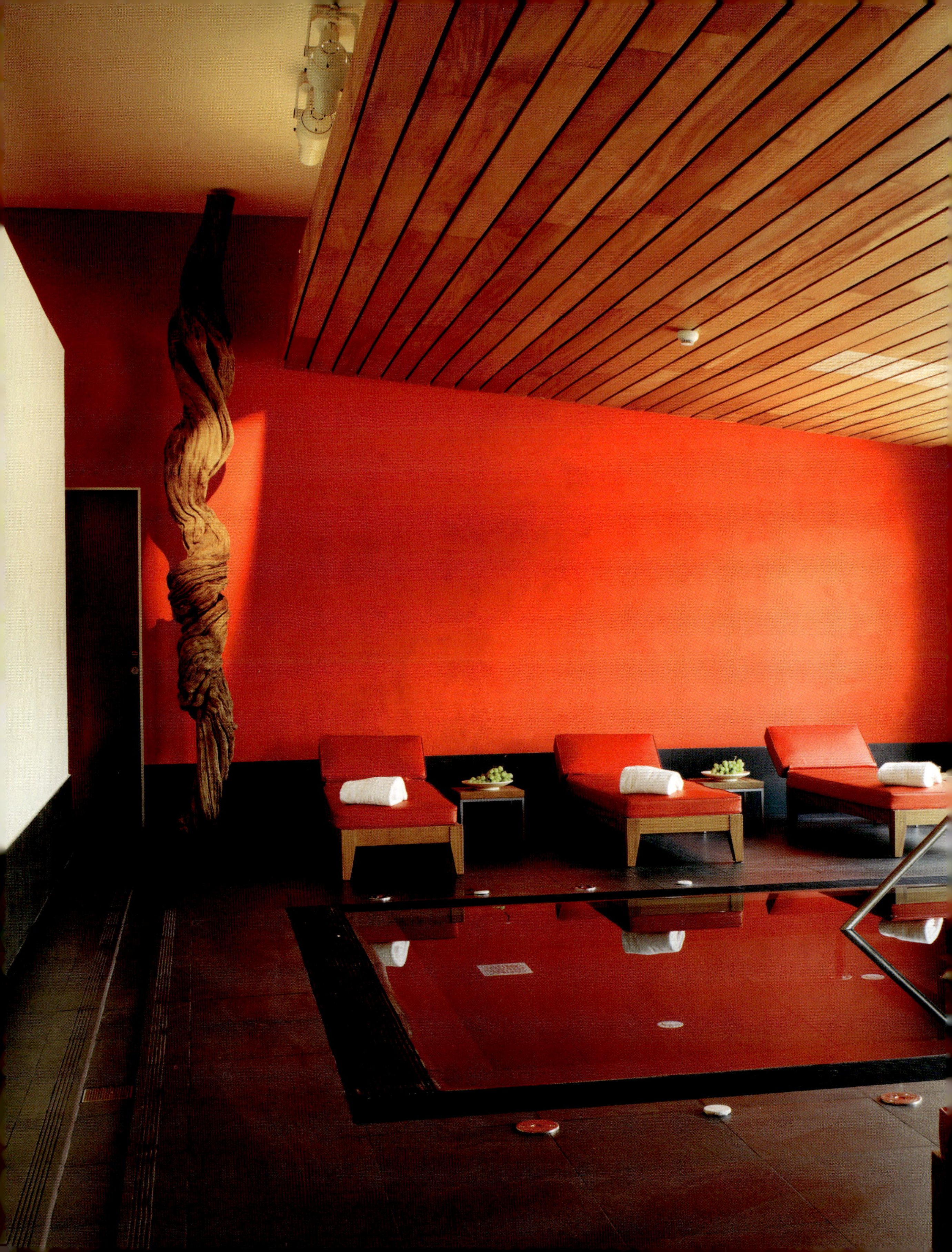

Spa at the Hotel Marqués de Riscal

Dieses vom französischen Vinotherapie-Anbieter Caudalie konzipierte Spa kombiniert den wohltuenden Effekt von Thermalwasser mit dem Extrakt der Weintraube. Die Therapien beinhalten Programme zur Entspannung, Gewichtsreduzierung, Revitalisierung, Stressbewältigung und Anti-Ageing. Das über eine Hängebrücke mit dem Hotel verbundene Spa verfügt über Hallenbad, türkisches Bad, Whirlpool, Erlebnisduschen, Fitnessbereich und 14 Kabinen für Schönheitsbehandlungen.

Caudalie, the French firm that specializes in wine therapy, was called in to build a spa that combines the benefits of thermal waters with the extracts of grapes and wine. Treatments include programs for relaxation, weight loss, invigoration, re-affirmation, anti-stress and anti-age. The spa is connected to the hotel by a suspended footbridge. It has an indoor pool, Turkish bath, cask baths, Jacuzzi, invigorating shower, fitness area and 14 cabins for beauty treatments.

Caudalie, la société française spécialiste de la vinothérapie, a fait construire au cœur de la célèbre Rioja espagnole un spa conjuguant les avantages de la thalassothérapie et les bienfaits des extraits de la vigne et du raisin. Les soins comprennent des programmes dédiés à la relaxation, à la perte de poids, à la revitalisation, ainsi que des programmes anti-stress et anti-âge. Le spa communique avec l'hôtel par une passerelle suspendue. Il comprend une piscine intérieure, un hammam, des bains barriques, un jacuzzi, une douche à jets d'eau de source revitalisante, une salle de fitness et 14 cabines pour les soins esthétiques.

De Franse, in wijntherapie gespecialiseerde firma Caudalie werd erbij gehaald om een bronnenbad te bouwen dat de voordelen van bronwater combineert met die van druiven- en wijnextracten. De behandelingen zijn gericht op ontspanning, gewichtsverlies, versterking en stressbestrijding. Een voetgangersbrug verbindt de thermen met het hotel. Je vindt er een binnenbad, Turks bad, wijntherapiebad, jacuzzi, fitnessruimte, douches en 14 cabines voor schoonheidsbehandelingen.

Rioja Alavesa, Spain

CAUDALIE

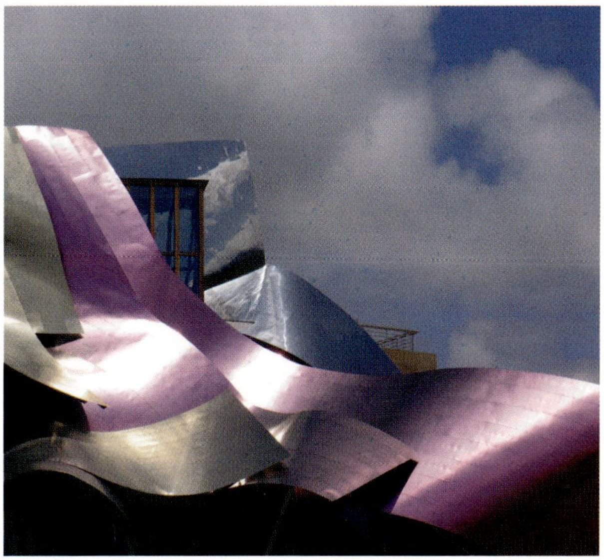

www.marquesderiscal.com

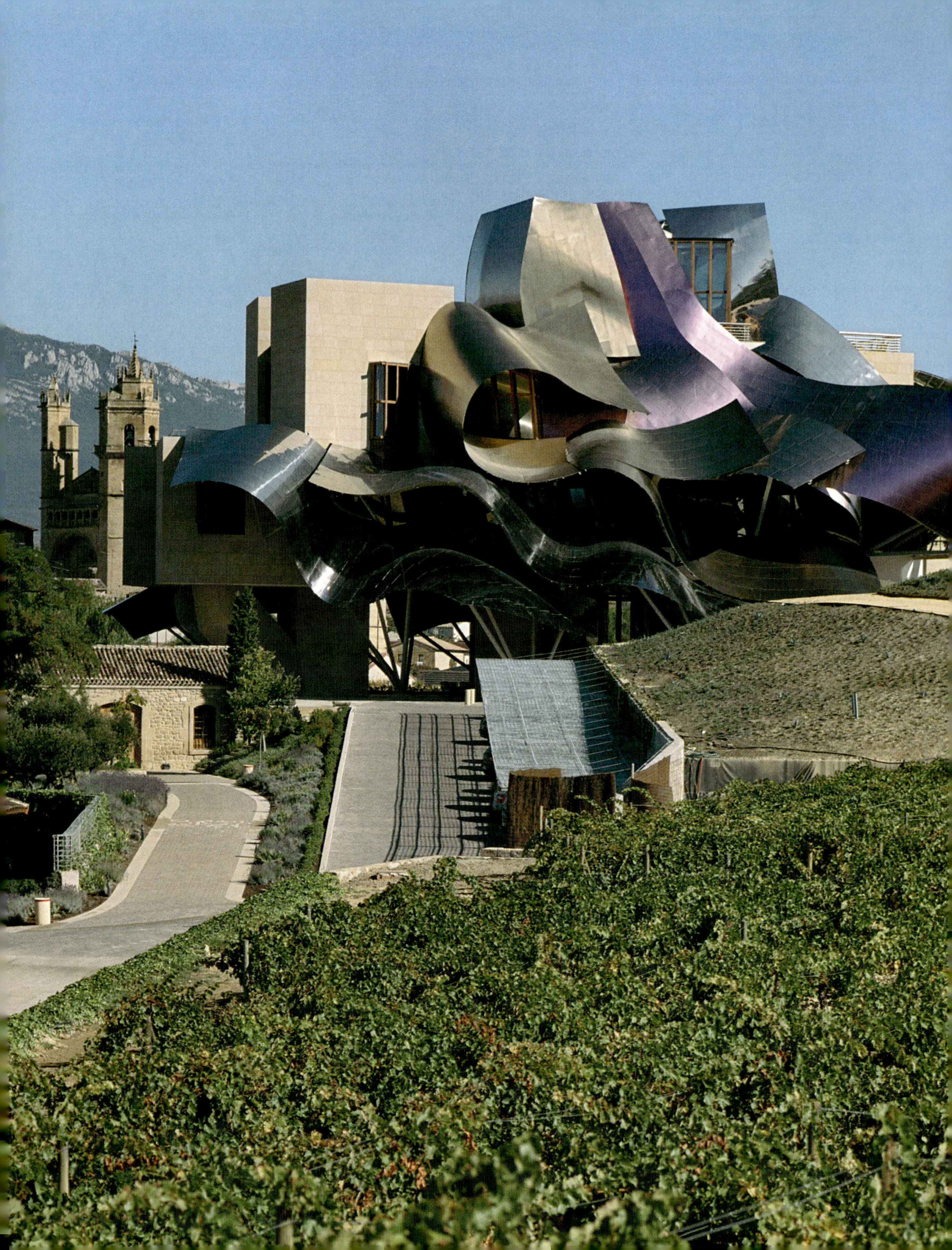

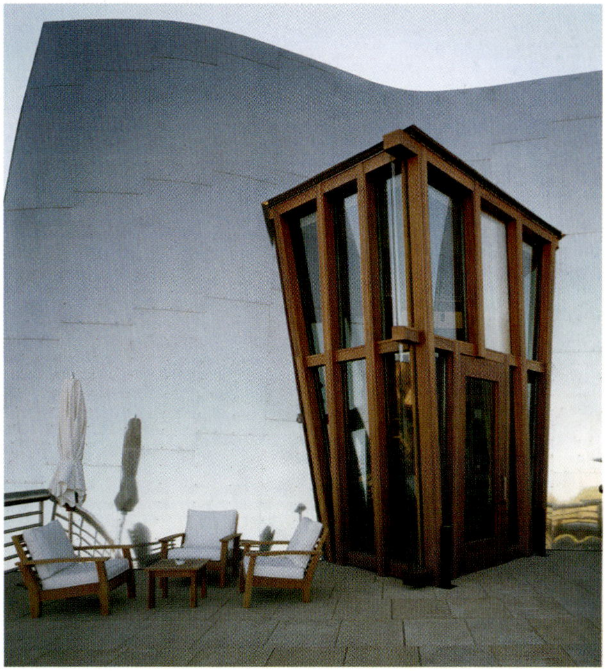

In dem beeindruckend gestalteten Dach des von Frank Gehry erbauten Gebäudes spiegeln sich Landschaft und Himmel.

The building constructed by Frank Gehry has views over the surrounding vineyards which are reflected on the Titanium bands on the roof.

Conçu par Frank Gehry, le bâtiment offre une vue sur les vignobles environnants, qui se reflètent dans les bandes de titane du toit.

Het door Frank Gehry ontworpen gebouw kijkt uit op wijngaarden, die weerspiegeld worden in de titanium dakranden.

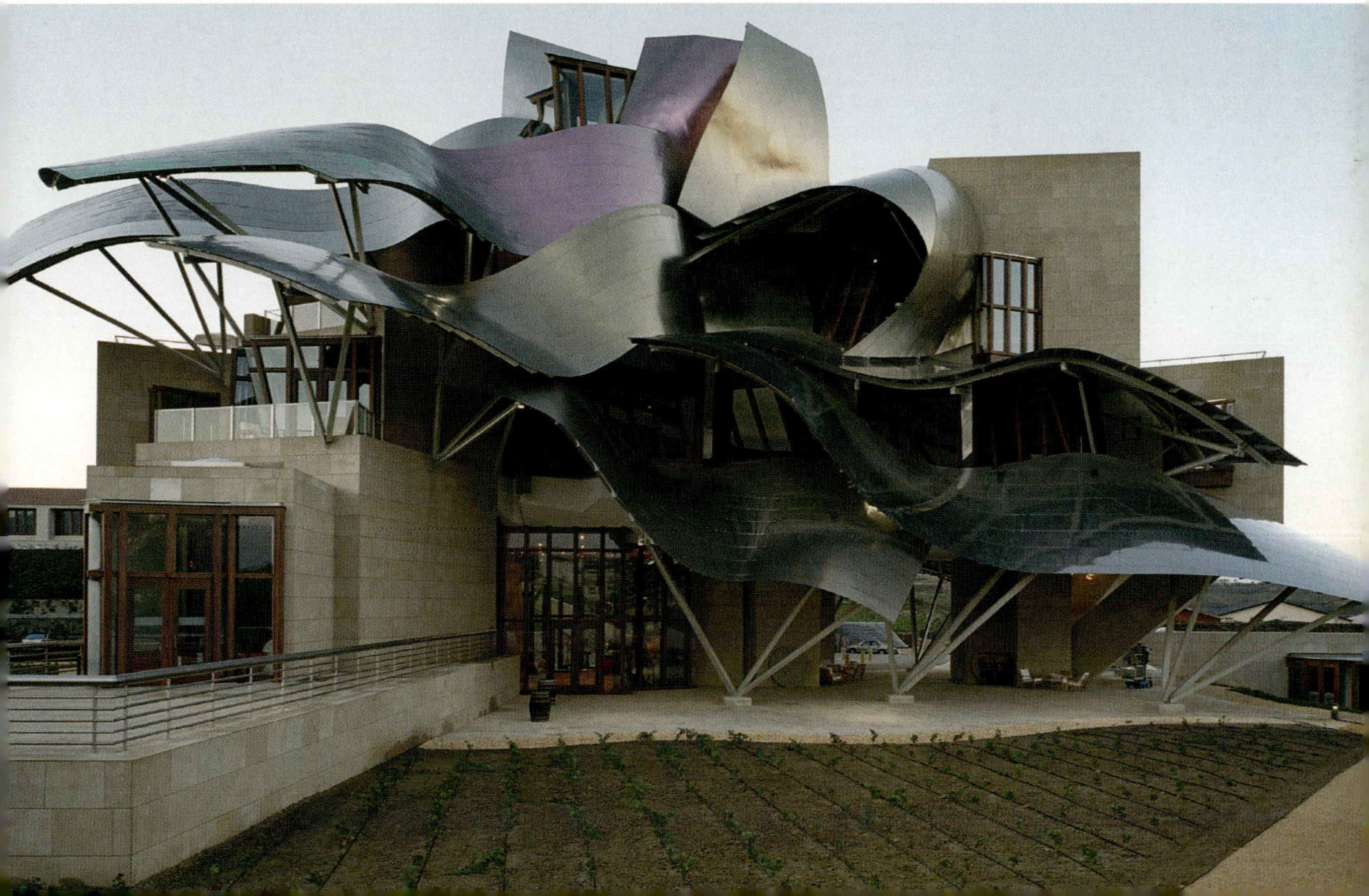

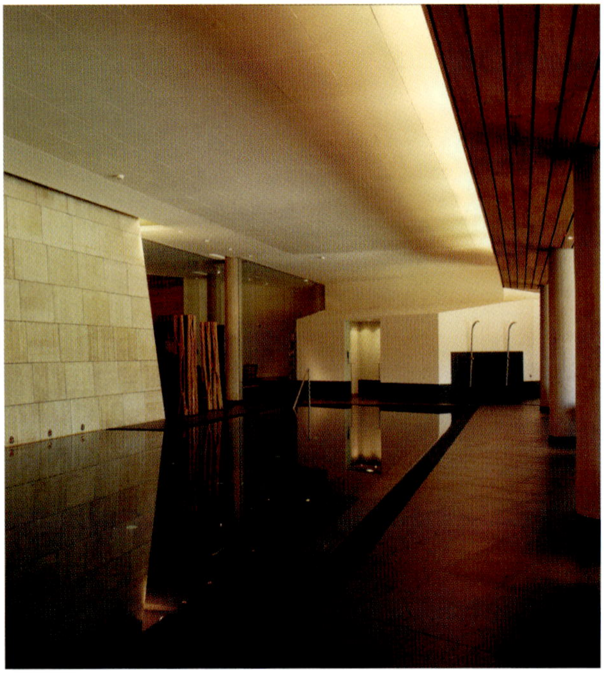

Das Spa besitzt ein Patent auf die Extraktion von Molekülen aus dem Traubenkern.

The spa has a patented formula for extracting molecules from the grape pit.

Le spa est détenteur d'une formule brevetée pour extraire la molécule OPC des pépins de raisin.

Dit ontspanningsoord gebruikt een gepatenteerde formule om bepaalde moleculen te onttrekken aan druivenpitten.

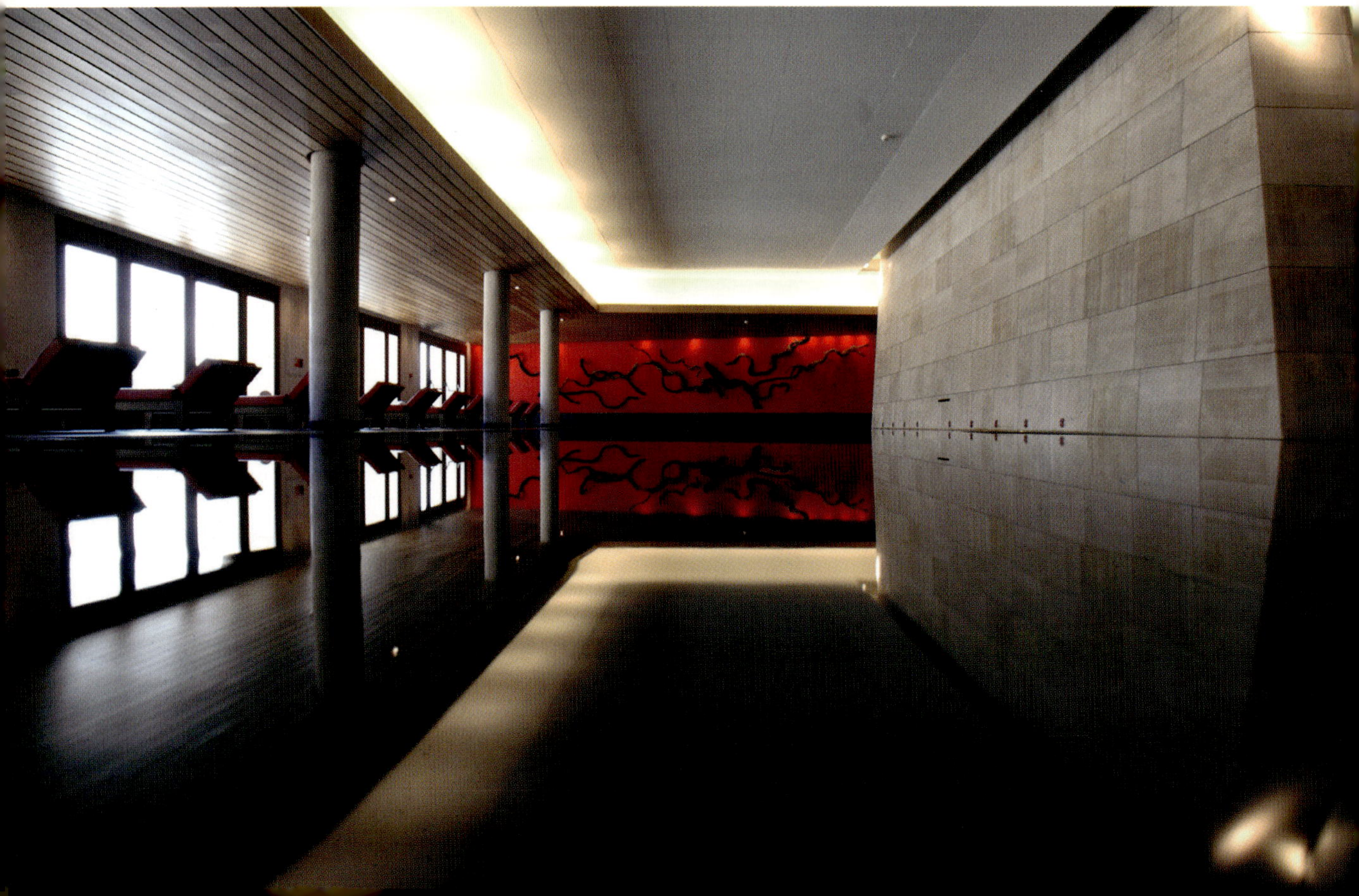

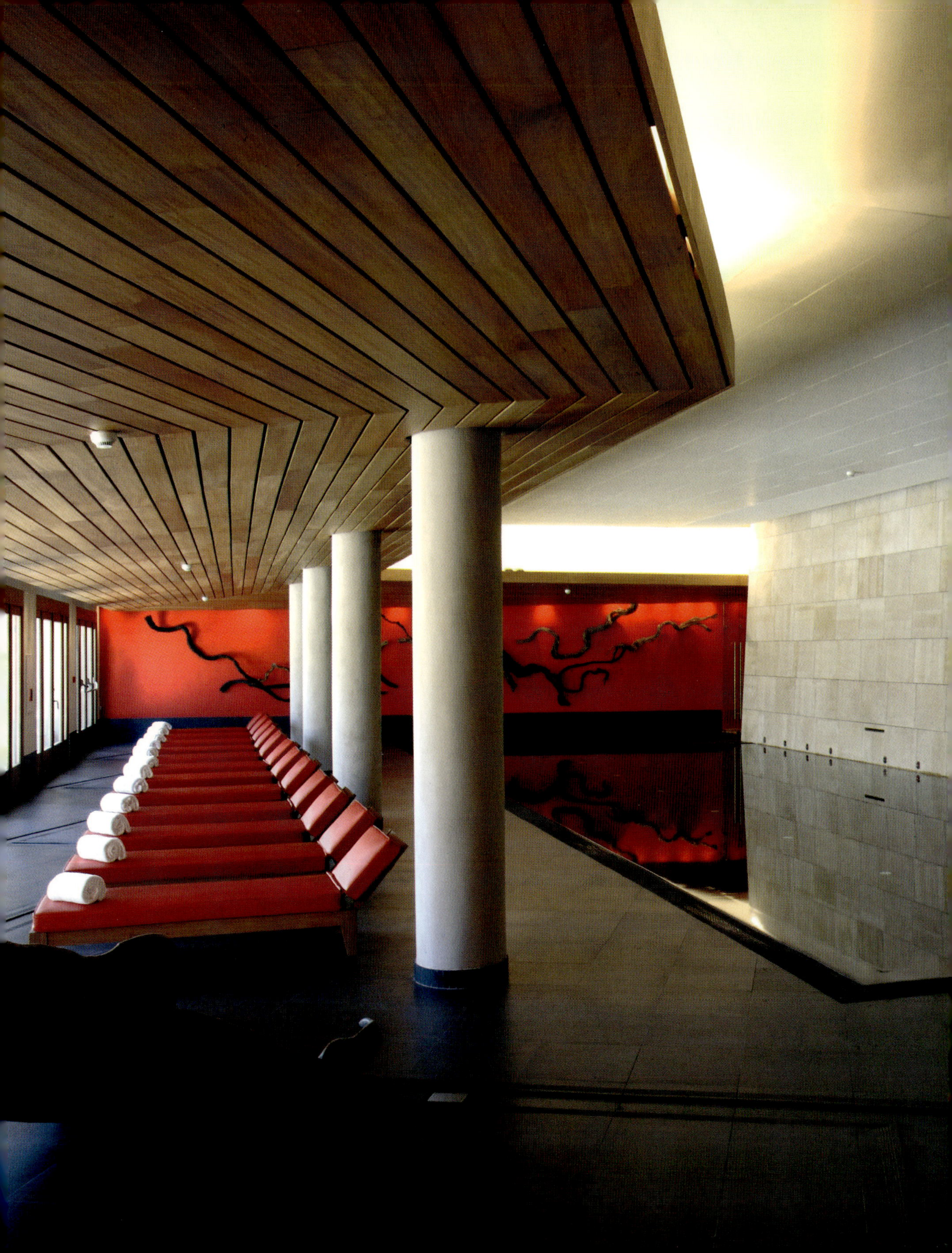

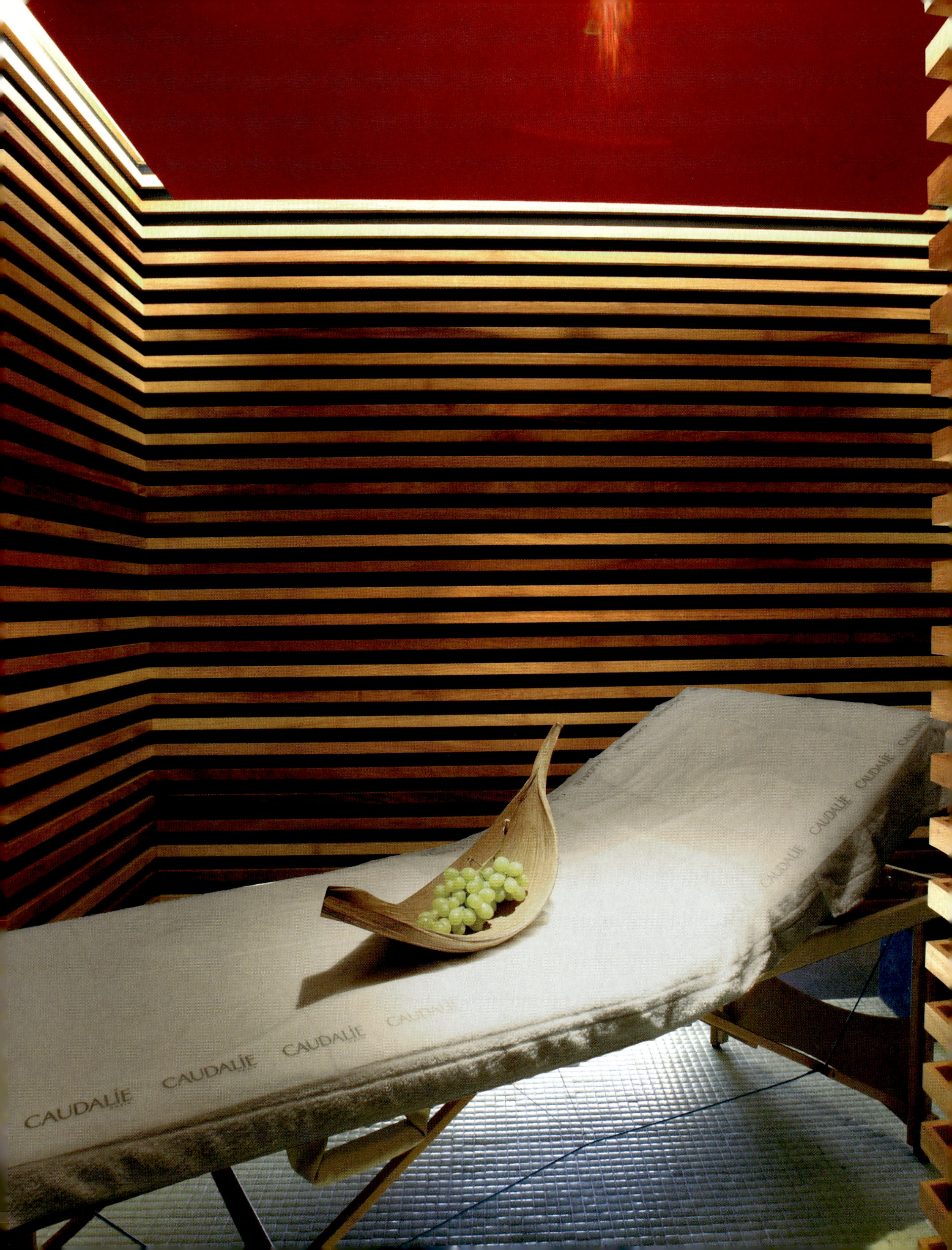
CAUDALIE
CAUDALIE
CAUDALIE
CAUDALIE
CAUDALIE
CAUDALIE
CAUDALIE

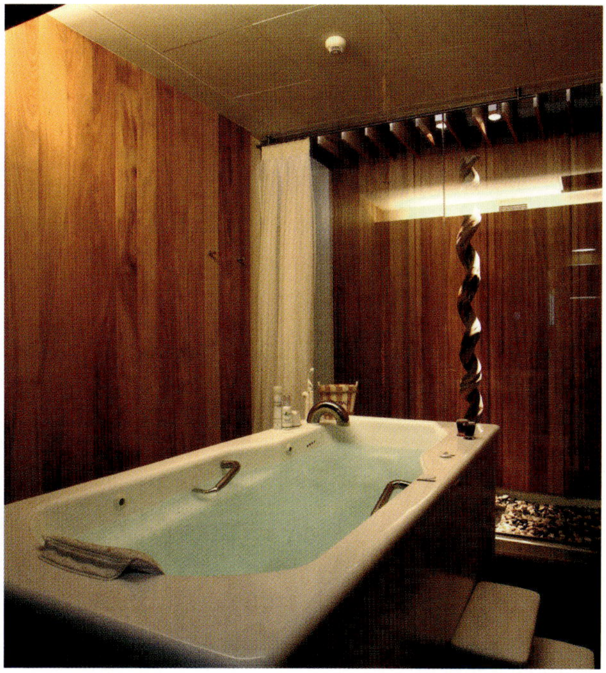

Schönheitsbehandlungen und Massageanwendungen werden in separaten Kabinen angeboten.

Beauty treatments and massage programs are offered in separated cabins.

Des soins de beauté et des programmes de massage sont prodigués dans de vastes cabines indépendantes.

Schoonheidsbehandelingen en massages worden aangeboden in aparte cabines.

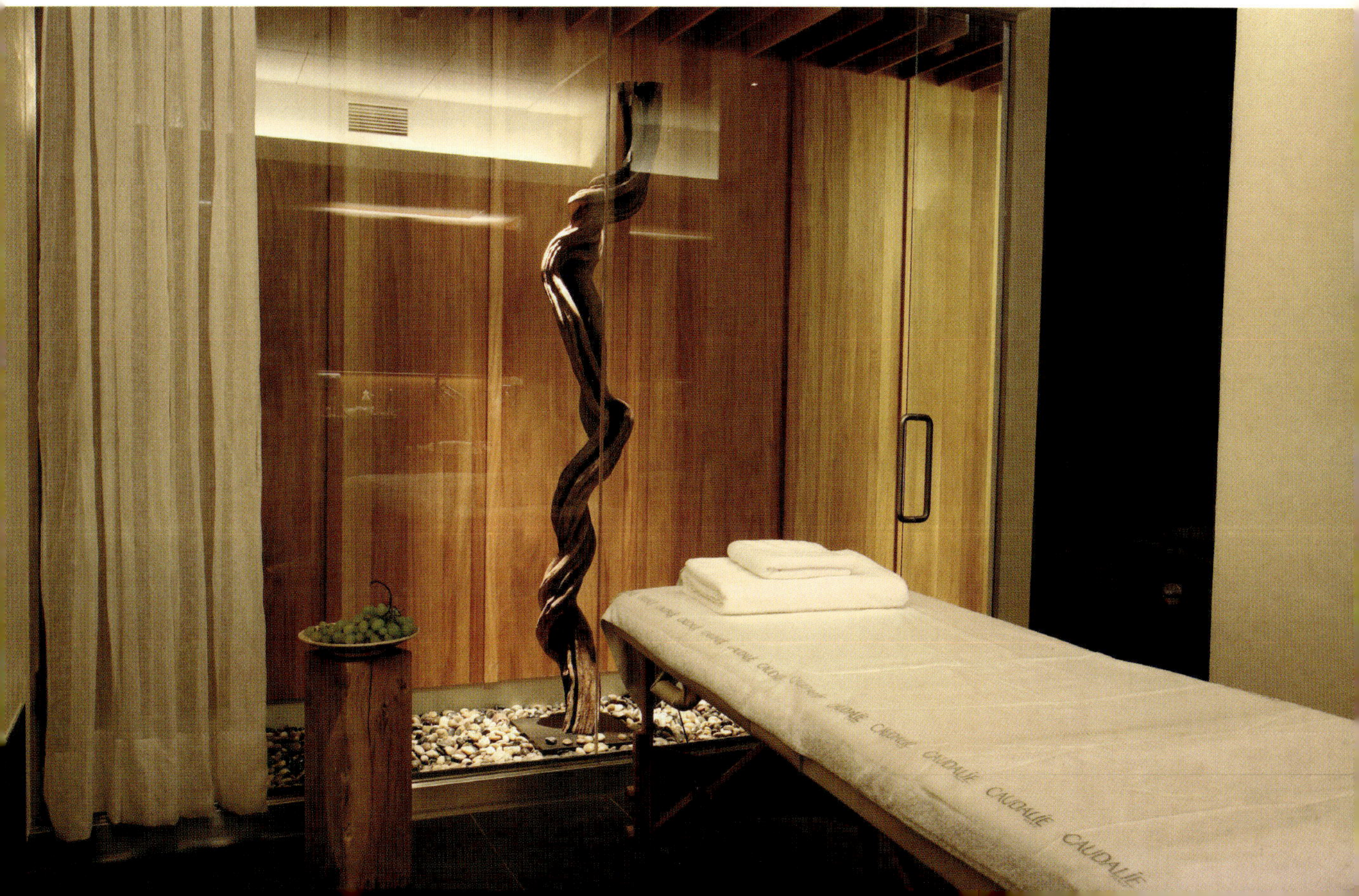

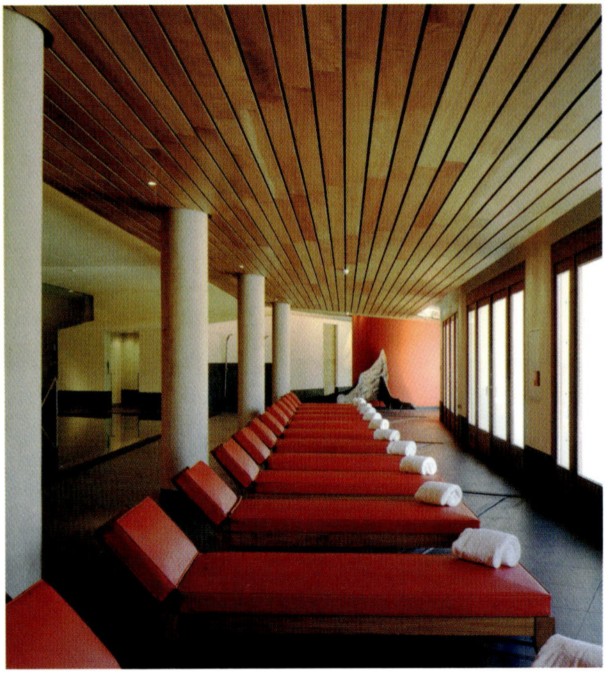

Die Inneneinrichtung zeigt direkten Bezug zu den Weinbergen, die das Gebäude umgeben.

The interior design refers directly to the vines that surround the building.

Le design intérieur s'inspire directement des vignes qui entourent le bâtiment.

Het interieur verwijst rechtstreeks naar de wijnranken die het gebouw omringen.

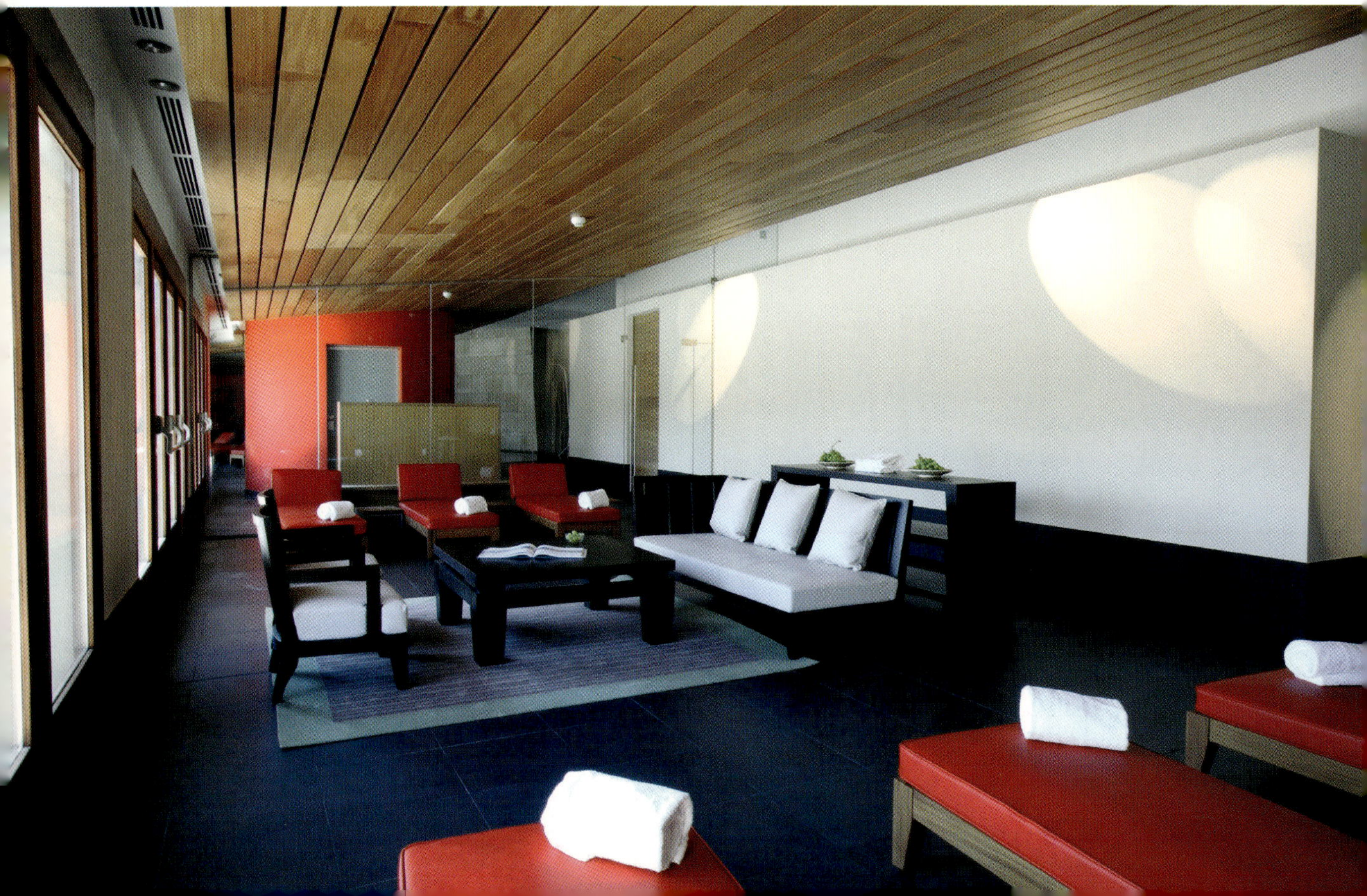

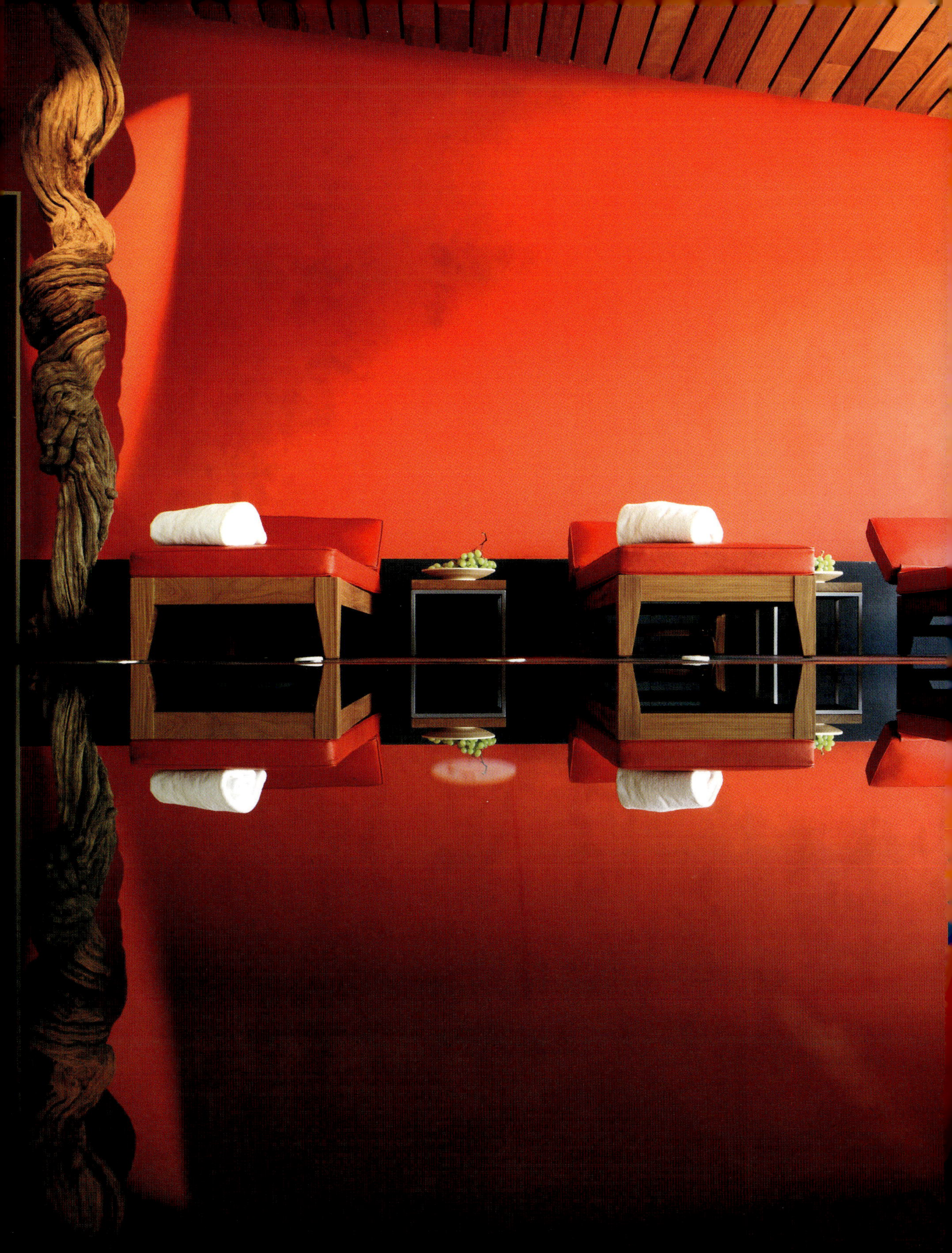

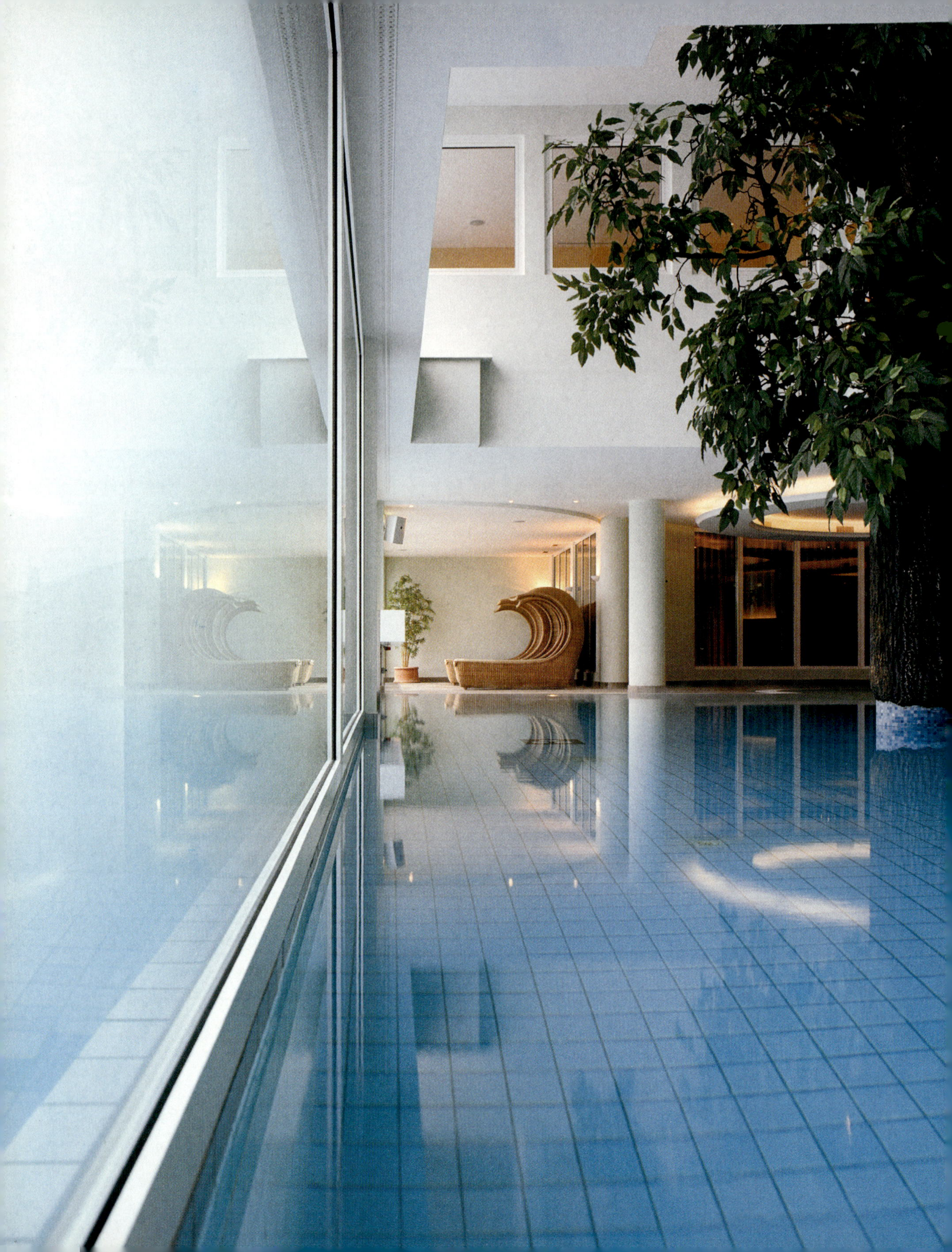

Akari Spa

Die 2.000 Quadratmeter große Anlage verteilt sich auf zwei Etagen. Die zweite Etage, welche die Thermal- und Beauty-Abteilungen beherbergt, verfügt über Saunen, Dampfbäder, Eisbrunnen und Erlebnisduschen. Das Erdgeschoss vereint die Bereiche Fitness & Sport sowie die Pools, zu denen auch ein beheizter Außenpool zählt, der mit der umliegenden Landschaft zu verschwimmen scheint.

The 21,500 square feet space is divided in two storeys. The second storey, which holds the thermal and beauty areas, has saunas, steam baths, ice fountain and invigorating showers. The ground level groups the facilities for fitness and the pools among which there is a heated one, located outside, that seems to fuse with the surrounding landscape, extending its imaginary boundaries towards the blue lagoon.

L'espace de 2.000 m² est le fruit de deux époques. Le rez-de-chaussée, plus ancien, regroupe l'espace fitness et les piscines. L'une d'entre elles, chauffée et située à l'extérieur, s'apparente à un lagon bleu où le paysage alentour vient « fondre » ses frontières imaginaires. La partie la plus récente, intégrant le spa et les espaces dédiés aux soins de beauté, est équipée de saunas, de hammams, d'une source glacée et de douches fortifiantes.

Het 2000 m² tellende oppervlak is verdeeld in twee verdiepingen. Op de bovenverdieping liggen de bronnenbaden en de ruimten voor schoonheidsbehandelingen, met sauna's, stoombaden, een ijsreservoir en verkwikkende douches. Beneden liggen de fitnessruimten en de zwembaden, waaronder een verwarmd buitenbad dat lijkt te versmelten met het omringende landschap en de blauwe lagune.

Feusisberg, Switzerland

HALTER ARCHITEKTEN
DESIGN: SCHLETTERER WELLNESS & SPA DESIGN

Photos © Hotz & Hotz

www.panoramaresort.ch

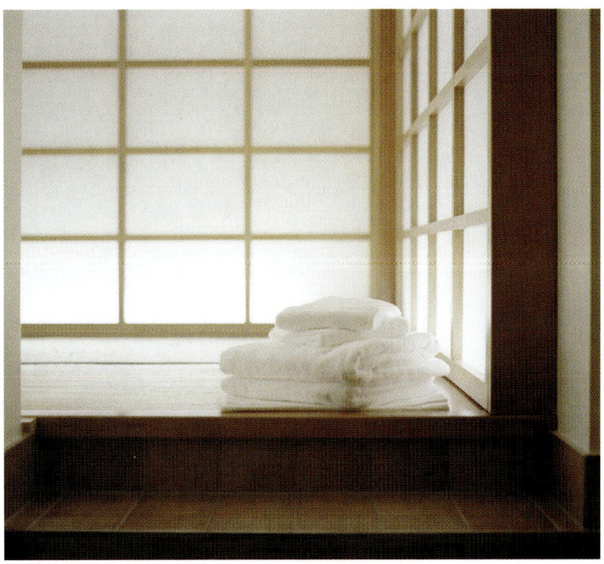

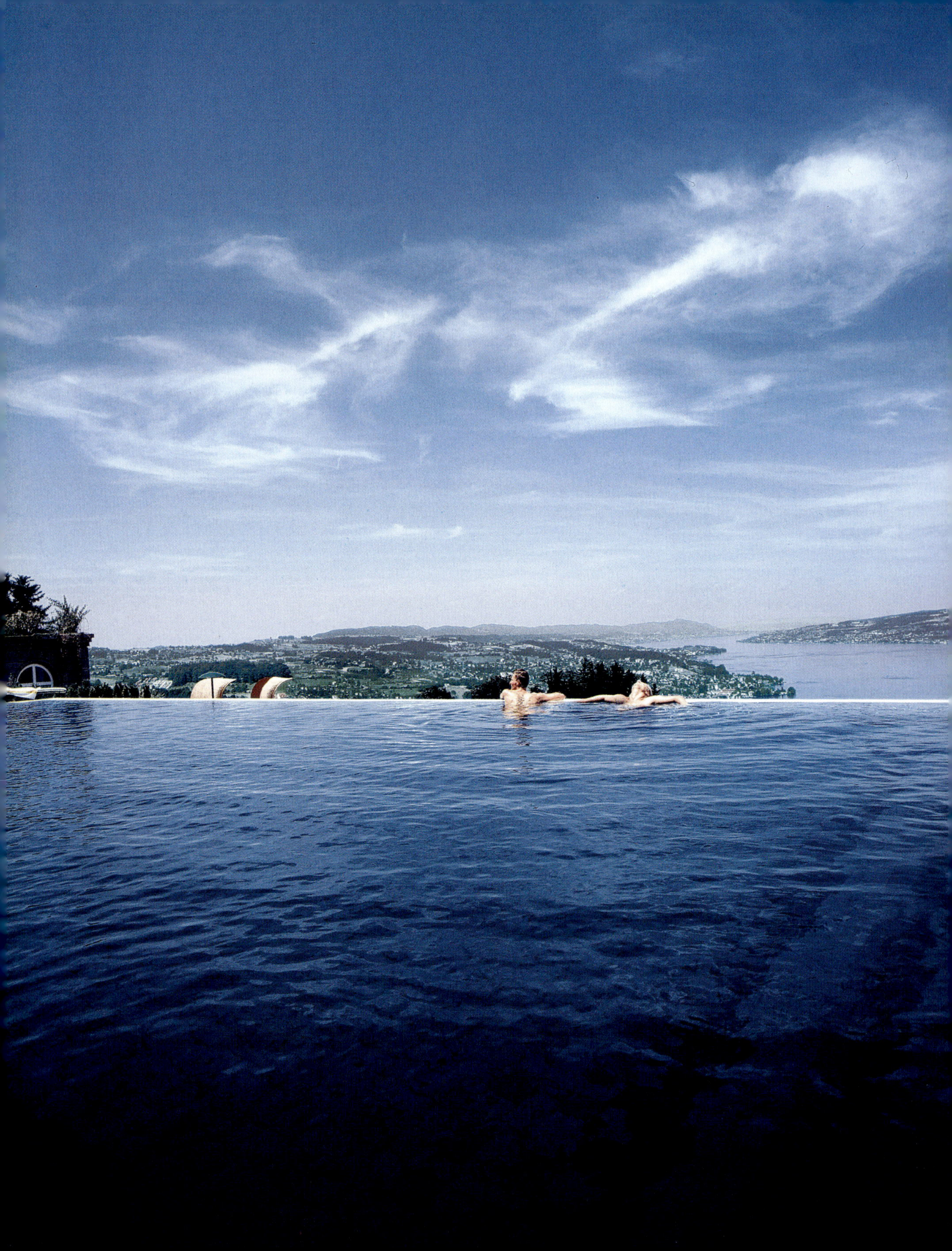

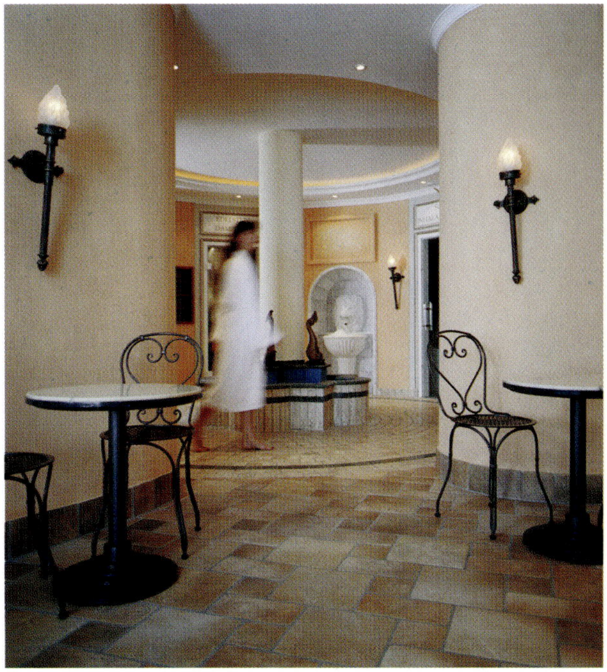

Pools, Saunen und Dampfbäder, Whirlpools, Fitnessbereich und ein Schönheitssalon bieten Sicht auf den Zürichsee.

Pools, saunas and steam rooms, whirlpool baths, fitness area and a beauty parlor offer views over Lake Zurich.

Piscines, saunas, hammams, bains bouillonnants, espace fitness et salons de beauté offrent autant de points de vue sur le lac Zurich.

Zwembaden, sauna's en stoomcabines, bubbelbaden, fitnessruimte en schoonheidssalon kijken uit over het Meer van Zürich.

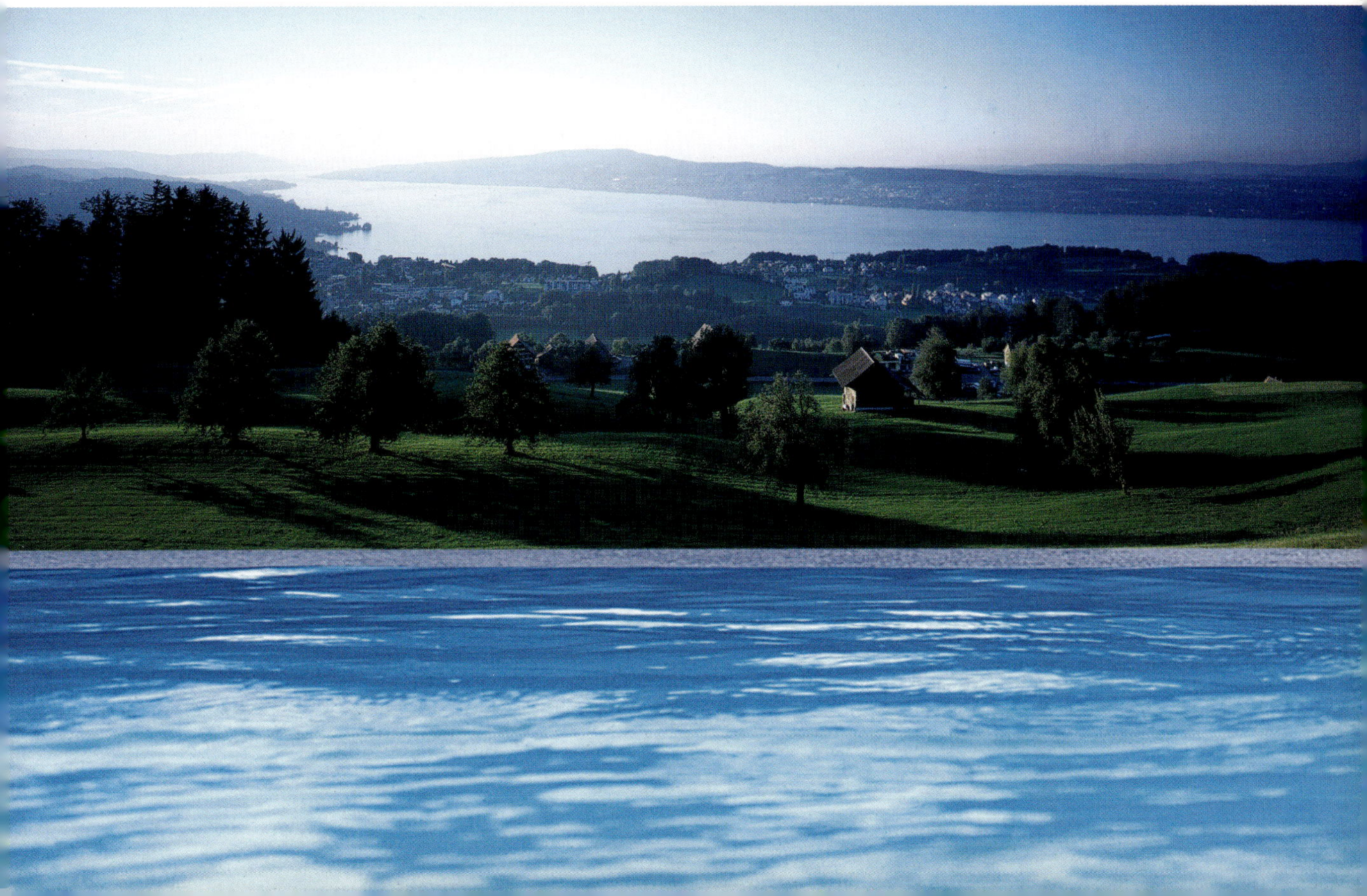

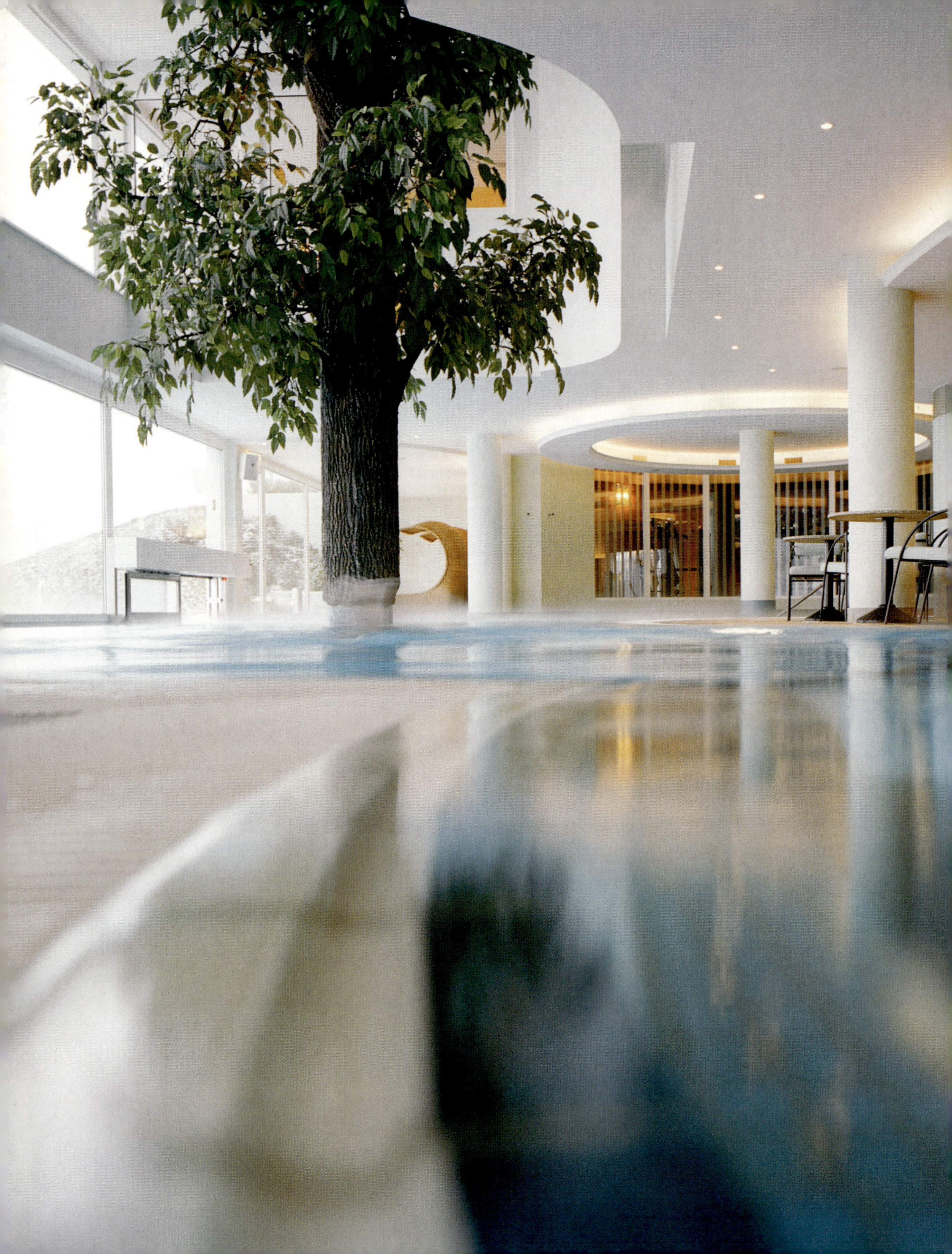

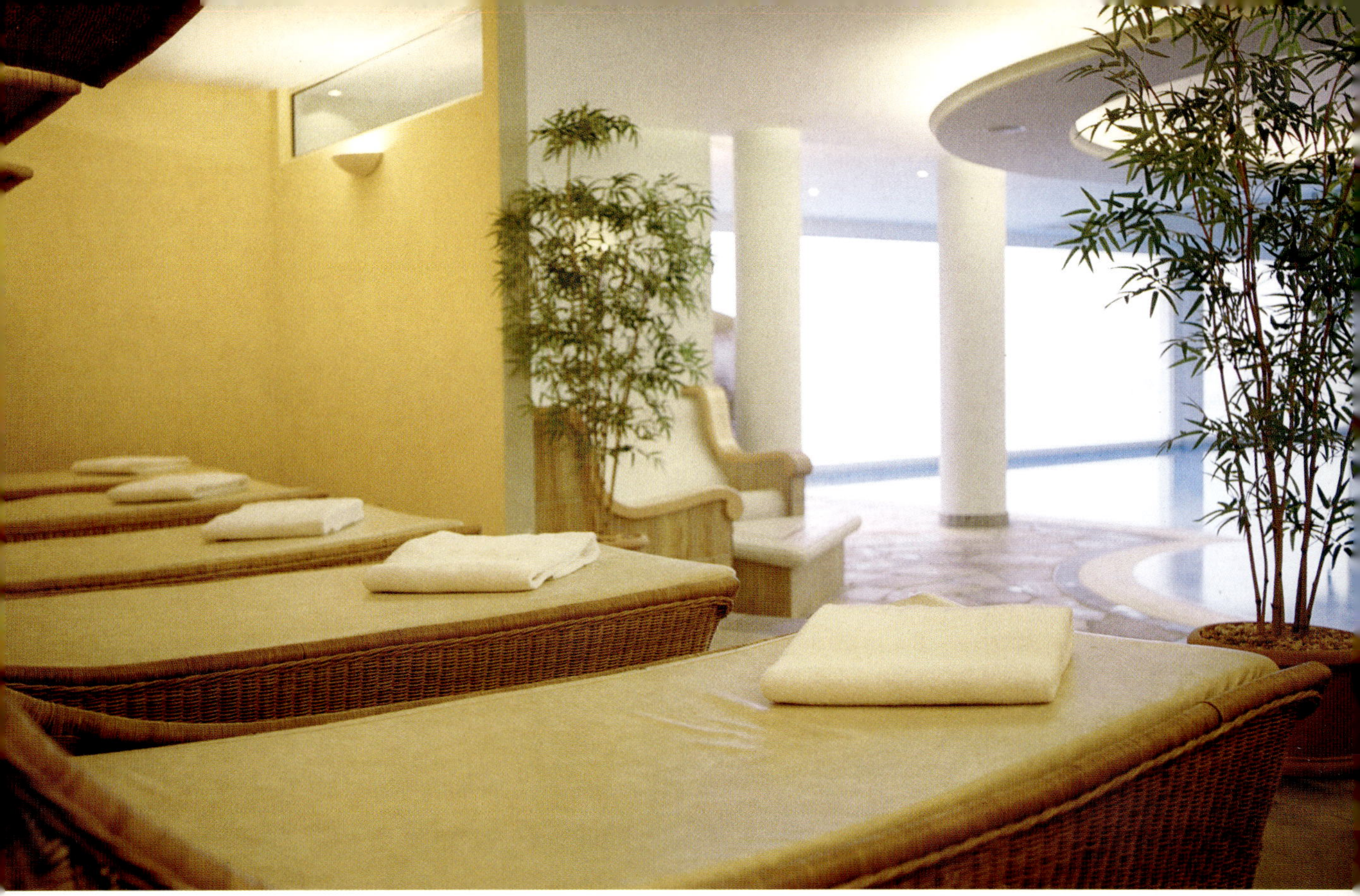

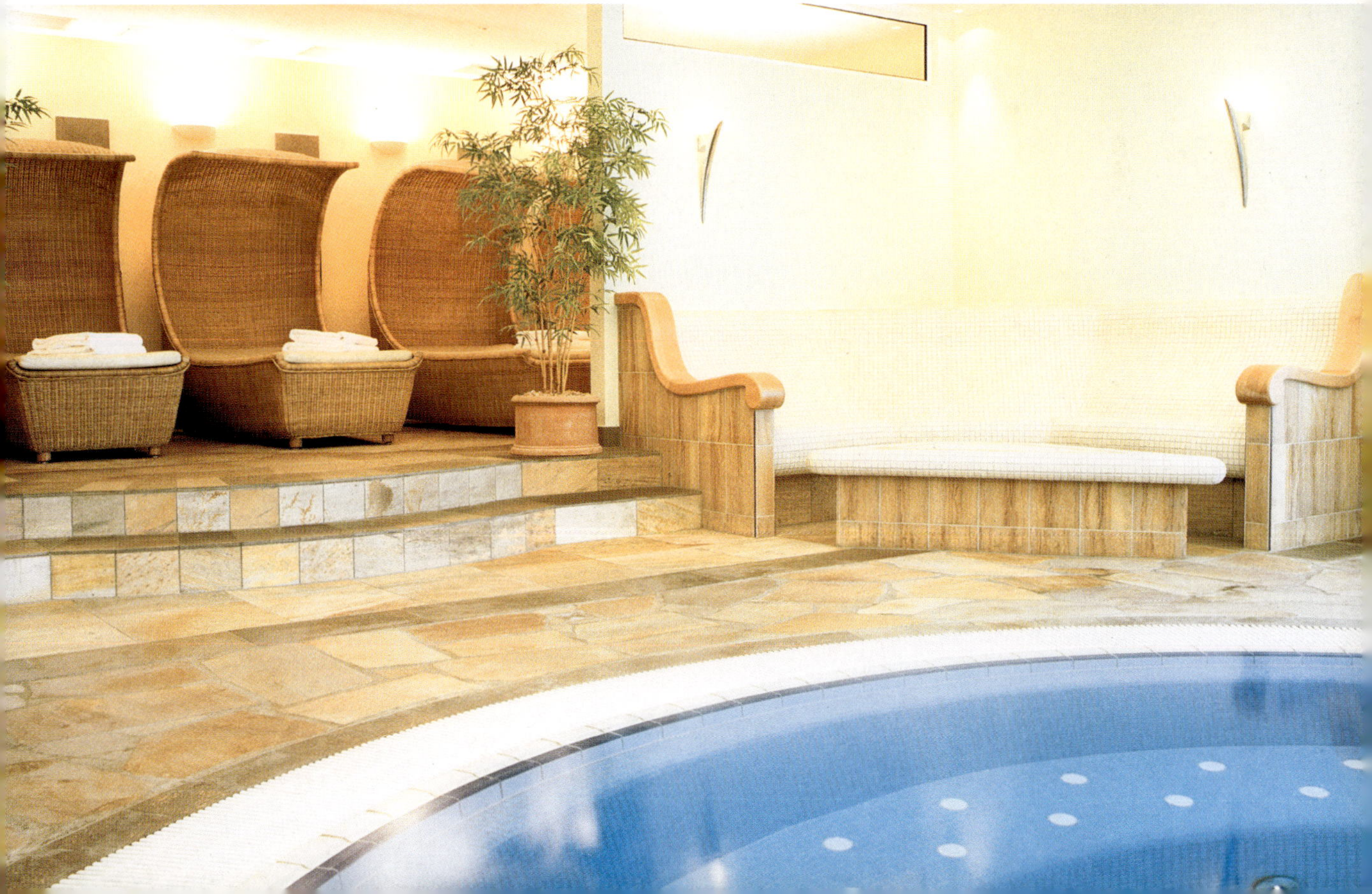

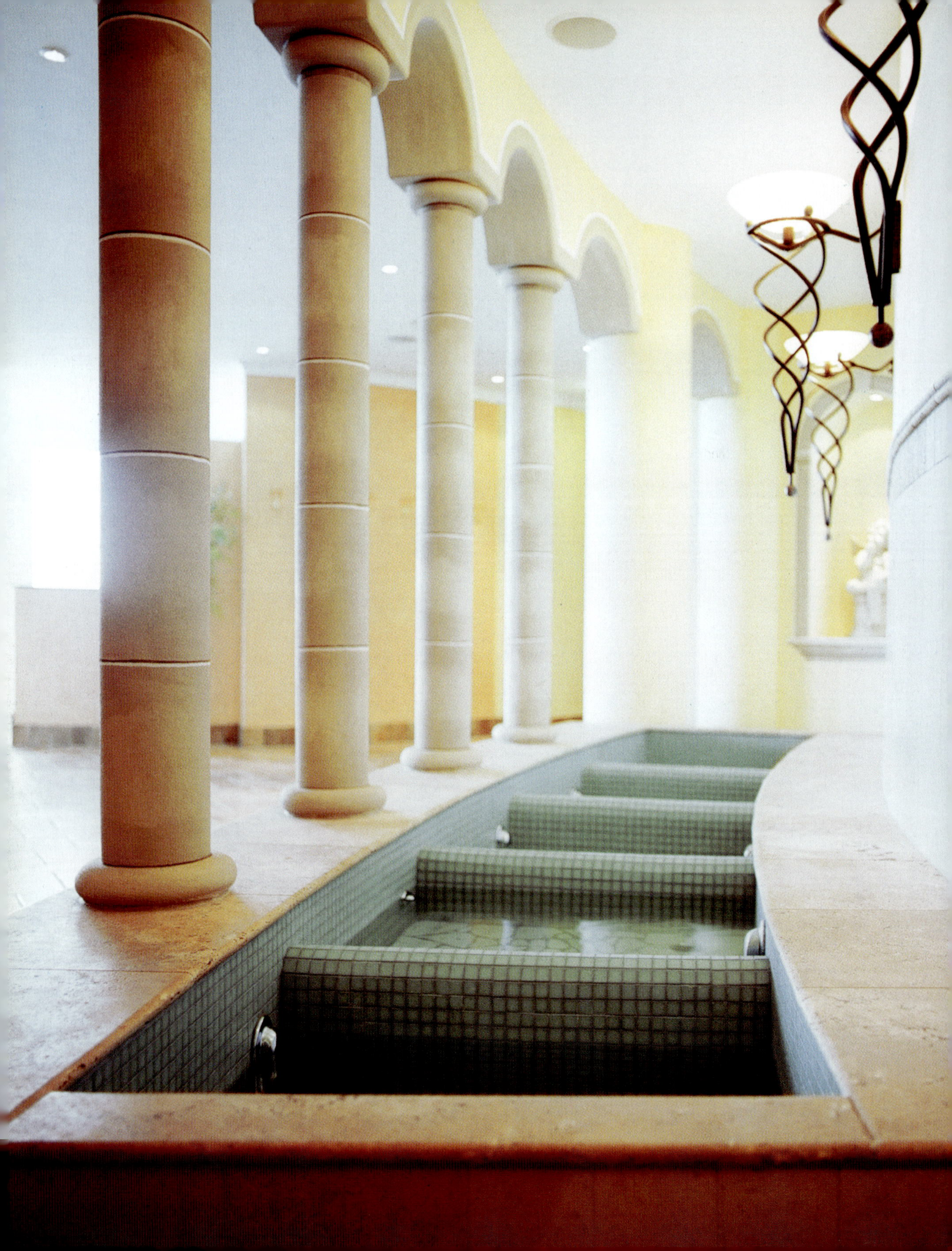

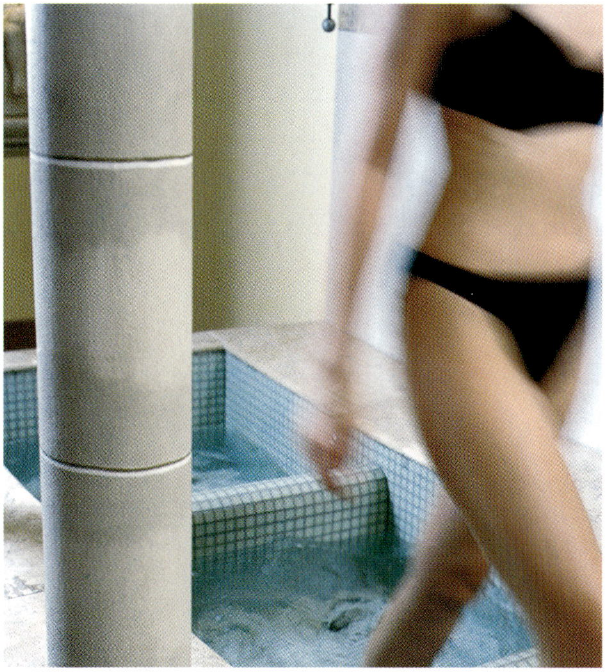

Die Innenbereiche zeichnen sich durch den aparten Mix mediterraner, asiatischer und moderner Stilelemente aus.

The interior areas are characterized by the convergence of Mediterranean, Asian and modern styles.

Les espaces intérieurs se caractérisent par un mélange des styles méditerranéen, asiatique et contemporain.

De interieurs worden gekenmerkt door een mengeling van mediterrane, Aziatische en moderne stijlen.

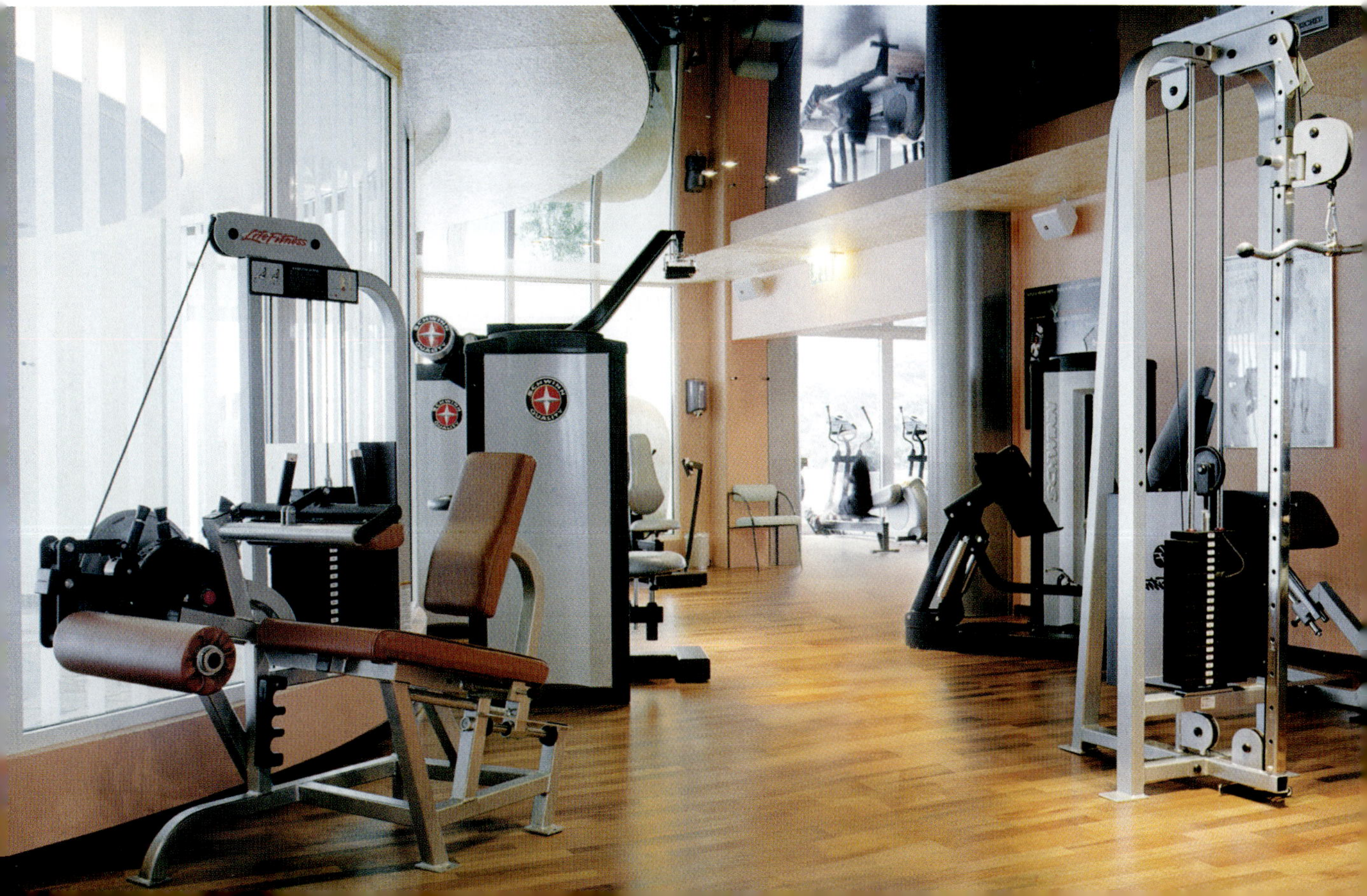

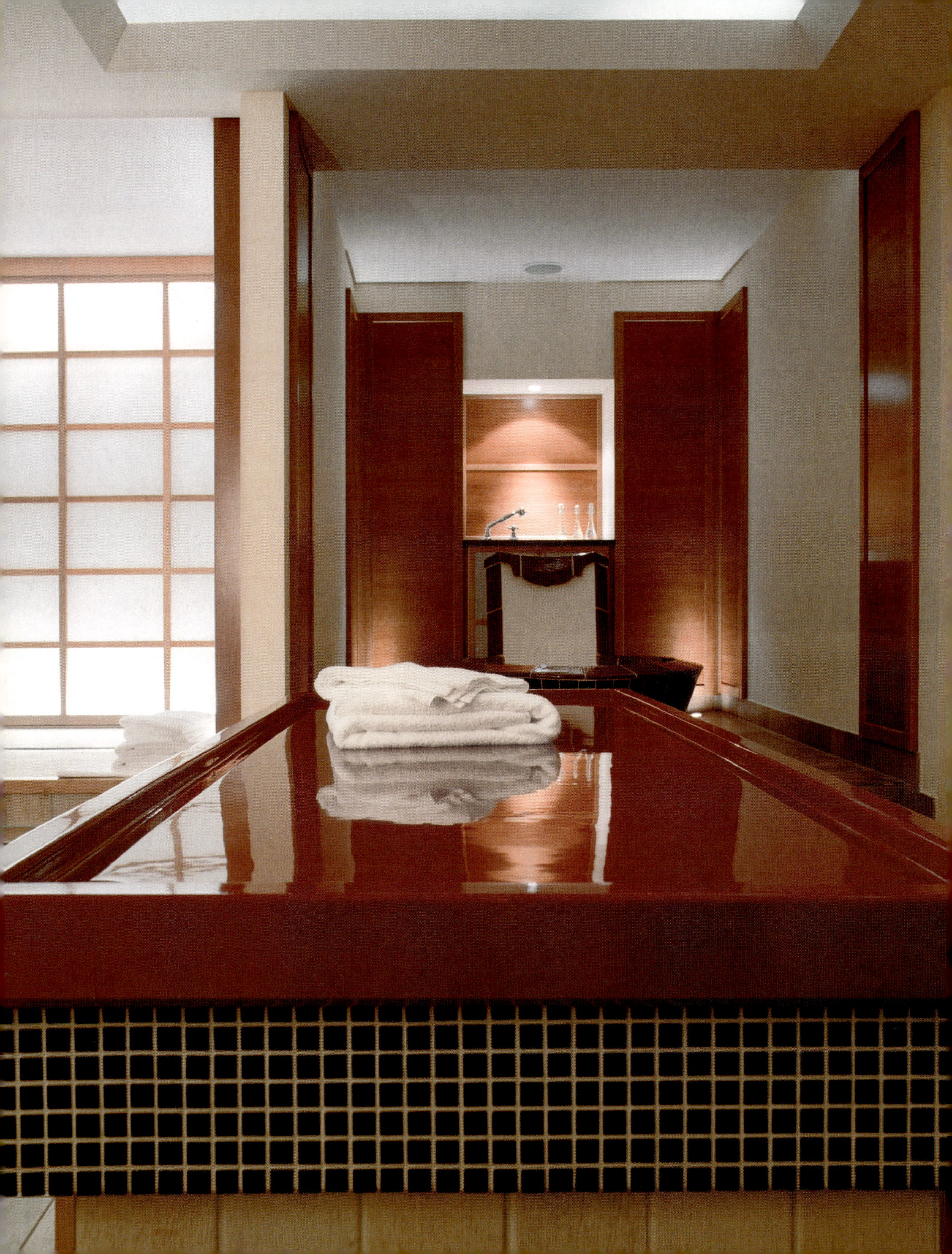

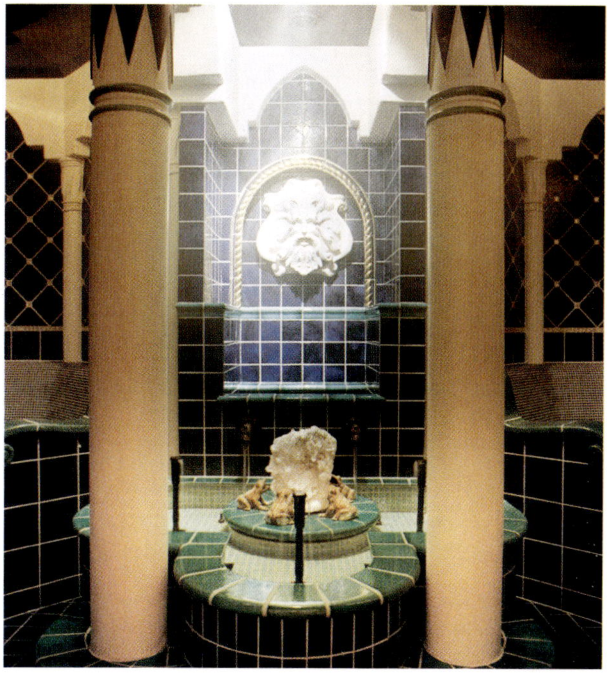

Schlafstörungen und Kopfschmerzen lassen sich gut mit Feuchtigkeit, Hitze und Kristallsteinen behandeln.

Humidity, 131 °F of temperature and the crystal rocks are useful for treating sleep disturbances and headaches.

L'humidité, la température de 48° Celsius et les cristaux de roches sont ici utilisés dans les traitements contre les troubles du sommeil et les migraines.

Met een hoge luchtvochtigheid, een temperatuur van 55 °C en rotskristallen worden slaapstoornissen en hoofdpijn behandeld.

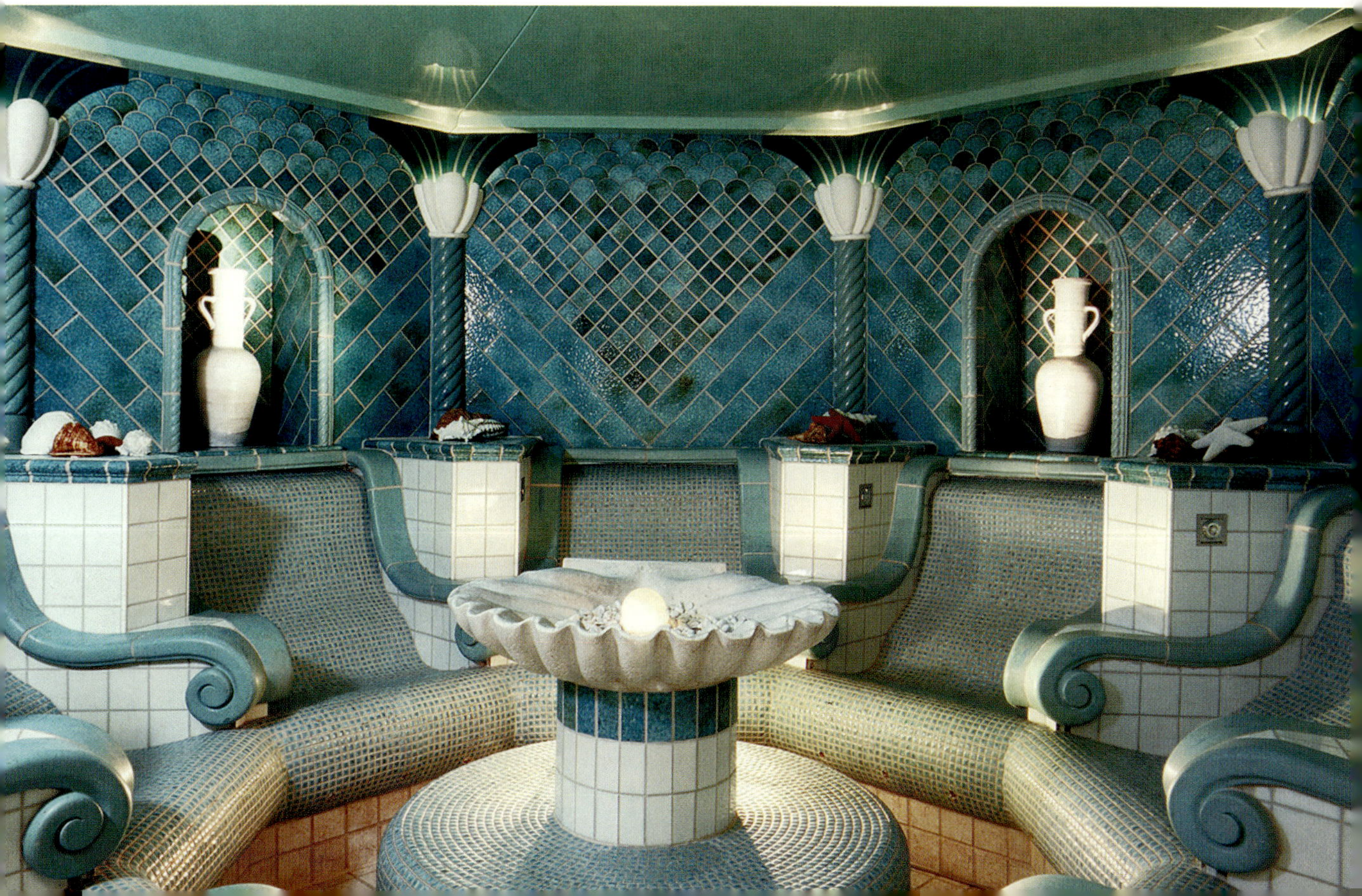

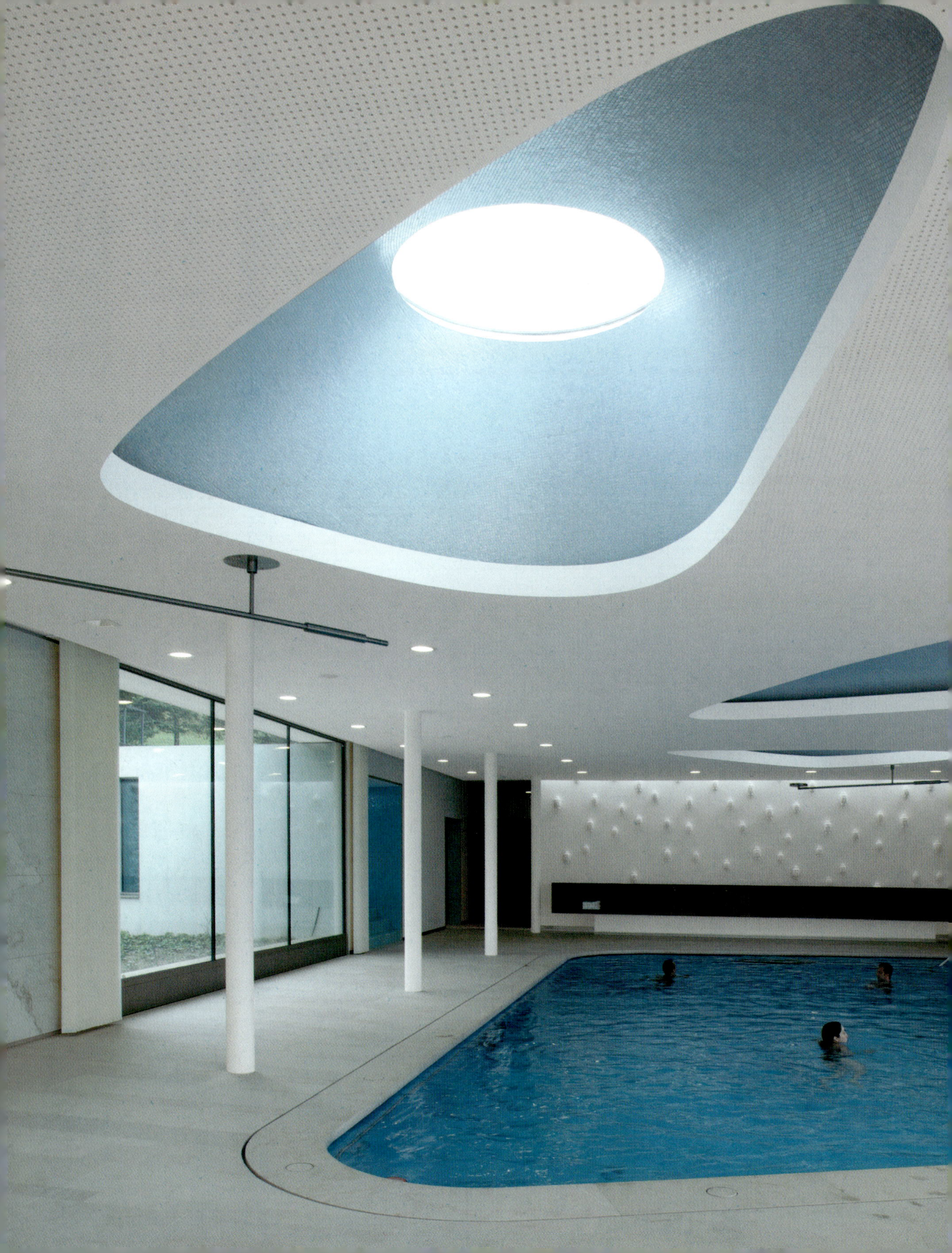

La Prairie Clinic Spa

Auf seinen drei Etagen beherbergt das Spa Rezeption und Aufnahmeraum, ein Restaurant, einen Nassbereich, Whirlpool und Sauna, die Schönheitsklinik, ein Thalassotherapiezentrum mit therapeutischem Salzwasserbecken und einen Fitnessraum. Das gesamte Gebäude ist von Tageslicht durchflutet, das durch die großen Fenster dringt. Restaurant und Terrasse bieten einen herrlichen Blick auf den kleinen Hafen von Basset, den See und die Alpen.

In its three floors the spa holds the reception and admittance room, a restaurant, a wet area, the Jacuzzi and the sauna, the beauty clinic, a thalassotherapy center with a therapeutic salt water pond, and a gymnasium. The whole building is bathed in intense natural light that comes in through all the openings connecting the outside with the pool. The restaurant and the terrace offer a magnificent view of the small harbor of Basset and the lake, as well as of the Alps.

Ce spa distribue sur trois niveaux une réception, un restaurant, un espace fraîcheur, un jacuzzi et un sauna, un institut de beauté, un centre de thalassothérapie pourvu d'un bassin d'eau salée, et un gymnase. Le bâtiment est baigné d'une lumière naturelle intense diffusée par toutes les ouvertures reliant l'extérieur à la piscine. Le restaurant et la terrasse offrent une vue magnifique sur le petit port de Basset et le lac, ainsi que sur les Alpes.

Dit kuuroord telt drie verdiepingen, met een receptie, een restaurant, baden, een jacuzzi met sauna, een schoonheidssalon, een centrum voor thalassotherapie met een therapeutisch zoutwaterbad en een sportruimte. Het hele gebouw baadt in intens daglicht, dat binnenvalt door openingen tussen zwembad en buitenlucht. Het restaurant en het terras bieden een schitterend uitzicht op het haventje van Basset, het meer en de Alpen.

Clarens, Switzerland

RICHTER & DAHL ROCHA ARCHITECTS

Photos © Yves André

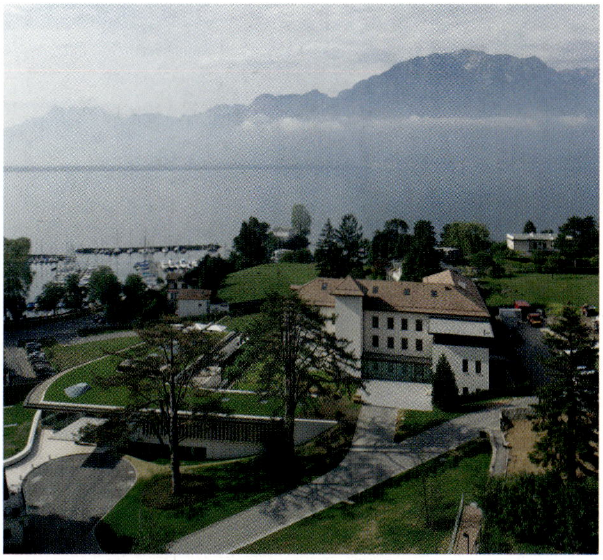

www.laprairie.ch

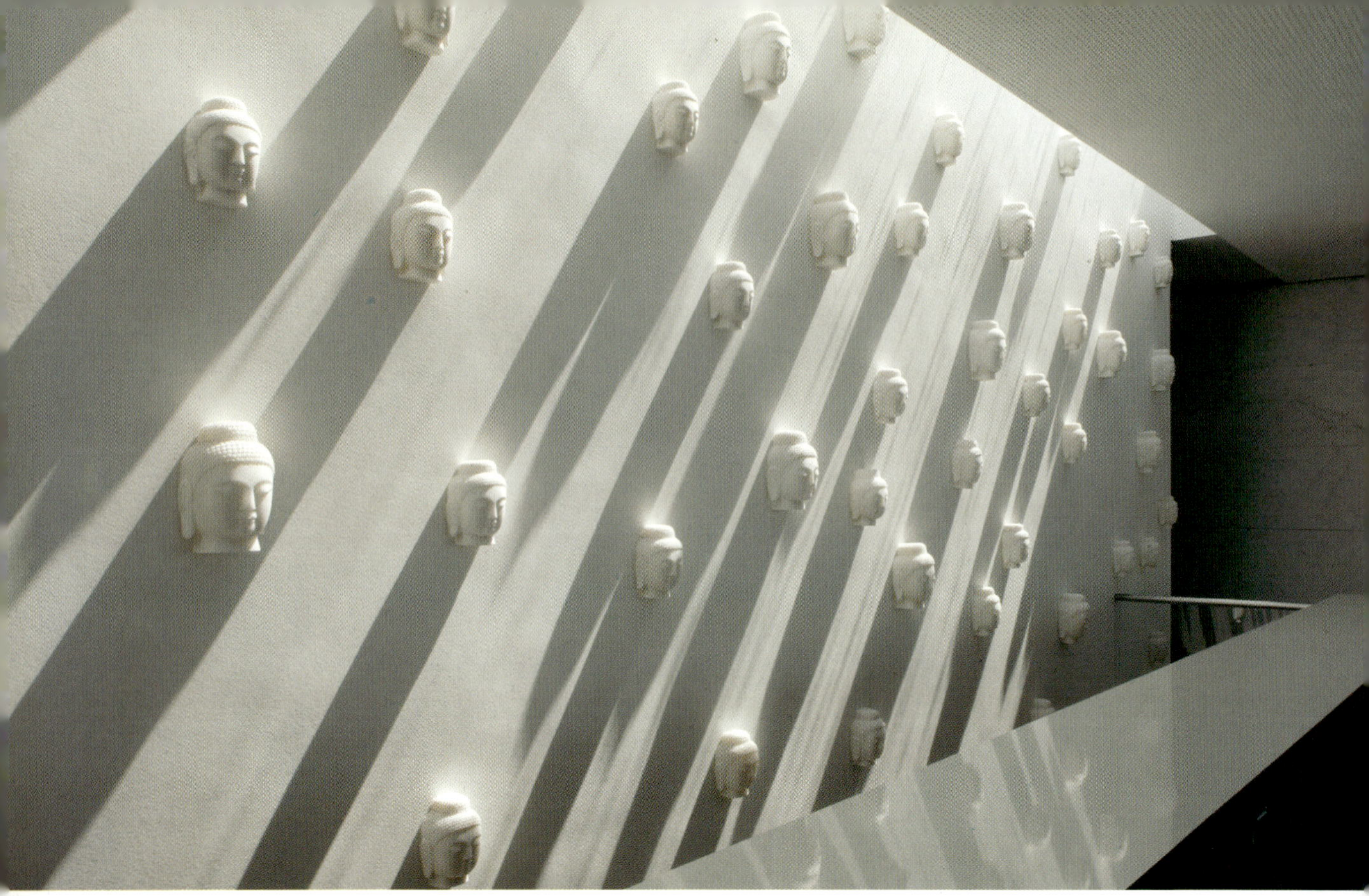
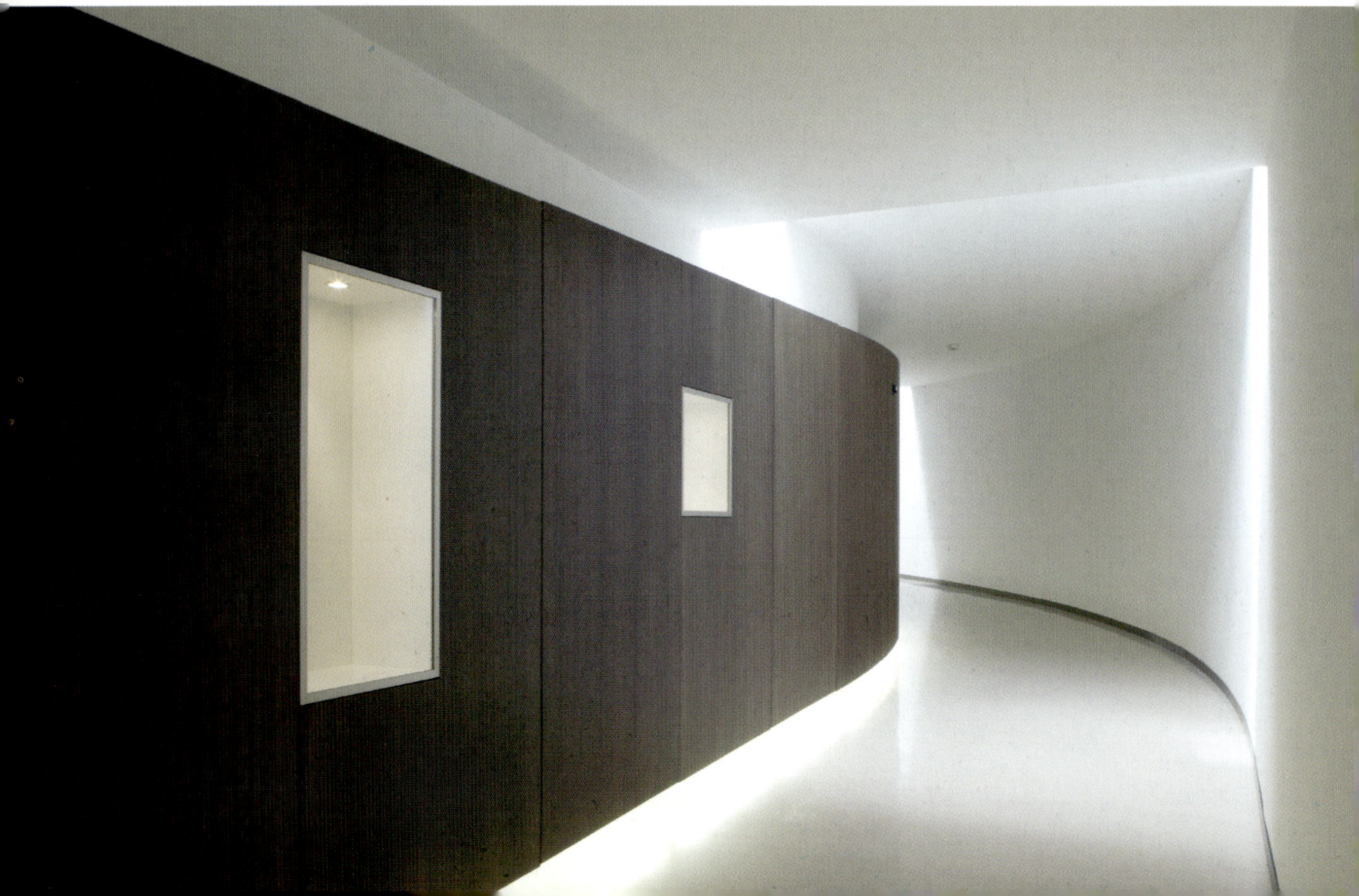

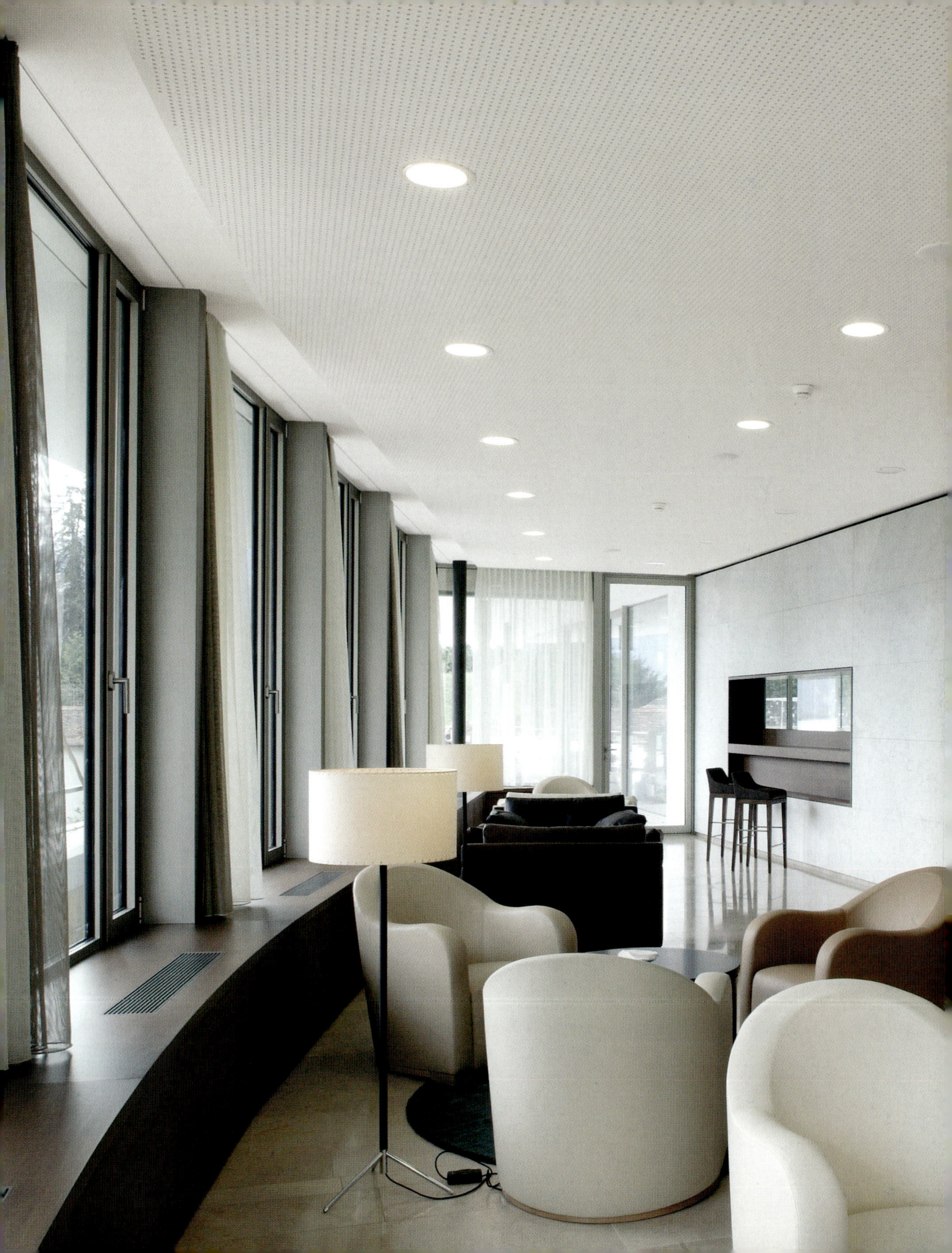

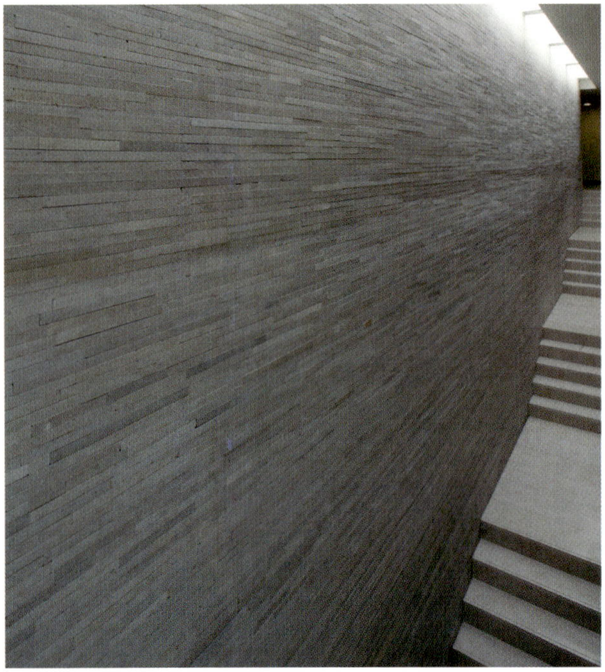

Im Thalassotherapiezentrum verspricht das Kaltwasserbecken den gleichen wohltuenden Effekt wie Meerwasser.

At the thalassotherapy center, the cold-water pool offers the same beneficial effects that sea water does for health.

Au centre de thalassothérapie, la piscine d'eau froide offre pour la santé les mêmes effets avantageux que l'eau de mer.

Het koudwaterbad in het centrum voor thalassotherapie biedt dezelfde gezondheidsvoordelen als zeewater.

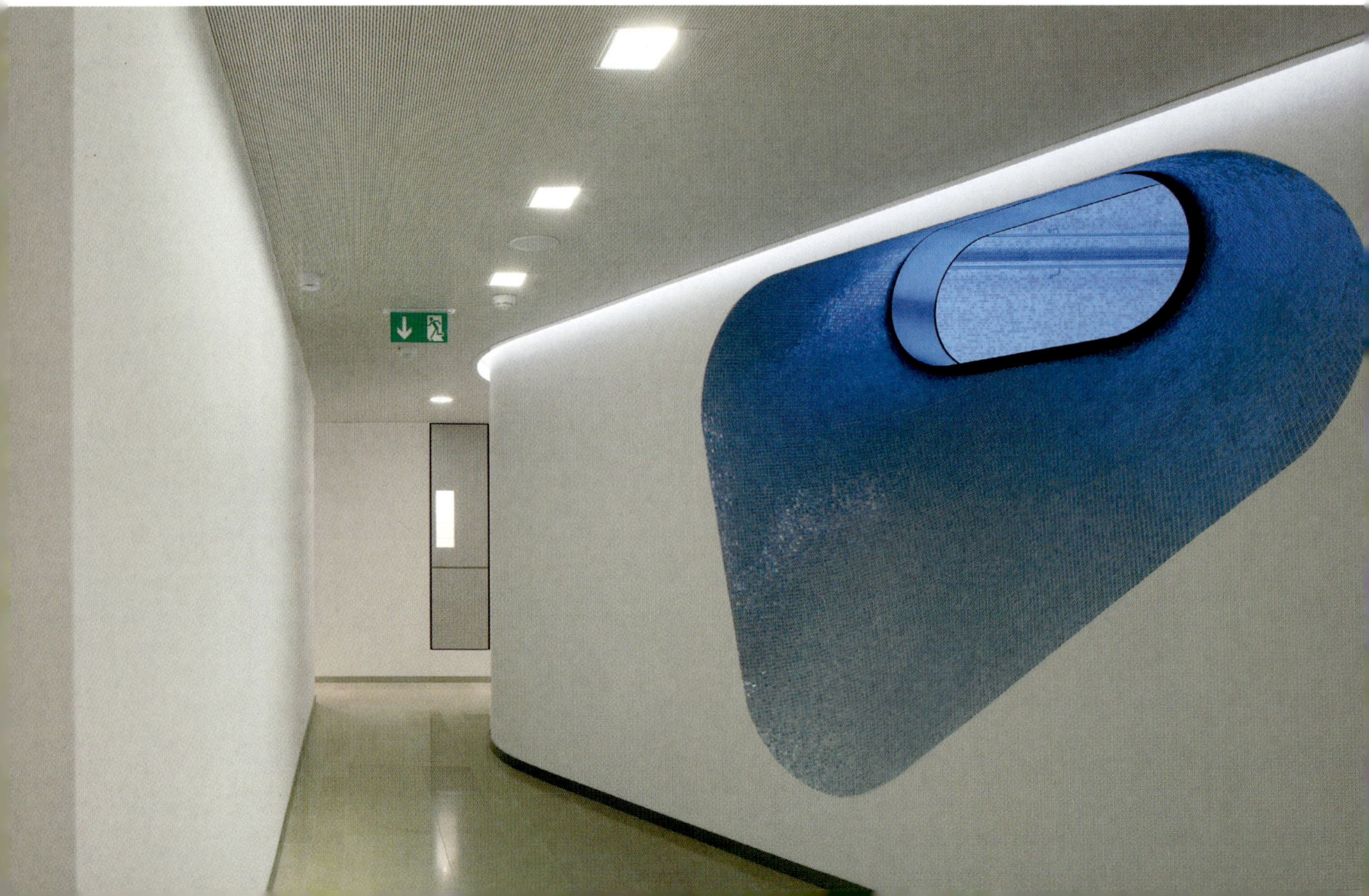

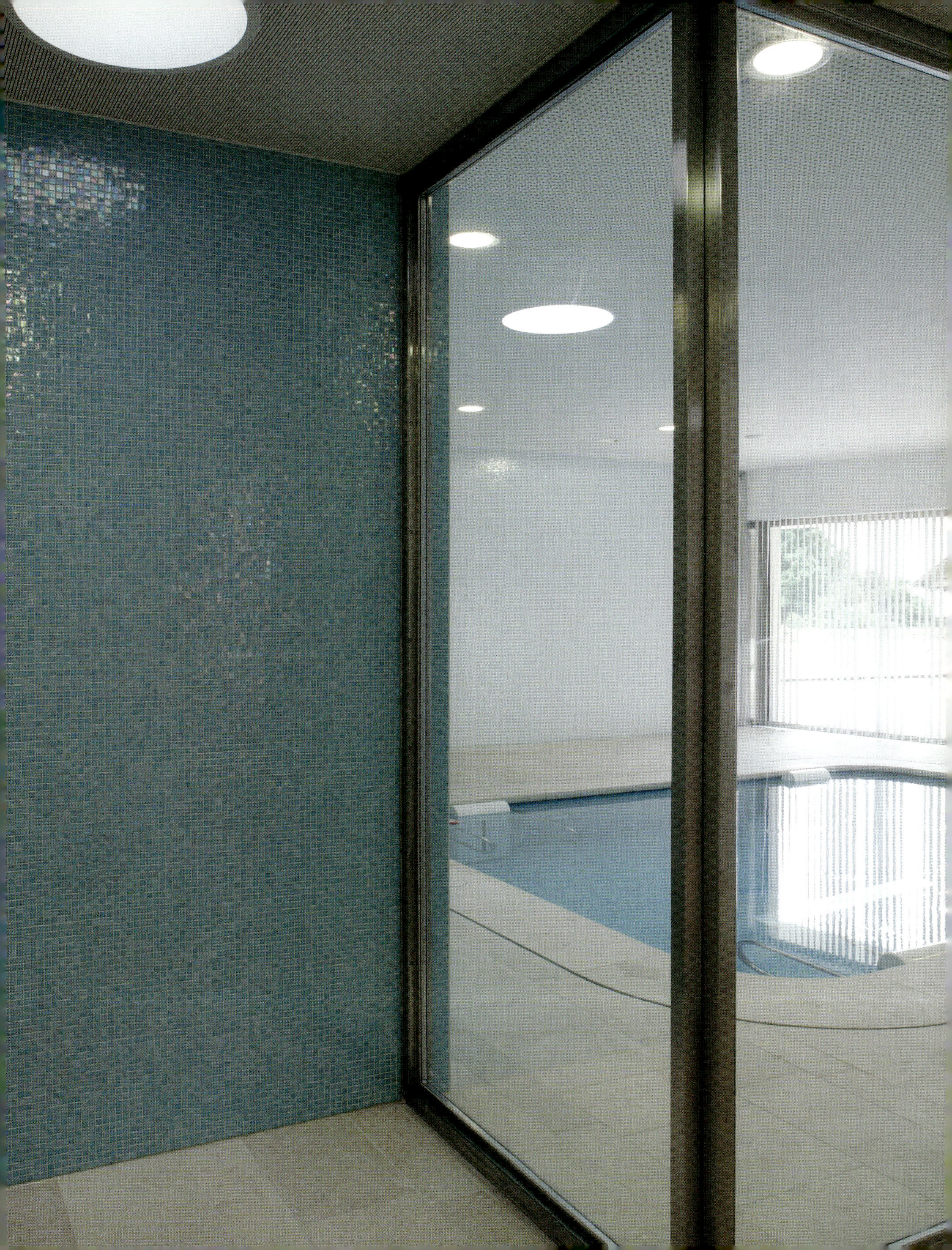

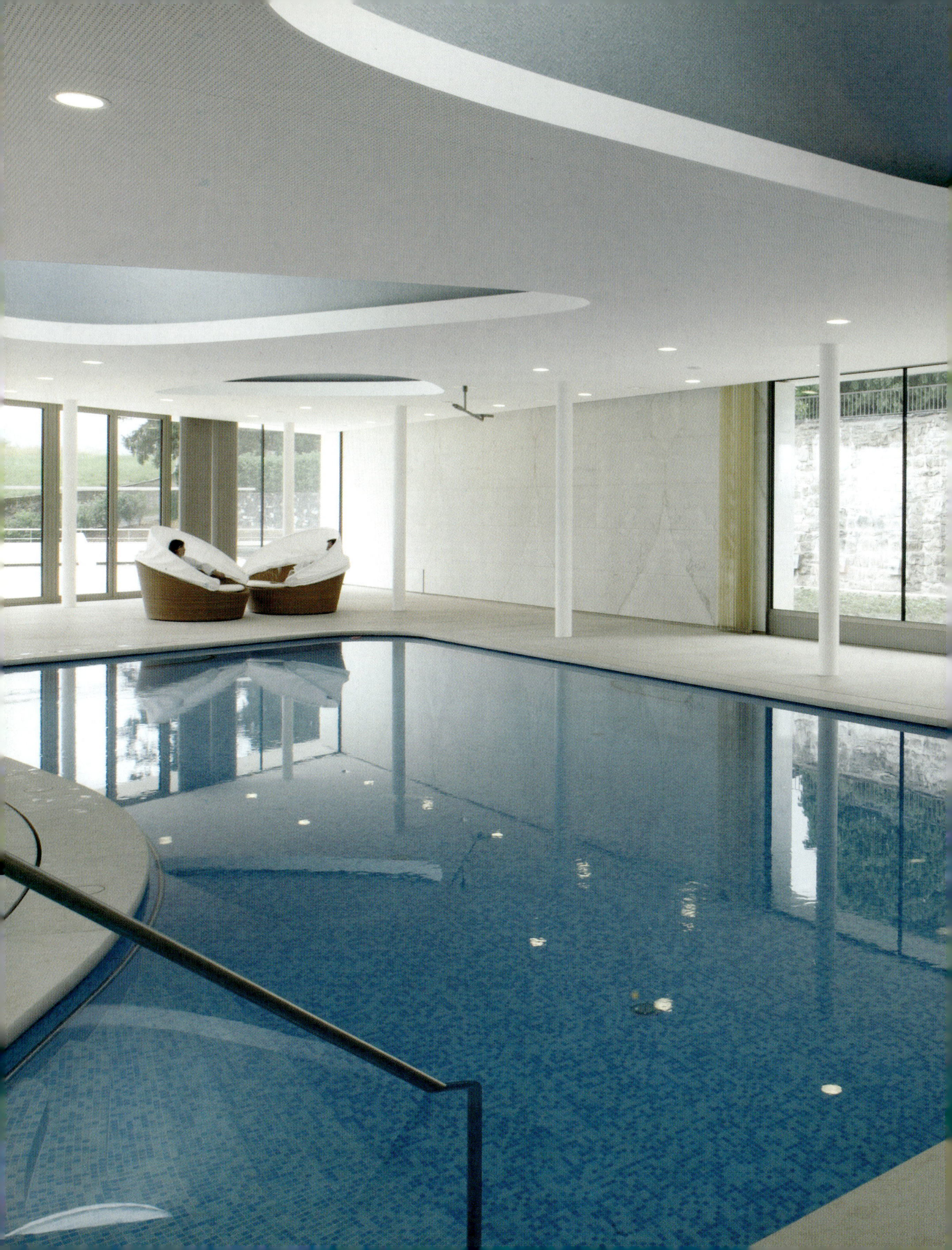

Die großen Öffnungen, die wie Schornsteine über dem Pool angeordnet sind, sorgen für helles natürliches Licht.

The great openings located like chimneys over the pool allow the bright natural light in.

De grandes ouvertures situées au-dessus de la piscine permettent à la lumière naturelle de pénétrer à l'intérieur du bâtiment.

De grote openingen die als schoorstenen boven het zwembad hangen, zorgen voor een mooie natuurlijke lichtinval.

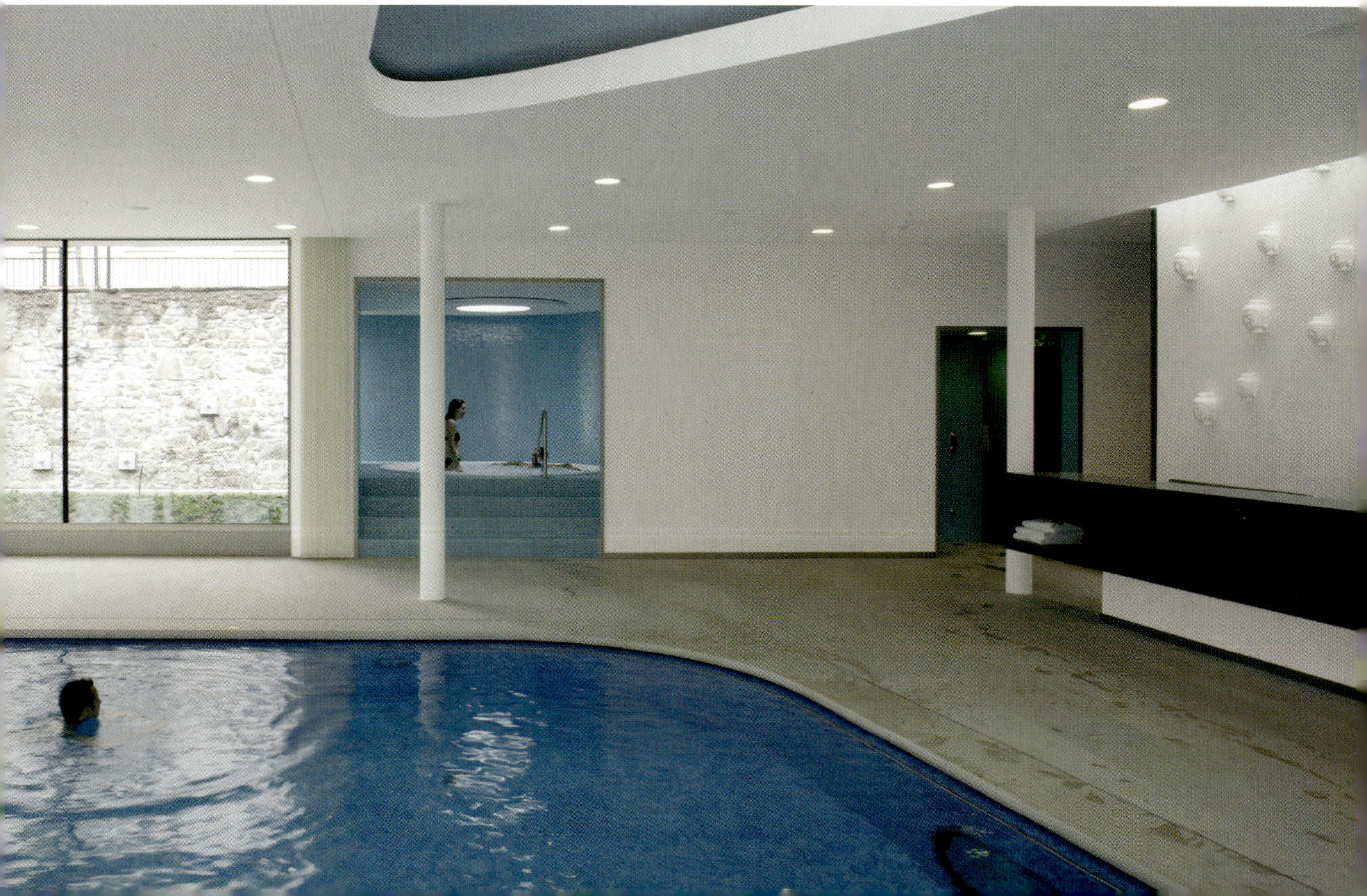

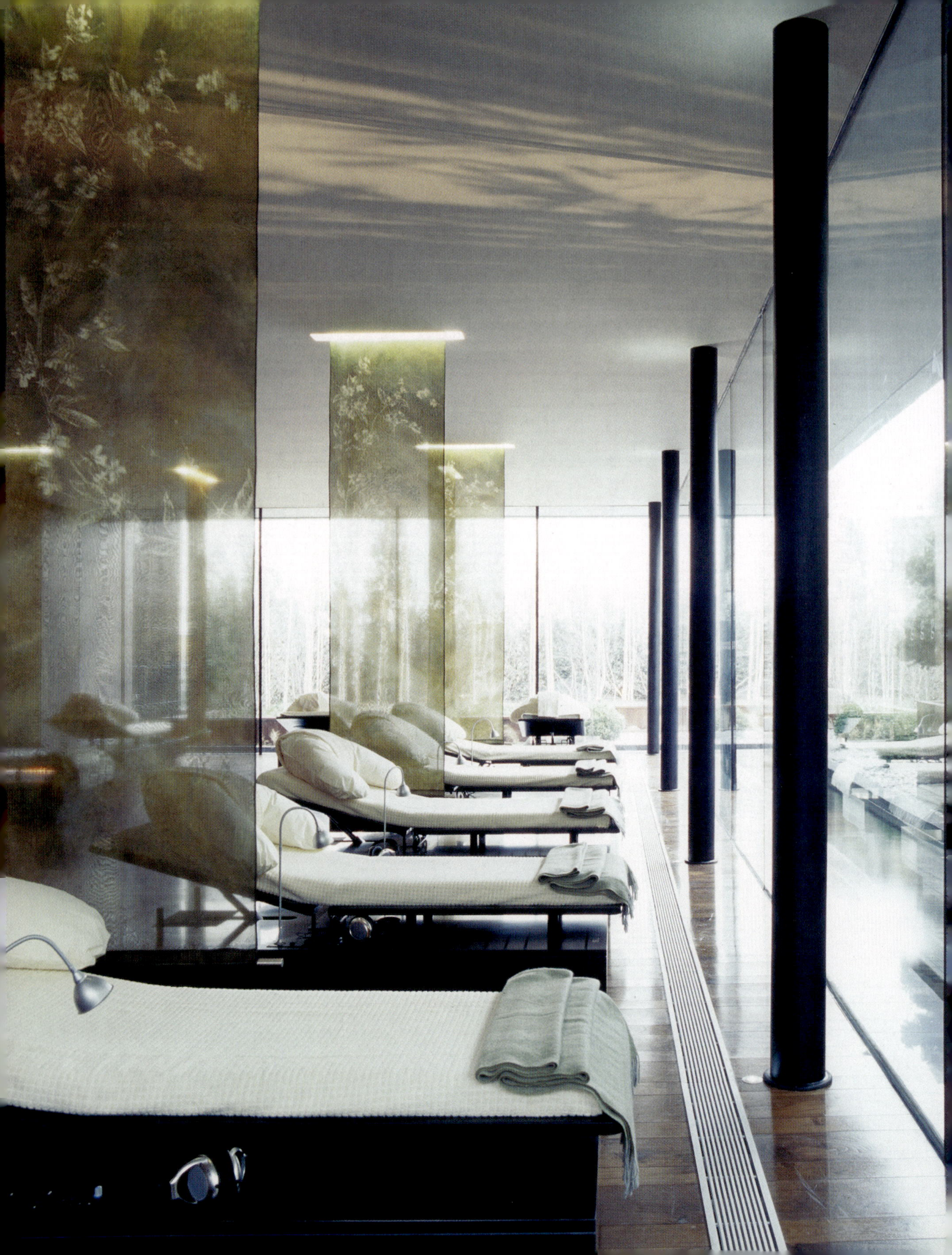

G Spa

Dieses Spa befindet sich in den oberen Etagen des spektakulären G Hotels im Herzen Irlands. In der ersten Etage befinden sich Nasszone, Wärmebäder, Tepidarium, Whirlpool, Steinsauna, Duschen und Eisbrunnen. Die zweite Etage beherbergt die Behandlungsräume, in denen die Verwendung natürlicher Substanzen zu Therapiezwecken oberstes Gebot ist. Der Entspannungsraum gewährt durch große Glasfenster Sicht auf einen japanischen Garten mit Bambus und weißen Steinen.

This spa occupies the top floors of the spectacular G Hotel placed in the heart of Ireland. The first floor holds the wet zone, the hot baths, the tepidarium, the whirlpool bath, the stone sauna, the showers and the ice fountains. The second floor holds the treatment rooms, where the use of natural substances for the therapies is mandatory. The relaxation room looks out through the large glass windows that allow one to see the Japanese garden with bamboo and white stones.

Ce spa occupe les derniers étages de l'étonnant hôtel G, situé à Galway, en plein cœur de l'Irlande. Au premier niveau se trouvent la zone fraîcheur, les bains chauds, les bains tièdes, le bain à remous, le sauna, les douches, et les fontaines glacées. Au second se situent les salles de soins ; l'utilisation de substances naturelles est systématique dans les thérapies prodiguées ici. Le salon de relaxation est tourné vers l'extérieur. De grandes baies vitrées permettent de voir le jardin japonais où se mêlent bambous et pierres blanches.

Dit kuuroord is gelegen op de bovenste verdiepingen van het spectaculaire G Hotel in het hart van Ierland. De eerste verdieping telt een zwembad, warme baden, het tepidarium, het whirlpoolbad, de stenen sauna, de douches en de ijsreservoirs. Op de tweede verdieping liggen behandelkamers waar uitsluitend natuurlijke ingrediënten gebruikt worden. De ontspanningsruimte kijkt via grote ramen uit op een Japanse tuin met bamboe en witte stenen.

Galway, Ireland

DOUGLAS WALLACE ARCHITECTS

Photos © G Hotel

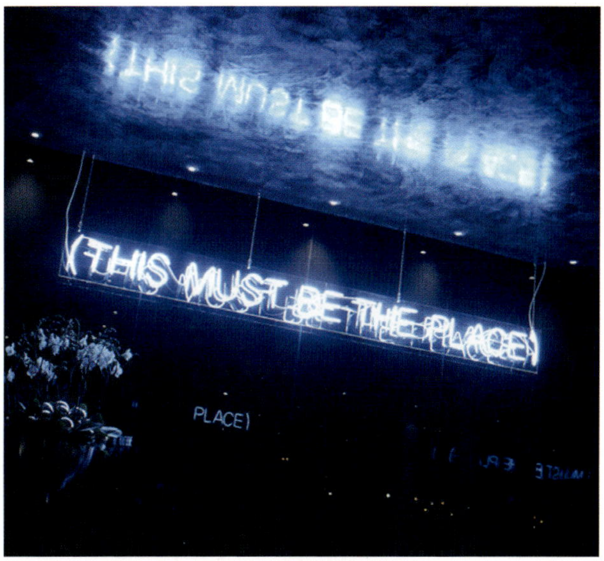

www.theghotel.ie

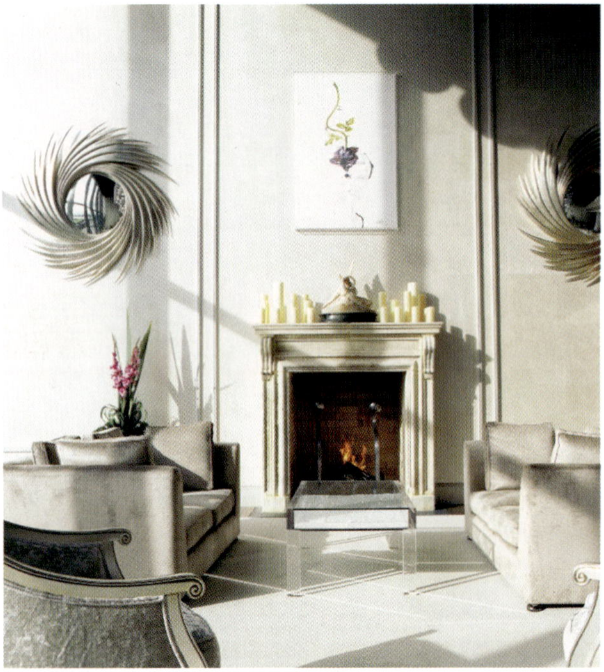

Der britische Designer Philip Treacy entwarf das Hotelinterieur.

The British designer Philip Treacy designed the hotel's interiors.

Le designer britannique Philip Treacy a conçu les espaces intérieurs de l'hôtel.

De Britse ontwerper Philip Treacy tekende voor de interieurs.

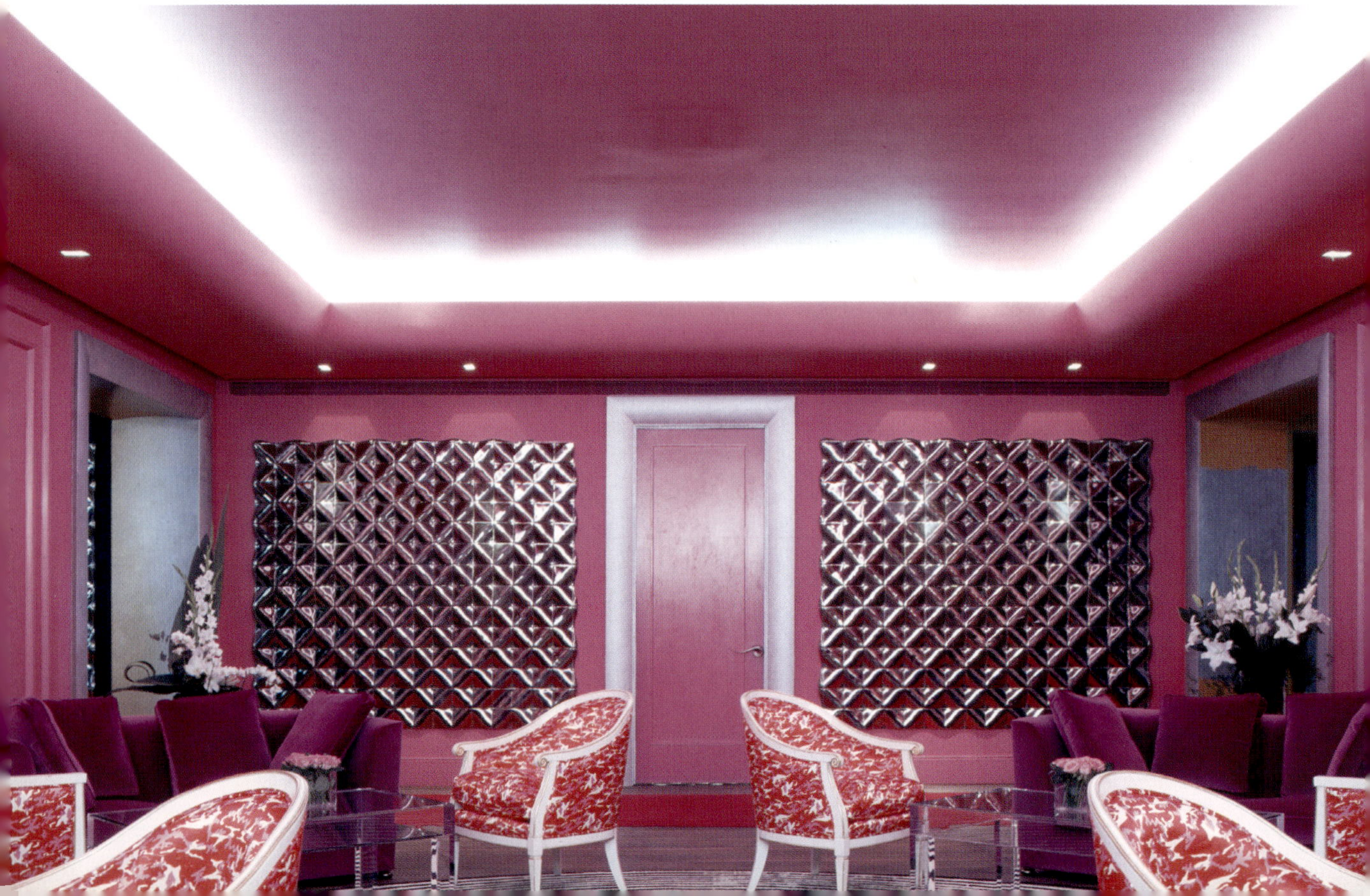

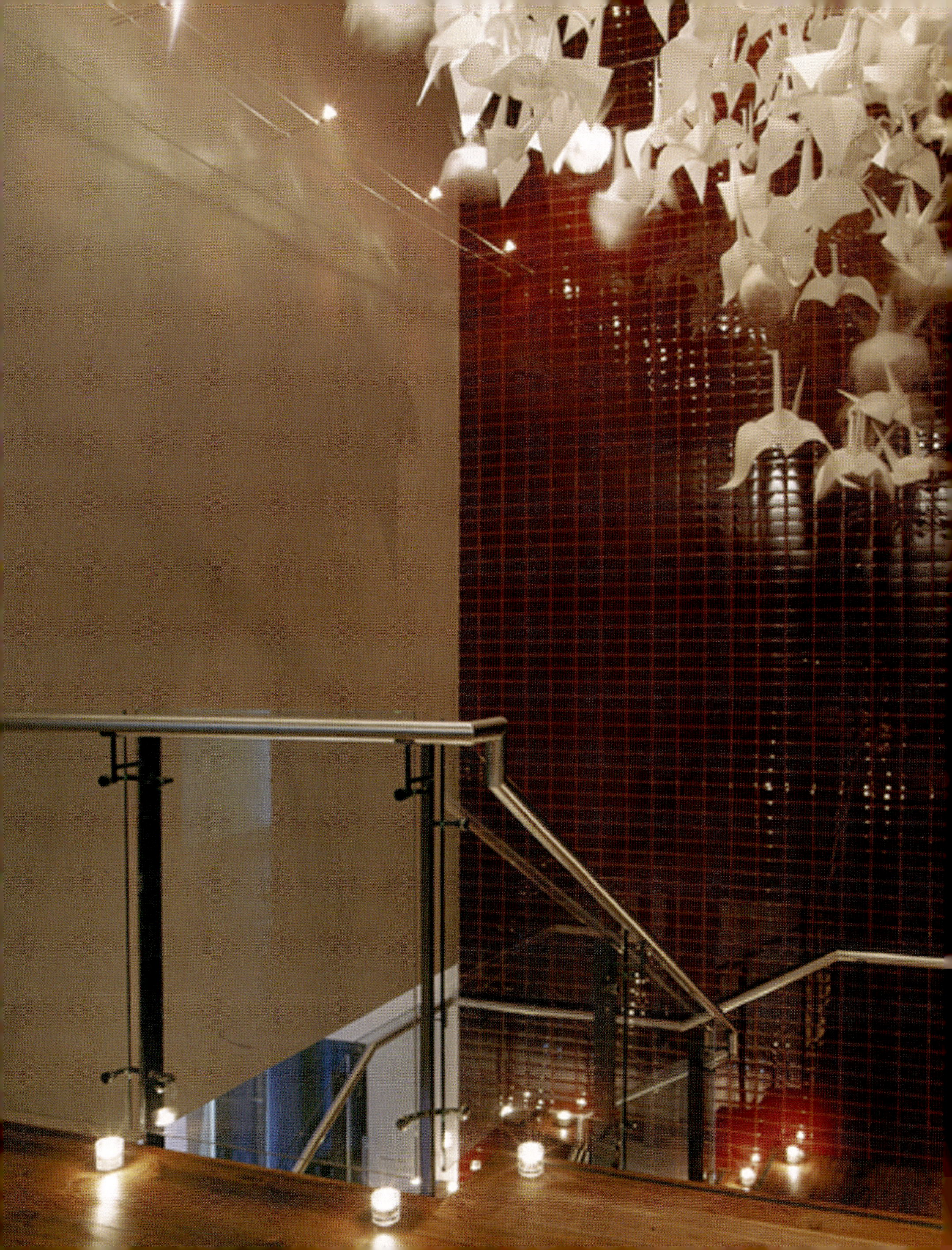

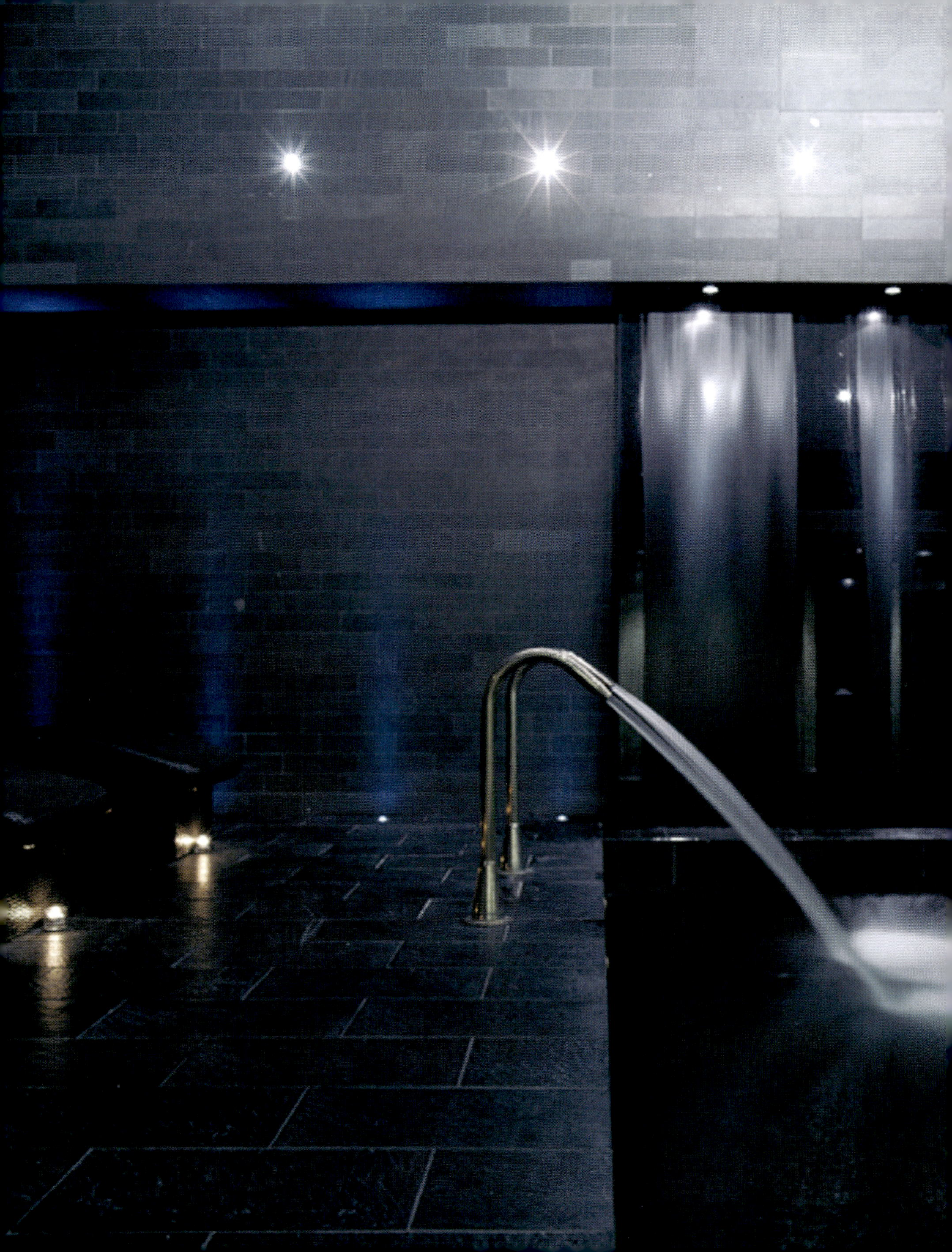

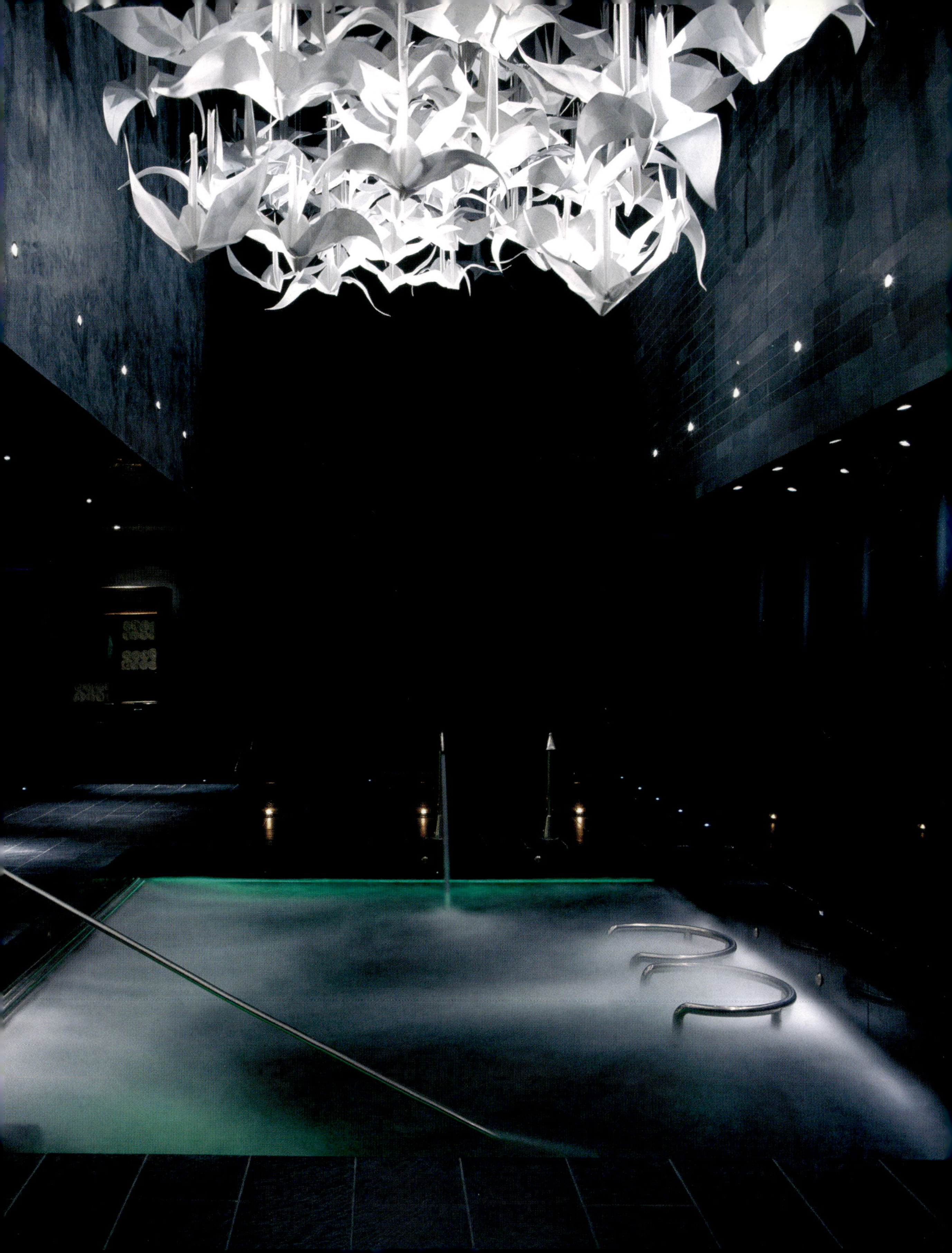

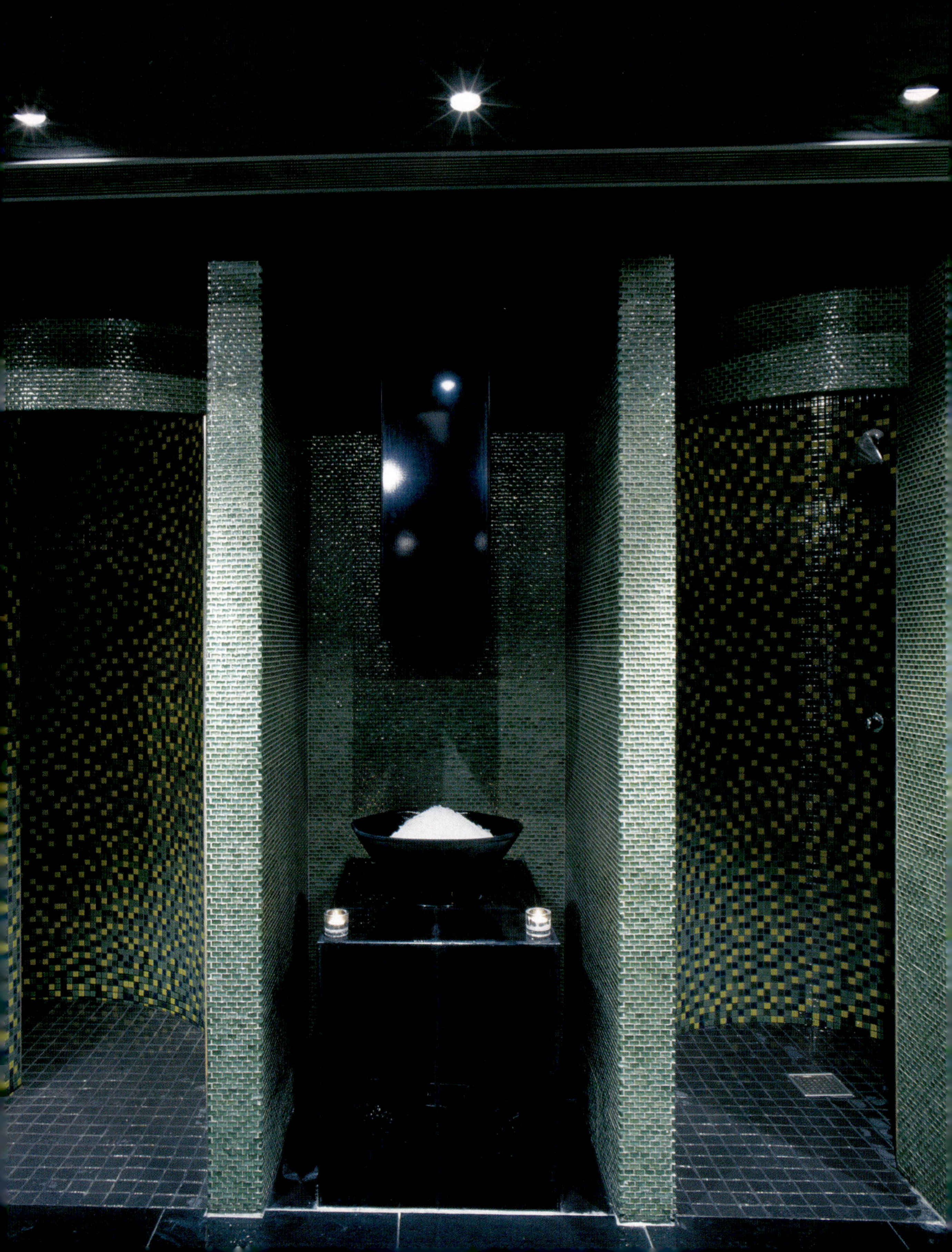

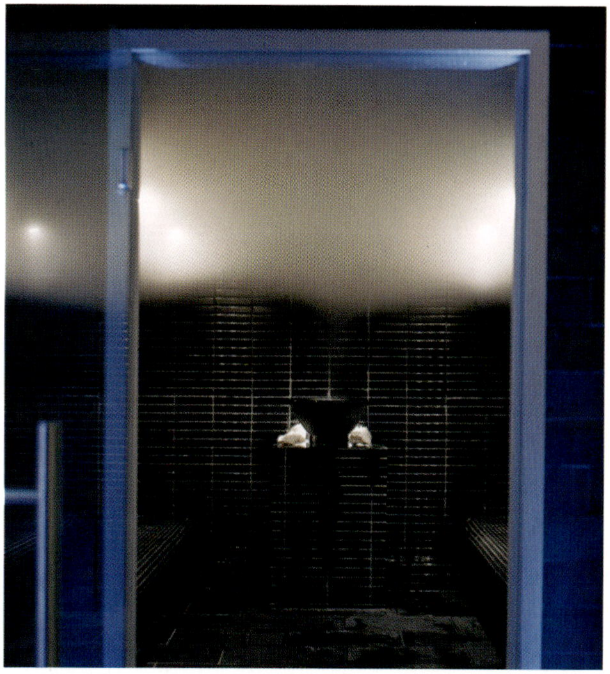

Der ganzheitliche Ansatz der Spa-Anwendungen zielt auf das Wohlbefinden von Körper und Geist.

Guided by holistic philosophy, the treatments offered by the spa are directed towards the wellbeing of the body and the spirit.

Inspirés de la philosophie holistique, les traitements offerts par le spa sont dédiés au bien-être du corps et de l'esprit.

De holistische behandelingen zijn gericht op welzijn voor lichaam en geest.

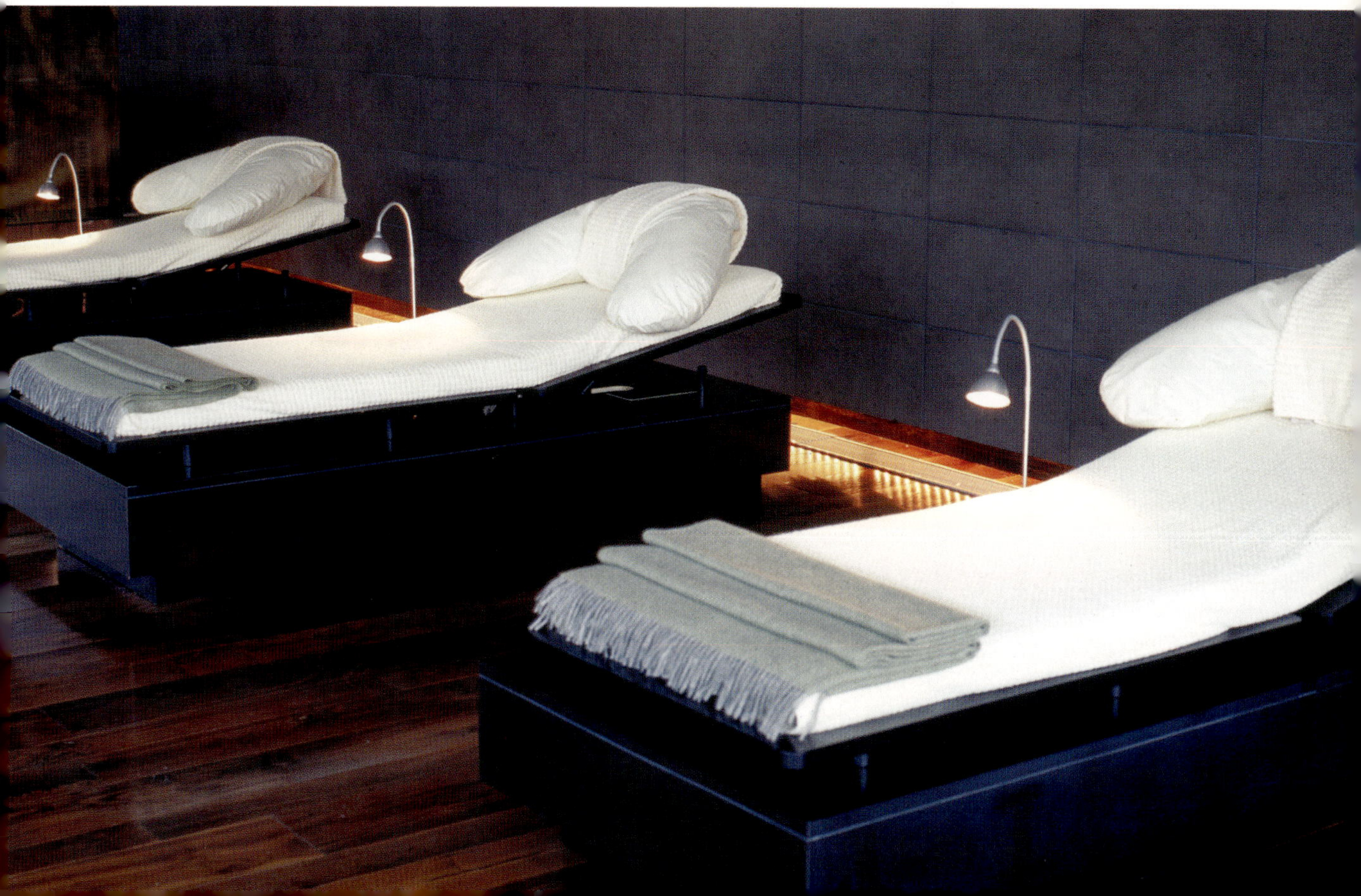

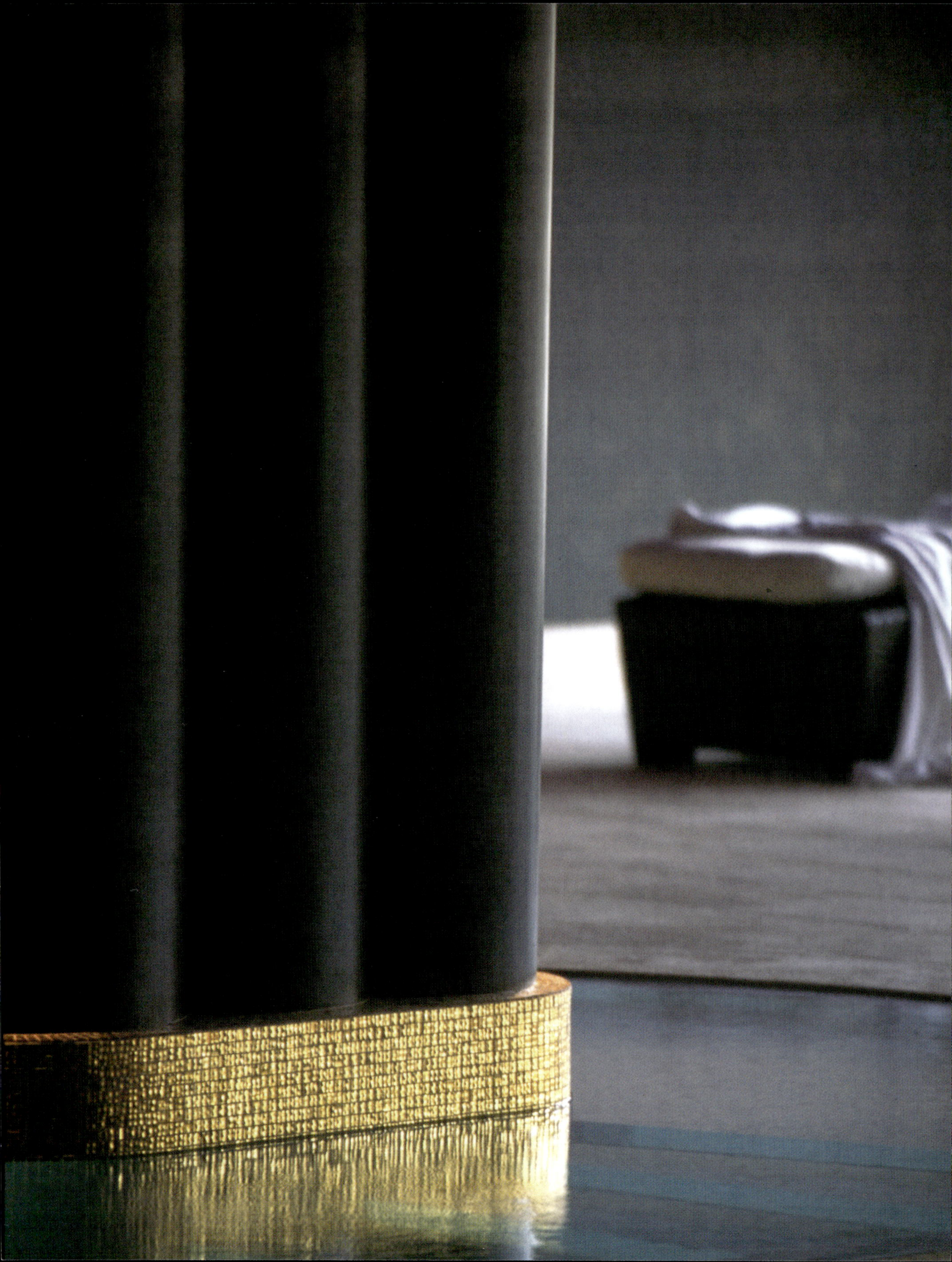

La Réserve

In dieser 2.000 Quadratmeter großen Anlage werden die Anwendungen auf jeden Gast individuell abgestimmt. Die Milch-, Öl-, Algen- und Honigbäder sind ebenso berühmt wie die gewichtsreduzierenden Massagen mit Crème aus brasilianischem Kaffee. Das Hallenschwimmbad bildet das Herz des Spas. Ergänzt wird es durch Außenpool, Sauna, Dampfbäder, Tennisplatz, Fitnessraum und eine Bar mit erfrischenden Getränken, die jeden Sport- und Erholungstag abrunden.

Within its 21,500 square feet there are personalized treatments designed for each guest. They are famous for their milk, oils, algae and honey baths, as well as for the massages to lose weight with Brazilian coffee cream. The indoor pool is the neuralgic center of the spa. It is complemented by the outside pool, the sauna, the steam baths, the tennis court, the gymnasium and a bar with invigorating drinks that complement a day dedicated to physical exercise and relaxation.

Au sein de ses 2.000 m^2, ce spa offre des traitements personnalisés, spécialement conçus pour chaque invité. Des soins célèbres tels que les bains de lait, d'huiles, d'algues ou de miel, ou encore les massages amincissants à la crème de café brésilien. La piscine intérieure est l'élément central de ce spa, complété par le bassin extérieur, le sauna, le hammam, le terrain de tennis, le gymnase, et le bar, dont les boissons fortifiantes viennent parfaire une journée consacrée à l'exercice physique et à la relaxation.

In deze 2000 m^2 tellende ruimte krijgen alle gasten een behandeling op maat. Dit kuuroord staat bekend om zijn baden met melk, oliën, algen en honing en massages met Braziliaanse koffiecrème om gewichtsverlies te bevorderen. Het binnenzwembad is het zenuwcentrum van de instelling. Verder zijn er nog een buitenzwembad, sauna, stoombaden, tennisbaan, fitnessruimte en een bar met verkwikkende drankjes die een dag van fysieke inspanning en ontspanning helemaal af maken.

Geneva, Switzerland

PATRICE REYNAUD, JACQUES GARCIA

Photos © Design Hotels

www.lareserve.ch

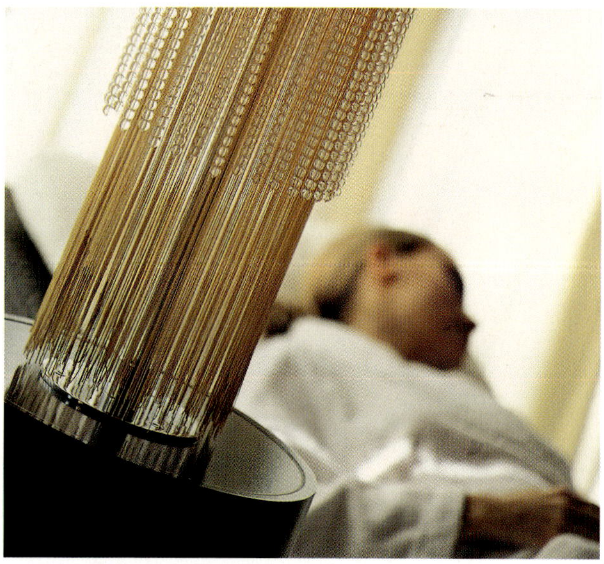

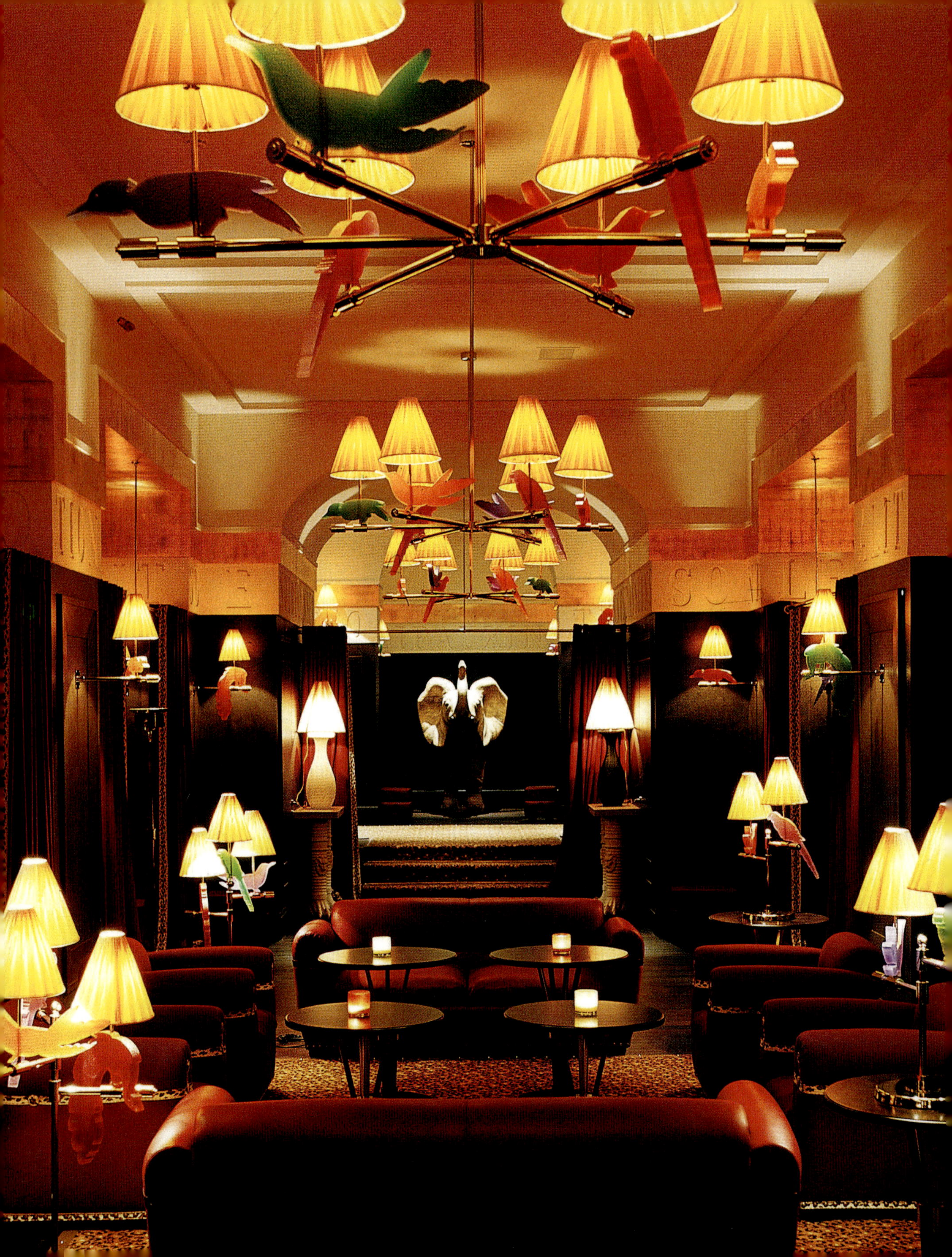

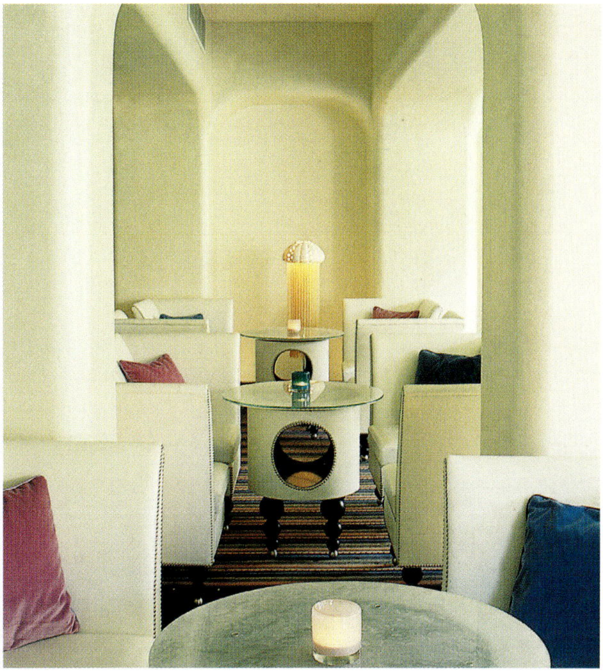

Eingebettet in eine Parklandschaft am Ufer des Genfer Sees liegt das Hotel La Réserve in friedlicher Abgeschiedenheit.

Located in a park, at the border of Lake Geneva, hotel La Réserve is a peaceful backwater.

Situé dans un parc au bord Lac Léman, l'hôtel La Réserve est un havre de paix.

Hotel La Réserve, gelegen in een park aan de oever van het Meer van Genève, staat garant voor rust.

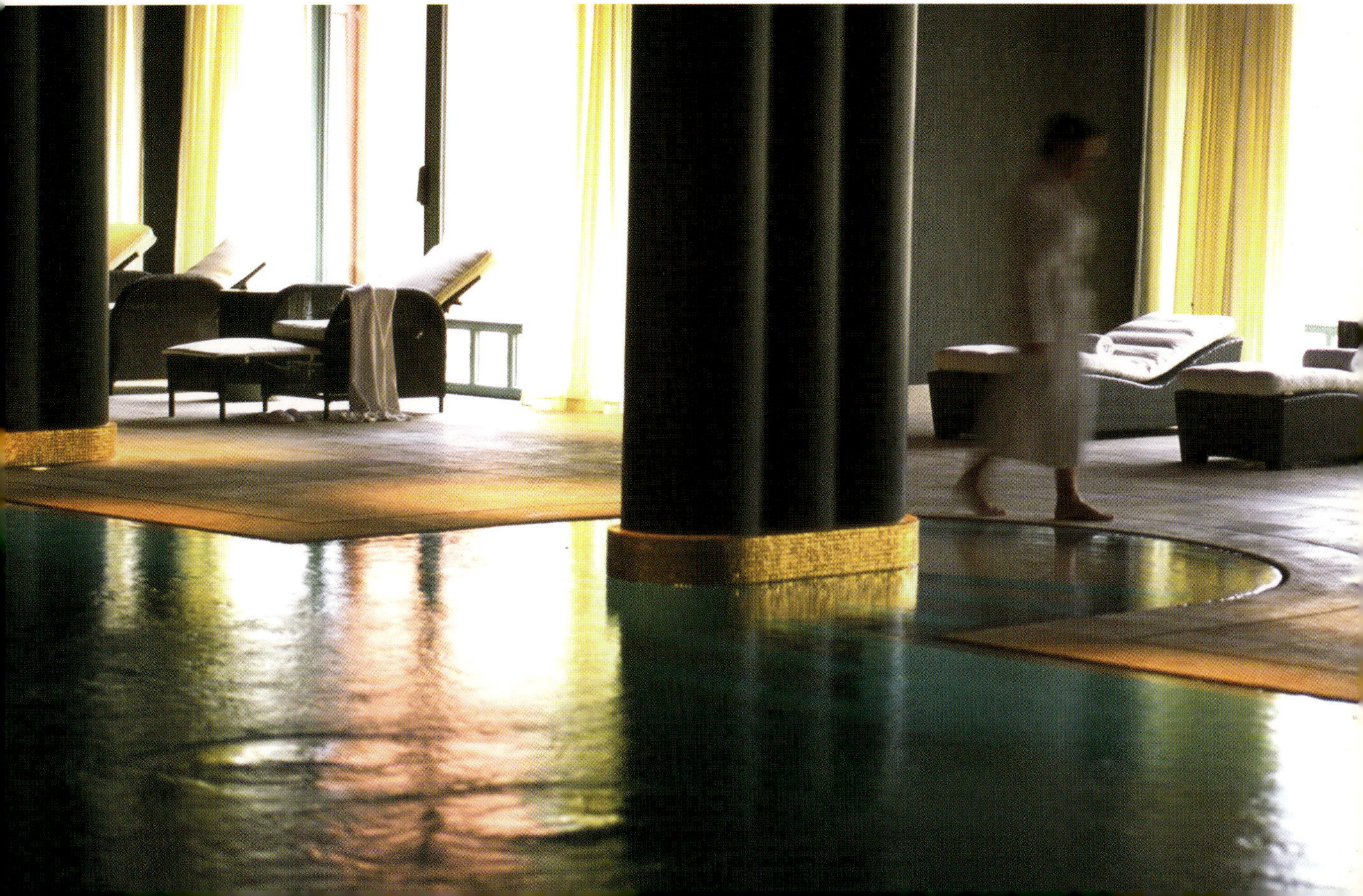

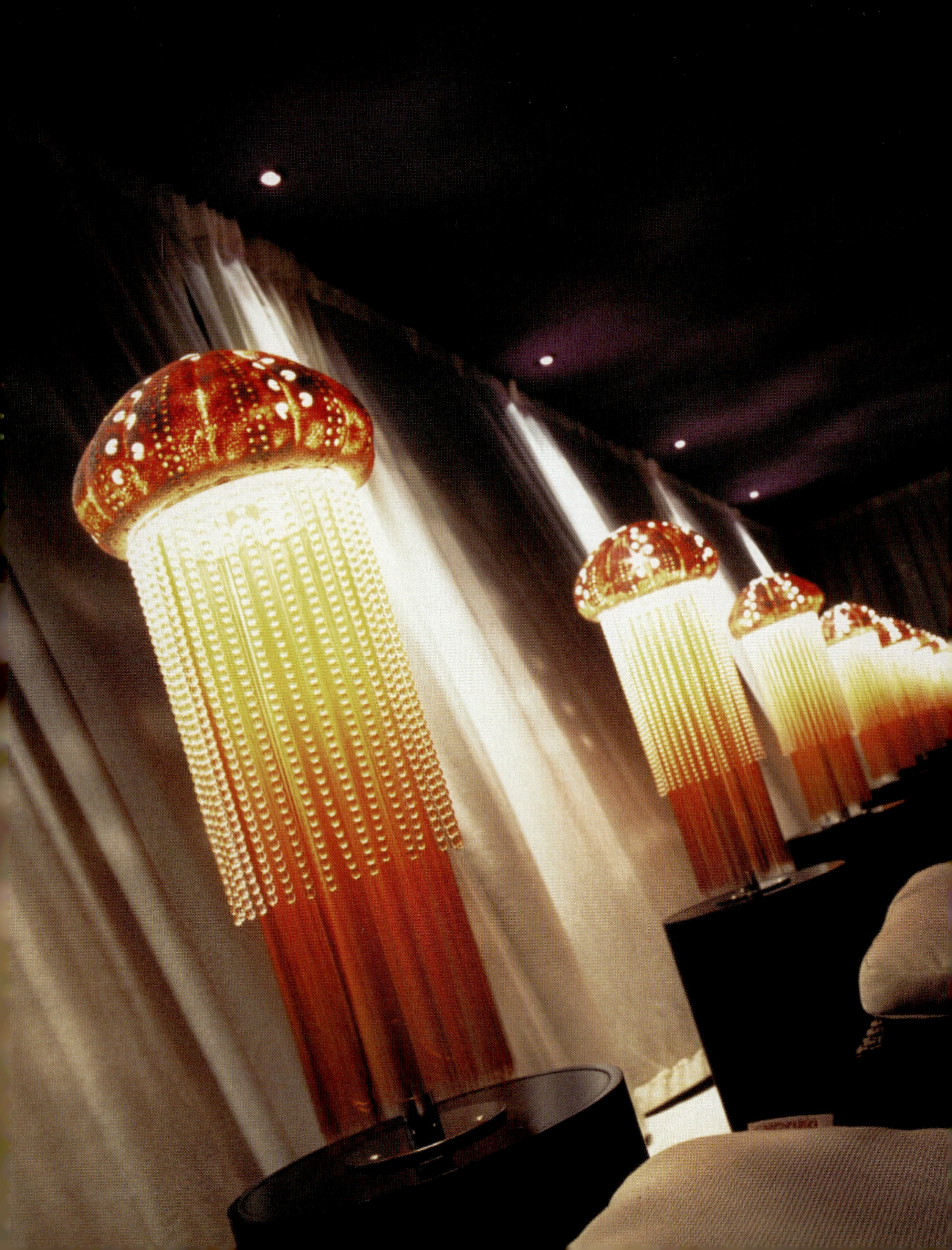

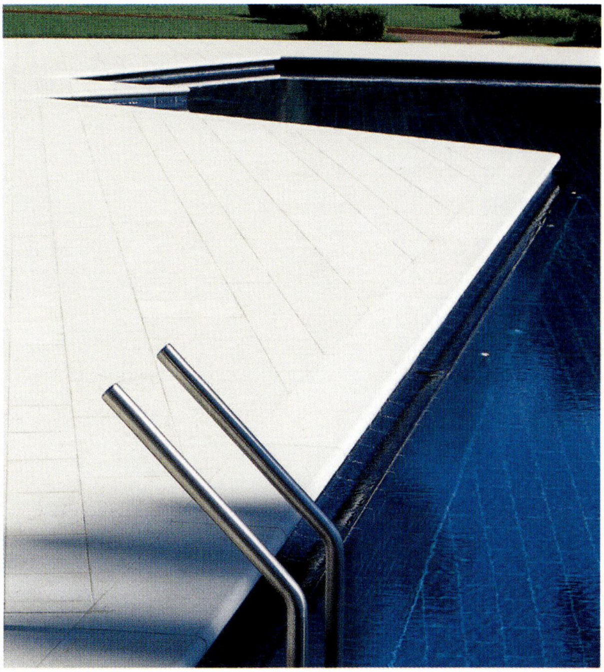

Die Therapien umfassen Bäder mit ätherischen Ölen, Algen, Honig und Gelée royale.

The therapies include baths with essences, oils, algae, honey and royal jelly.

Les thérapies incluent des bains à base d'essences naturelles, d'huiles essentielles, d'algues, de miel, et de gelée royale.

De therapieën omvatten onder andere baden met oliën, extracten, algen, honing en koninginnegelei.

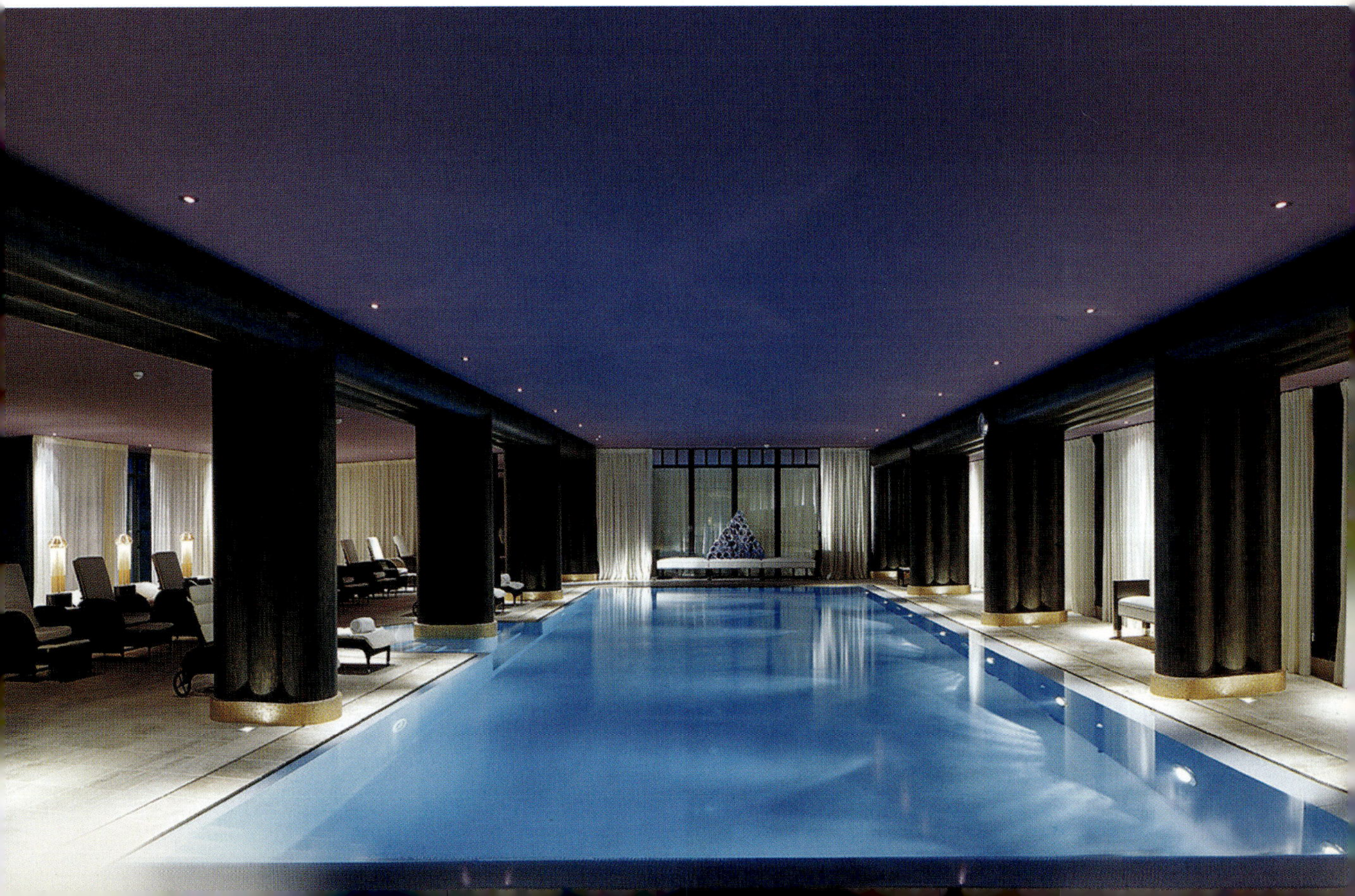

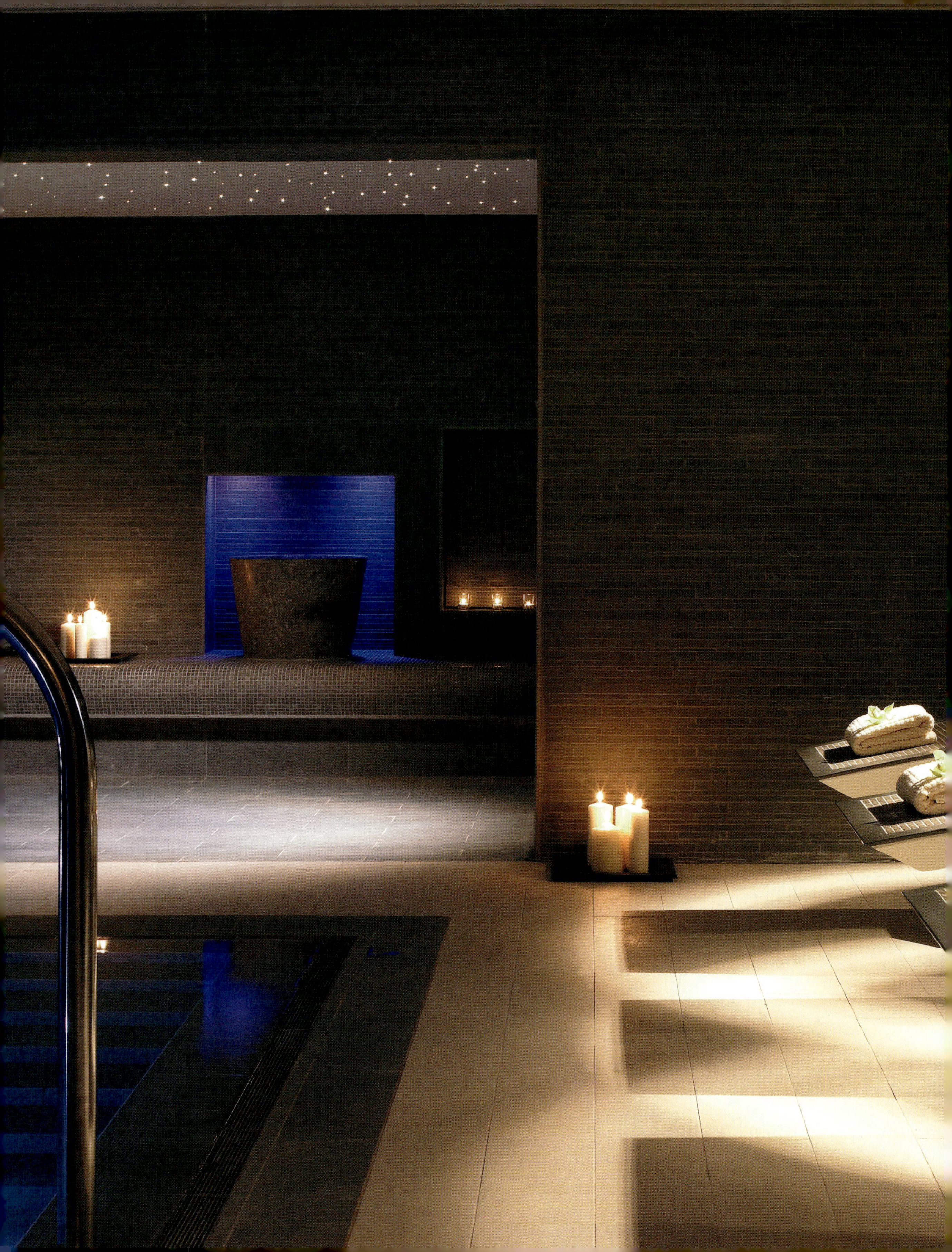

Maryborough Hotel and Spa

Dieses Spa ist Teil des Maryborough Hotels, das die Eigenschaften eines Landhauses mit denen eines modernen Hotels vereint. Ein großer Wasserfall dominiert das Zentrum des Spas und ebnet sich seinen Weg durch die Glasmauern, die den Behandlungsbereich von Dampfbädern und Pool trennen. Saunen, türkische Bäder sowie Eiskabinen sind durch eine funkelnde Decke, die einen Sternenhimmel simuliert, optisch miteinander verbunden.

This spa is part of the Maryborough hotel, an establishment that brings together the characteristics of a country house and those of the contemporaneous hotel industry. A great waterfall dominates the center of the spa and runs through the glass walls that separate the treatment area from the steam baths and the pool. Saunas and Turkish baths, as well as ice cabins, are visually connected by a twinkling ceiling that simulates a sky full of stars.

Ce spa fait partie de l'hôtel Maryborough, un établissement qui allie tous les avantages d'une hôtellerie contemporaine au charme d'un manoir. Au centre du spa, un mur d'eau attire le regard, glissant le long des parois vitrées qui séparent la zone de soins du hammam et de la piscine. Les saunas et les bains turcs, ainsi que les cabines d'eau glacée, sont visuellement reliés par un plafond scintillant simulant un ciel étoilé.

Dit etablissement maakt deel uit van het Maryborough Hotel, dat de eigenschappen van een landelijk hotel paart aan die van een modern resort. Het badgedeelte wordt gedomineerd door een grote waterval, die door de transparante muren stroomt die de behandelruimten scheiden van de stoombaden en het zwembad. Sauna's, Turkse baden en ijscabines zijn visueel met elkaar verbonden door middel van een fonkelend plafond, dat een sterrenhemel imiteert.

Cork, Ireland

MICHELE SWEENEY/OPPERMANN ASSOCIATES

Photos © Andrew Bradley

www.maryborough.com

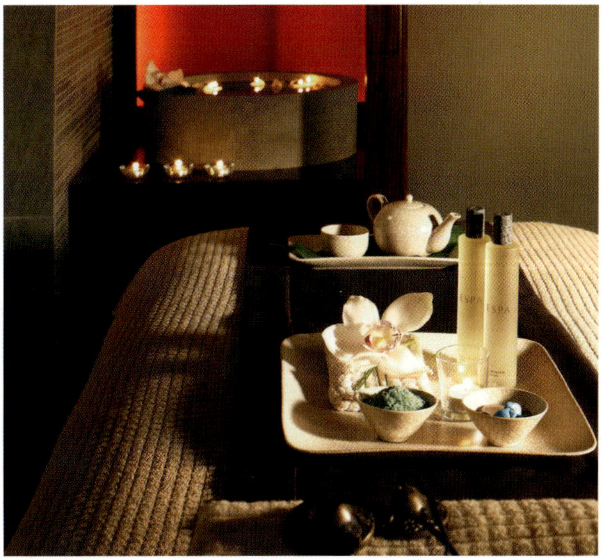

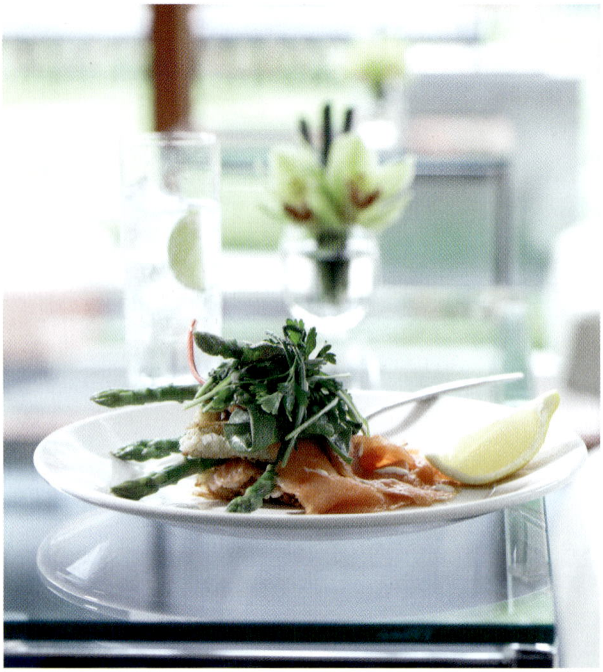

Die Therapien sind durch östliche und westliche Heil- und Entspannungstechniken inspiriert.

Therapies are inspired in healing and relaxation techniques, originated in the East and the West.

Les thérapies sont inspirées des techniques de relaxation et de guérison pratiquées autant en Asie qu'en Occident.

De therapieën zijn geïnspireerd op genezende en ontspannende technieken uit het Oosten en Westen.

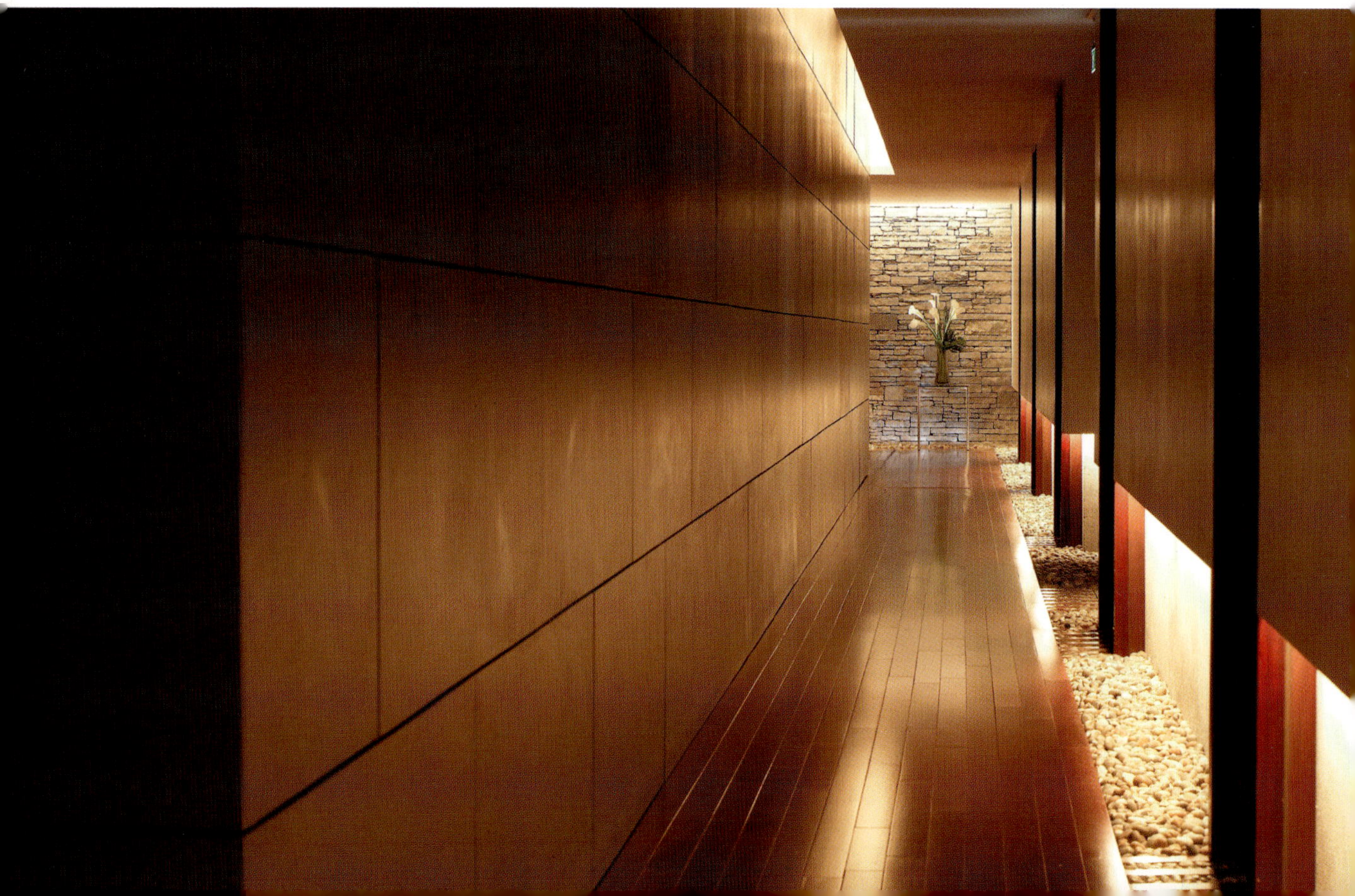

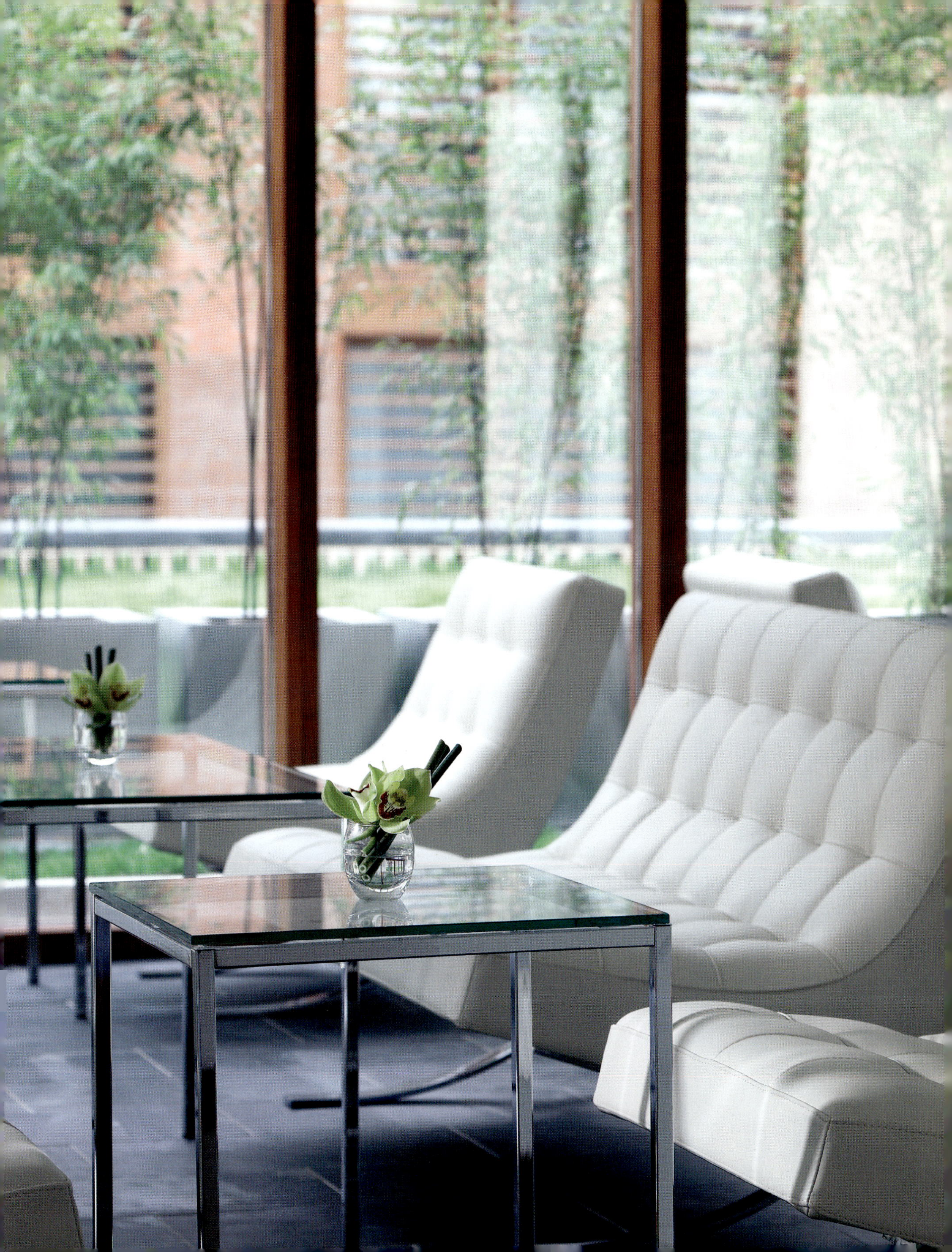

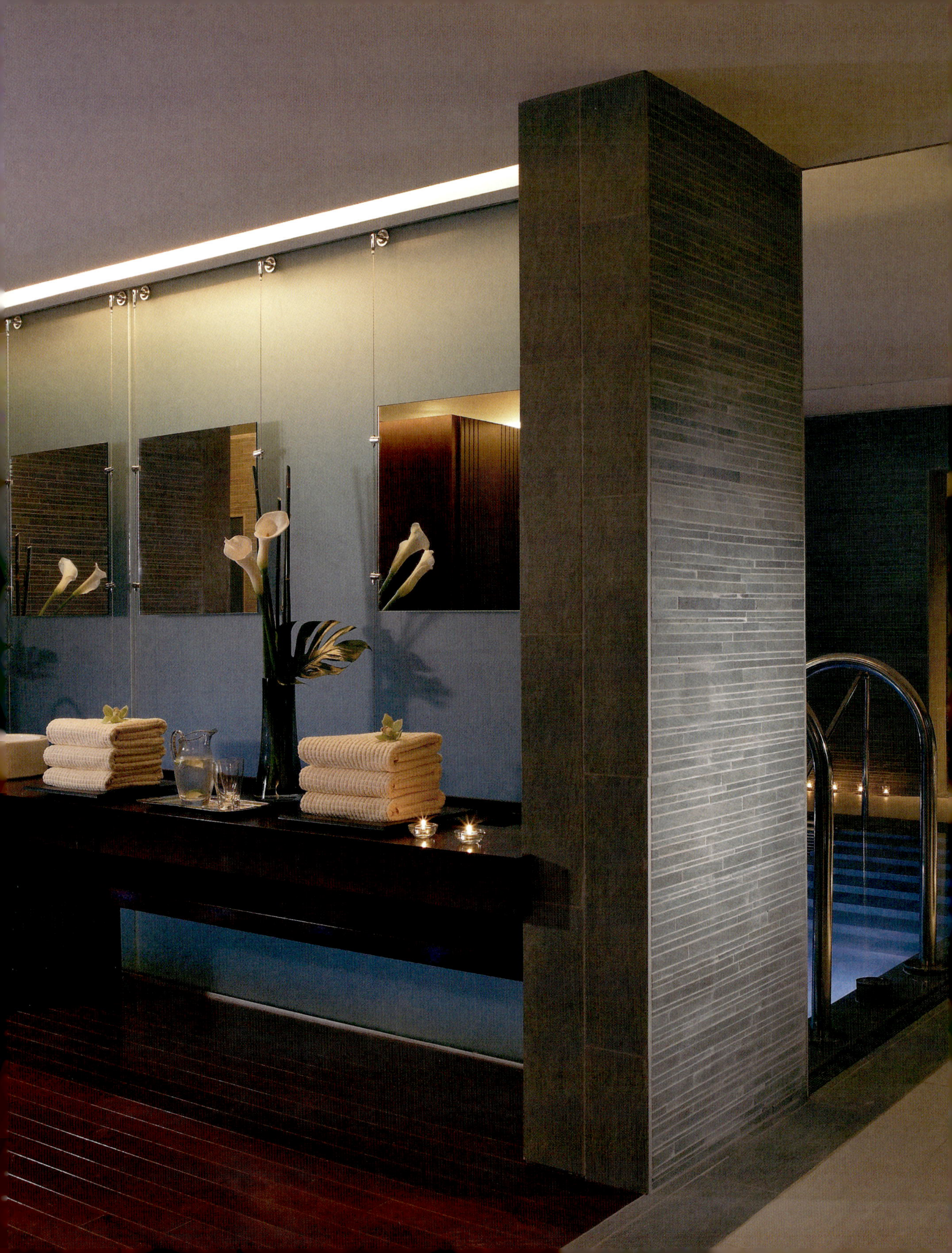

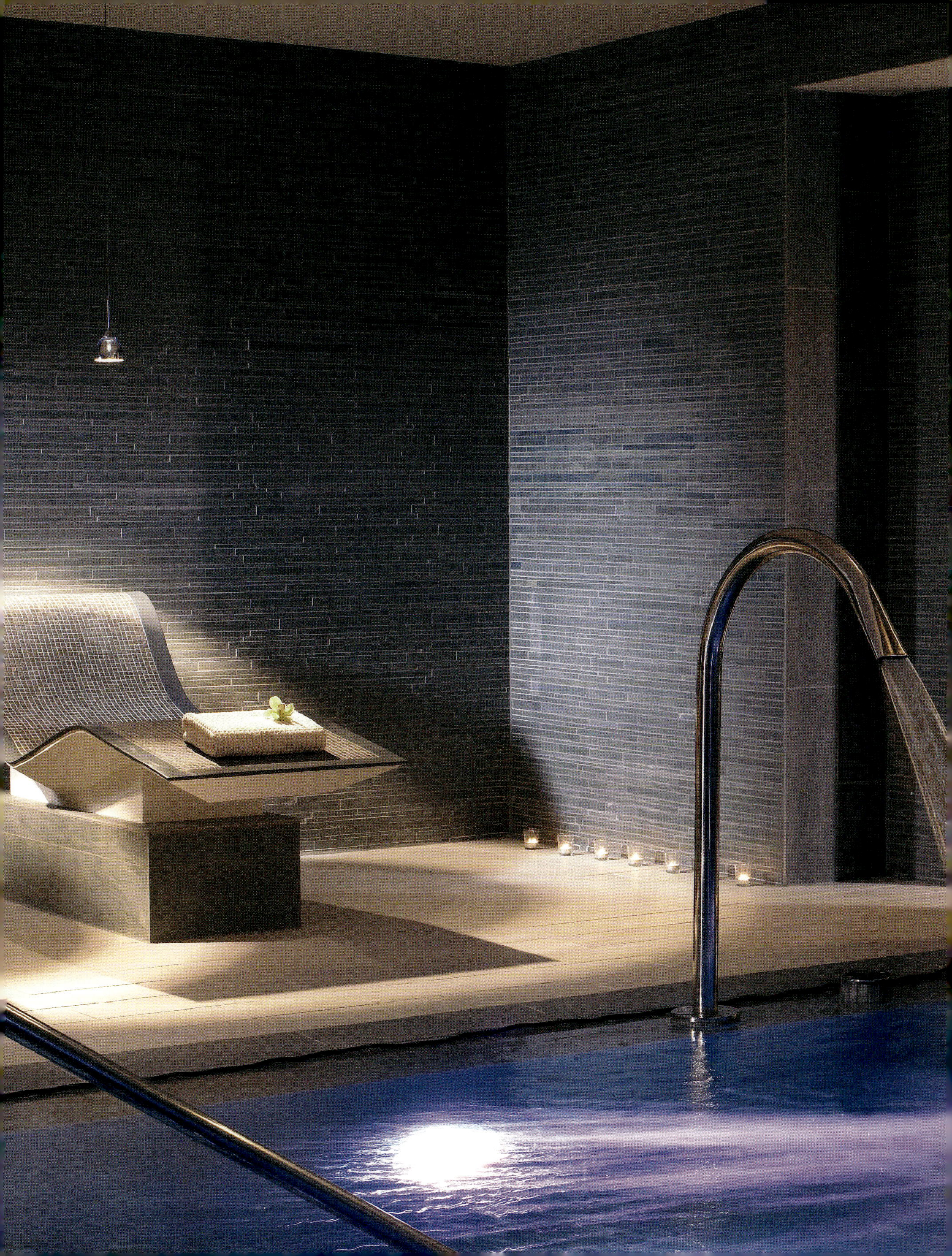

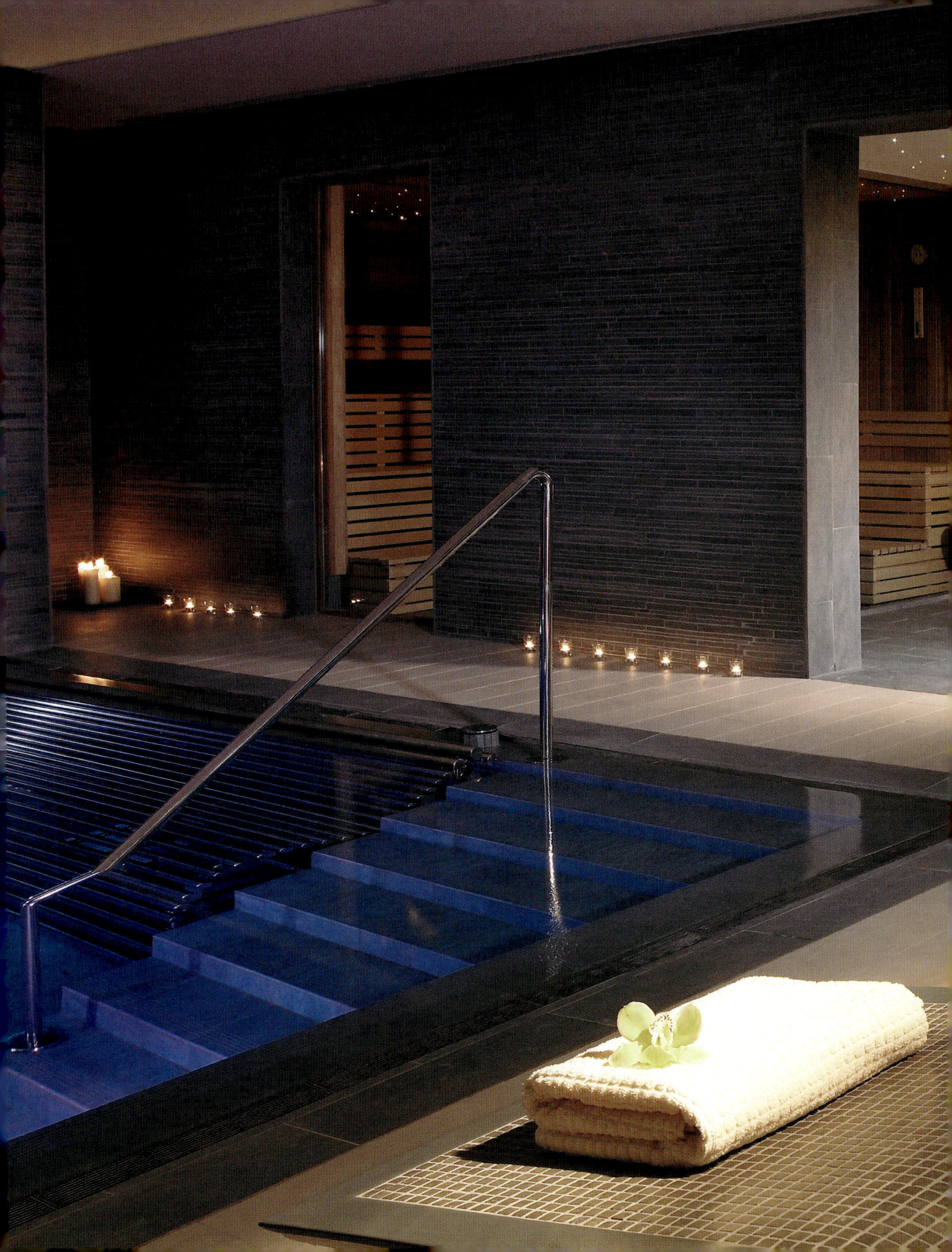

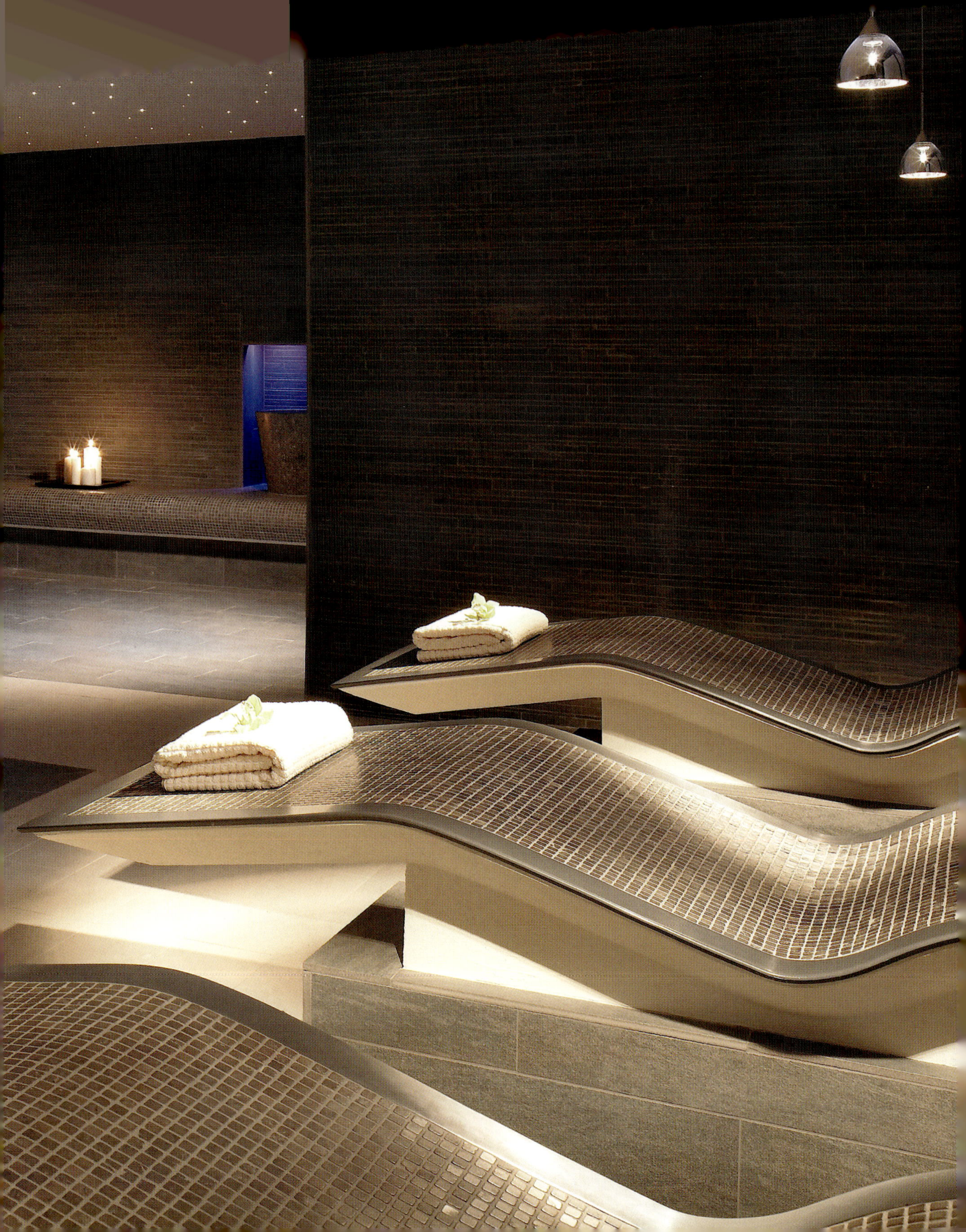

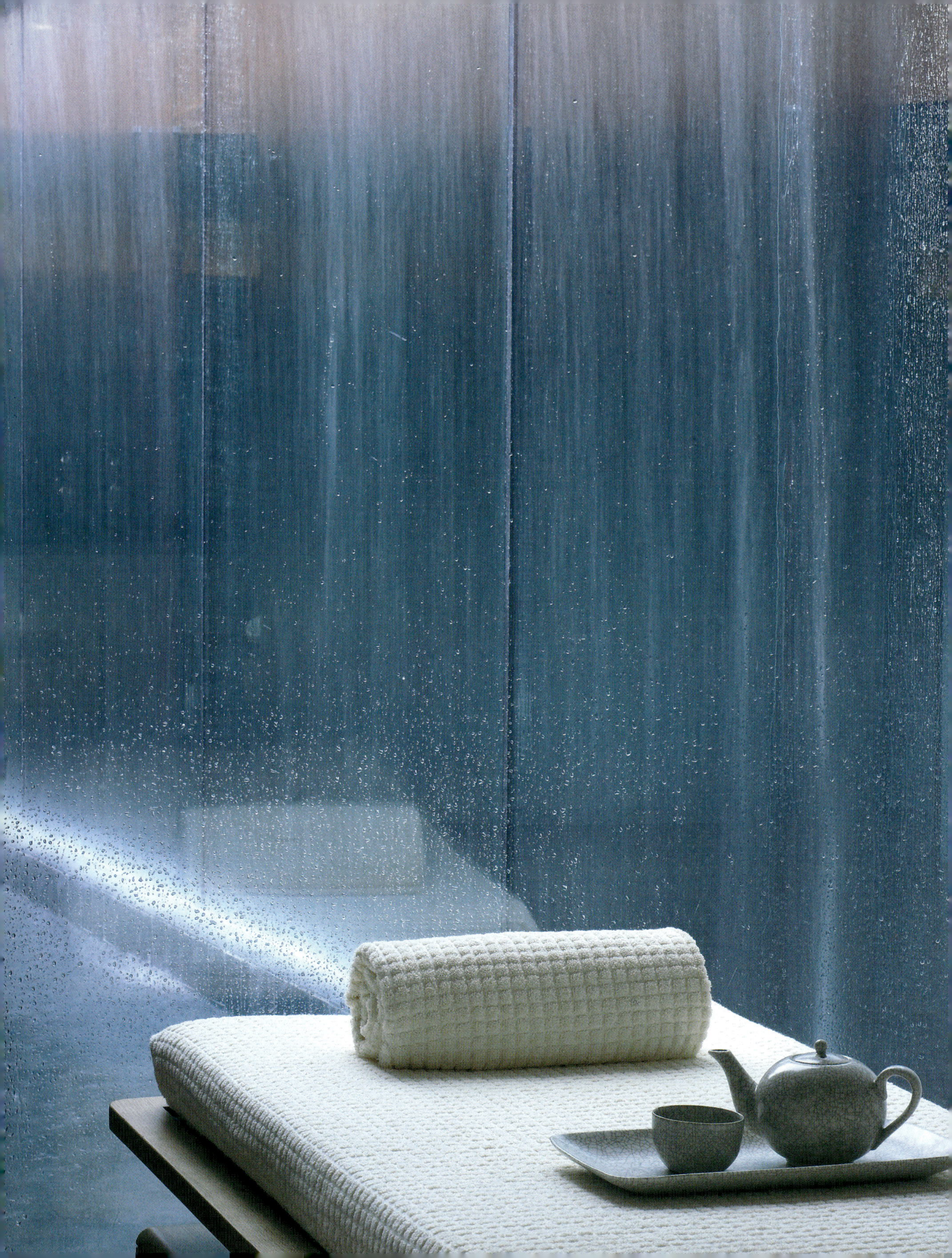

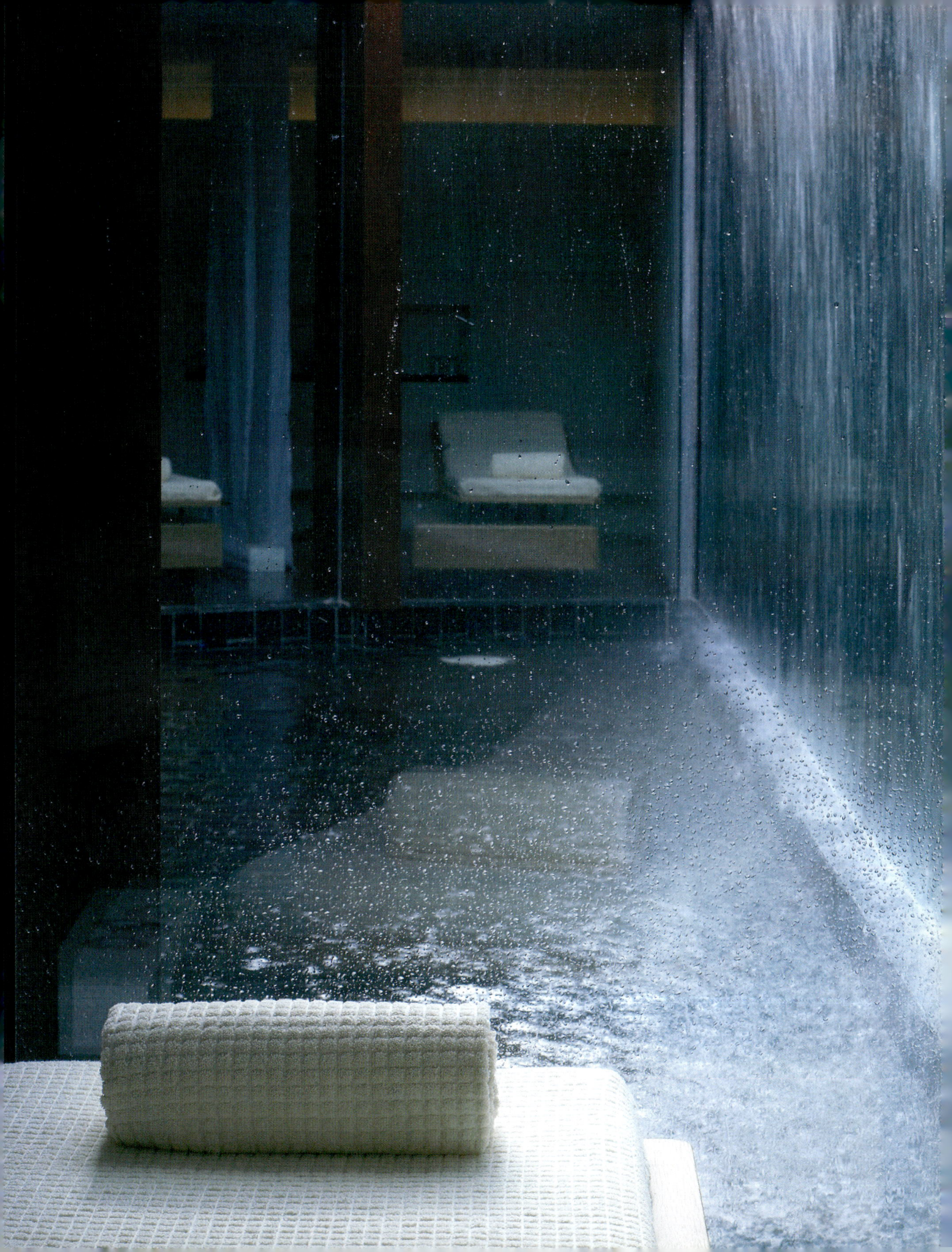

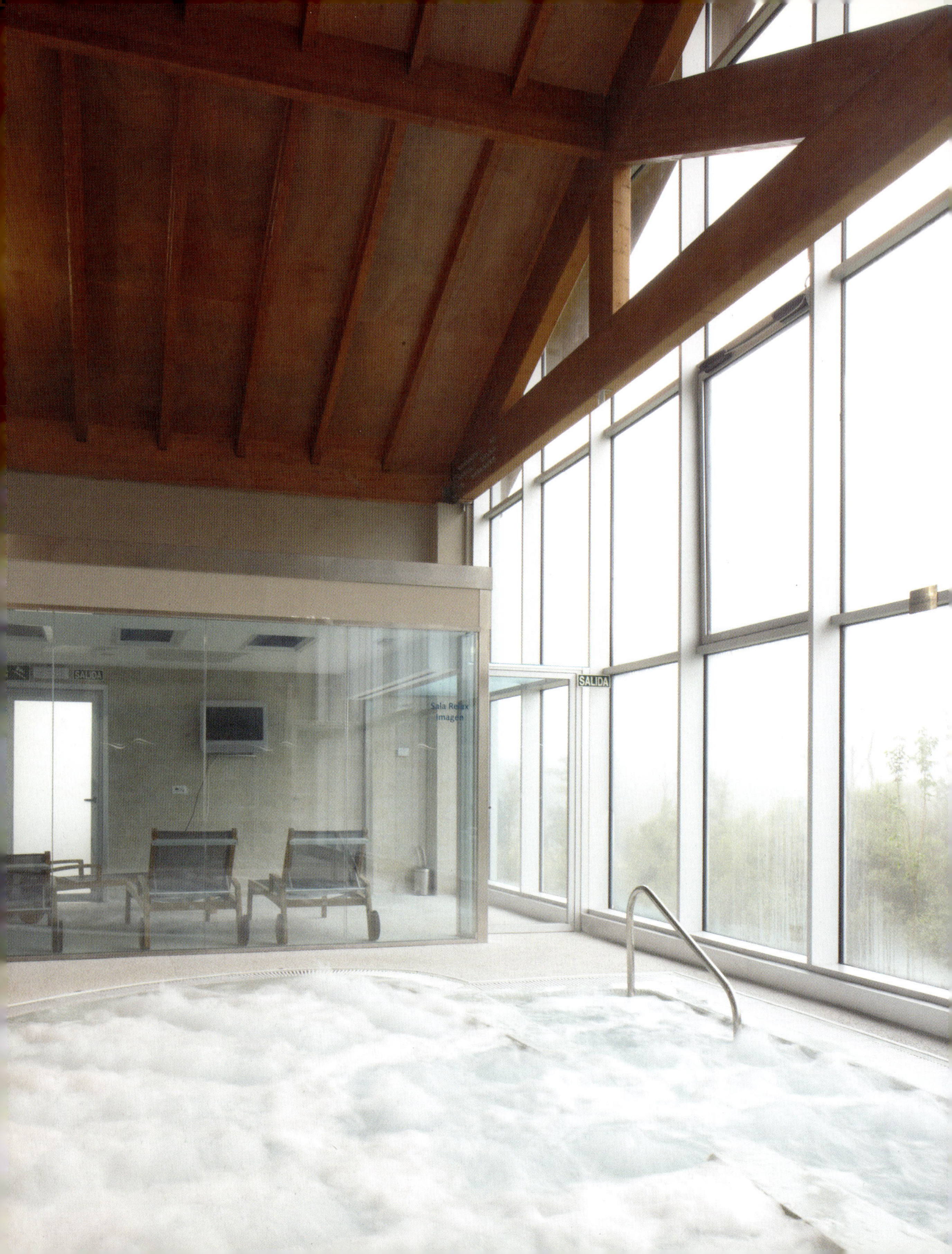
SALIDA
SALIDA

Spa Termas de Villalba

Auf 2.100 Quadratmetern bietet dieses Spa einen großzügigen Thermo-Wellness-Bereich mit römischen Thermalbädern, finnischer Sauna, türkischem Bad, Aroma- und Farbtherapiebehandlungen, Hot-Stone-Therapie und Nebelduschen. Im therapeutischen Bereich werden die Gäste mit revitalisierenden und erholsamen Wickelbehandlungen, Algenkompressen, ätherischen Ölbädern, Schlammpackungen, Vichy-Duschen und Entspannungsmassagen verwöhnt.

The 22,600 square feet of facilities are divided in two areas. The thermo-recreational area, composed of the Roman thermal baths, the Finnish sauna, the Turkish bath, the aromatherapy, chromotherapy treatments, the warm stones walk and the mist showers. At the therapeutic area they apply bandages and algae compresses, essential oils and mud, as well as Vichy showers with relaxing massages, ideal to eliminate stress and revitalize the organism.

Les 2.100 m² d'équipements sont répartis en deux zones. Le centre thermo-ludique est dédié aux thermes romains, au sauna finlandais, au bain turc, à l'aromathérapie, à la chromothérapie, aux promenades sur pierres chaudes, et aux douches brumisantes. Dans la partie réservée aux soins thérapeutiques, le spa propose des masques et des enveloppements d'algues, d'huiles essentielles et de boue, ainsi que des massages sous douche d'affusion, la prestation idéale pour évacuer le stress et revitaliser l'organisme.

De ruim opgezette faciliteiten zijn verdeeld in twee gebieden. Het thermale en recreatieve gedeelte, dat bestaat uit Romeinse baden, een Finse sauna, een Turks bad, aromatherapie en chromotherapie-behandelingen, een warm stenenpad en neveldouches. In het therapeutische gedeelte wordt gewerkt met windsels en algenkompressen, etherische oliën en modder. Verder zijn er Vichydouches en ontspannende massages, ideaal tegen stress en verkwikkend voor lijf en leden.

Galicia, Spain

FADESA TECHNICAL OFFICE

Photos © Jordi Escandell

www.tesal.com

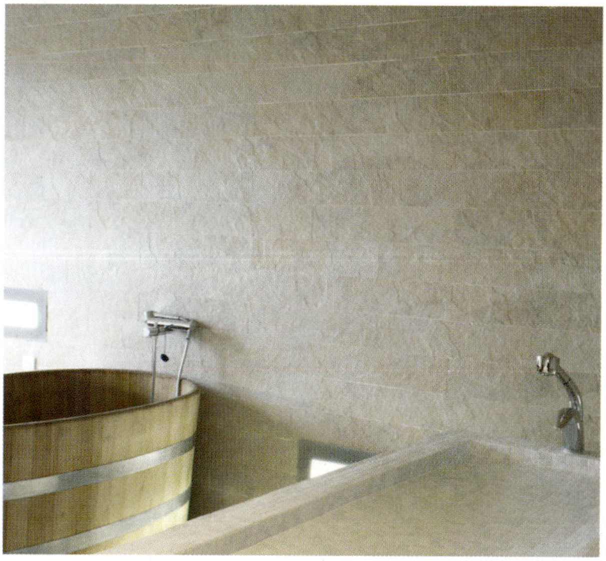

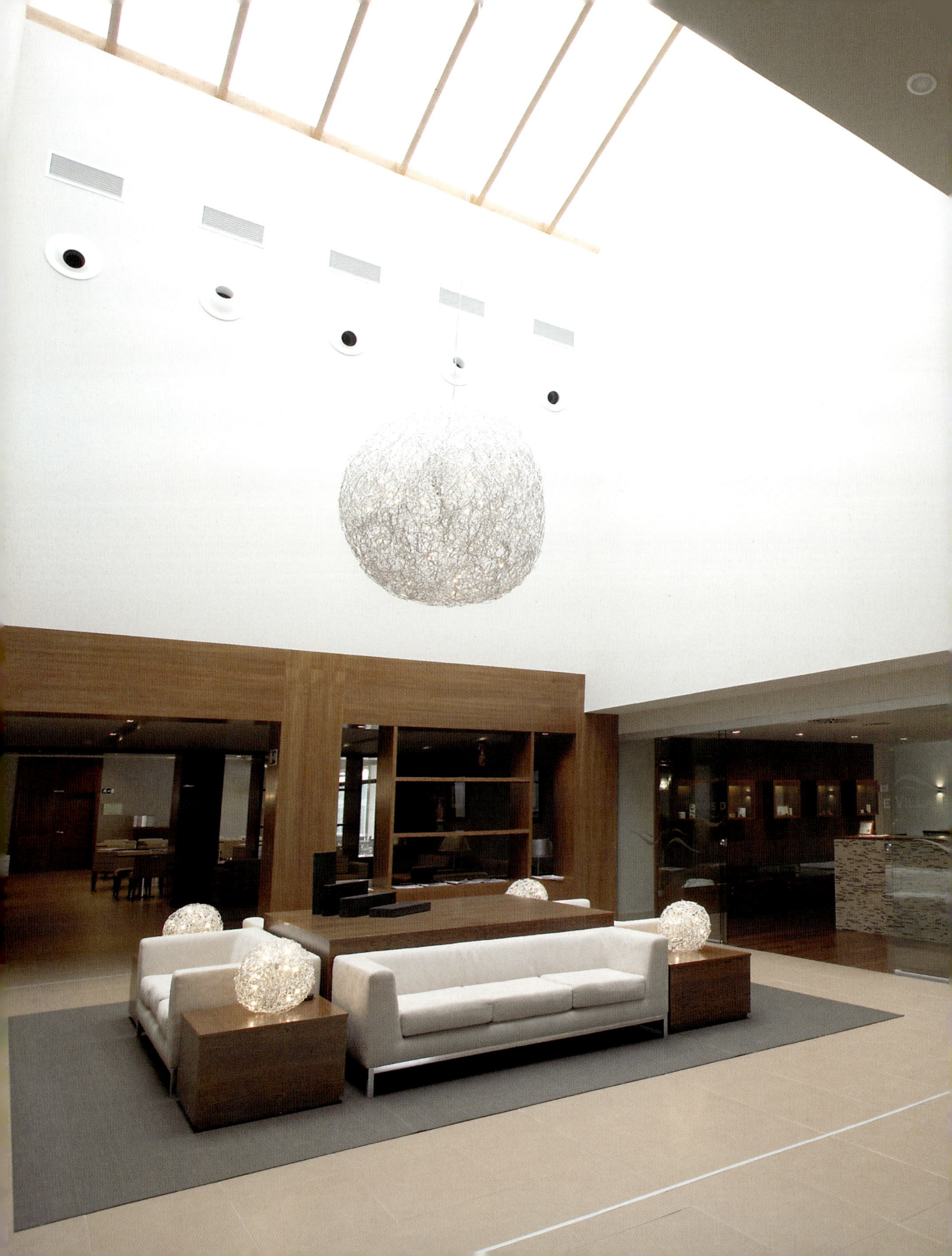

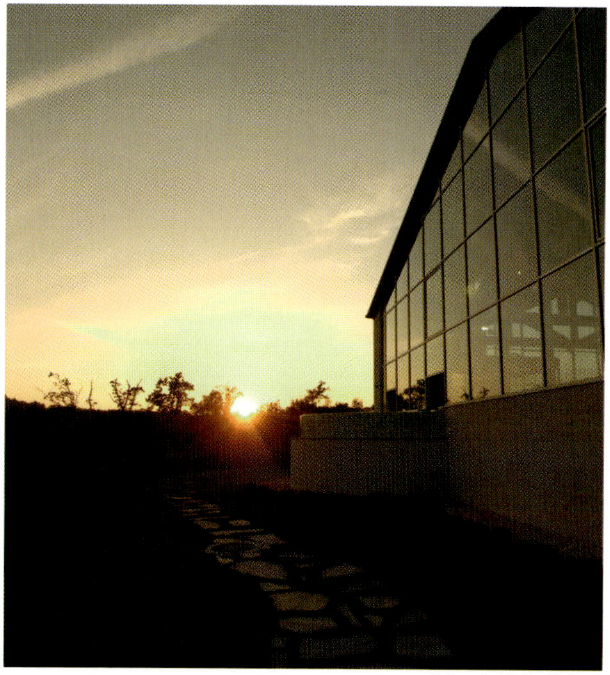

Charca do Alligal, der Ort, an dem sich dieses beeindruckende Spa befindet, ist für seine Thermalquellen bekannt.

Charco do Alligal, where this fabulous spa is located, is well known because of the thermal properties of its waters.

Ce superbe spa est situé à Charca do Alligal, bien connu pour les propriétés thermales de ses eaux.

Charco do Alligal, waar dit fraaie kuuroord ligt, staat bekend om de heilzame eigenschappen van het lokae bronwater.

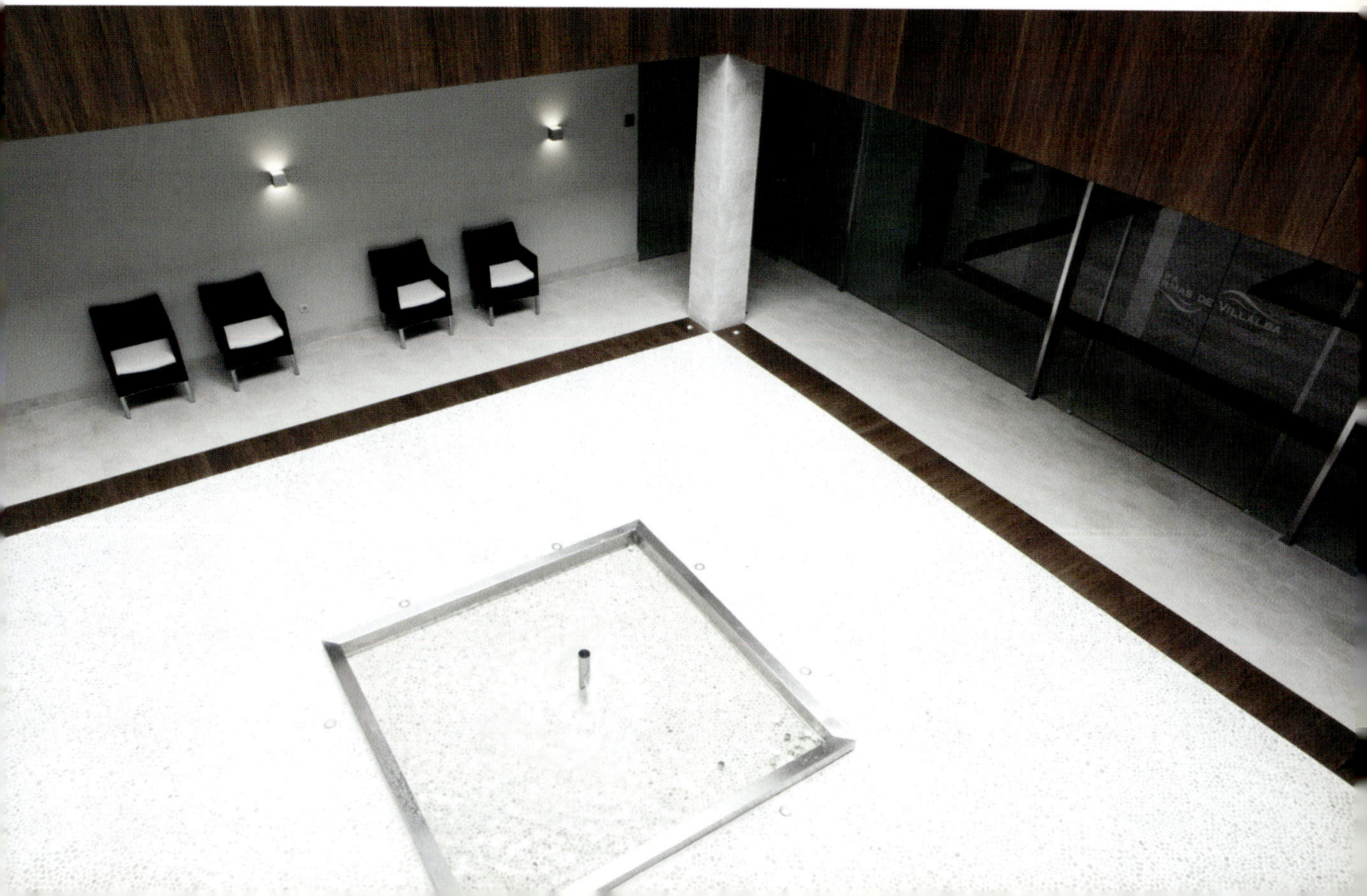

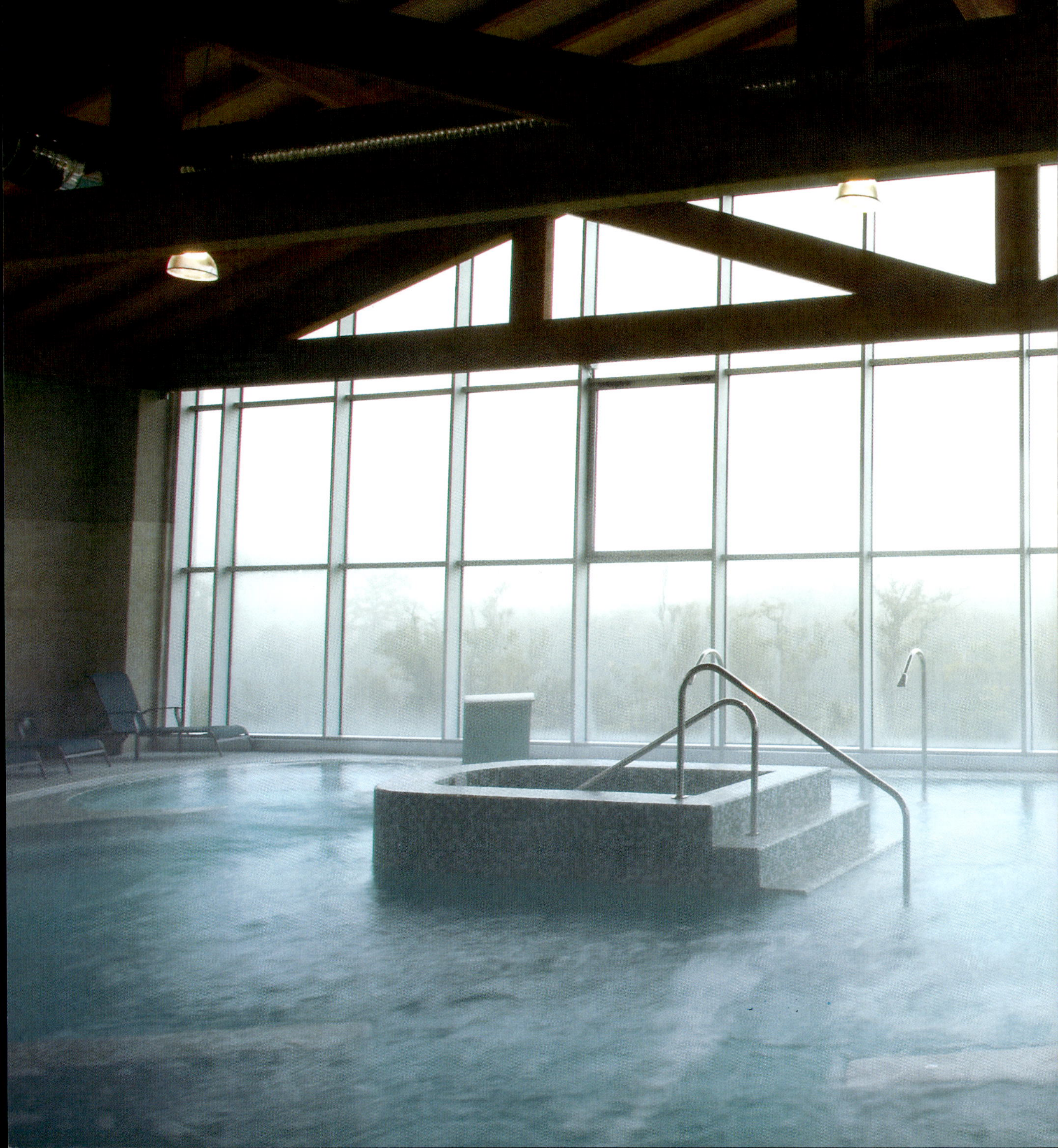

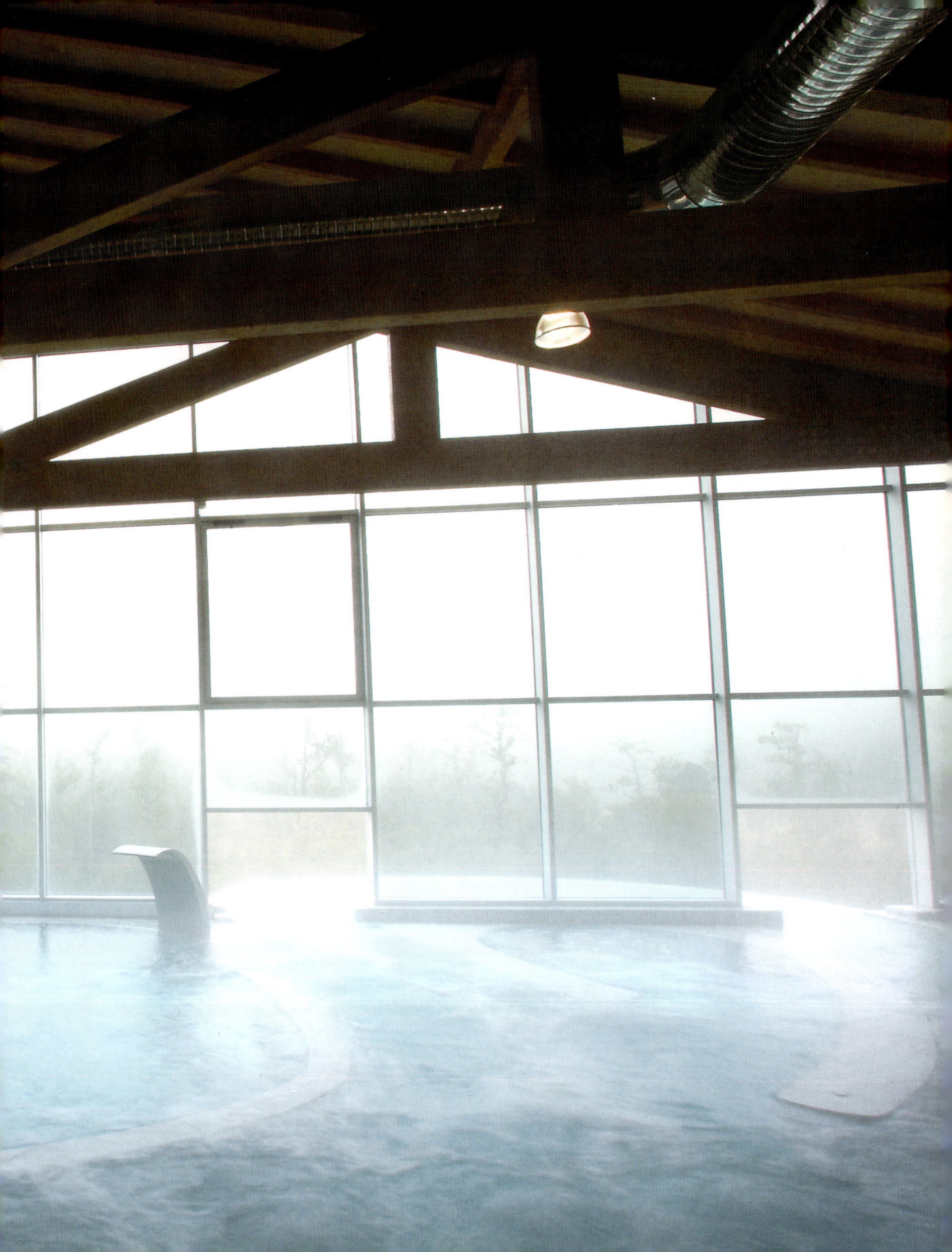

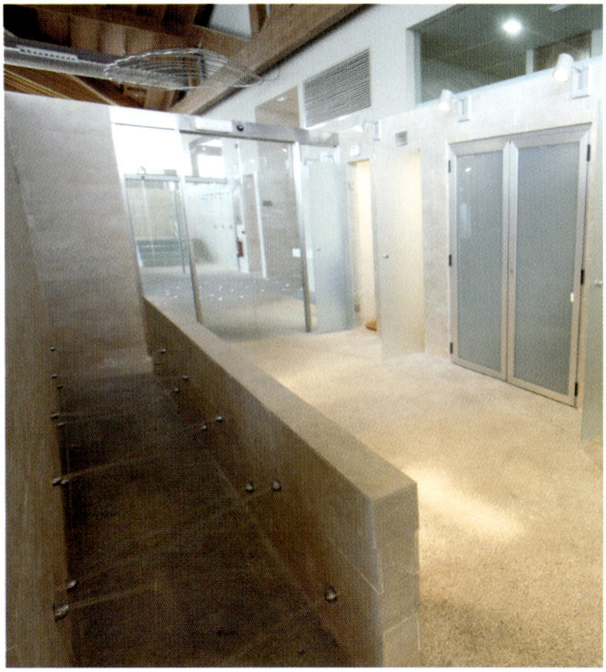

VIP-Kunden haben Zugang zu Exklusivanwendungen im „Wooden Font Cloister" und „Great Cloister".

VIP customers have access to exclusive treatments like the "Wooden Font Cloister," and the "Great Cloister."

Les clients VIP ont accès à des traitements exclusifs comme le « Wooden Font Cloister » , ou le « Great Cloister » .

Belangrijke gasten hebben toegang tot behandelingen met allerlei exotische namen.

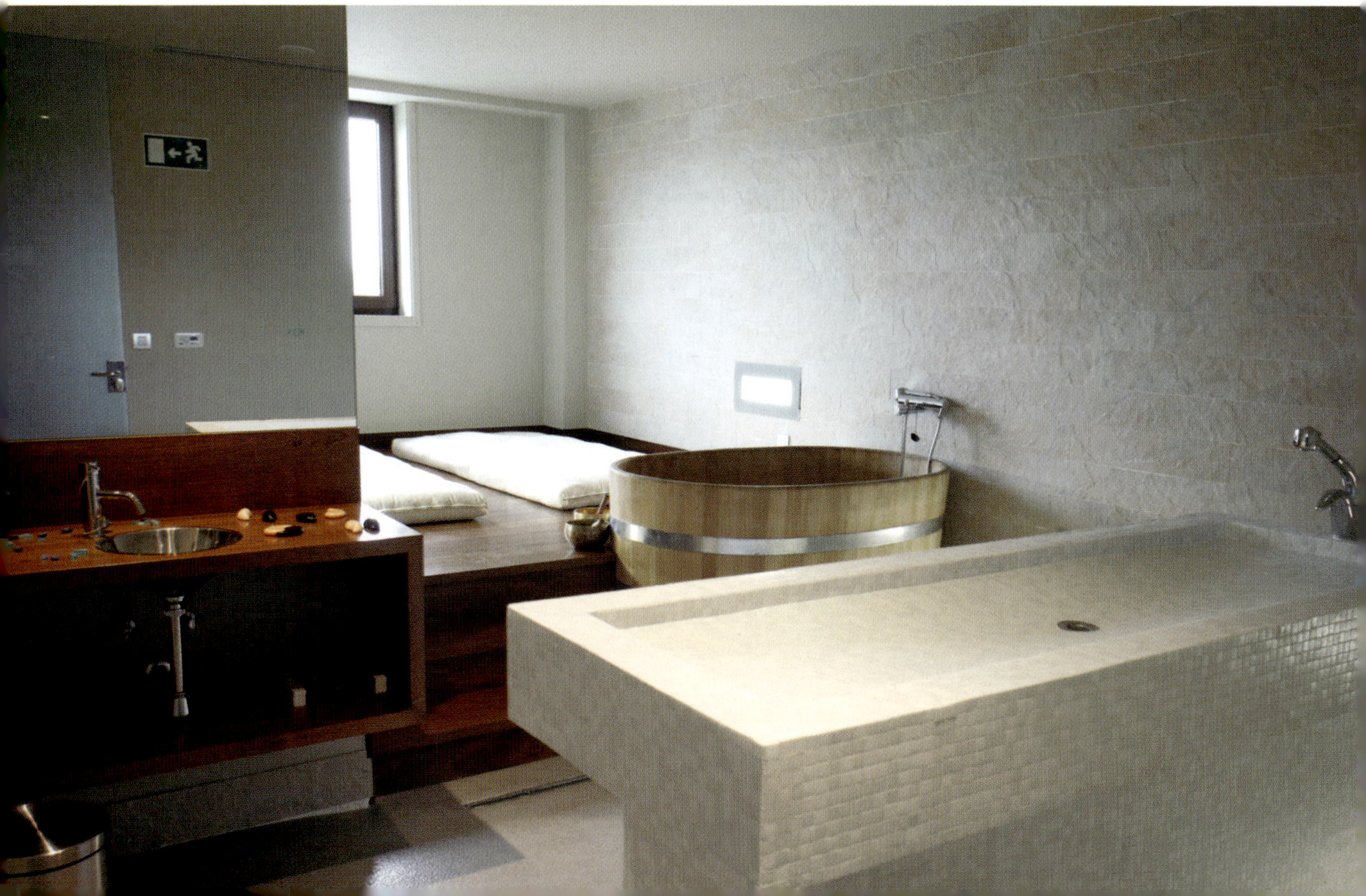

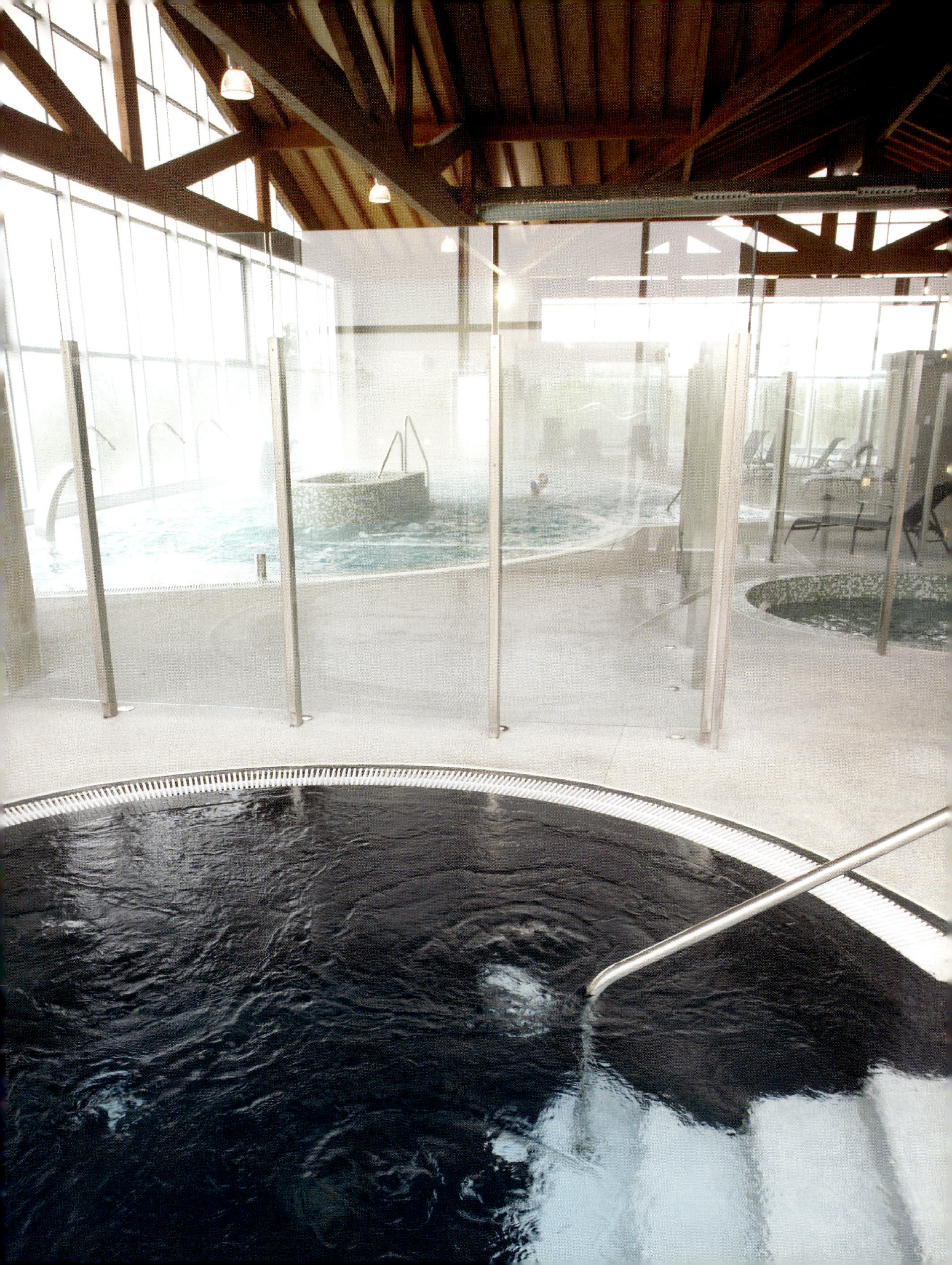

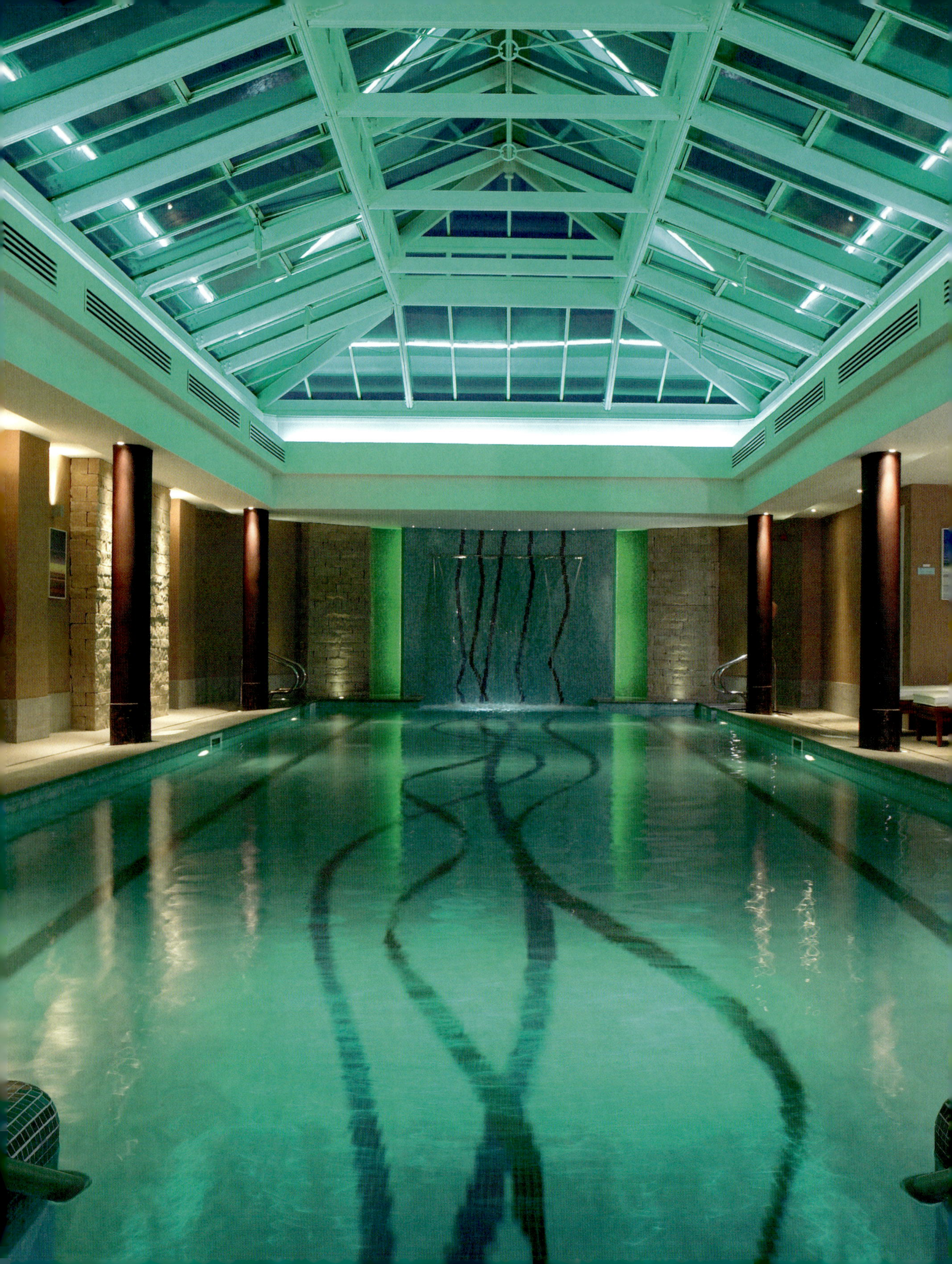

Kohler Waters Spa

Dieses Spa gehört zum Old Course Hotel, einem alten Herrenhaus, das 2004 renoviert wurde. Rings um den Pool befinden sich 11 Behandlungsräume und eine Thermal-Suite mit Whirlpool, Kaltwasserbecken, Sauna, Duschen und einer Kabine mit japanischen Dampf- und Salzbädern. Es gibt Fitnessräume und eine Dachterrasse mit einem Heißwasserbecken, das acht Personen Platz bei herrlichem Blick auf Golf-Greens und Nordsee bietet.

The building of the Old Course Hotel was renovated in 2004. The works conserved the original style of the manor house. Around the pool there are 11 treatment rooms and a thermal suite that has a whirlpool bath, a cold water pool, a cabin offering Japanese steam and salt baths, a sauna and showers. The fitness rooms and a terraced roof with a hot water bathtub, suitable for eight people and from which it is possible to see the golf course and the North Sea.

Le bâtiment du Old Course Hotel a été rénové en 2004. Les travaux ont conservé le style original de ce manoir écossais. Autour de la piscine, on ne compte pas moins de 11 cabines de traitements et une suite thermale équipée d'un bain à remous, une piscine d'eau froide, une cabine de sauna japonais et de bains salés, un sauna, et des douches. Les salles de remise en forme ainsi que la terrasse du toit, dotée d'un jacuzzi pouvant accueillir huit personnes, offrent un joli panorama sur le terrain de golf et sur la mer du Nord.

Het gebouw van het Old Course Hotel is in 2004 gerenoveerd, waarbij de originele landhuisstijl behouden is gebleven. Rondom het zwembad liggen 11 therapieruimten en een thermale afdeling met bubbelbad, koudwaterbad, een cabine met Japanse stoom- en zoutbaden, een sauna en douches. Verder zijn er nog fitnessruimten en een dakterras met een achtpersoons badkuip met uitzicht op de golfbanen en de Noordzee.

St Andrews, Fife, Scotland

CORPORATE EDGE

Photos © Kohler Waters Spa

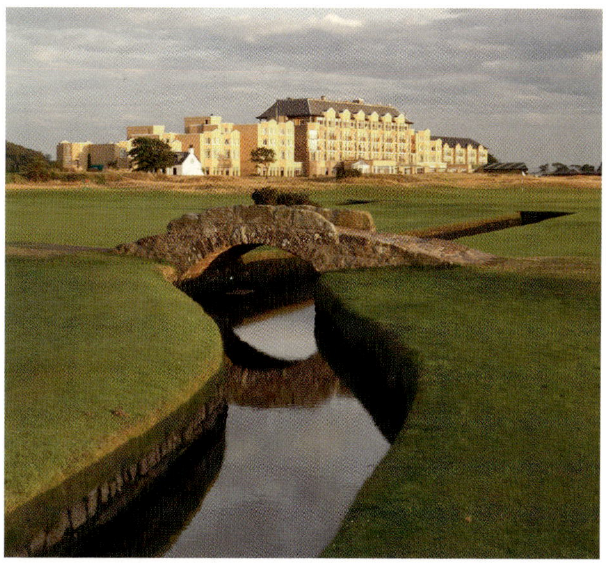

www.oldcoursehotel.co.uk

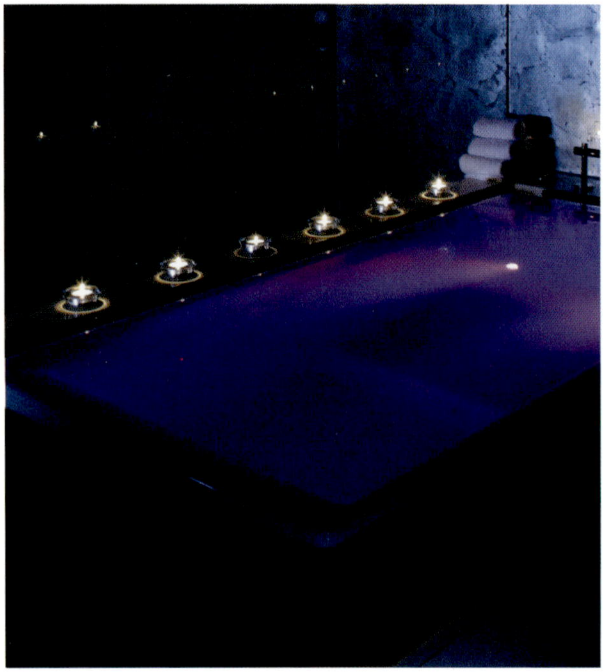

Die Spa-Anwendungen dienen der Remineralisierung des Körpers durch den Einsatz von Meerwasser.

The spa treatments are directed towards the remineralization of the body through the use of sea water.

Les traitements délivrés par ce spa sont consacrés à la revitalisation du corps grâce aux vertus de l'eau de mer.

De thermale behandelingen zijn gericht op remineralisering van het lichaam met behulp van zeewater.

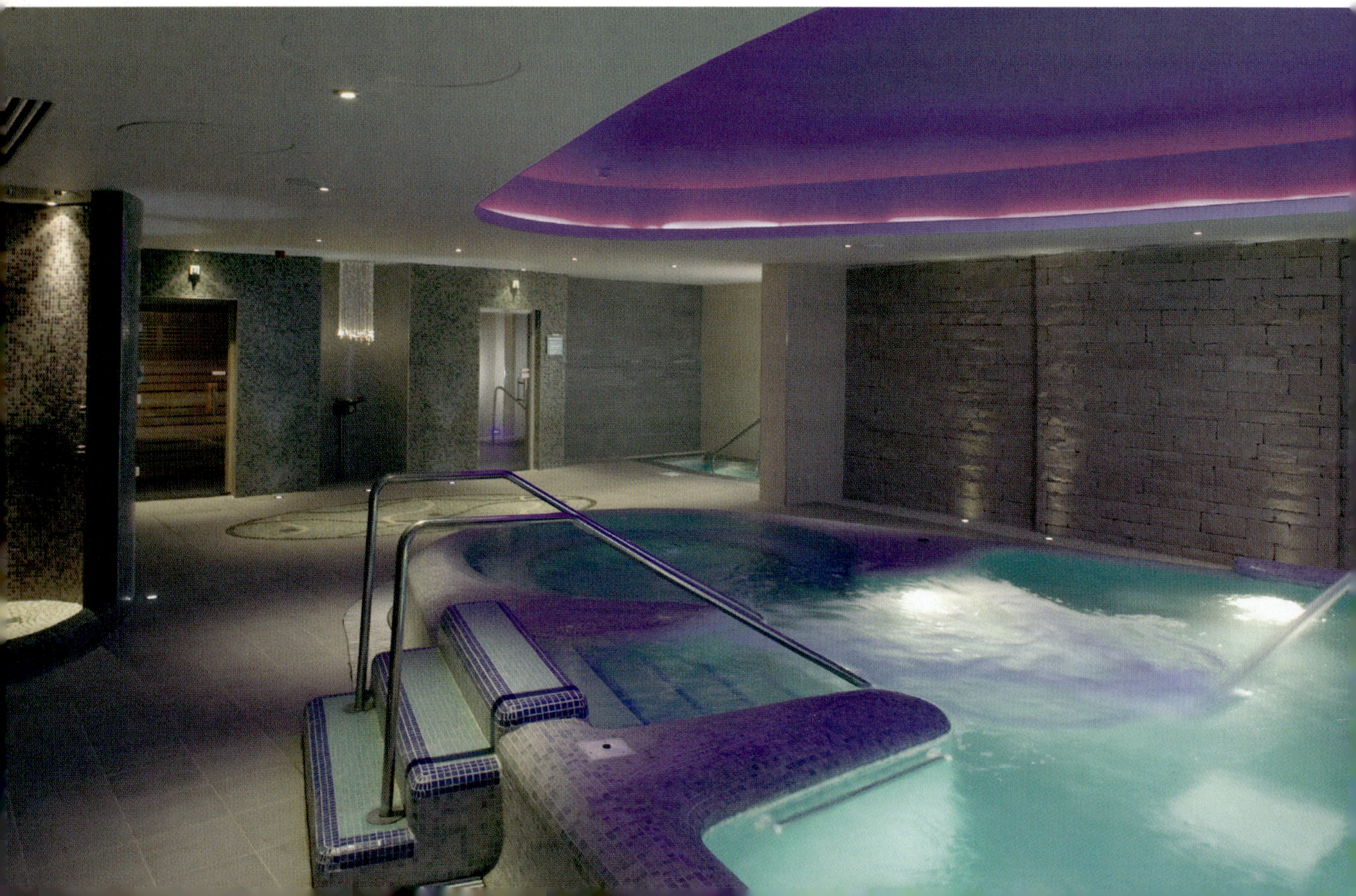

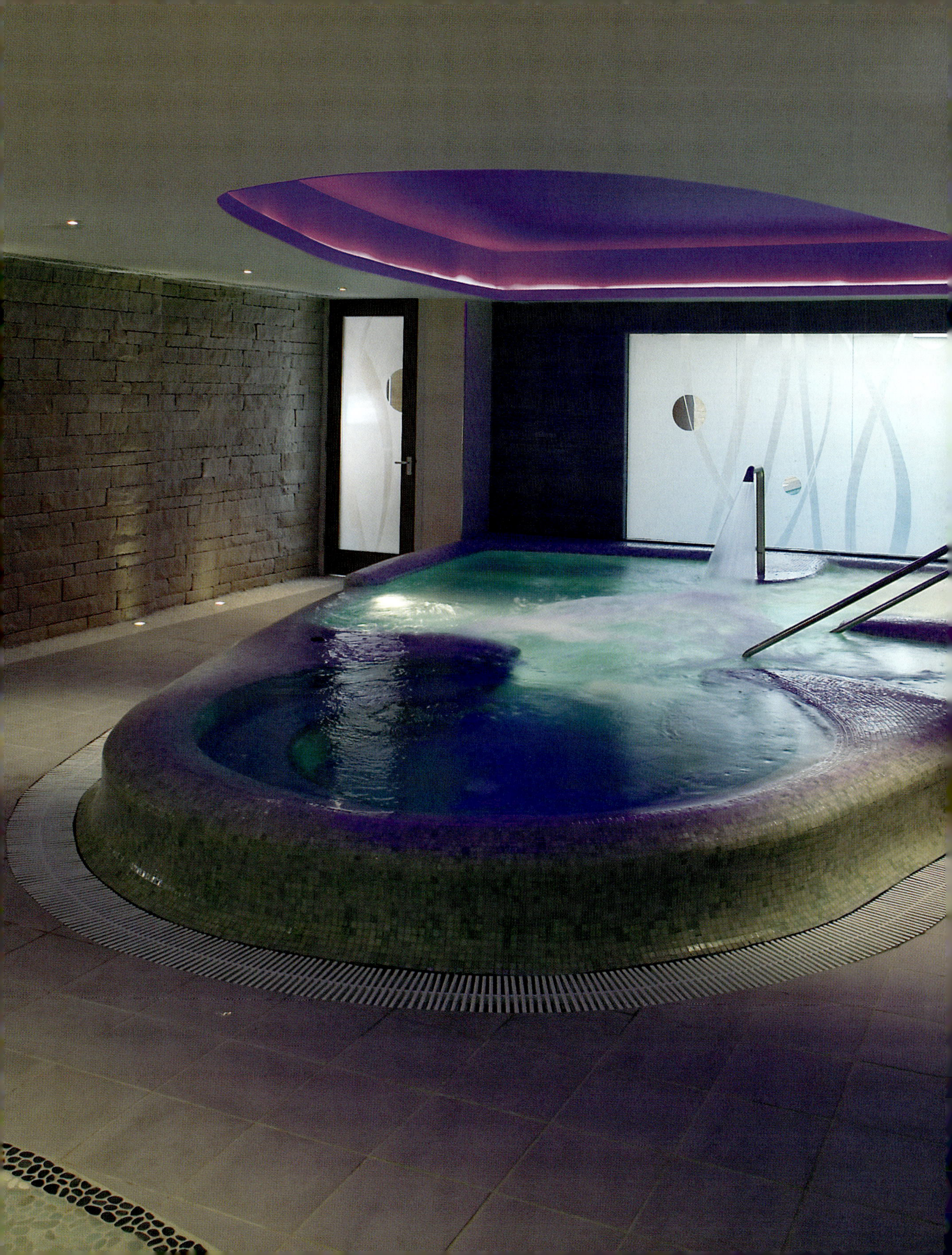

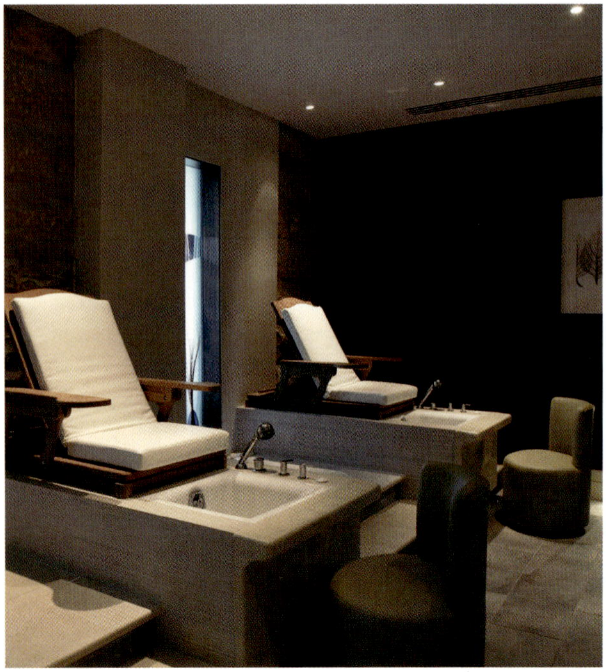

Die Dachterrasse verfügt über ein Heißwasserbecken mit Platz für acht Personen.

The deck on the terrace has a bathtub big enough for eight people.

La terrasse possède un jacuzzi pouvant accueillir huit personnes.

Op het dakterras staat een badkuip voor acht personen.

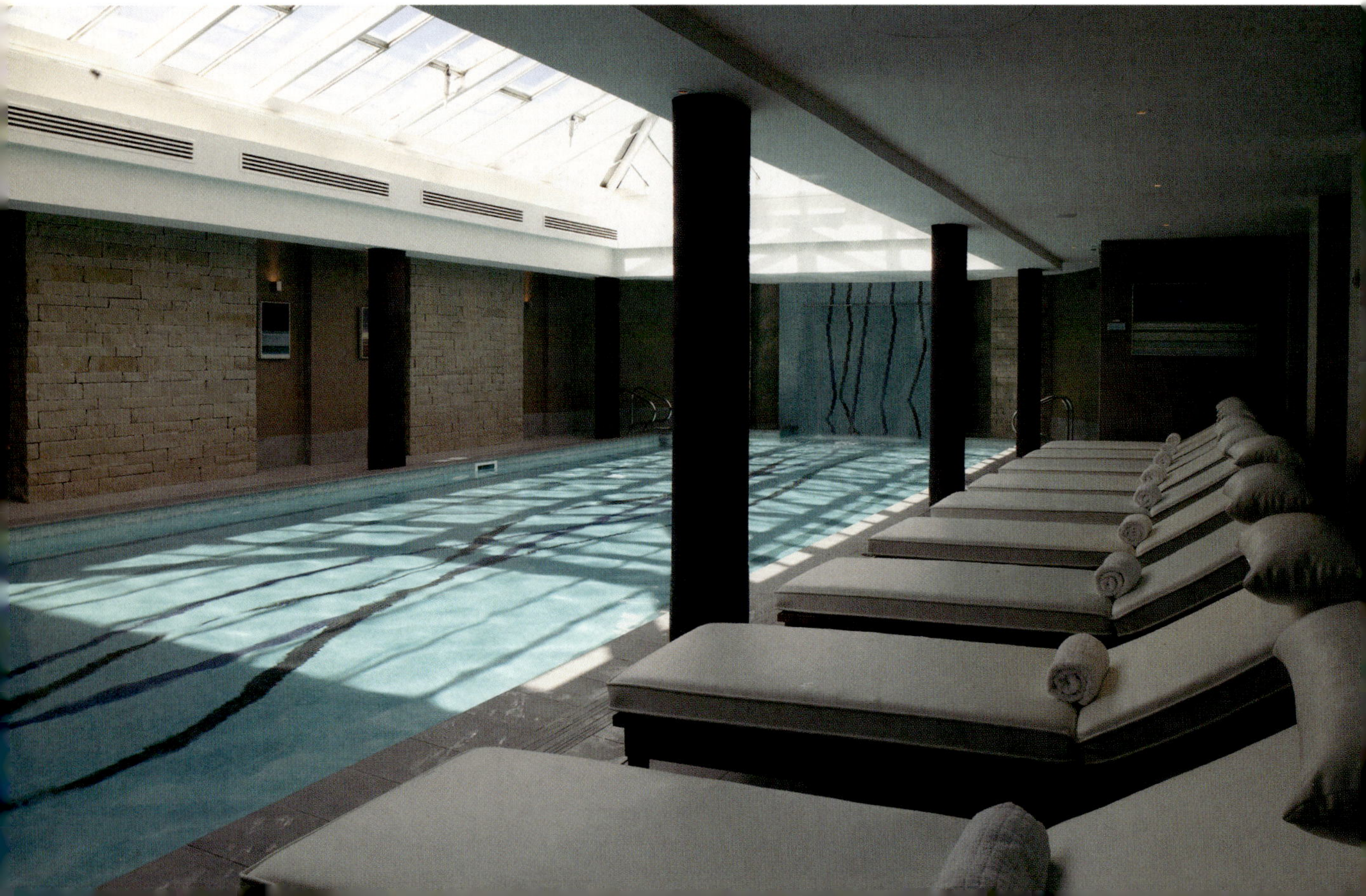

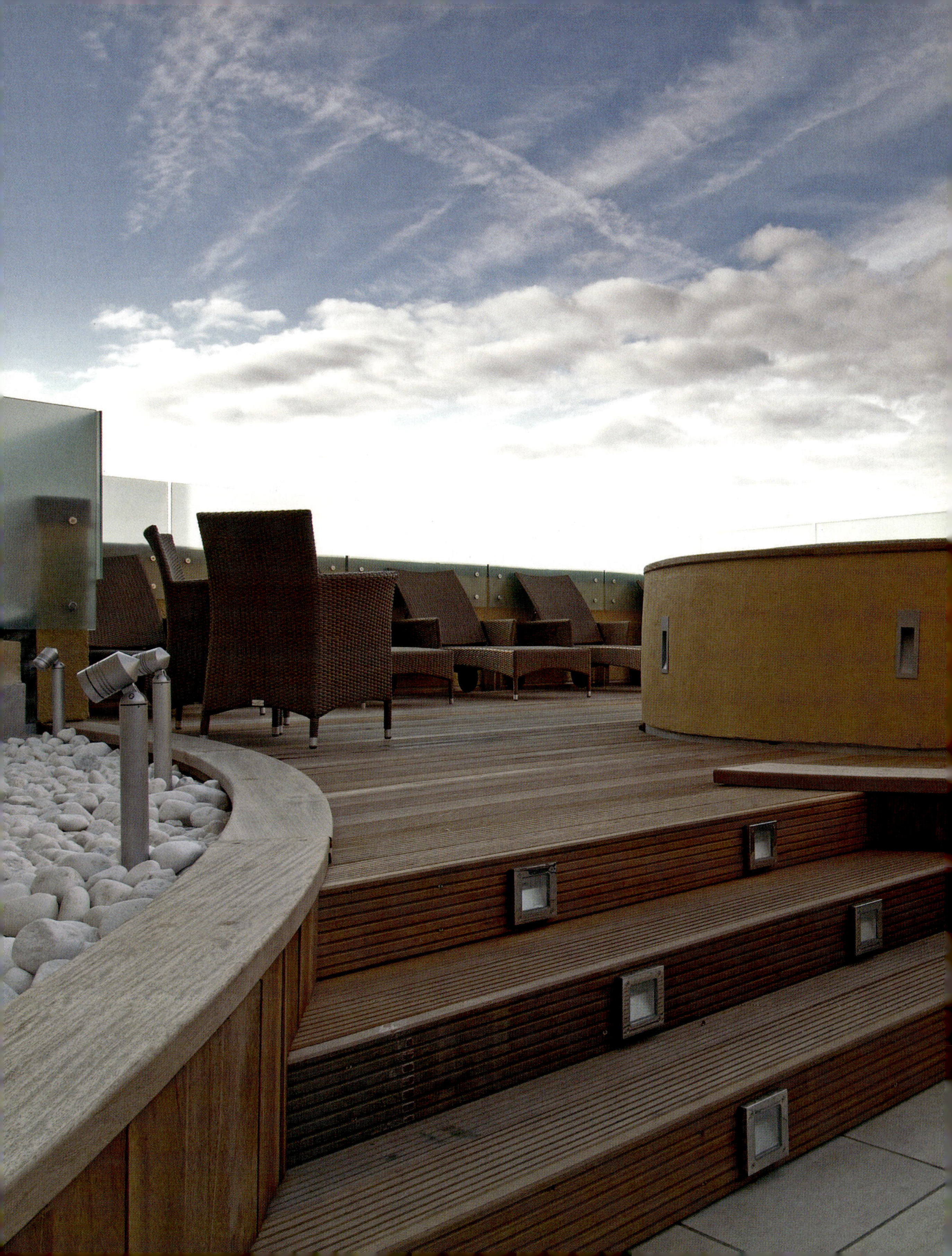

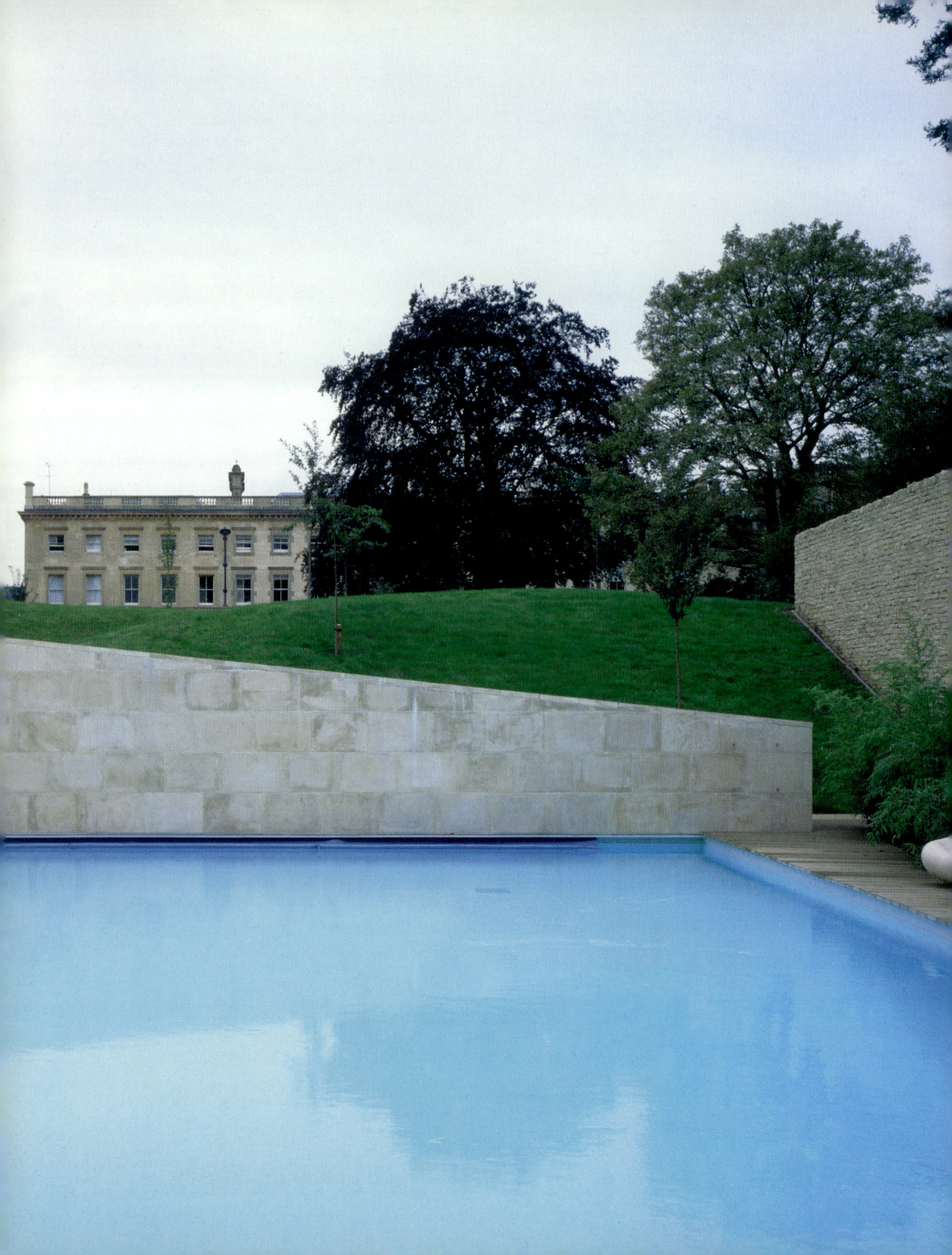

C-Side

Bei diesem Spa-Konzept war die Einbettung in die Landschaft genauso wichtig wie die Gestaltung des Gebäudes. Das in einem der Gärten gelegene Spa wird durch einen großen Pool, drei Mauern und einen Zaun begrenzt. Die Einrichtungen, zu denen Sauna, Dampfbad, Fitnessraum und Hallenbad gehören, sind unterirdisch angelegt. Der minimalistische Stil und der Blick auf die Gärten verleihen der Anlage eine friedliche Ruhe, die sich gleich beim ersten Betreten offenbart.

This spa, named C-Side, has been conceived as a space framed within the landscape more than as a building. Located in one of the gardens, its boundaries are formed by a large pool, three walls and a fence. The facilities, including sauna, steam bath, gymnasium and indoor pool, are in the basement. The minimalist style and the views of the gardens instill a calm that is perceived from the moment of entering the precincts.

Le C-Side a été conçu pour s'intégrer dans le paysage comme une construction spécifique. L'espace du spa, situé dans un des jardins, est délimité par une vaste piscine, trois murs et une rampe d'accès. Les équipements – le sauna, le hammam, le gymnase et la piscine intérieure –, sont situés au sous-sol. Le style épuré et la vue sur les jardins confèrent immédiatement une ambiance de sérénité dès que l'on pénètre dans son enceinte.

Het kuuroord C-Side is meer ontworpen als een omkaderde ruimte binnen het landschap dan als een gebouw. Het is gelegen in een tuin en wordt begrensd door een groot zwembad, drie muren en een hek. De faciliteiten, waaronder een sauna, stoombad, fitnessruimte en binnenbad, bevinden zich in de kelder. De minimalistische inrichting en het uitzicht op de tuinen doordesemen de ruimte met een rust die de bezoeker al tegemoetkomt als hij het terrein betreedt.

Gloucestershire, United Kingdom

DE MATOS STOREY RYAN LTD

Photos © David Grandorge, Bill Burlington

www.cowleymanor.co.uk

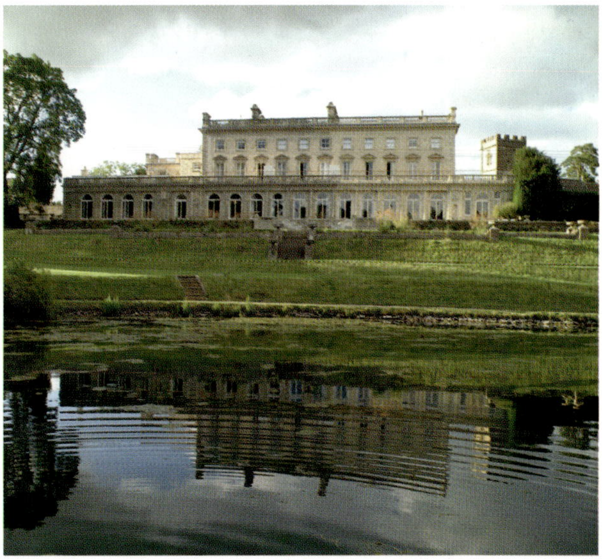

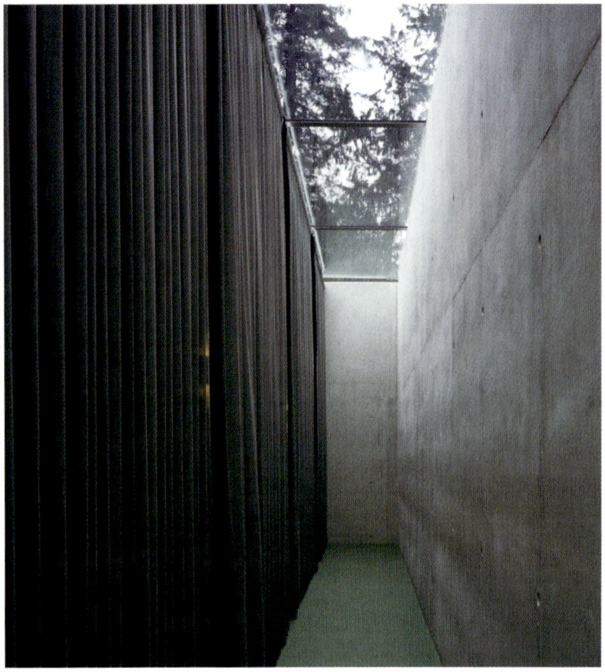

In der Mitte des Gartens laden zwei beheizte Pools, ein Innen- und ein Außenpool, zum Verweilen ein.

Located in the middle of the garden, the two heated pools, one inside one outside, invite relaxation.

Situées au milieu du jardin, les deux piscines chauffées, l'une à l'intérieur, l'autre à l'extérieur, invitent la relaxation.

De twee verwarmde zwembaden midden in de tuin, een binnenbad en een buitenbad, nodigen uit tot ontspanning.

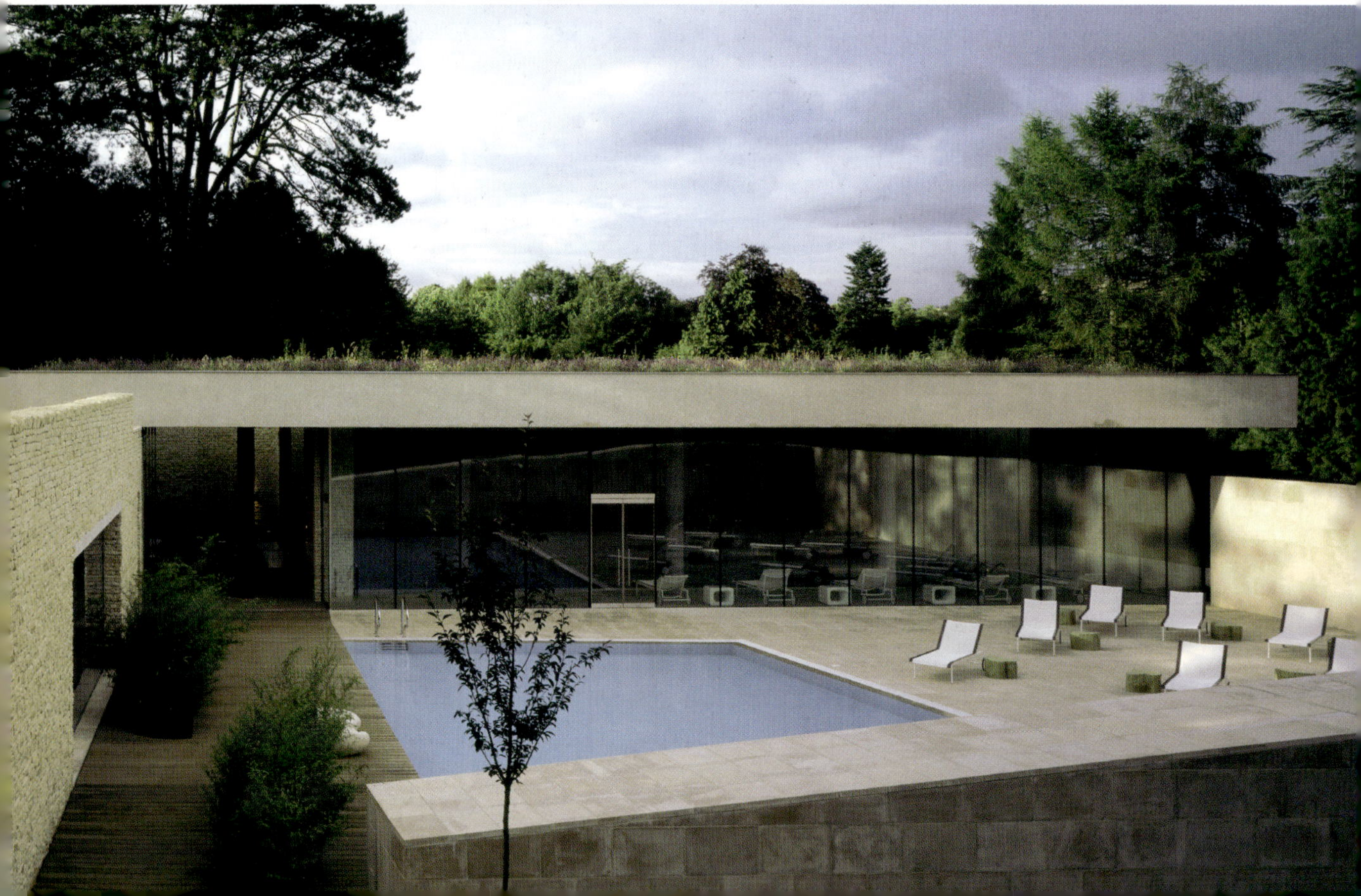

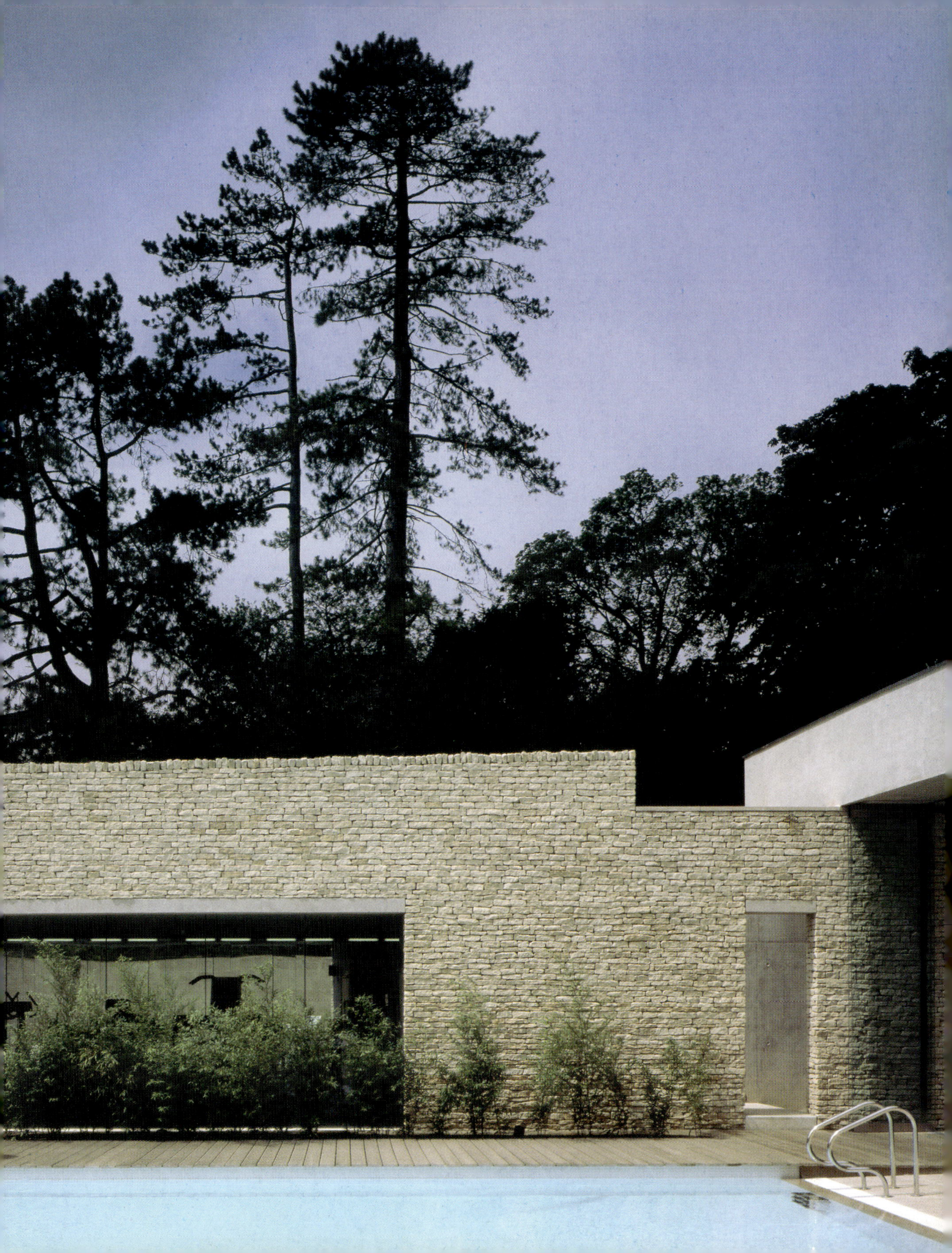

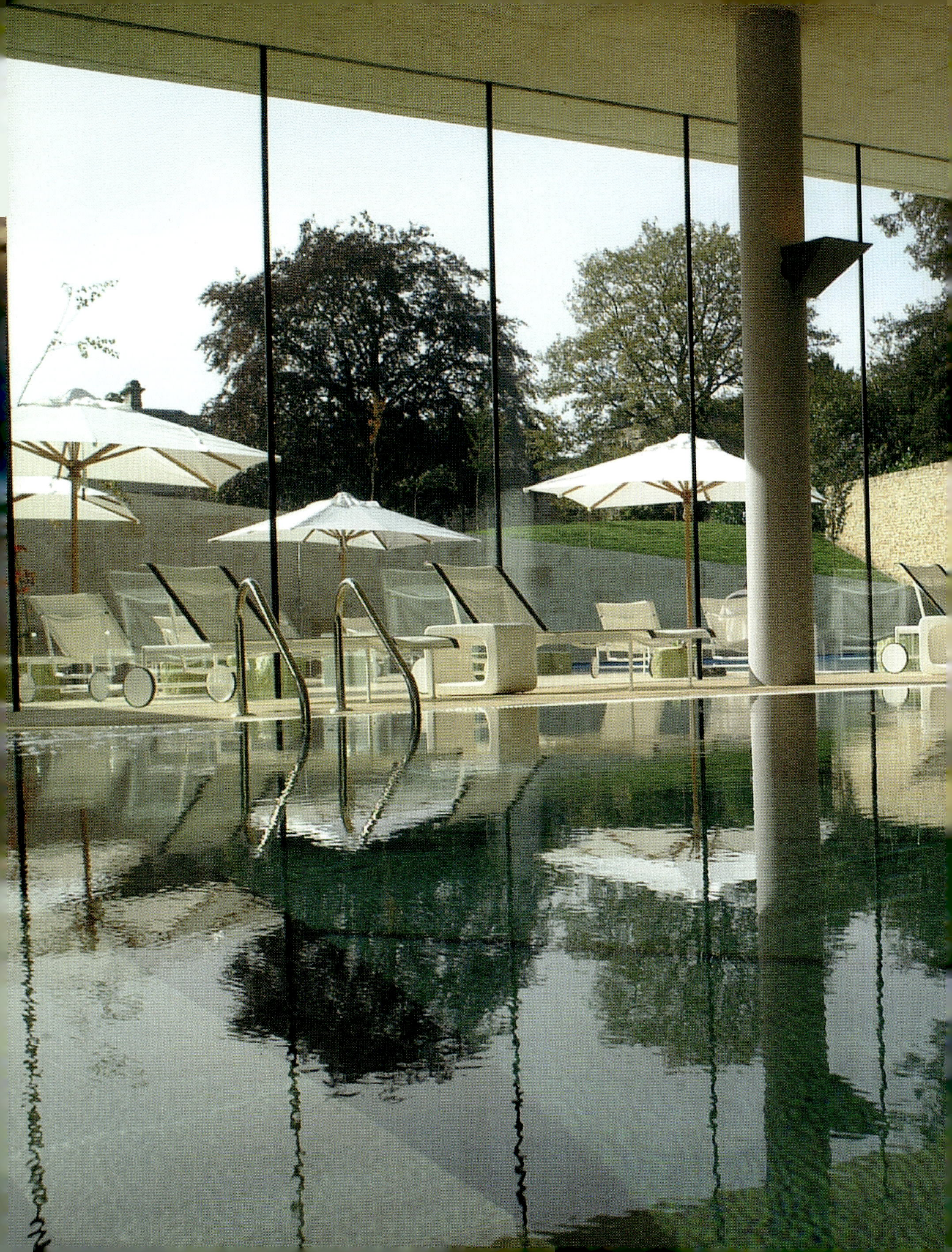

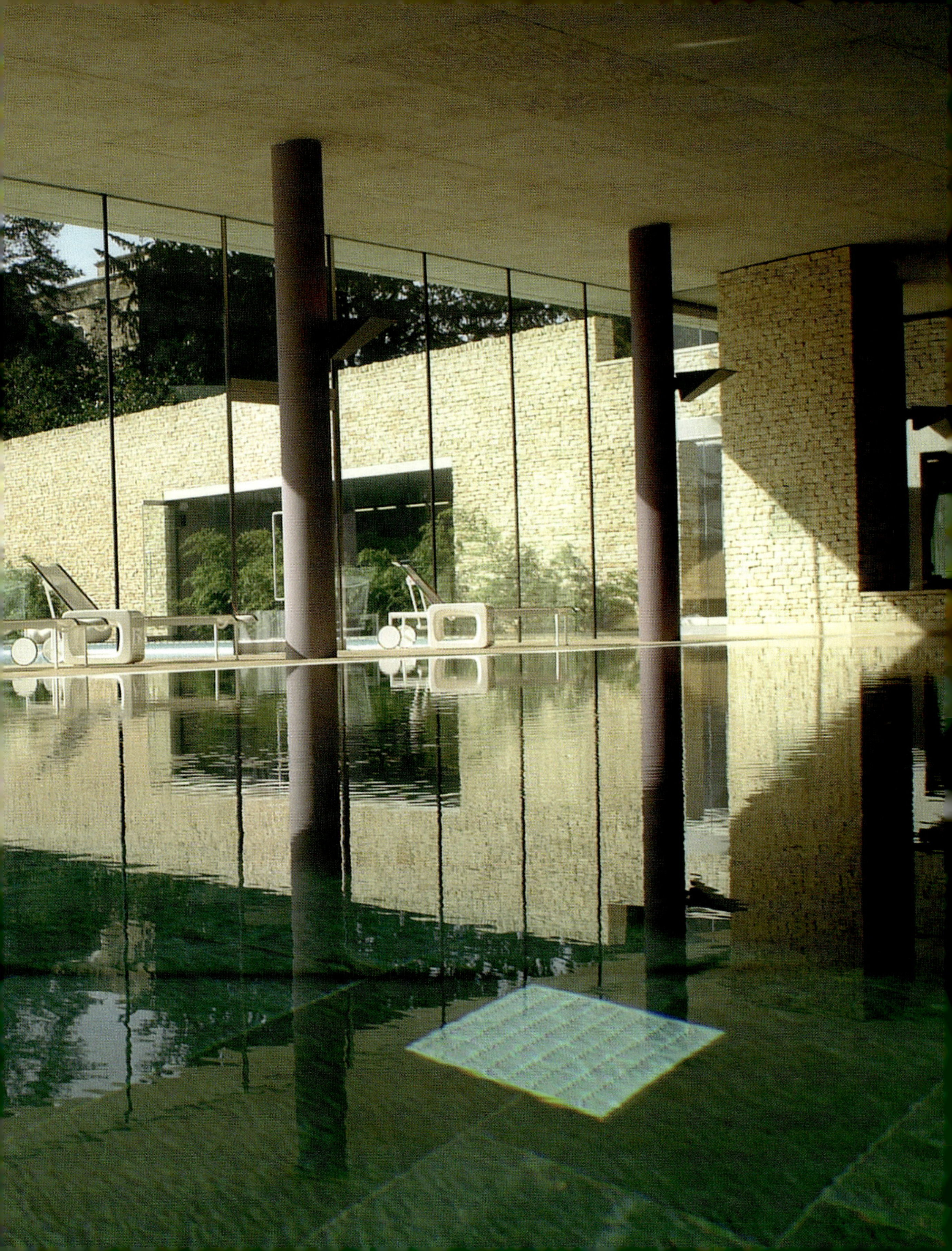

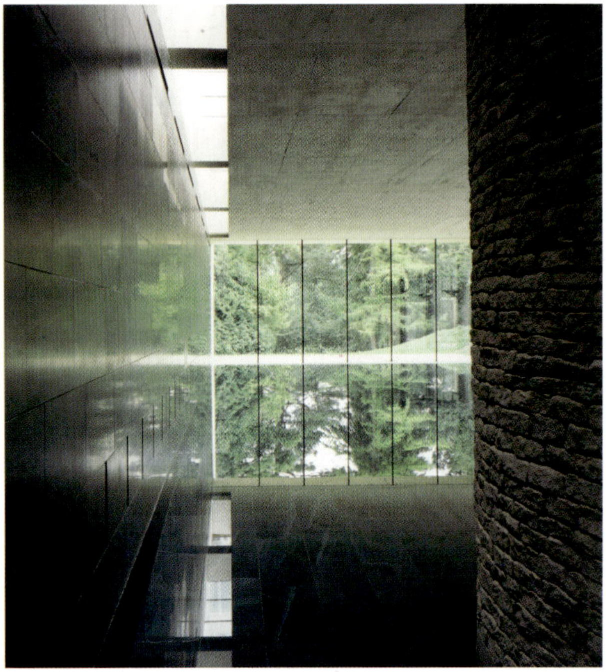

Das Spa ist Teil des Cowley Manor Hotels, dessen Interieur nach modernen ästhetischen Kriterien neu gestaltet wurde.

The spa is part of the Cowley Manor hotel, the interior of which has been renovated with contemporary esthetic criteria.

Le spa fait partie du Cowley Manor Hotel, dont l'intérieur a été rénové selon les critères de l'esthétique contemporaine.

De badinrichting maakt deel uit van hotel Cowley Manor, dat vanbinnen is gerenoveerd volgens moderne stijlopvattingen.

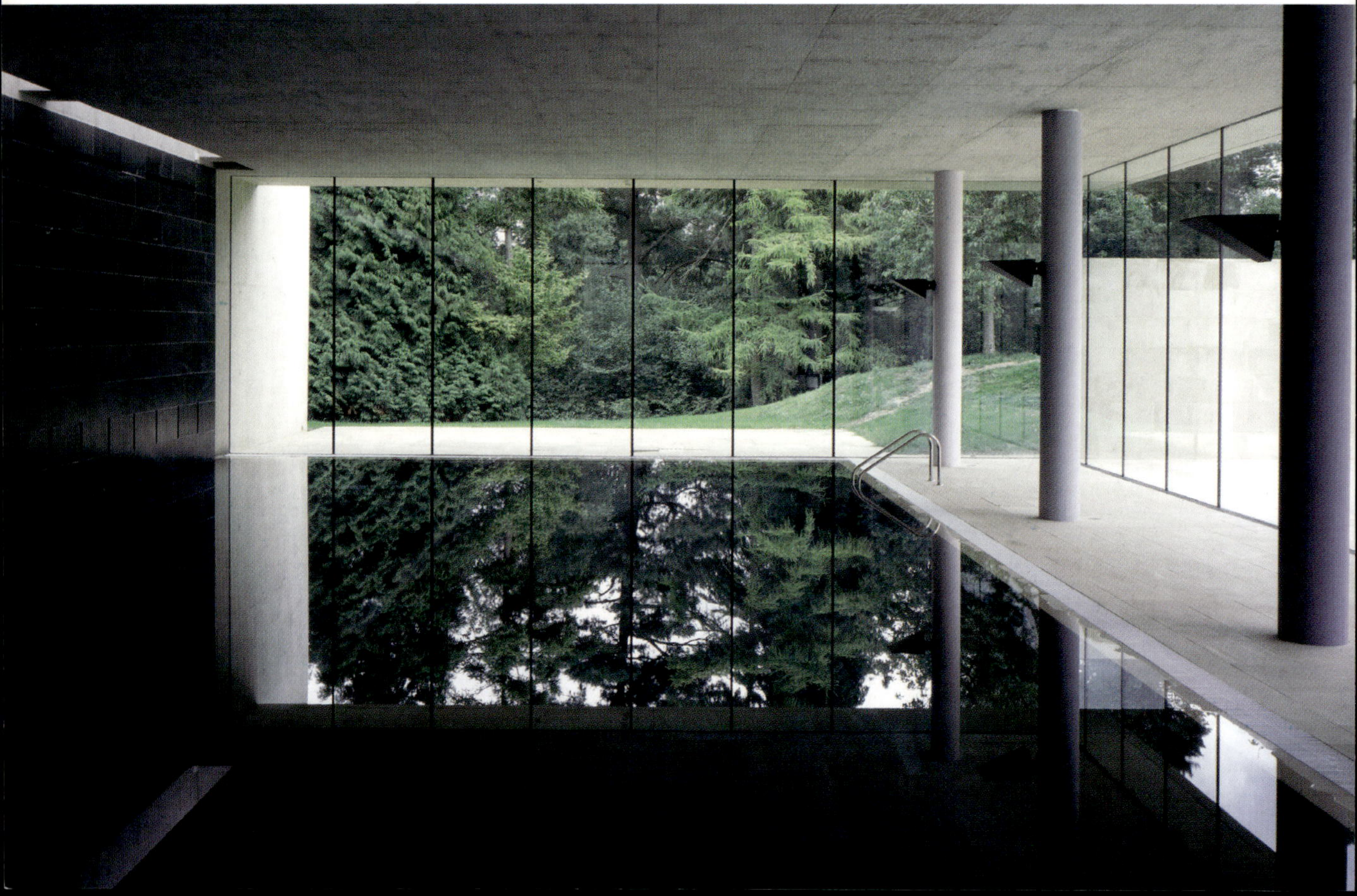

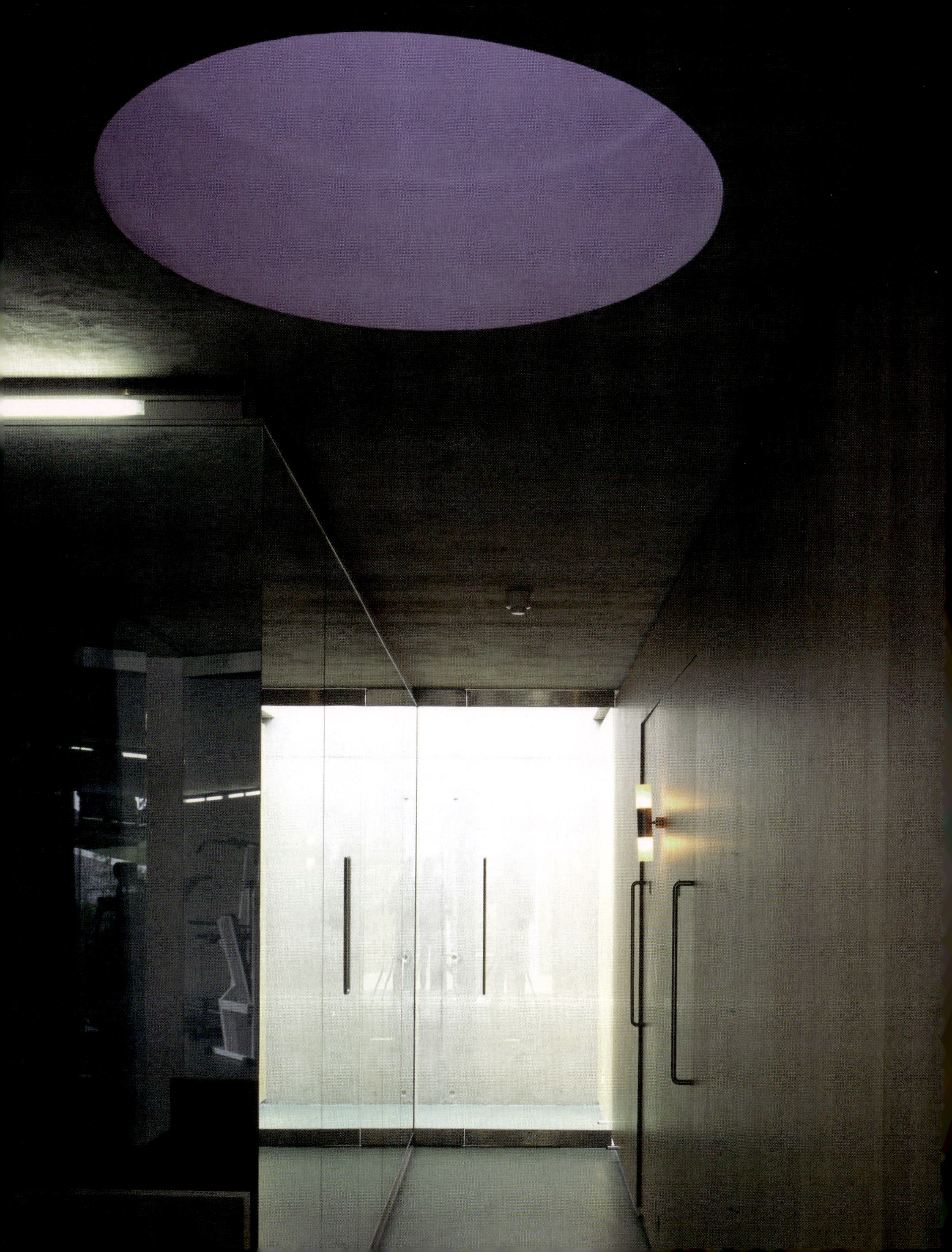

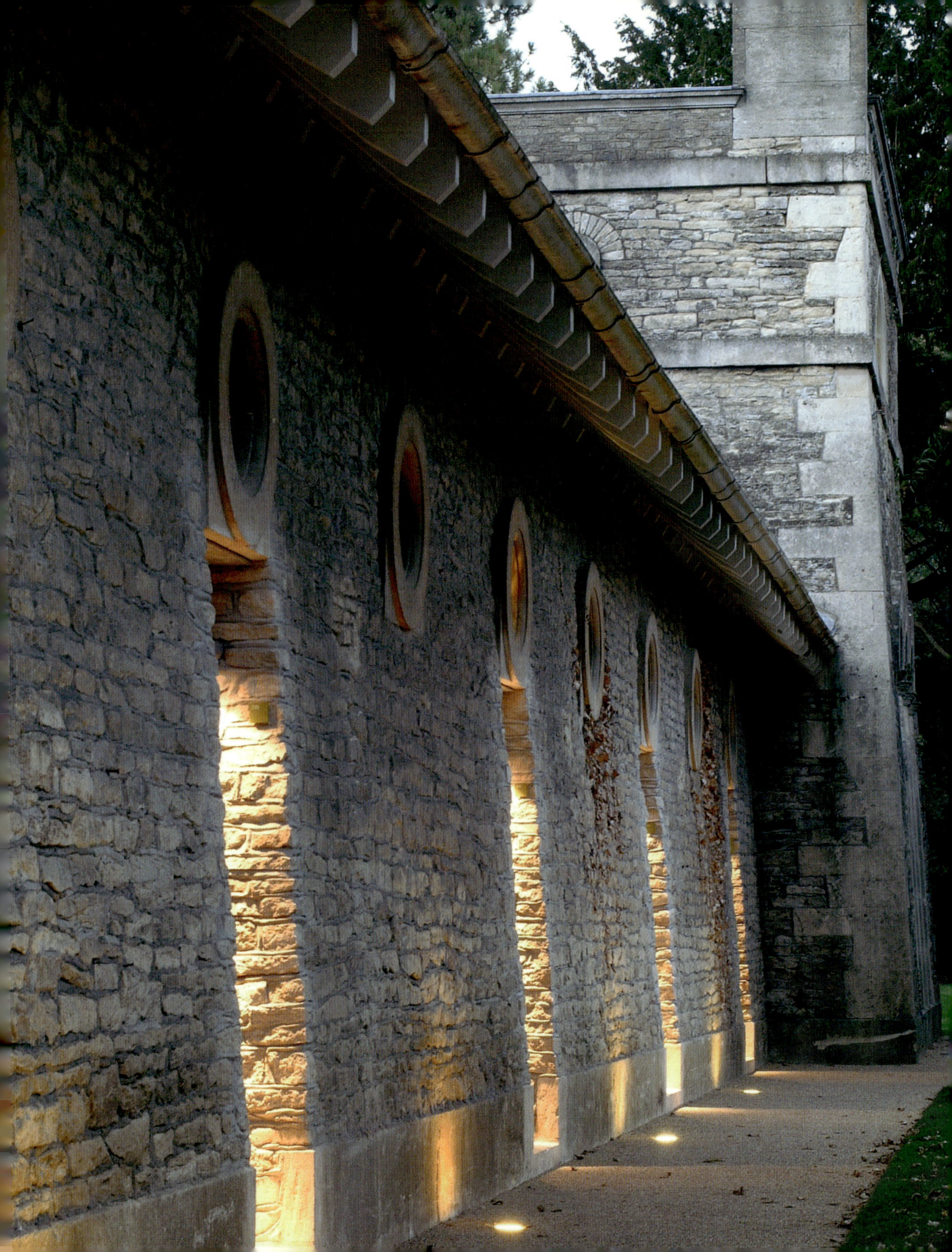

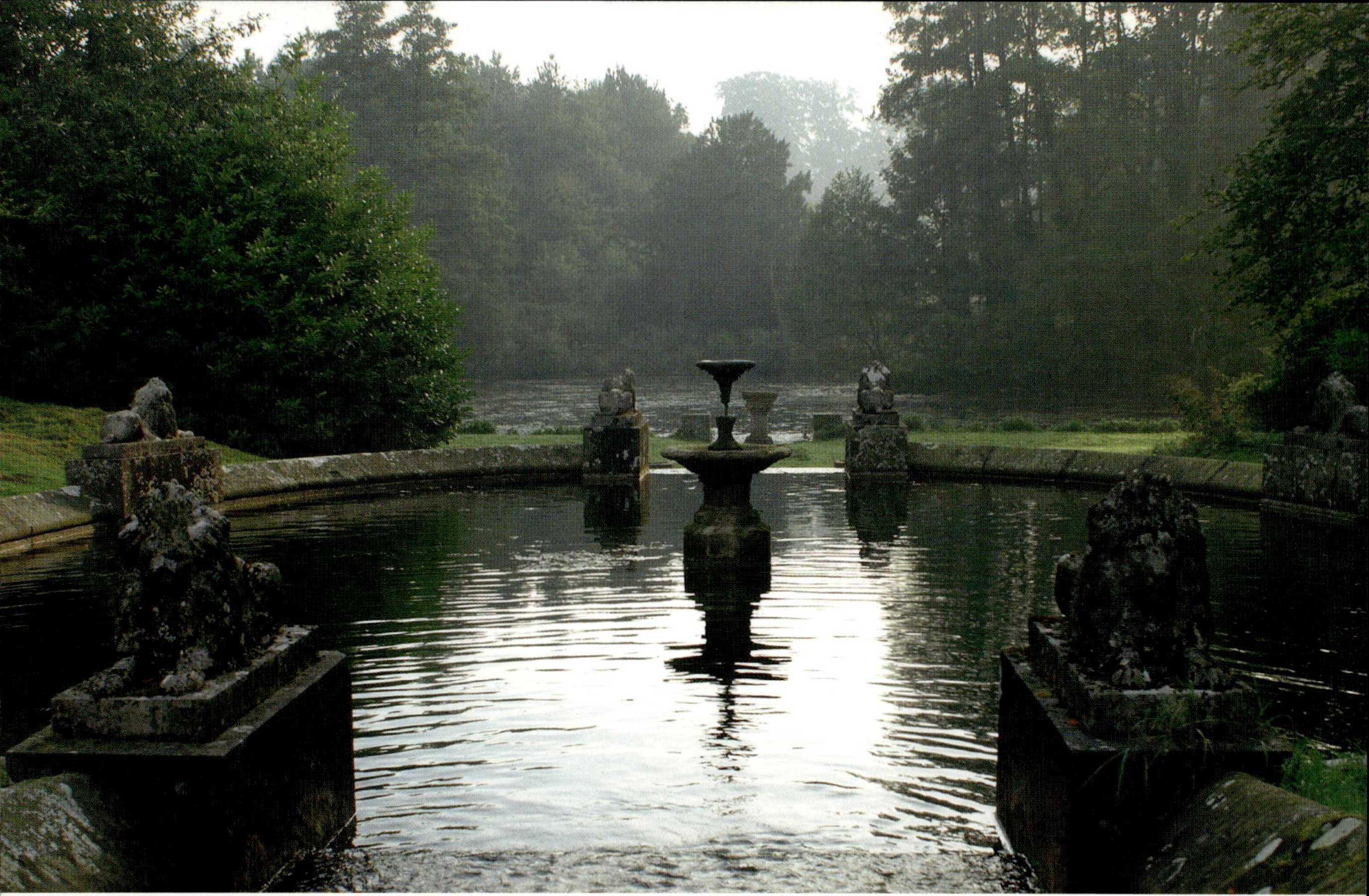

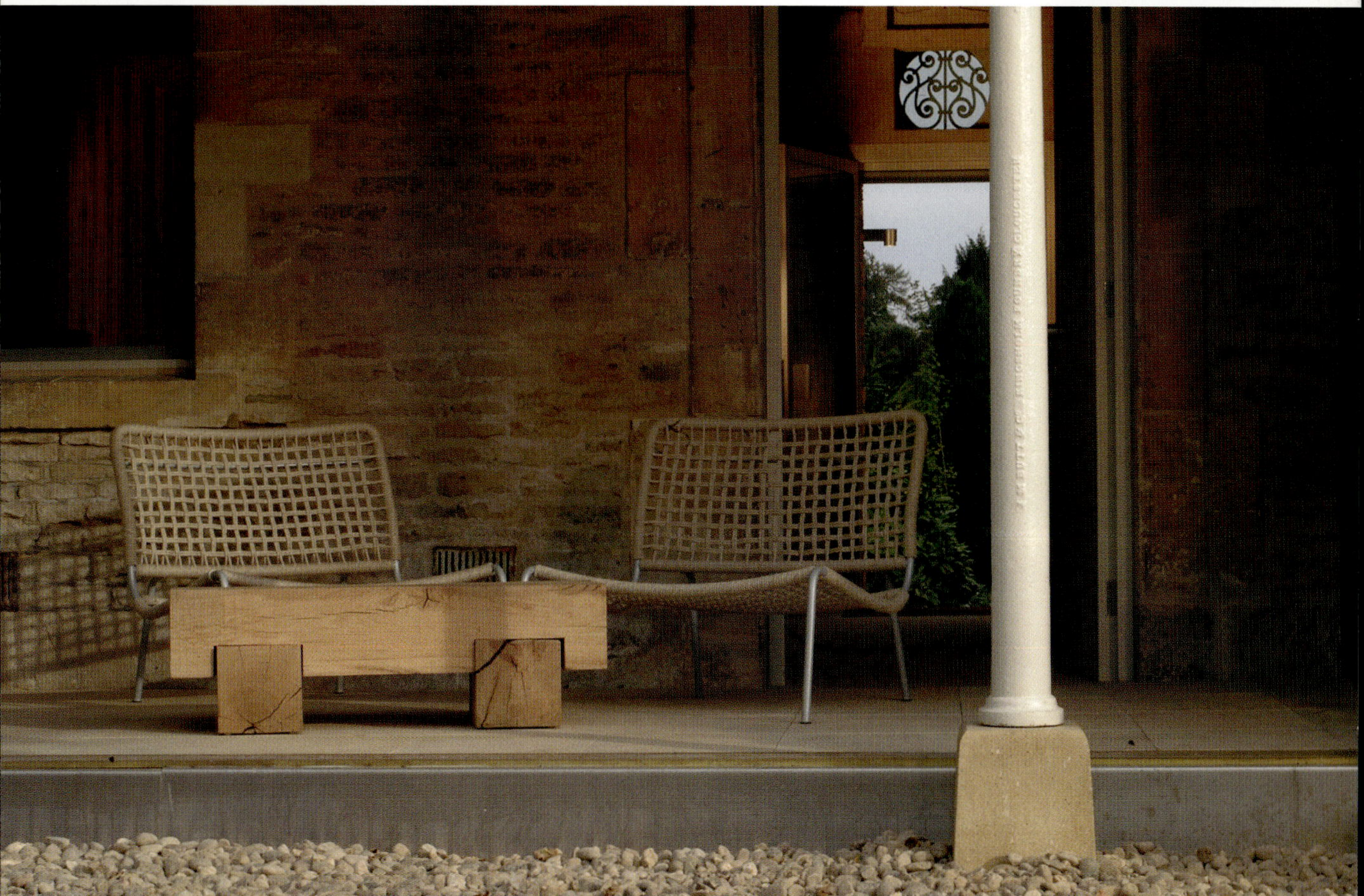

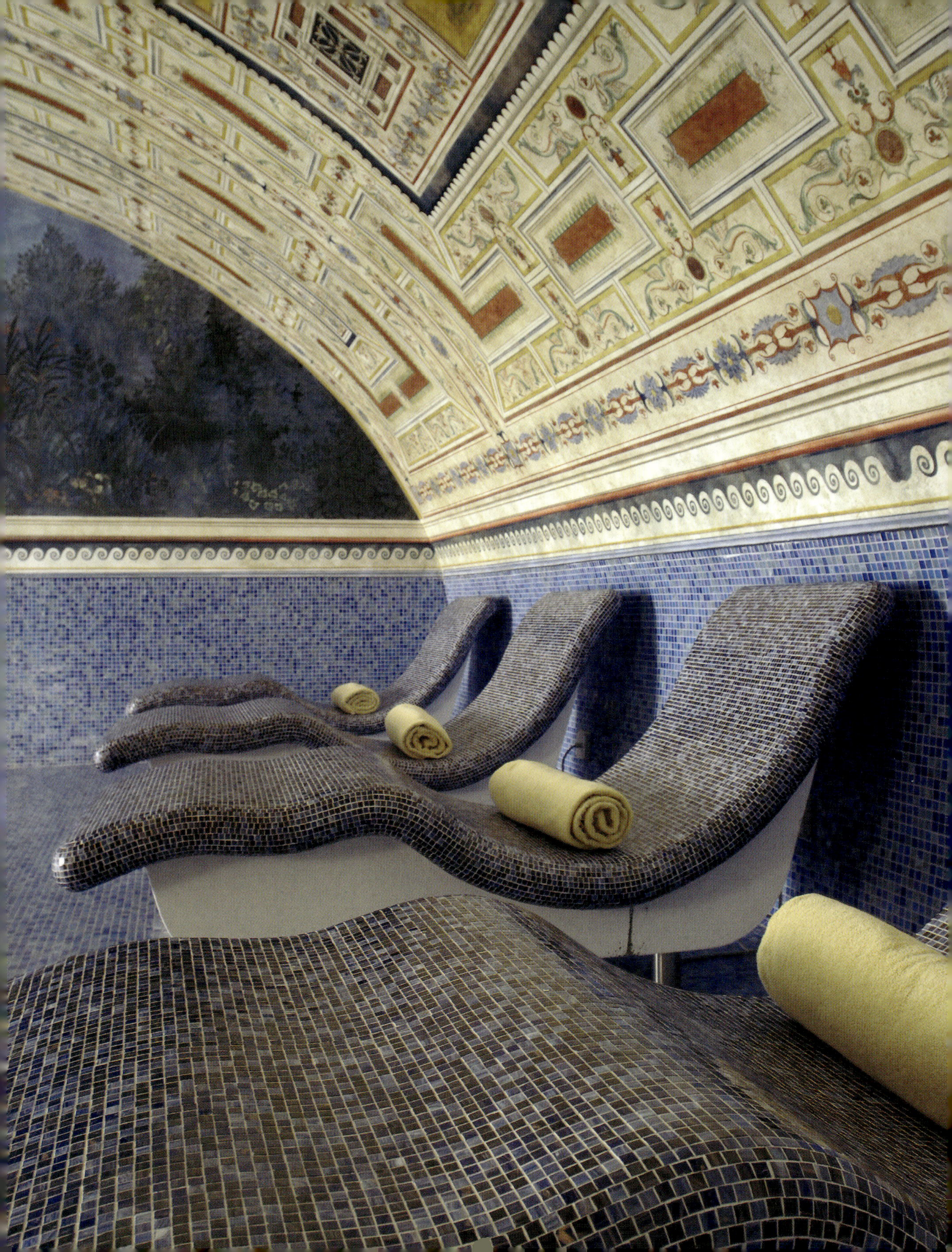

Spa at the Byblos Art Hotel

Dieses Spa erinnert an die Ästhetik römischer Bäder und pompejischer Malerei. Der Whirlpool greift die elegante Form des Impluviums der Patrizierhäuser auf. Die blau-goldenen Bodenmosaiken wirken opulent, ohne sich dem Betrachter aufzudrängen. Dem zentralen Nassbereich angegliedert sind das türkische Bad und die Sauna; dazu kommen Whirlpool- und Fitotherapiekabinen sowie weitere Räume für Massagen und Schönheitsbehandlungen.

This spa is associated to the aesthetics inspired by Roman baths and Pompeian painting. Therefore, the whirlpool bath is elegantly shaped like the impluvium of patrician houses, and the blue and golden mosaics that cover the pavement appeal to opulence without giving up intimacy. Attached to this central wet area are the Turkish bath and the sauna; also cabins with whirlpool baths and those for fitotherapy, and other rooms where massages and esthetic treatments are carried out.

Ce spa est associé à une esthétique inspirée par les thermes romains et les fresques de Pompéi. Ainsi, le bain à remous est élégamment dessiné comme l'impluvium des maisons antiques et les mosaïques bleu et or qui couvrent le sol évoquent l'opulence, tout en préservant une certaine intimité. Dans cette même zone centrale se trouvent le hammam et le sauna, les cabines de jacuzzis et de traitements phytothérapeutiques, ainsi que d'autres salons dédiés aux massages et soins esthétiques.

Dit badcomplex is duidelijk geïnspireerd op de Romeinse badhuizen en schilderingen uit Pompeji. Het bubbelbad is een elegante variant op het impluvium uit Romeinse patriciërshuizen en de blauw met gouden mozaïekvloeren scheppen een sfeer van overvloedige weelde zonder aan intimiteit te verliezen. Naast deze centrale ruimte liggen het Turkse bad en de sauna, cabines met bubbelbaden en ruimten voor fytotherapie, massages en schoonheidsbehandelingen.

Corrubbio, Italy

ATELIER MENDINI

Photos © Henri Dal Olmo

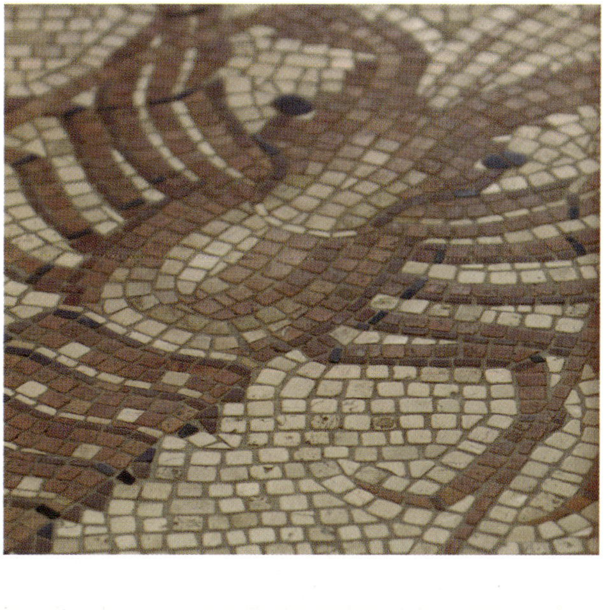

www.byblosarthotel.com

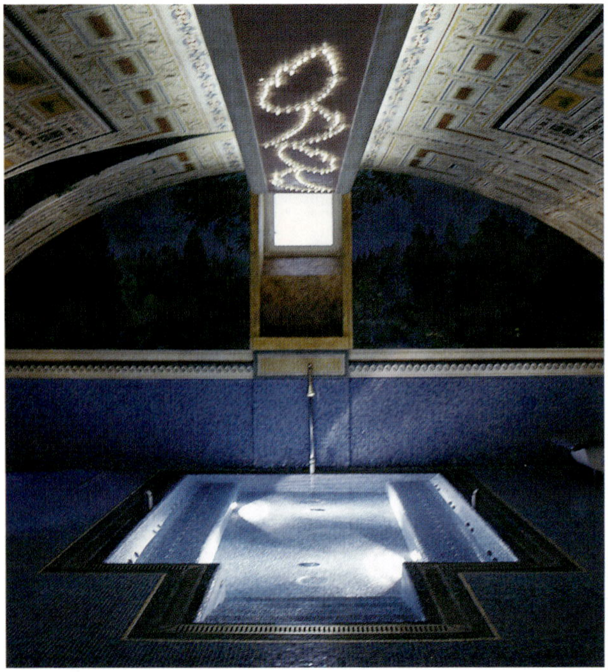

Die reich bebilderten Wände sind durch pompejische Malerei inspiriert.

Pompeian painting inspires the profusion of images on the walls.

Les nombreuses peintures qui décorent les murs sont directement inspirées des fresques de Pompéi.

De Pompejaans aandoende muurschilderingen zijn rijk aan beelden.

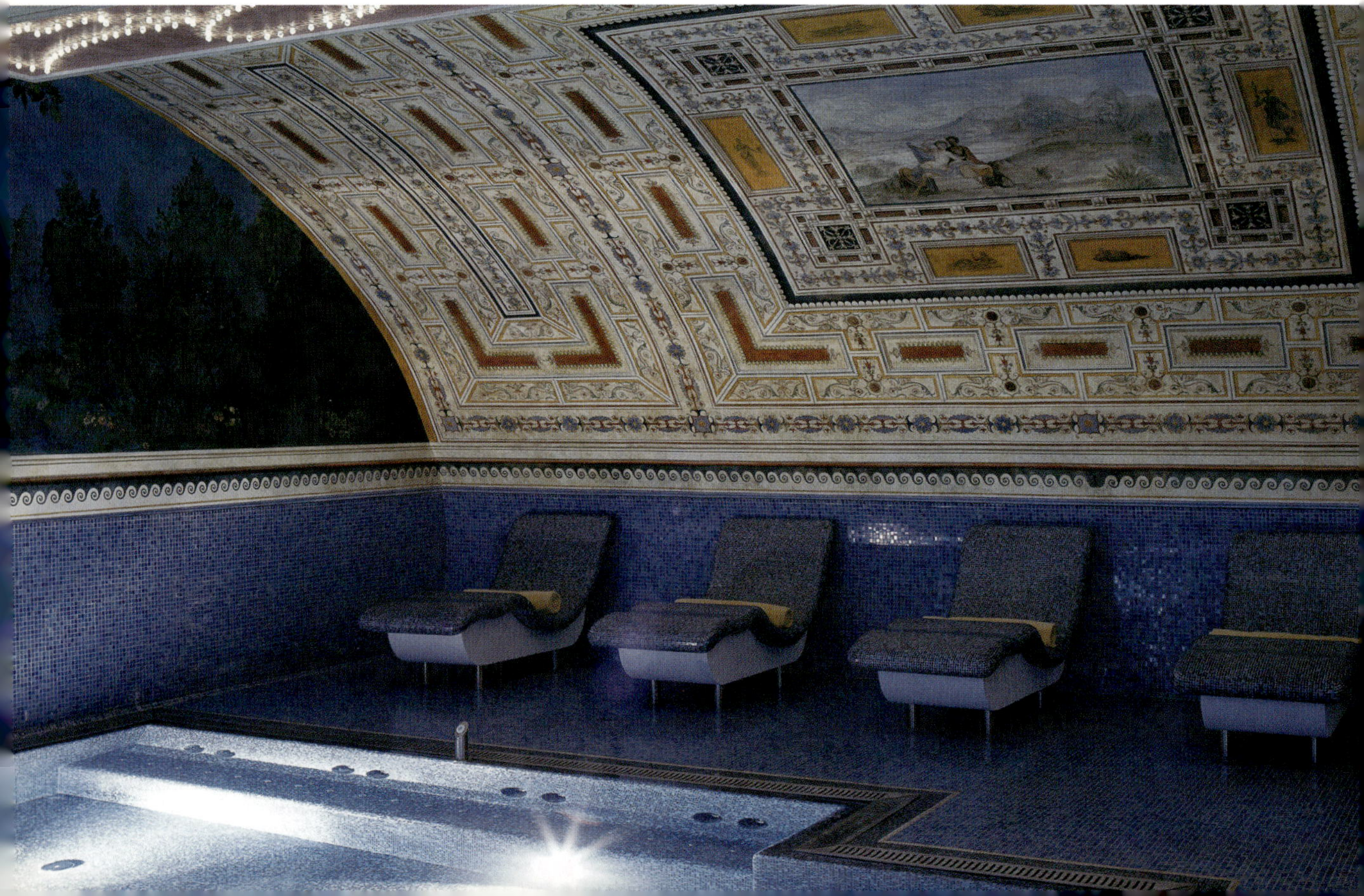

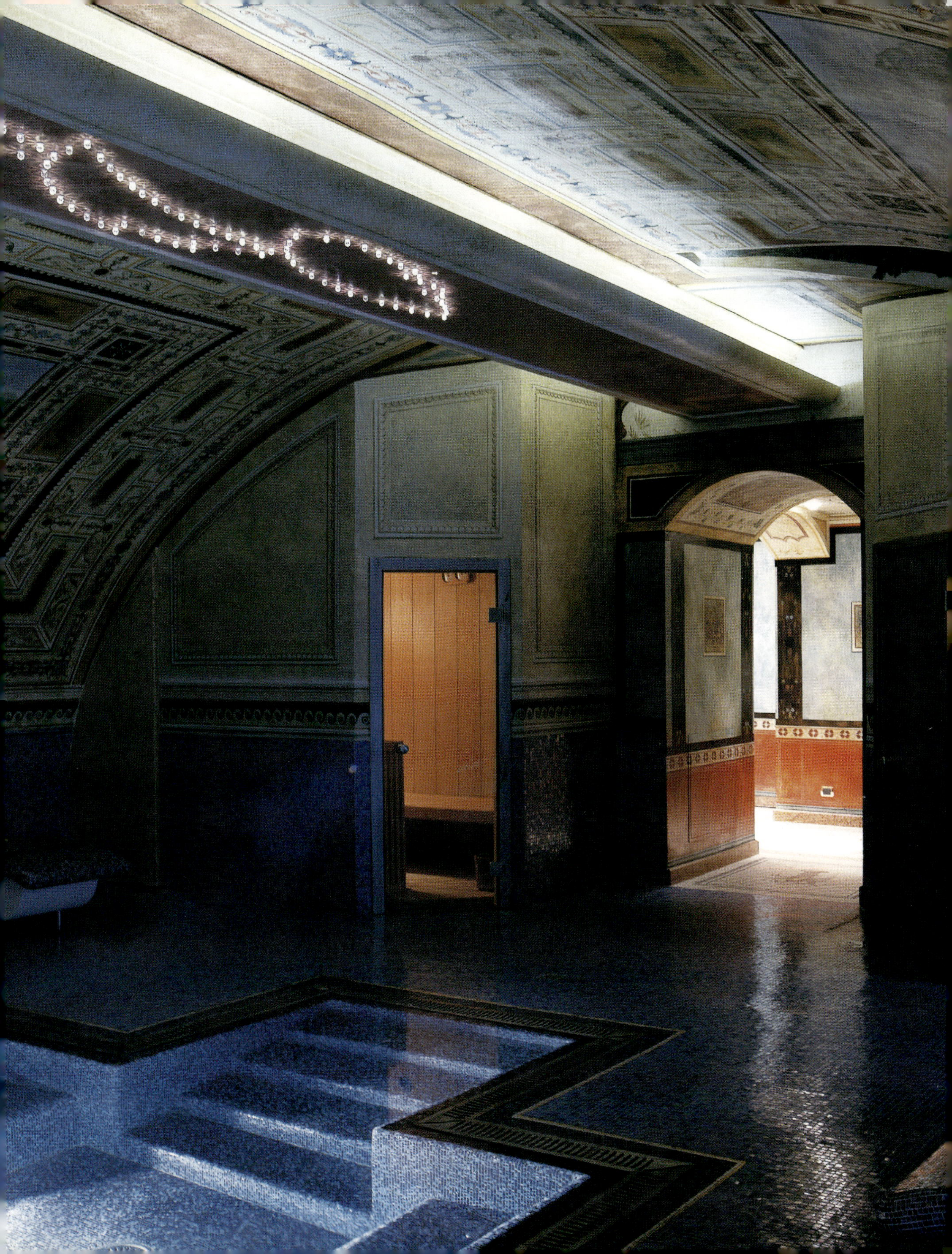

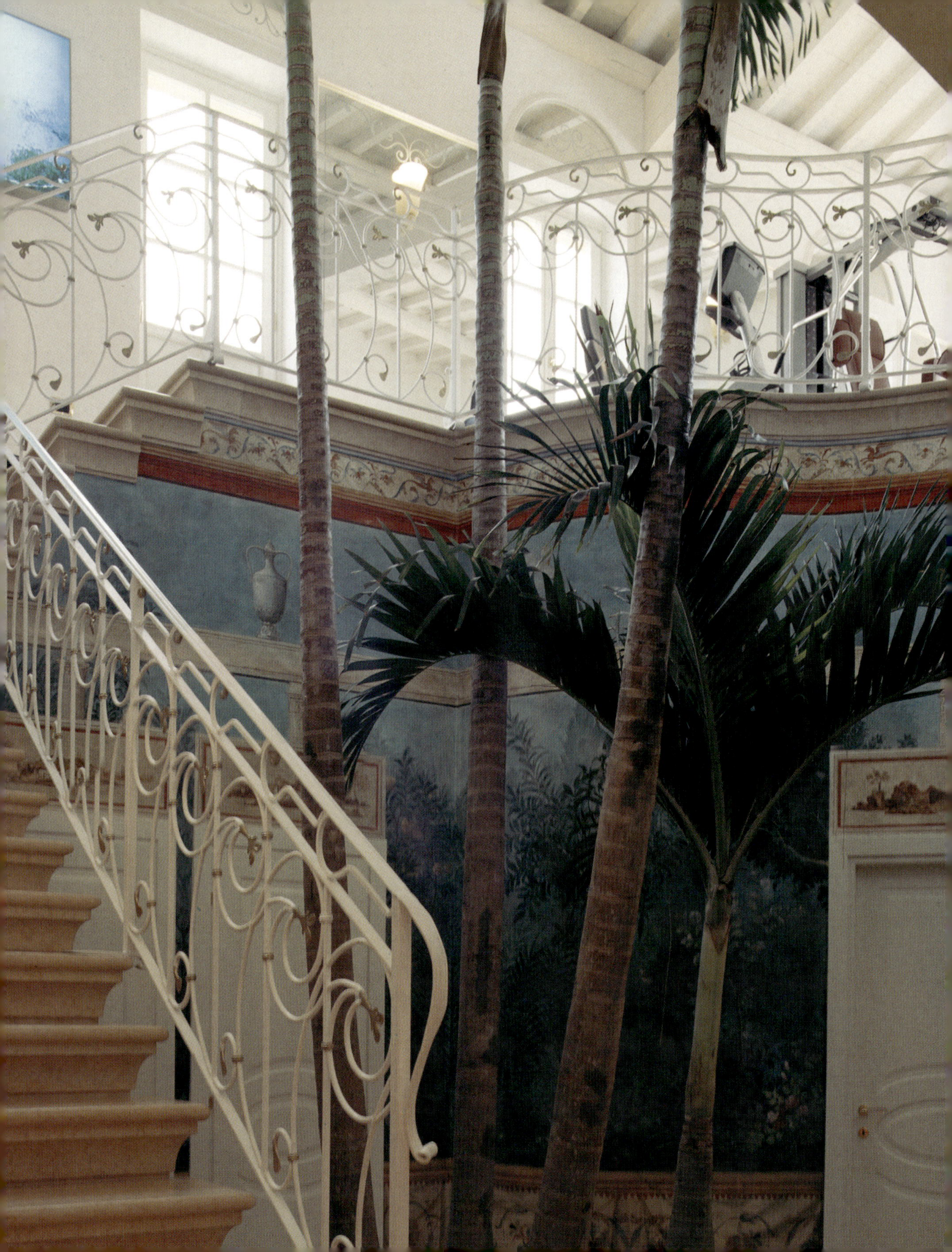

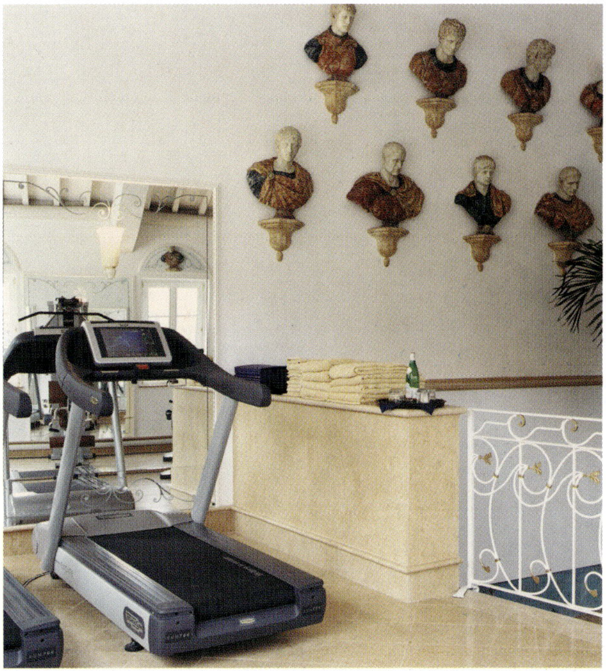

Das Hotel Byblos zeigt Werke bedeutender zeitgenössischer Künstler.

Hotel Byblos holds works by the most prominent contemporary artists.

L'hôtel Byblos présente les œuvres des artistes contemporains les plus en vue.

Hotel Byblos heeft werken van prominente moderne kunstenaars in huis.

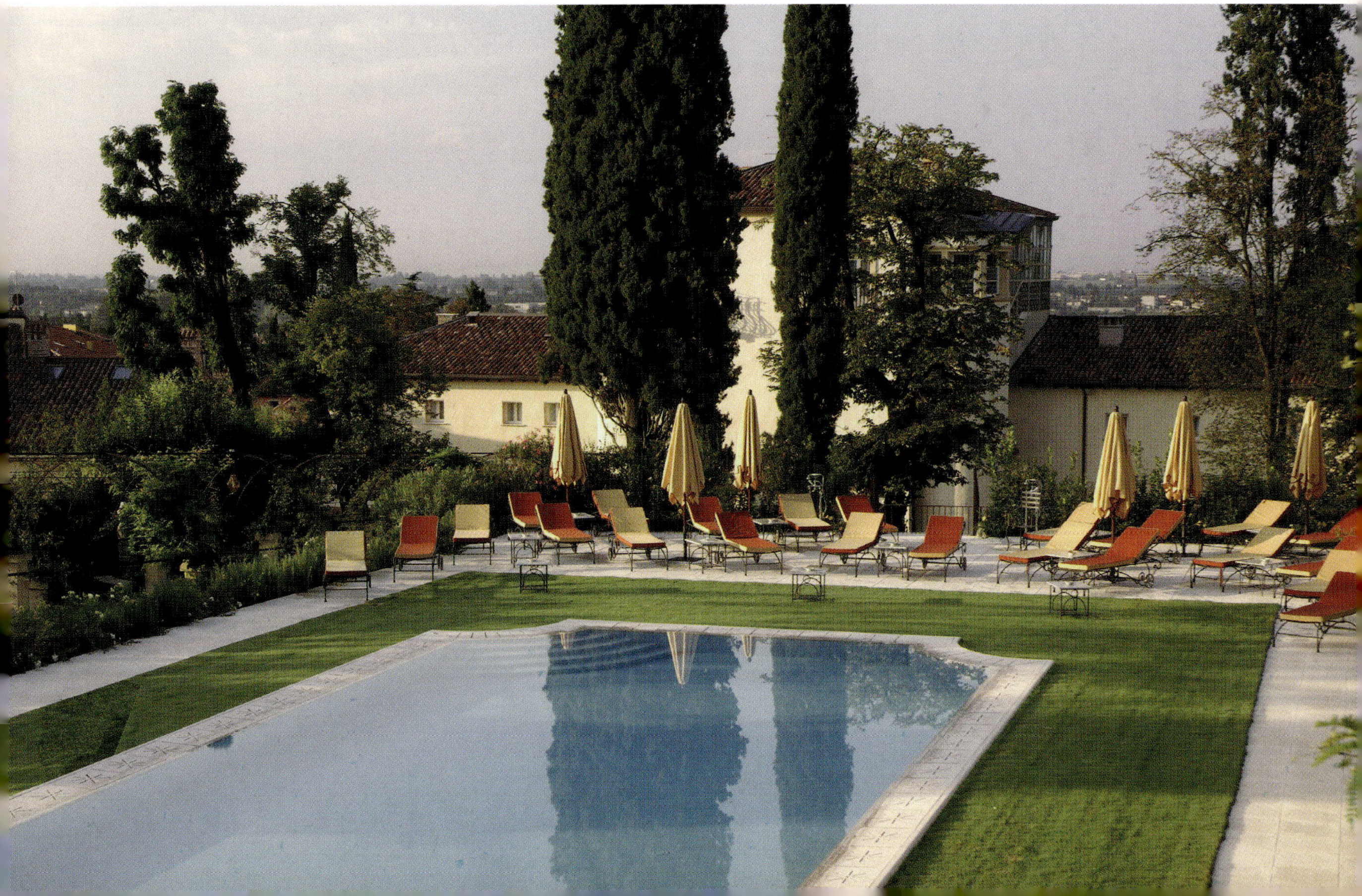

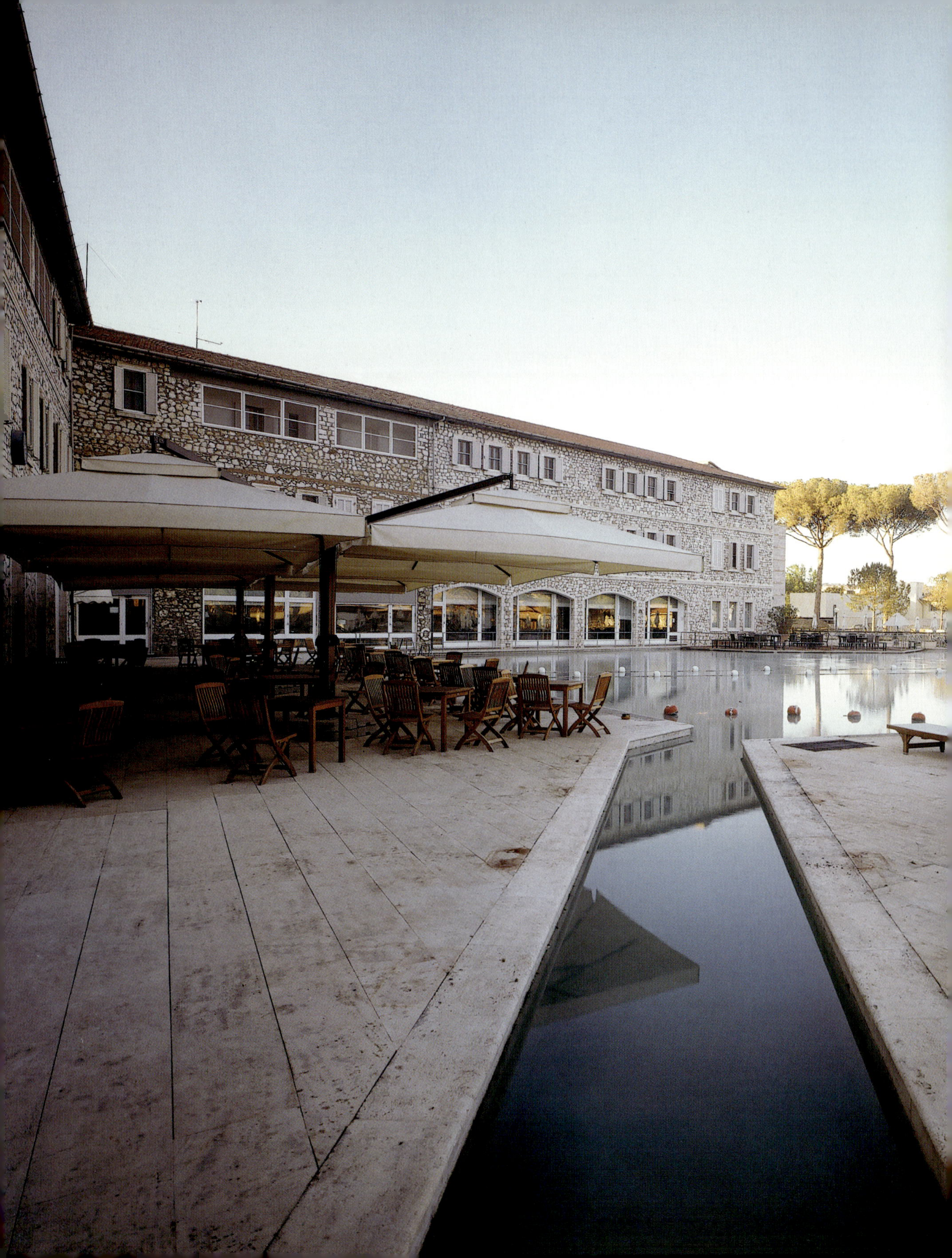

Terme di Saturnia Spa & Golf Resort

Abseits vom Großstadtstress lebt in dieser Therme die Idylle der toskanischen Landschaft auf. Warme schwefelhaltige Quellen sprudeln hier seit über 3.000 Jahren aus dem Erdinneren. Die vier Thermalbecken locken mit Wasserfällen, Whirlpools und einem Warm- und Kaltwasserparcours. Mit 60 Kabinen bietet das Spa ein breitgefächertes Therapiespektrum mit Massagen, Schönheitsbehandlungen, Thermalanwendungen, Physiotherapie, Diät-, Ernährungs- und Fitnessprogrammen.

Far from city stress, the Saturnia thermal baths summarize the calm of the Tuscan countryside. Warm and sulfurous waters gush from its springs, kept inside the earth for over 3,000 years. The four thermal pools include waterfalls, Jacuzzis and cardiovascular circuits of cold and hot water. The 60 spa cabins offer a wide variety of therapies that range from massages to beauty treatments, thermal and physiotherapy cures, diets, nutrition programs and fitness.

Loin du stress de la ville, les bains thermaux du Saturnia incarnent à merveille le calme de la campagne toscane. De ses sources jaillissent des eaux chaudes et sulfureuses, conservées sous terre depuis plus de 3.000 ans. Les quatre piscines thermales incluent des chutes d'eau, des jacuzzis ainsi que des parcours de stimulation cardiaque et de circulation sanguine. La station thermale, dotée de 60 cabines, offre un large éventail de thérapies et soins : massages esthétiques, cures thermales, cures d'amincissement, programmes de nutrition et de remise en forme.

De thermaalbaden van Saturnia, ver verwijderd van grootsteedse stress, belichamen de rust van het Toscaanse landschap. Warm, zwavelhoudend water dat ruim 3000 jaar in de grond heeft gezeten, borrelt op uit de bronnen. De vier baden zijn voorzien van watervallen, jacuzzi's en circuits met koud en warm water die de bloedsomloop stimuleren. De 60 cabines bieden tal van therapieën, variërend van massages tot schoonheidsbehandelingen, fysiotherapie, voedingsprogramma's en fitness.

Maremma, Italy

STUDIO TECNICO DI ARCHITETTURA
LORENZO BELLINI

Photos © Alessandro Ciampi, Federico Cedrone

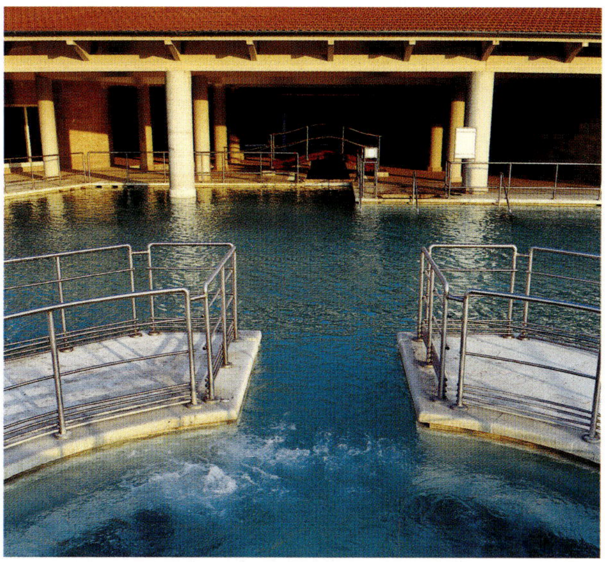

www.termedisaturnia.it

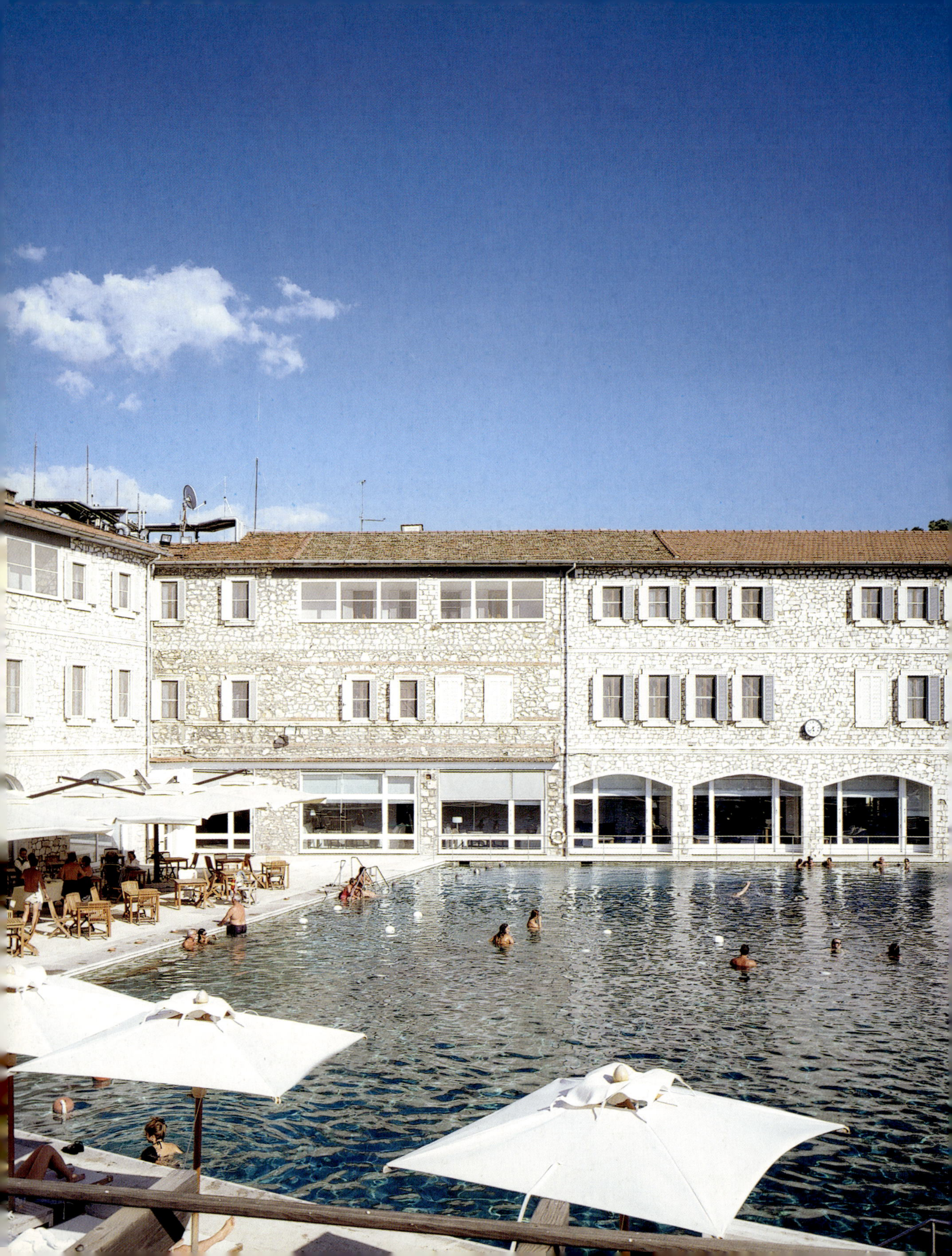

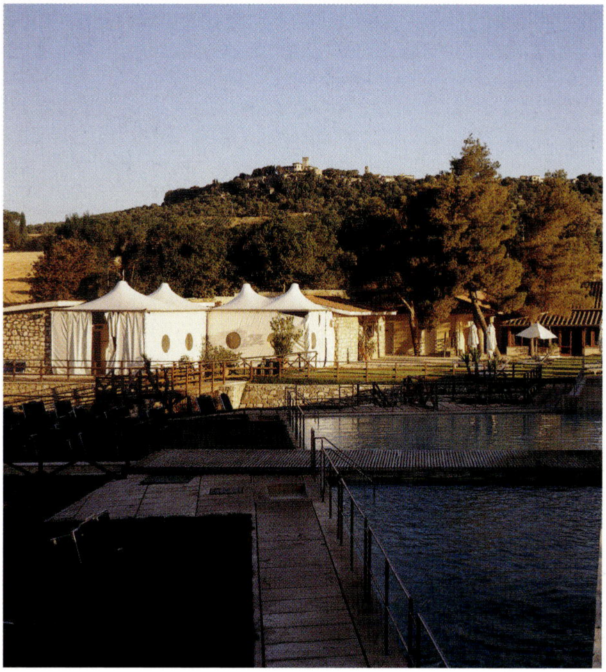

Römisches Bad und Sauna sind mit dem Thermalbrunnen des Wasserparks verbunden.

The Roman bath and sauna are connected with the thermal fountain at the water park.

Le bain romain et le sauna sont reliés au bassin aquatique par la source thermale.

Het Romeinse bad en de sauna staan in verbinding met de minerale bron in het waterpark.

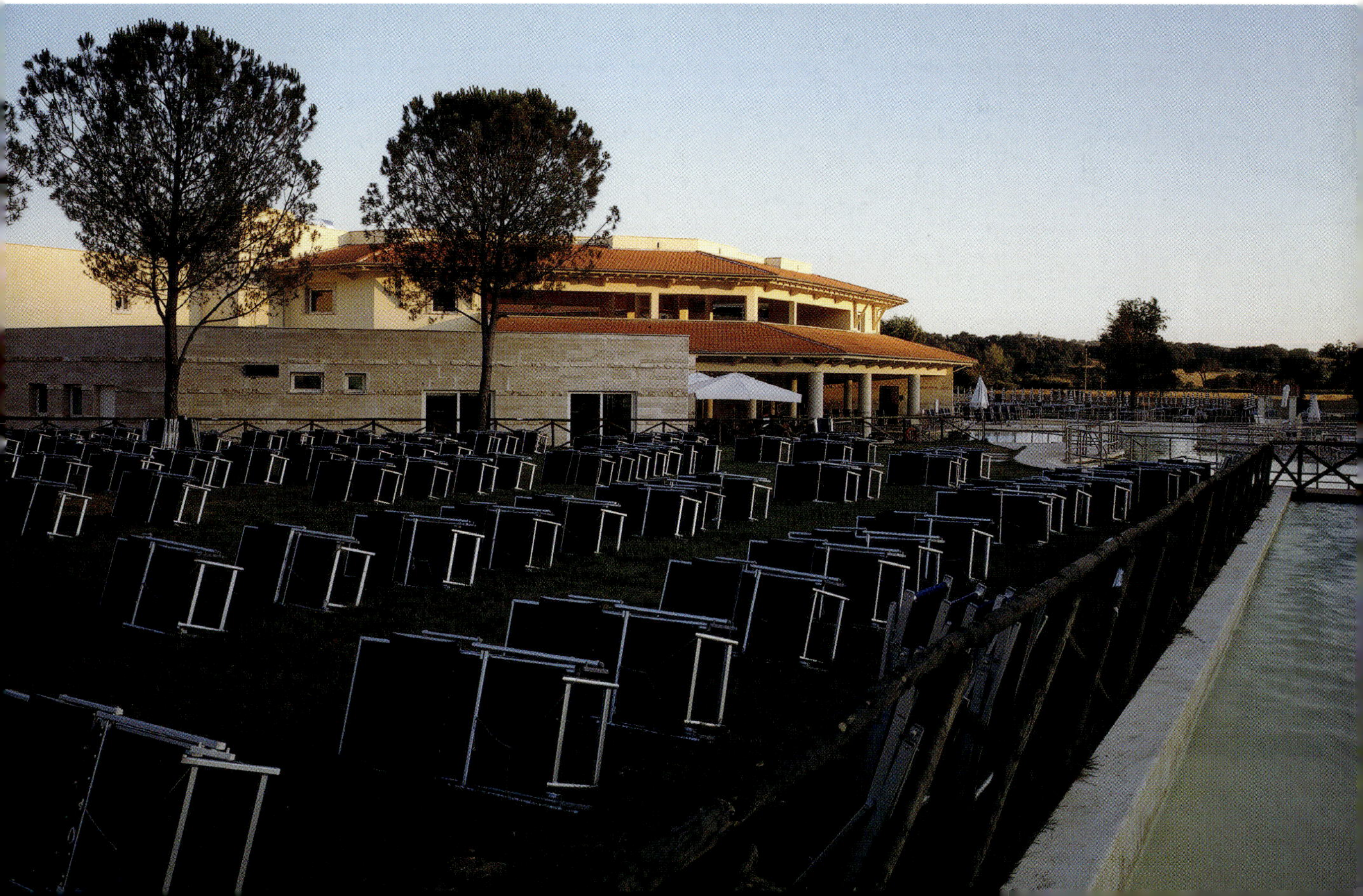

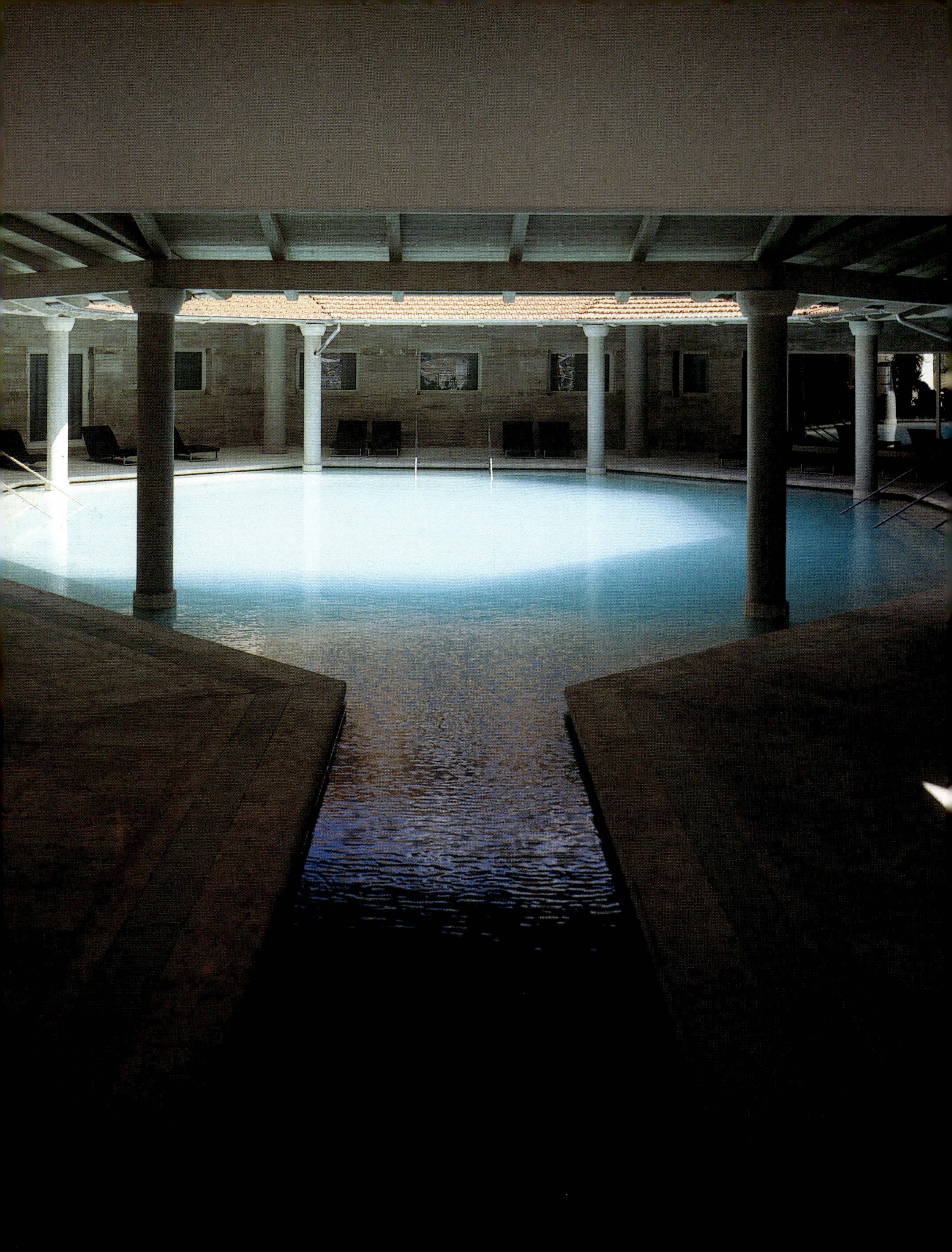

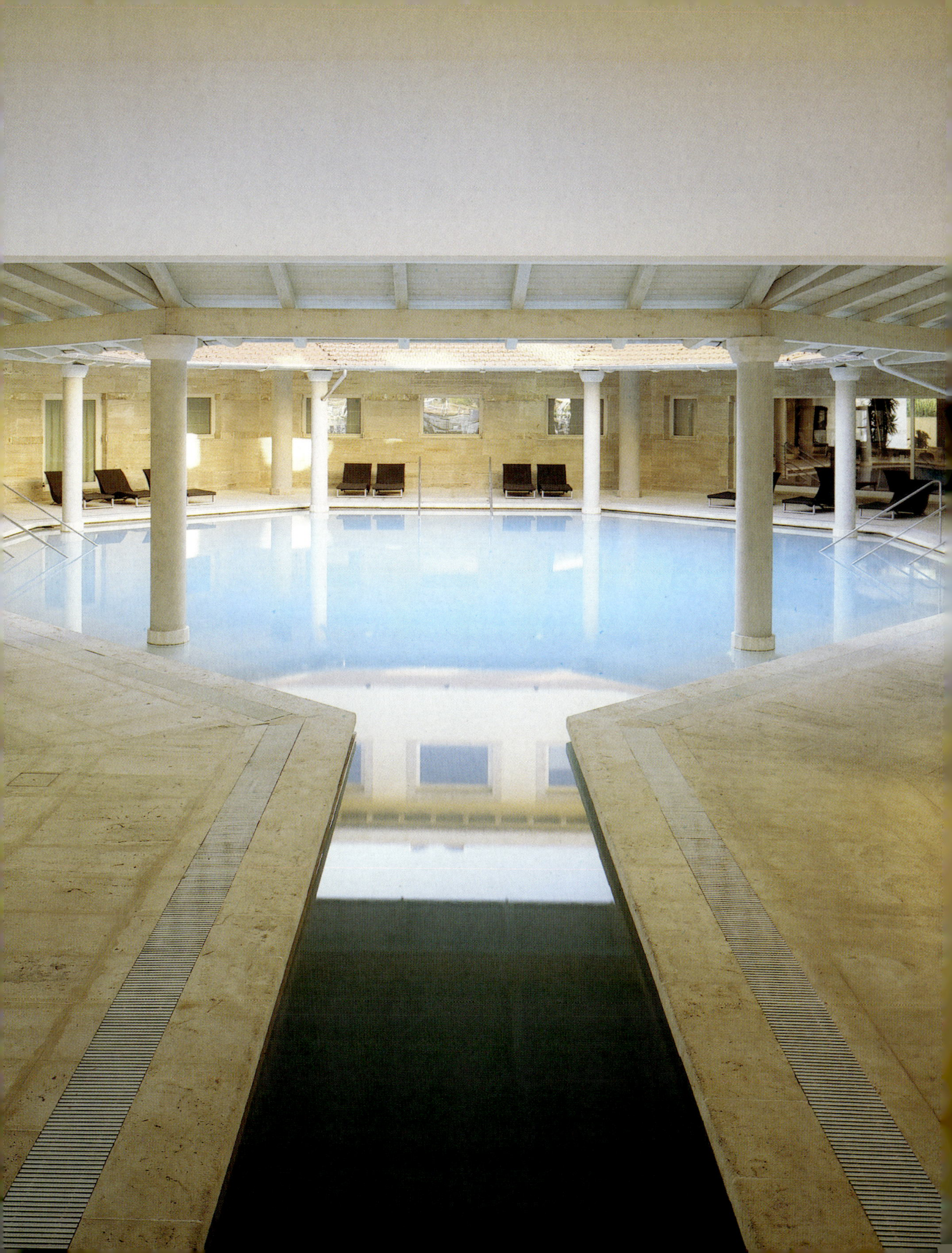

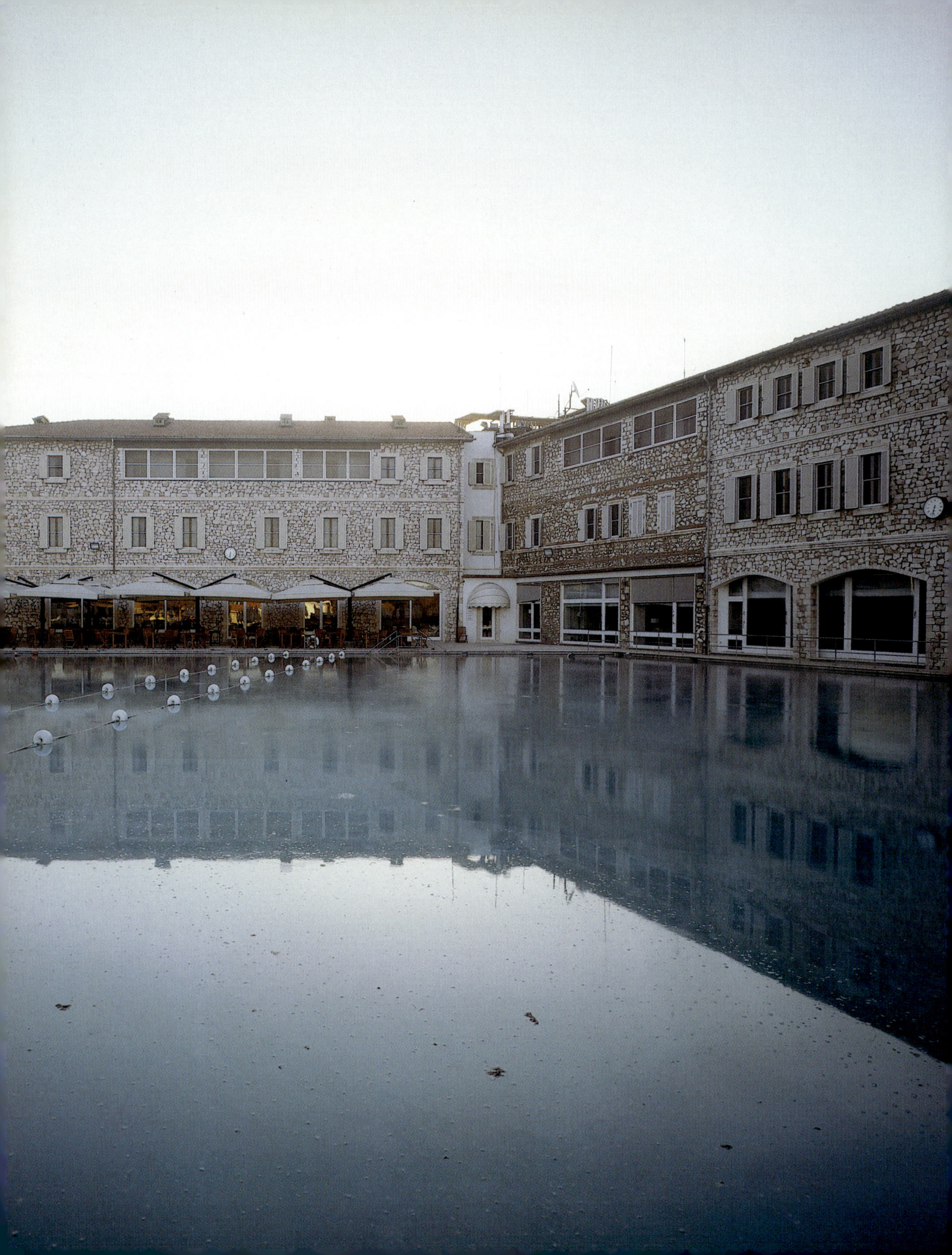

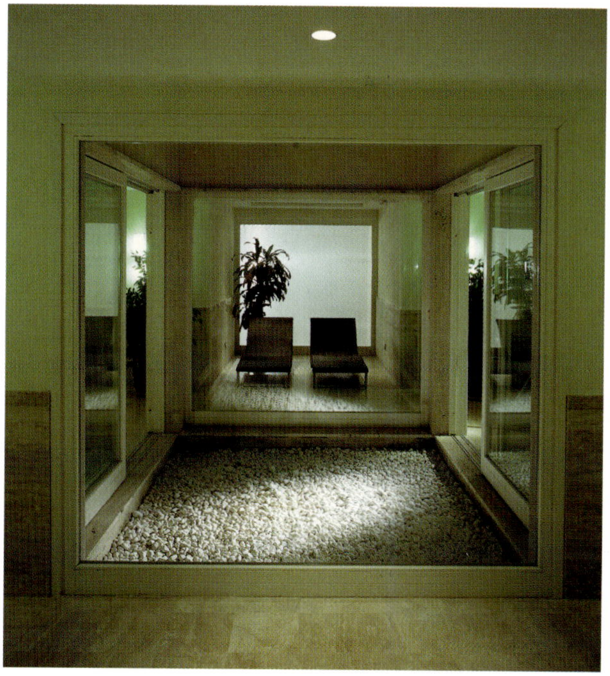

Das Thermalwasser fließt mit einer Geschwindigkeit von 800 Litern pro Sekunde bei konstanter Temperatur von 37´C.

The thermal waters flow at a pace of 800 liters per second and at a constant temperature of 99 °F.

Les eaux thermales ont un débit de 800 litres par seconde et ont une température constante de 36° Celsius.

Het bronwater komt met 800 liter per seconde en een constante temperatuur van 37 °C aan de oppervlakte.

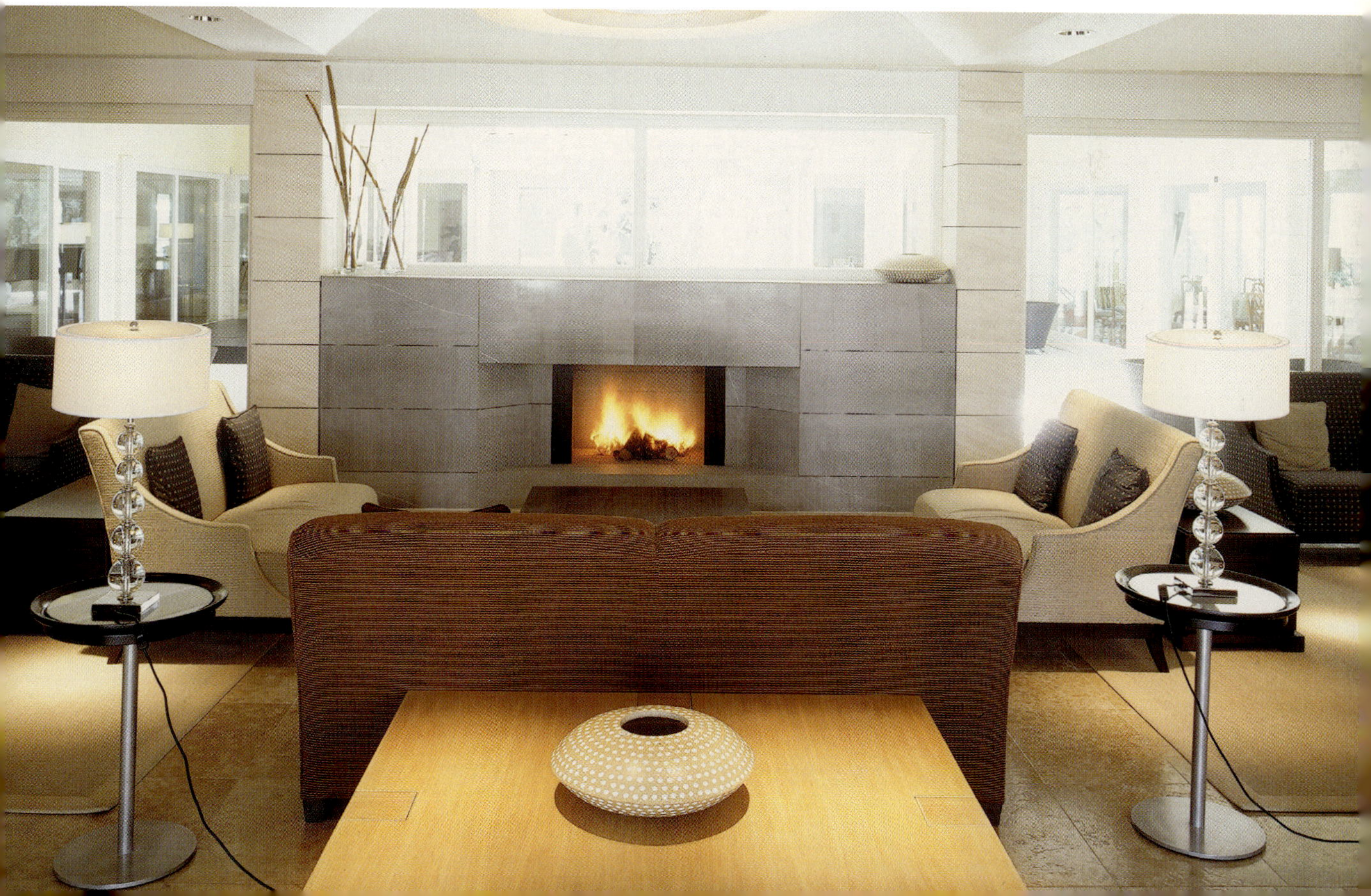

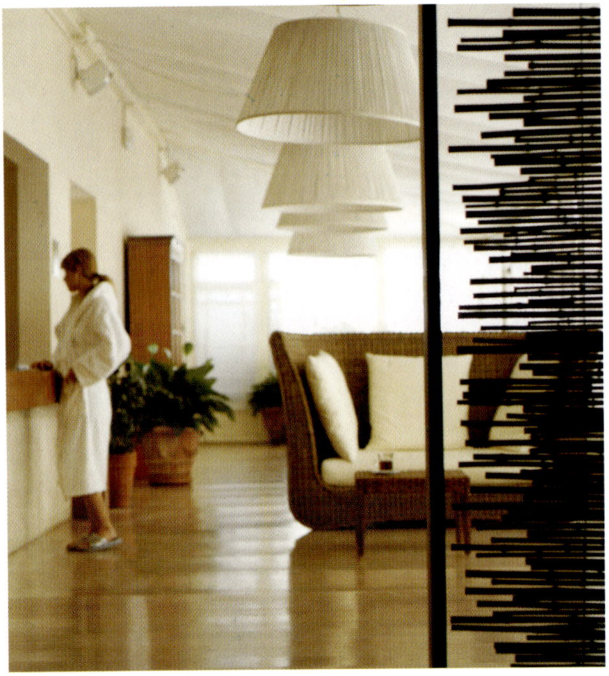

Der vollständig renovierte Komplex beherbergt ein elegantes Hotel, das Spa, Thermalquellen und einen Golfplatz.

The totally renovated complex includes an elegant hotel, a spa, thermal springs and a golf course.

Le complexe, totalement rénové, comprend un hôtel de grand standing, un spa, des sources thermales et un terrain de golf.

Het gerenoveerde complex omvat een stijlvol hotel, een kuurinrichting met thermale bronnen en een golfbaan.

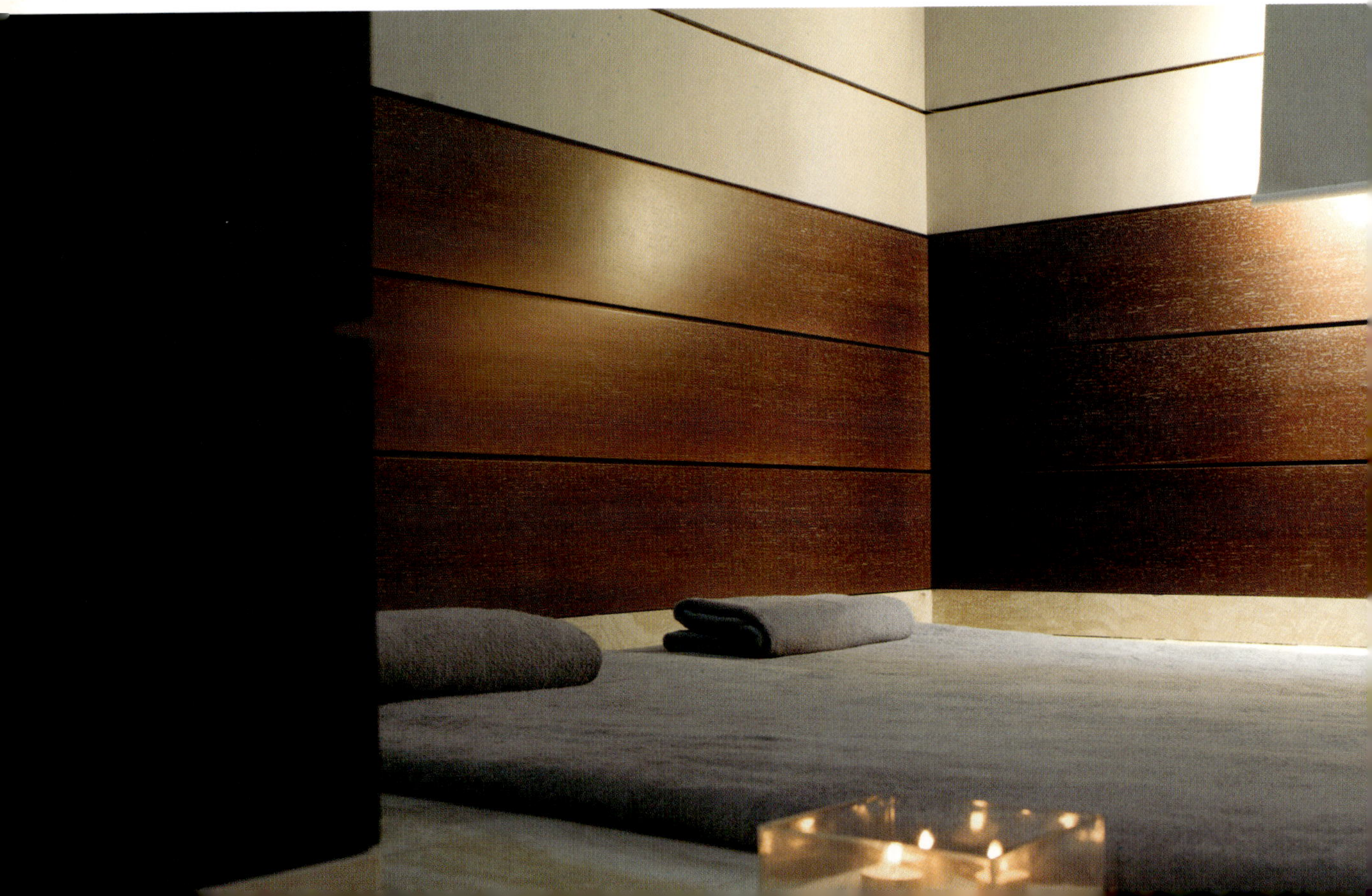

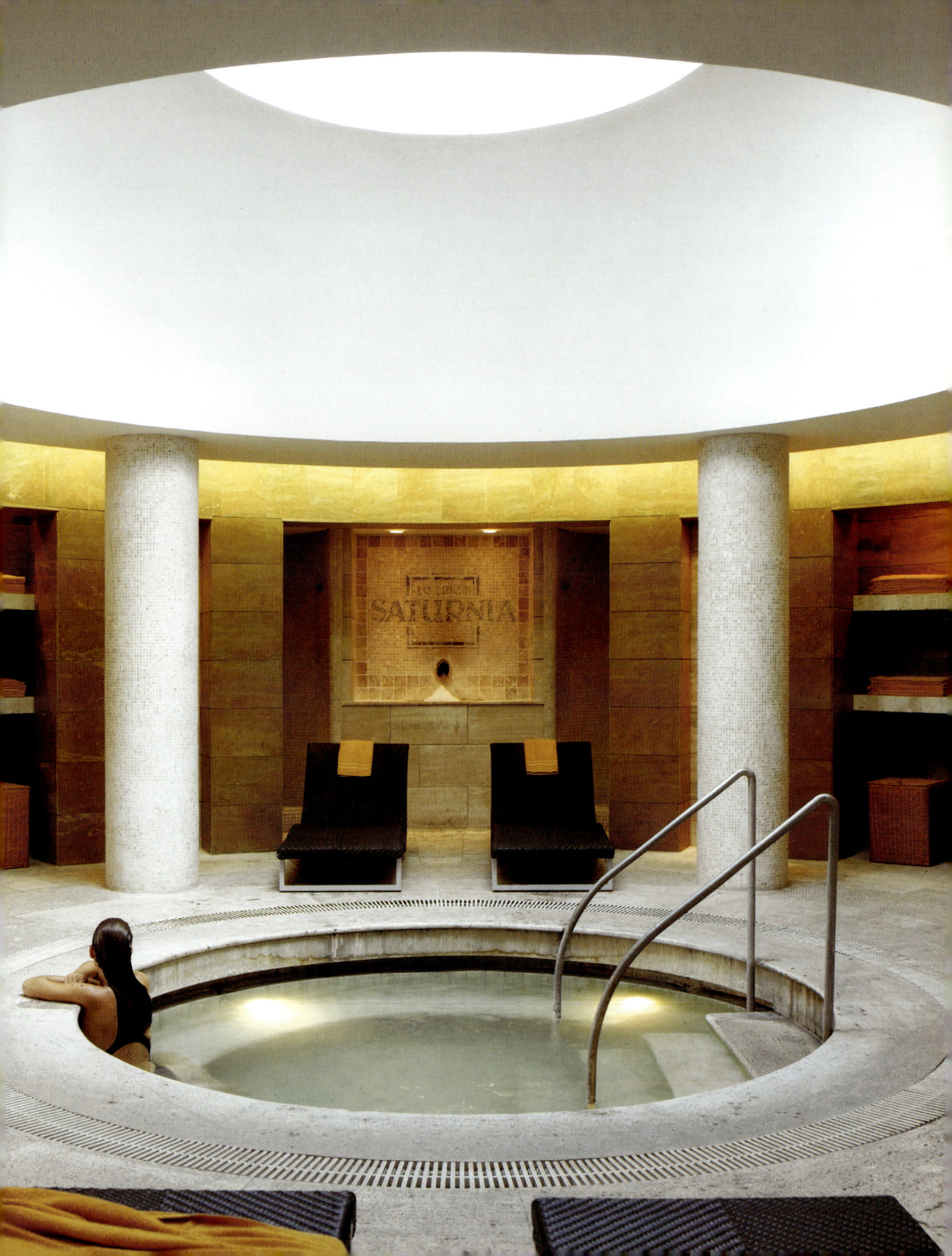
SATURNIA

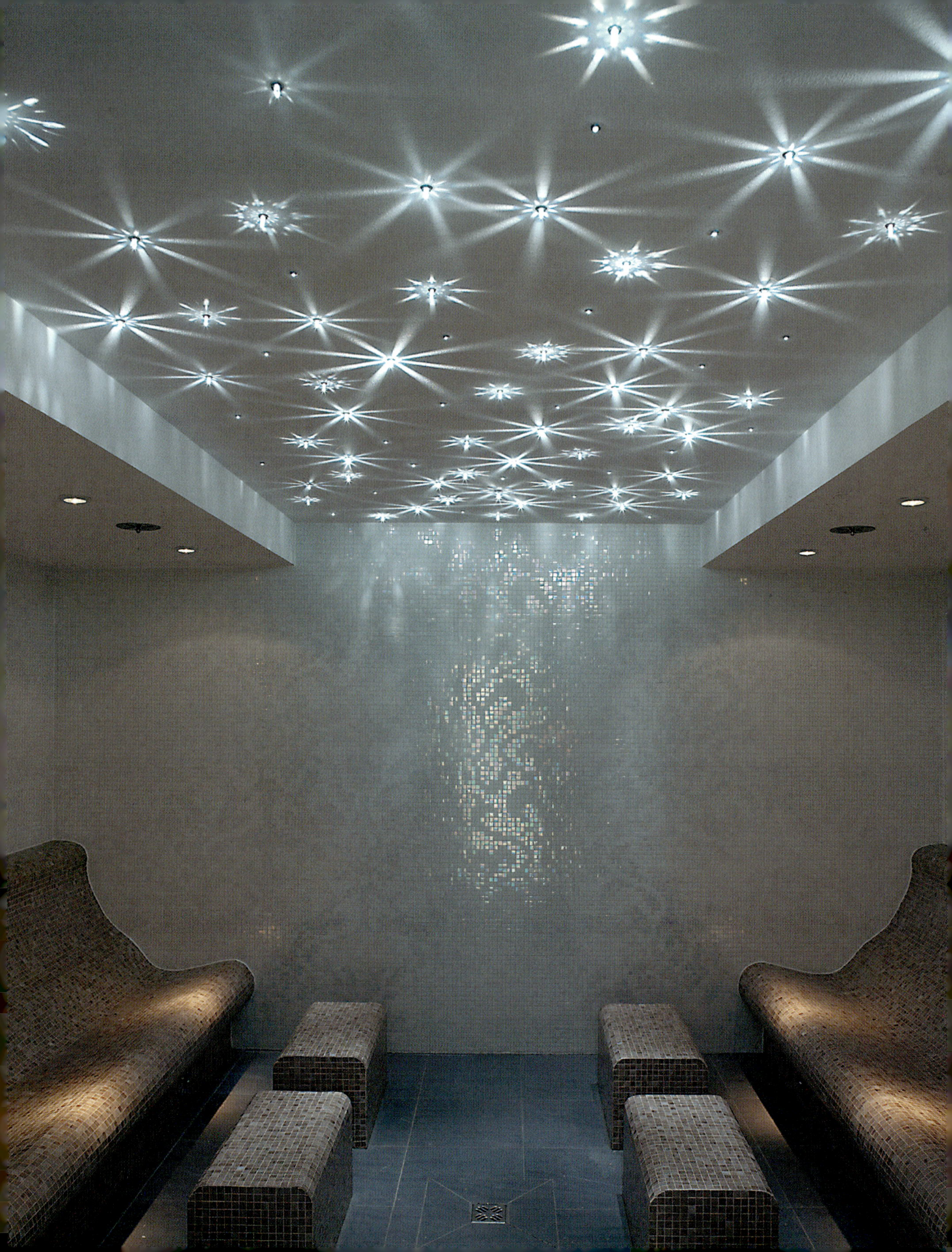

Balance Resort Stegersbach

Dieses Hotel Spa bietet seinen Gästen durch großzügige Glasfassaden einen herrlichen Blick auf die Landschaft. Das Spa gliedert sich in zwei große Bereiche: Dampfzone und Wasserzone. In der ersten Zone umfasst das Behandlungsspektrum neben Kräuterdämpfen und finnischer Sauna auch Aromatherapie, Laconium und Kabinen zur Aquameditation. Die zweite Zone verfügt über einen Pool mit Wasserfall, in welchem Unterwasser- und Whirlpoolmassagen angeboten werden.

This hotel spa has been provided with glass facades that allow the visitor to enjoy the spectacular all round views. The spa is divided in two major areas: the steam zone and the water zone. The first one holds a wide variety of treatments going from herbal vapors to the Finnish sauna, aromatherapy, the laconium and the cabins for aqua-meditation. The second area consists of an edgeless pool, which has a waterfall and where underwater and whirlpool massages are offered.

Les façades de verre de l'hôtel permettent au visiteur d'apprécier la vue spectaculaire sur les alentours. Le spa est divisé en deux secteurs majeurs. Le premier privilégie la vapeur, proposant un éventail de soins, allant des brumisations d'herbes jusqu'au sauna finlandais, en passant par l'aromathérapie, le laconium et les cabines pour l'aqua-méditation. Le deuxième espace est dédié aux traitements par l'eau, il comprend une piscine à débordement, agrémentée d'une cascade, où l'on peut s'offrir des massages aquatiques et des bains bouillonnants.

Dit kuurhotel is voorzien van glazen wanden waardoor de bezoeker de omgeving kan bewonderen. De kuurinrichting is verdeeld in twee afdelingen: de stoomzone en de waterzone. De eerste zone biedt een heel scala aan behandelingen: kruidendampen, een Finse sauna, aromatherapie, een laconium en cabines voor aquameditatie. De tweede zone bestaat uit een uitgestrekt zwembad met een waterval, waar onderwater- en whirlpoolmassages worden aangeboden.

Stegersbach, Austria

ARCHISPHERE ARCHITECTS AND DESIGNERS | DESIGN: SCHLETTERER WELLNESS & SPA DESIGN

Photos © Andi Bruckner

www.balance-resort.at

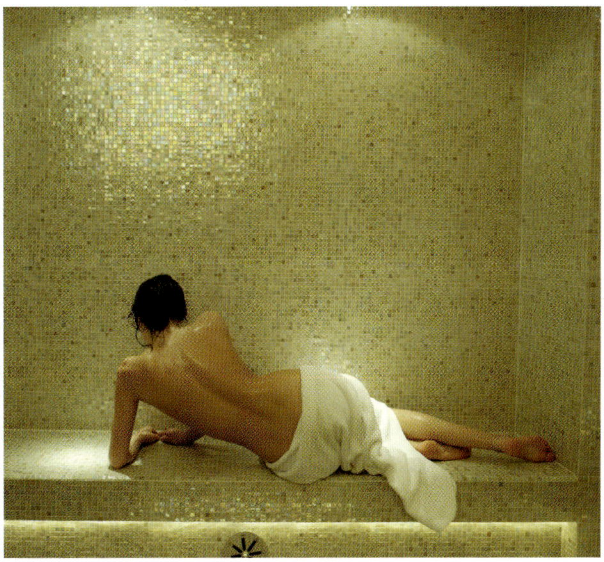

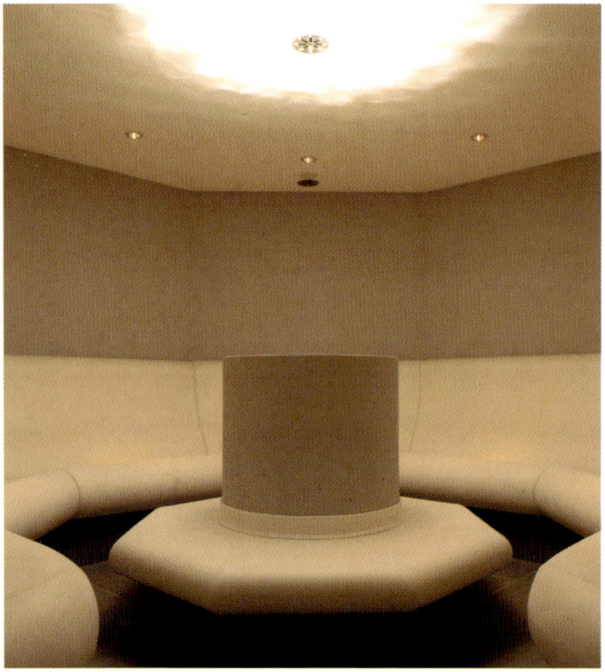

Nach seiner vollständigen Renovierung feierte das Spa im Balance Resort Stegersbach 2004 seine Wiedereröffnung.

The spa at the Balance Resort Stegersbach reopened in 2004 after a thorough renovation.

Le spa Balance Resort Stegersbach a réouvert en 2004, après une rénovation complète.

Het bronnenbad van het Balance Resort Stegersbach heropende in 2004 na een grondige renovatie.

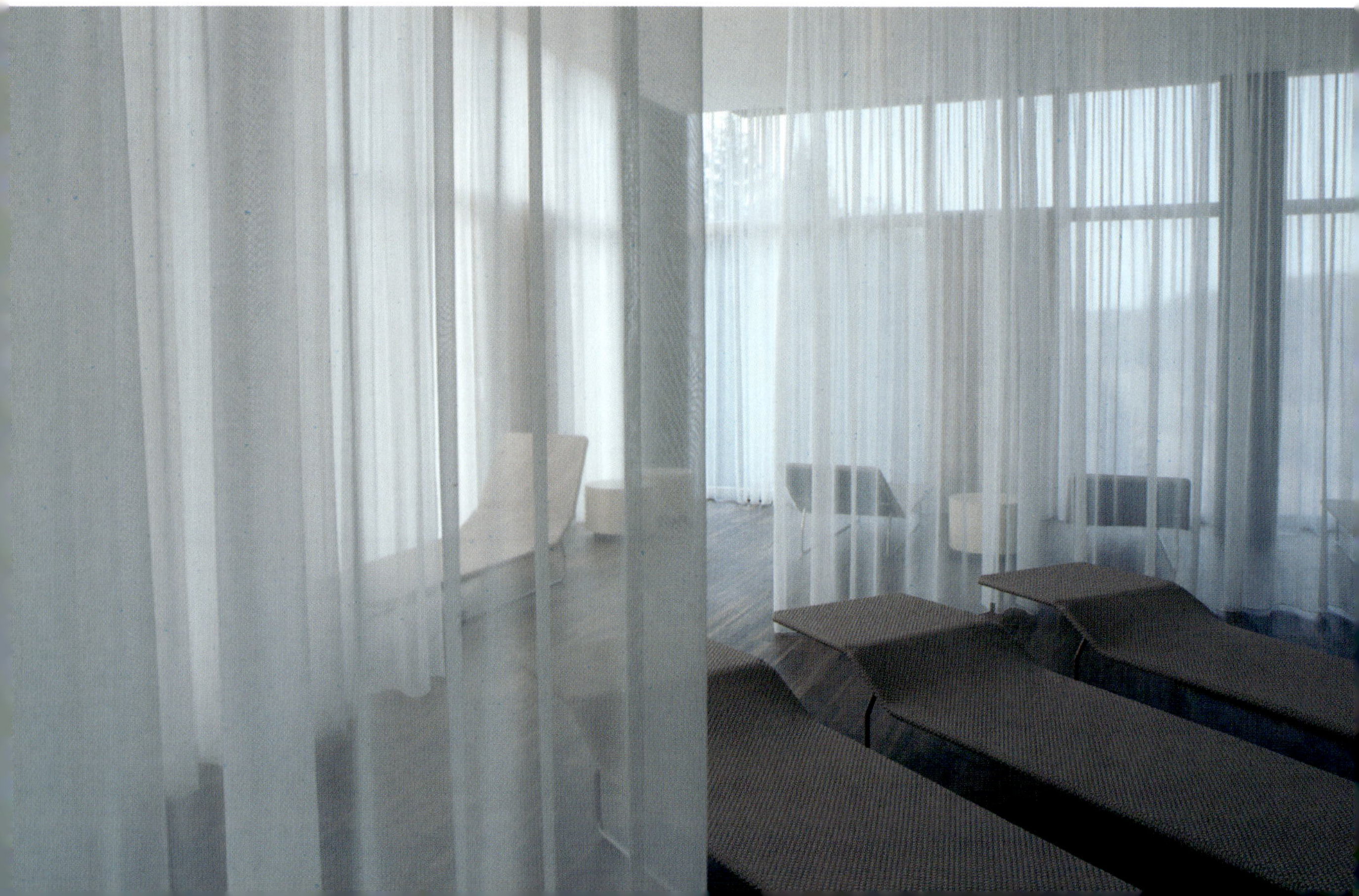

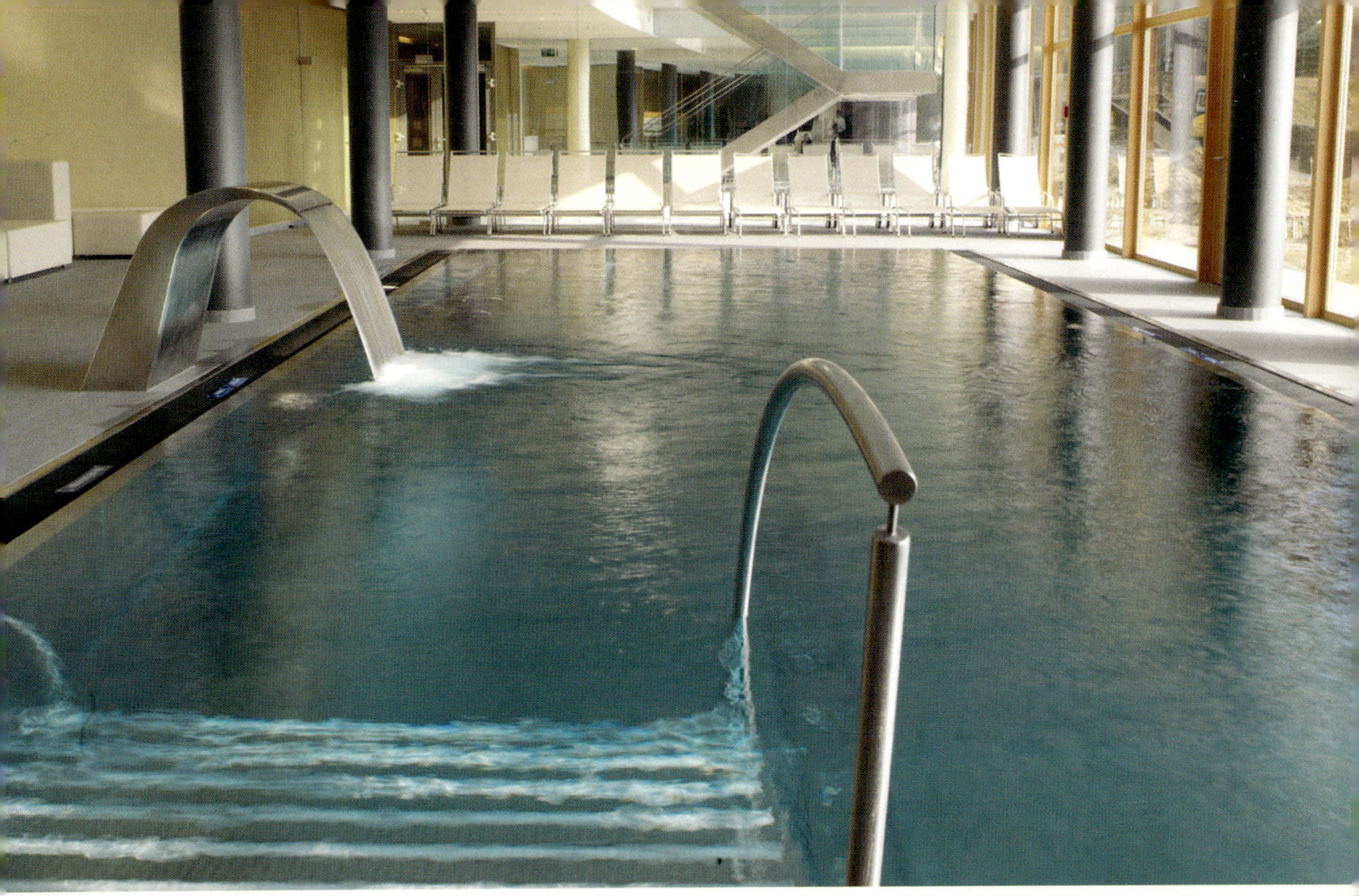

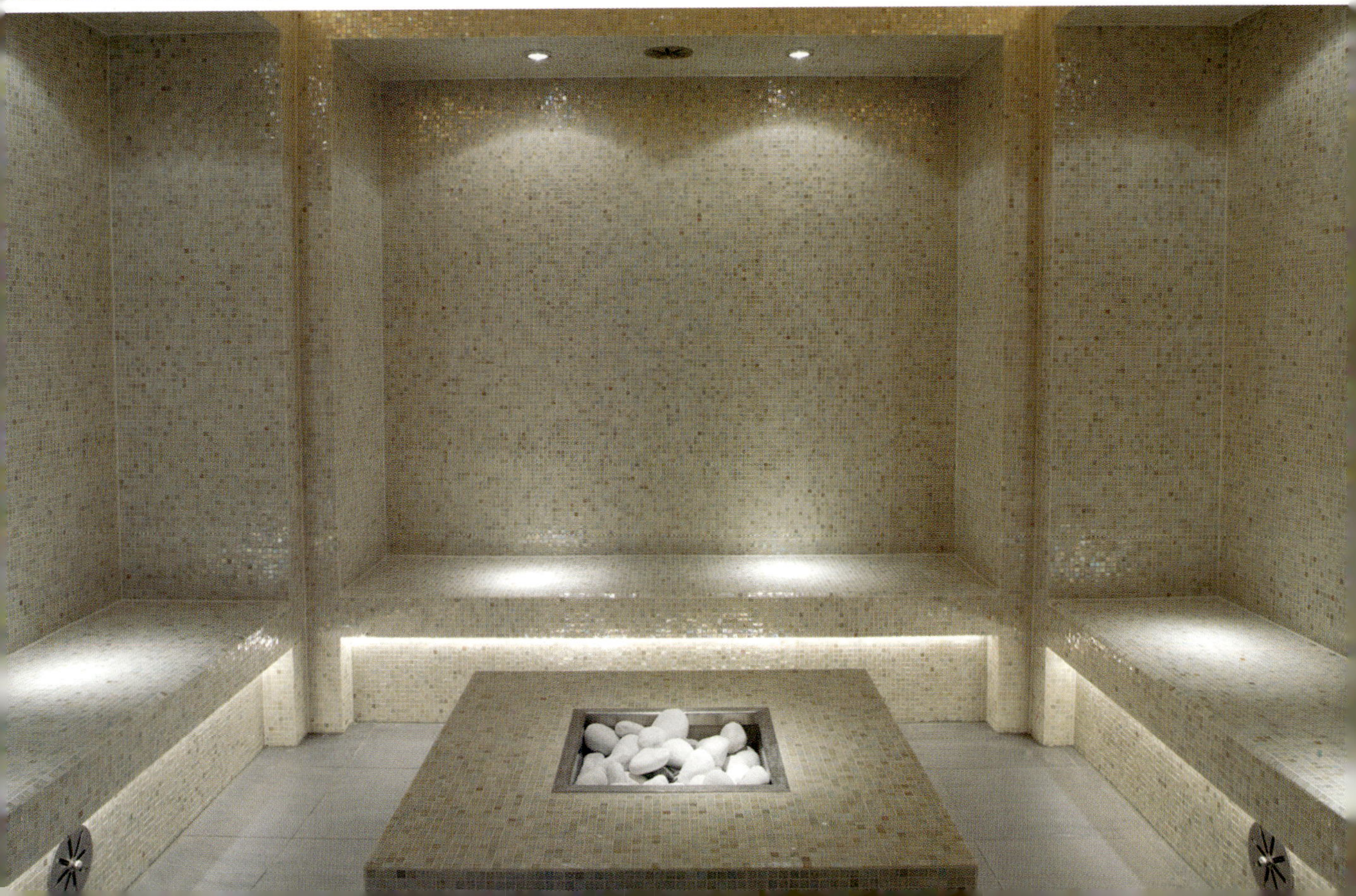

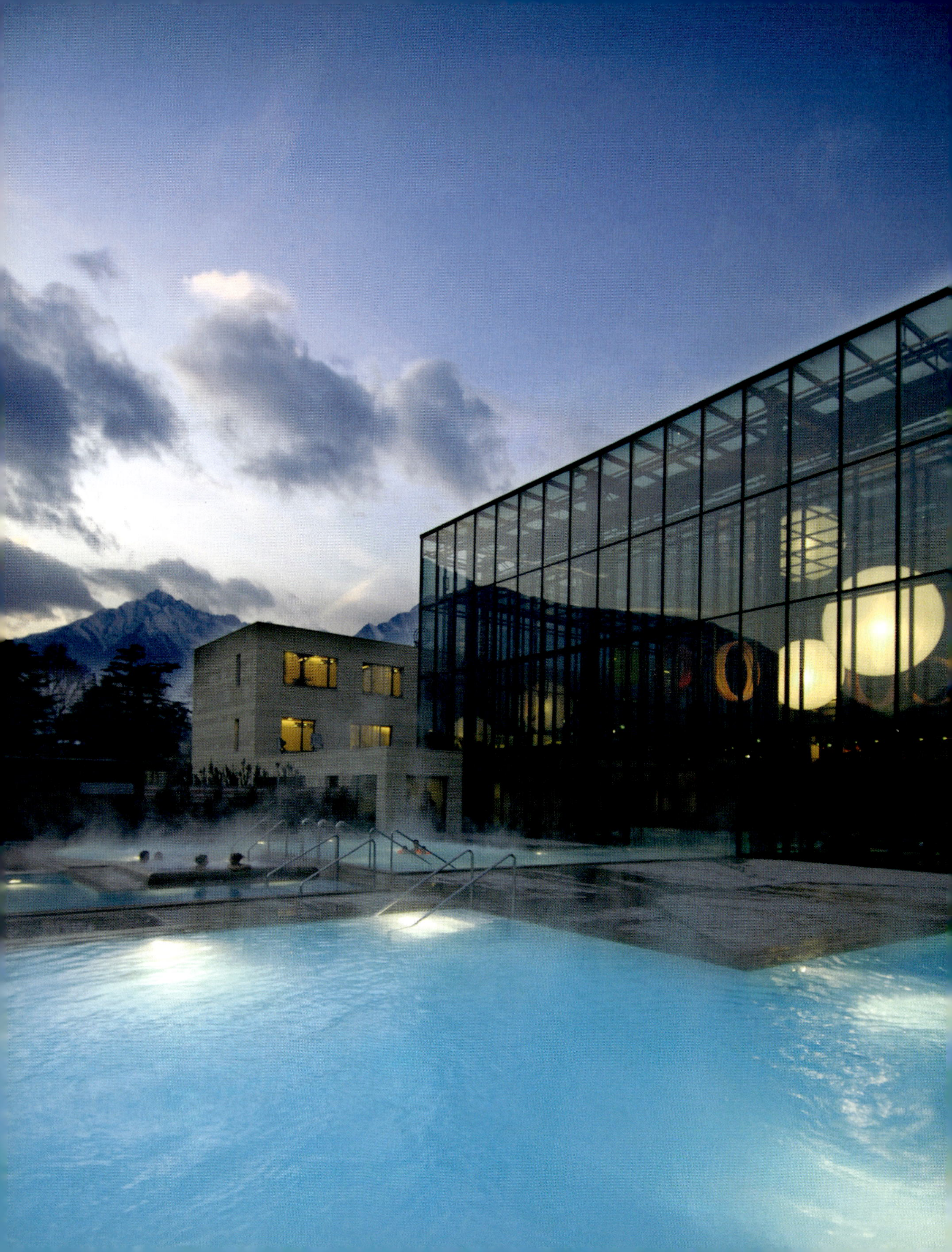

Merano Thermal

Die offene Struktur dieses Spas ist von der weitläufigen Parklandschaft mit 13 Freiluftbecken geprägt. Zentrales Gebäude ist ein großer Glaskubus mit Blick auf die nahe gelegenen Berge. Trotz ihrer beachtlichen Größe vermittelt die Therme überall ein Gefühl von Behaglichkeit. Eine sorgfältige Farb- und Materialauswahl zeichnet die verschiedenen Bereiche aus. Indirekte Beleuchtung trägt ebenfalls zu der entspannten und intimen Atmosphäre bei.

Its open structure is defined by the great park, that surrounds it and that holds 13 outside pools. The central building is a great glass cube, through which it is possible to see the nearby mountains. Despite the large size of the thermal baths, in all the areas there is a feeling of coziness that responds to a careful selection of natural materials and colors that define the different areas and the indirect light that harmonizes so well with relaxation and privacy.

La structure dégagée de ce spa est délimitée par le grand parc qui l'entoure et qui comporte treize piscines d'extérieur. Le bâtiment principal est un grand cube de verre, d'où l'on peut admirer les montagnes voisines. Malgré l'imposante taille des bassins thermaux, la sensation de confort est omniprésente. Cela procède tout autant du choix judicieux de matériaux naturels et de couleurs spécifiques aux différentes zones, que de la lumière indirecte favorisant relaxation et intimité.

Het luchtige gebouw wordt sterk gedefinieerd door het grote omringende park met dertien buitenbaden. Het centrale gebouw is een grote glazen kubus vanwaaruit de nabijgelegen bergen te zien zijn. Ondanks de afmetingen van de bronnenbaden behouden alle ruimten een sfeer van gemoedelijkheid, dankzij een nauwgezette keuze voor natuurlijke materialen en kleuren die de verschillende ruimten typeren. Het indirecte licht, dat ontspanning en privacy bevordert, werkt daar ook aan mee.

Merano, Italy

MATTEO THUN

Photos © Gionata Xerra

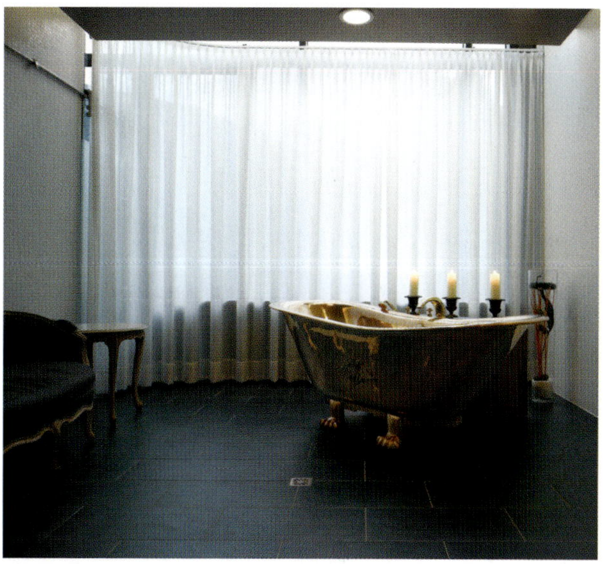

www.termemerano.com

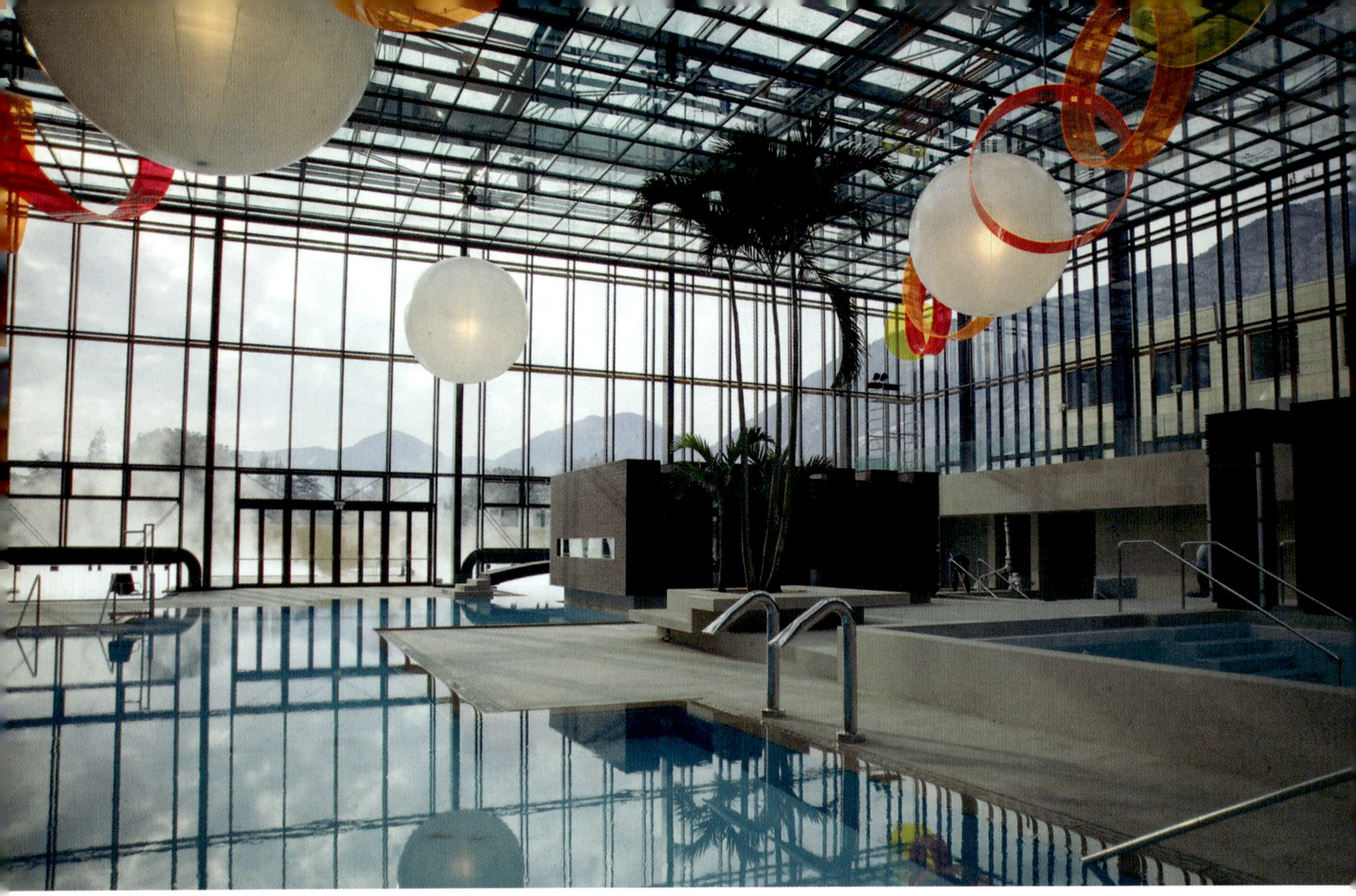

Auf dem Wasser und auf dem Glas spiegeln sich die bunten Scheiben und Kugeln, die an der Decke hängen.

The discs and spheres that hang from the ceiling rotate freely and reflect their colors on the water and the glass.

Les sphères et les disques suspendus au plafond tournoient librement et reflètent leurs couleurs sur l'eau et le verre.

De roterende schijven en bollen aan het plafond werpen een kleurig schijnsel op het water en het glas.

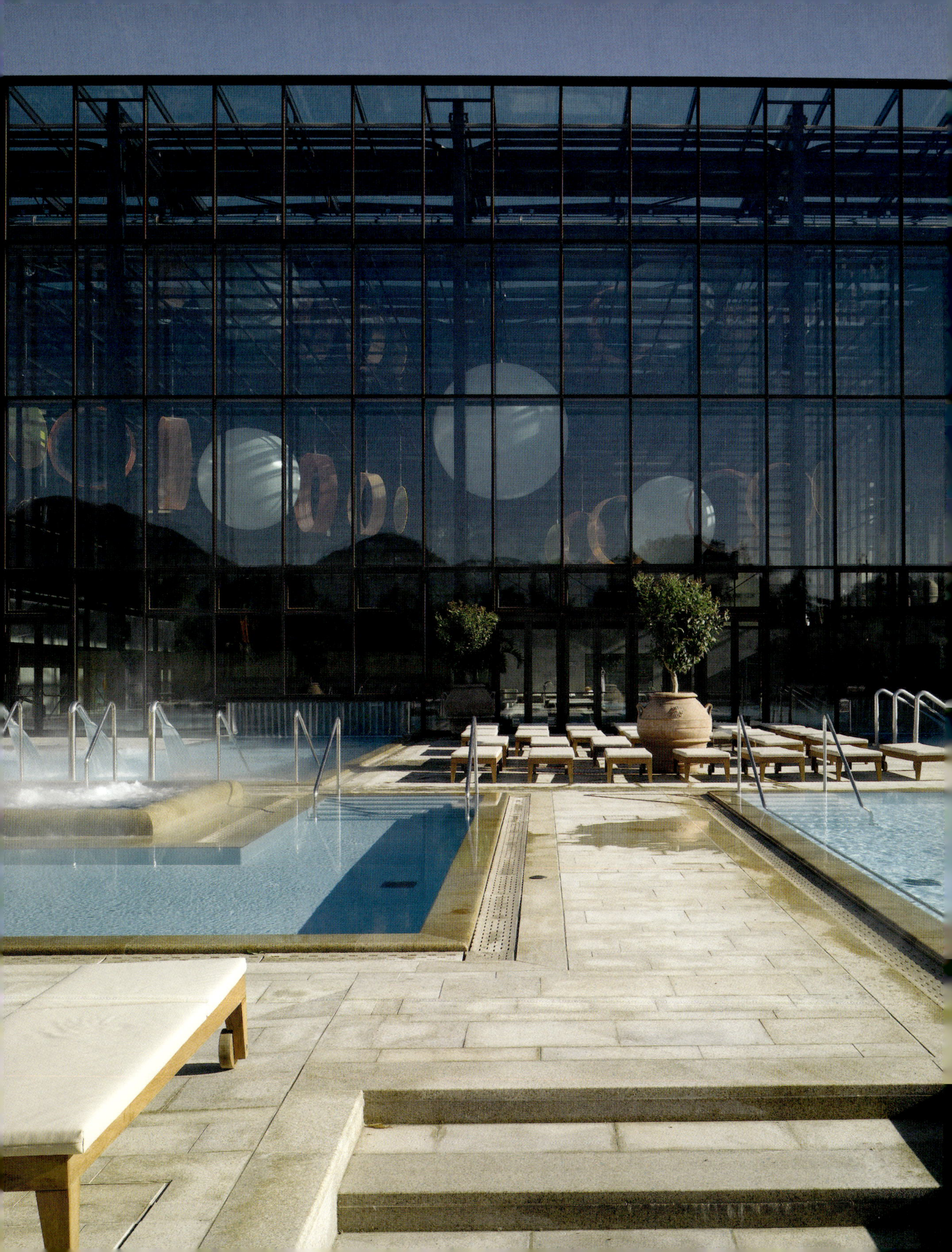

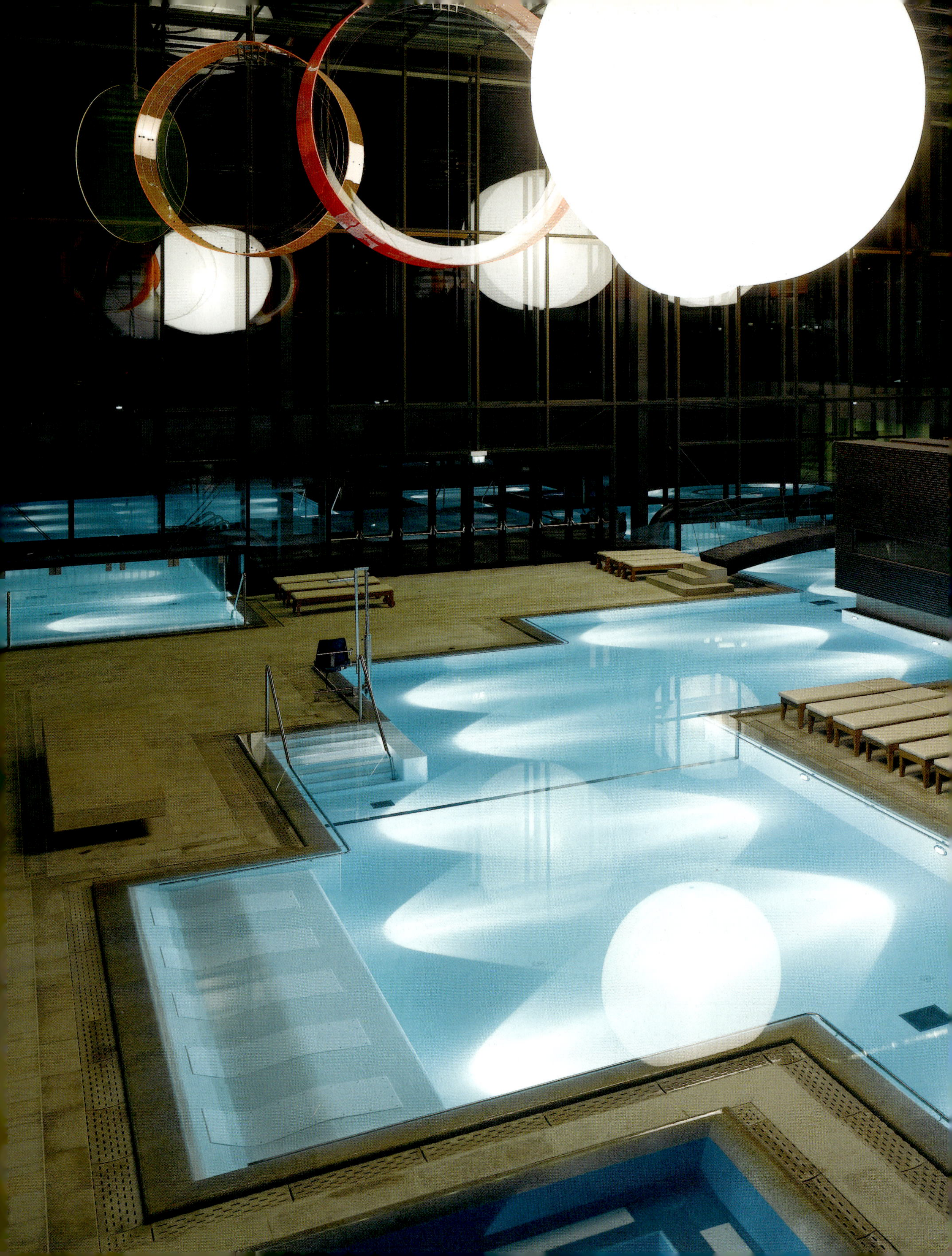

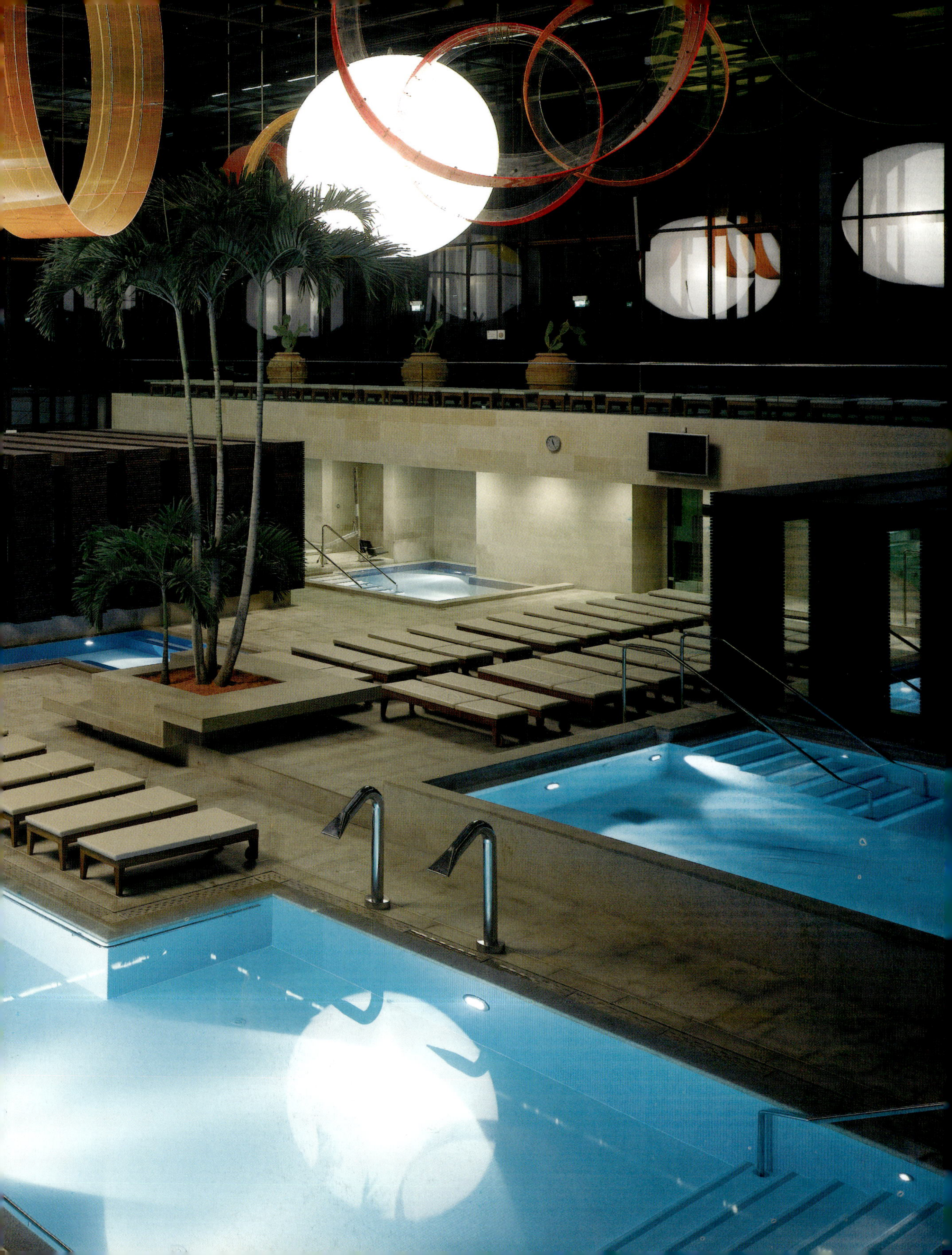

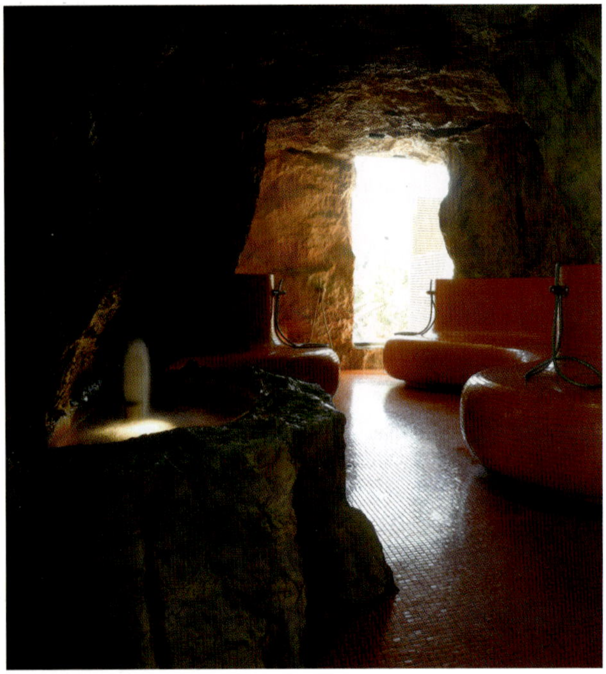

Jedem der Spa-Bereiche ist eine bestimmte Farbe zugeordnet, die für die hier angebotene Behandlung steht.

Each of the different spa areas has a special color in harmony with the treatment to which it is destined.

Chacun des secteurs du spa est défini par une couleur spécifique, en harmonie avec le type de traitements auxquels il est dédié.

Alle afzonderlijke afdelingen hebben een eigen kleur die past bij de behandeling die er gegeven wordt.

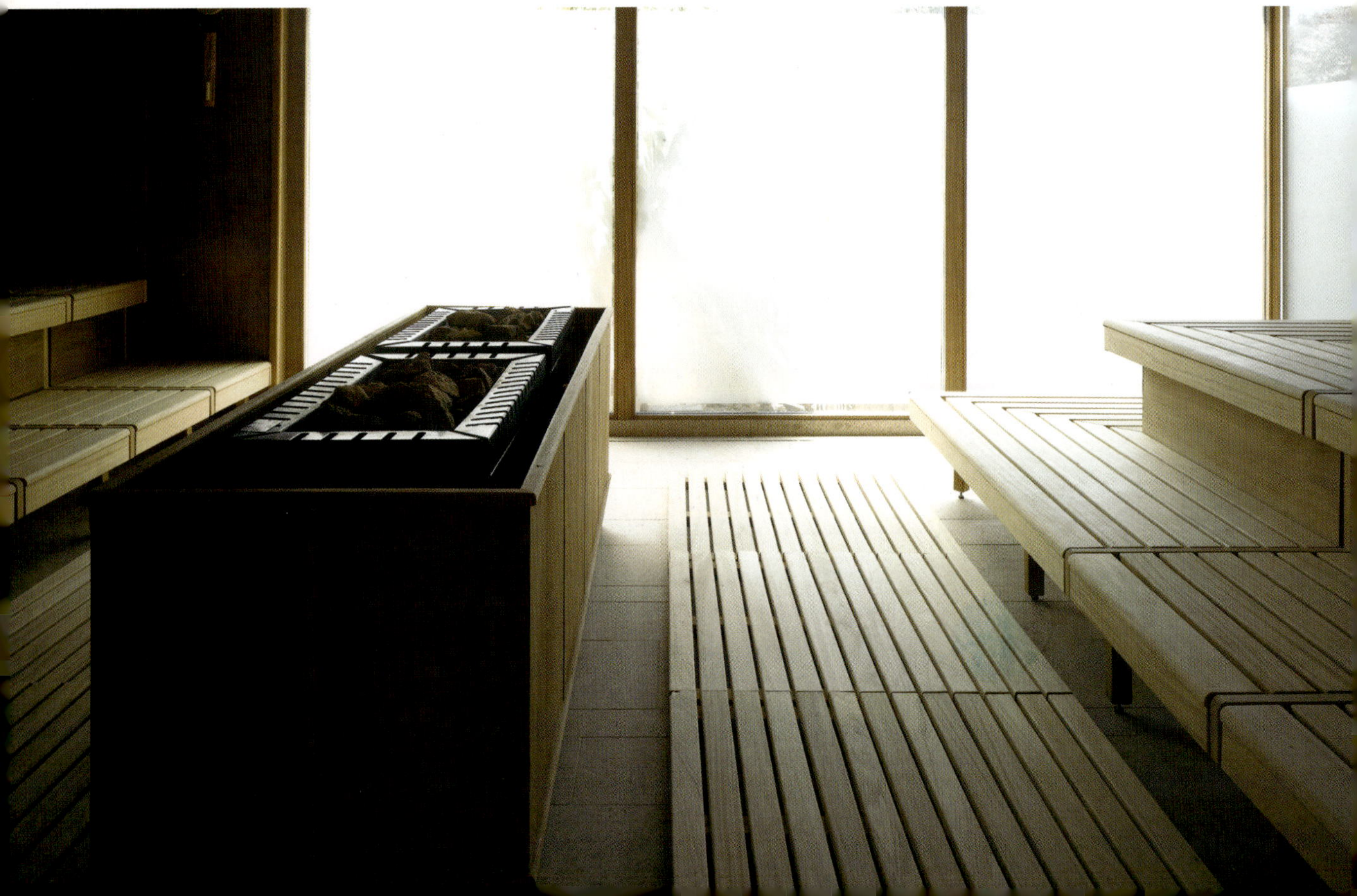

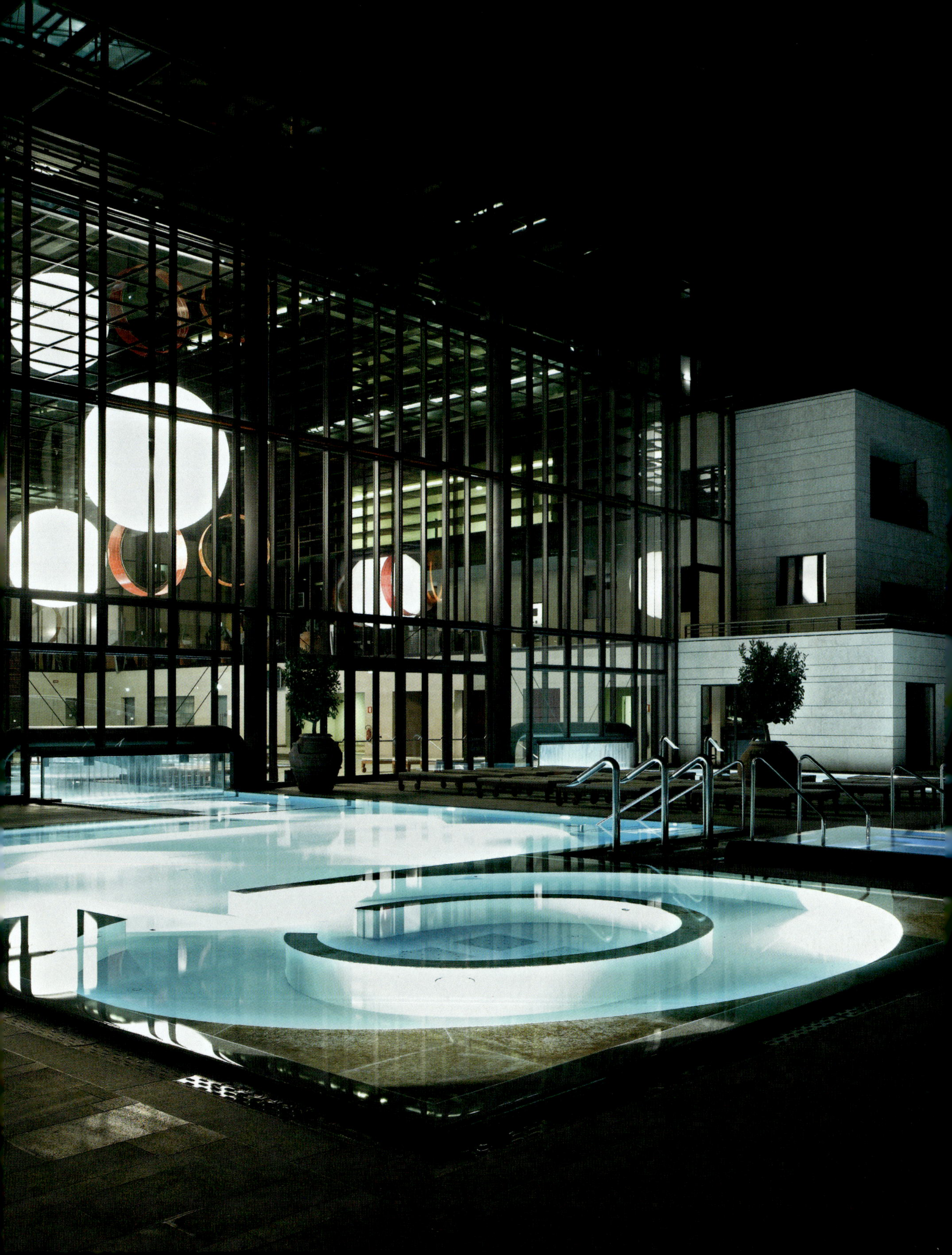

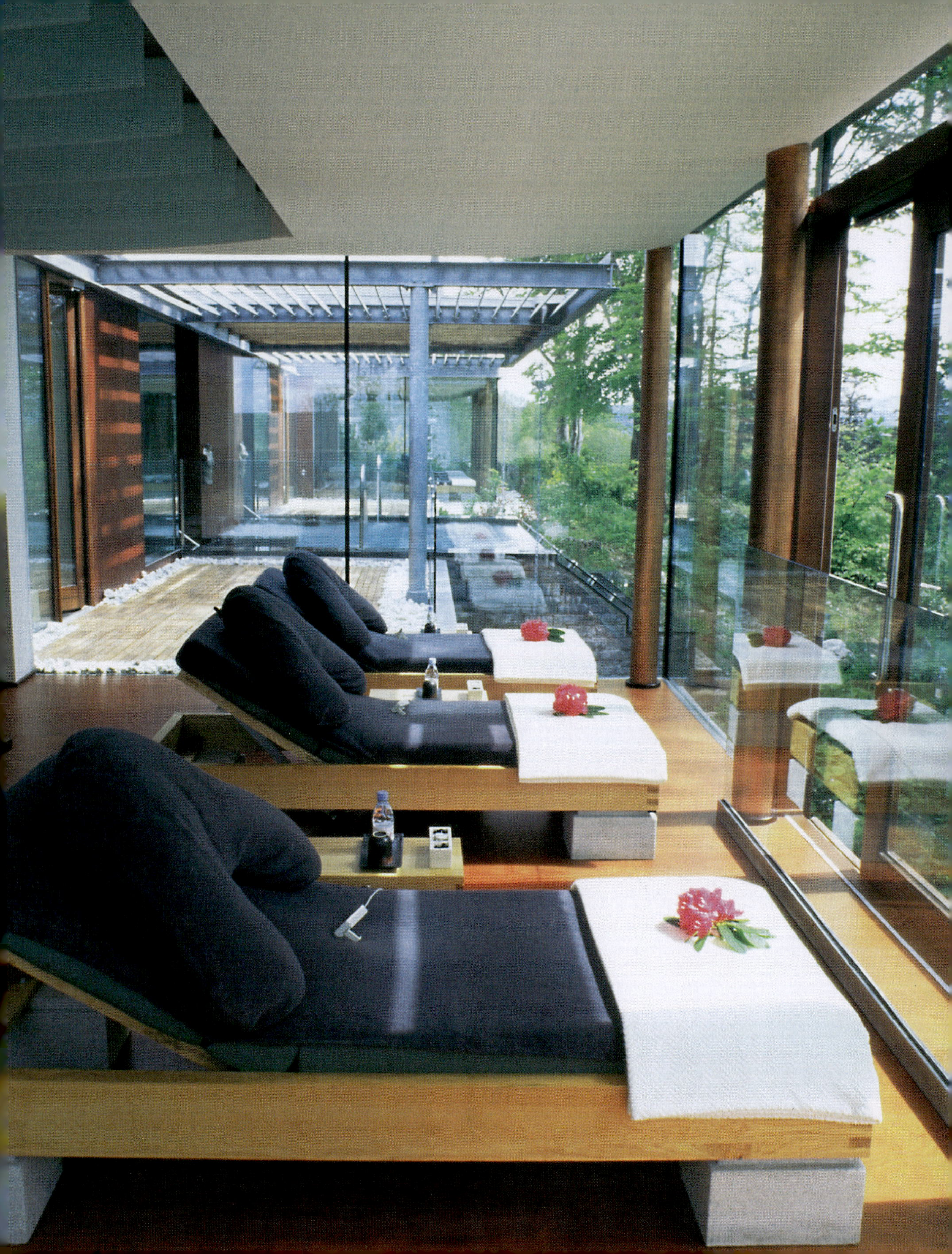

Sámas Spa

Der Aufenthalt im Sámas Spa ist als reinigende Reise angelegt. Die Stationen führen den Besucher durch Thermal-Suiten, Entspannungsräume, Meditationsflächen, Gärten mit Privatpools und einen Hauptpool, der mit der umliegenden Landschaft zu verschwimmen scheint. Natürliche Materialien wie Holz und Steine, Glaswände, die die Grenzen zur umgebenden Landschaft aufheben und das einzigartige Grasdach verwandeln dieses Spa in einen wahren Natur- und Erholungstempel.

The Sámas Spa is set as a journey towards purification. Their treatments will take the visitor through thermal suites, relaxation rooms, areas for meditation, gardens with private pools and a main pool that seems to overflow on the surrounding landscape. The use of natural materials like wood and stone from the area, the glass walls that blur the limits with the surroundings and the grass roof turn this building into a temple of nature and relaxation.

Le spa Sámas est une invitation à la purification. Le visiteur peut bénéficier de divers soins au sein des suites thermales, des salons de relaxation, des espaces pour la méditation et des jardins, agrémentés de bassins privés et d'une piscine principale semblant s'écouler à l'infini au creux du paysage. Le choix de matériaux naturels locaux comme le bois et la pierre de la région, les murs de verre qui estompent les frontières avec le paysage alentour, et le toit recouvert de pelouse, font de ce bâtiment un temple dédié à la nature et à la relaxation.

De Sámas Spa is opgezet als een zuiveringstraject. De behandelingen voeren de bezoeker mee door bronnenbaden, ontspanningskamers, meditatieruimten, tuinen met privébaden en een groot zwembad dat lijkt te vervloeien met het omringende landschap. De natuurlijke bouwmaterialen, zoals plaatselijke hout- en steensoorten, de glazen wanden die het gebouw naadloos doen overgaan in de omgeving en het grasdak vormen samen een heiligdom voor natuur en ontspanning.

Kenmare, Ireland

MICHELE SWEENEY/OPPERMANN ASSOCIATES

Photos © Sámas Spa

www.samaskenmare.com

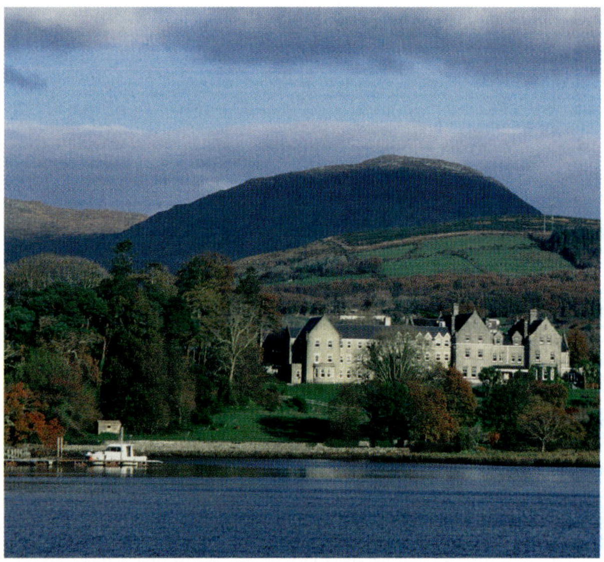

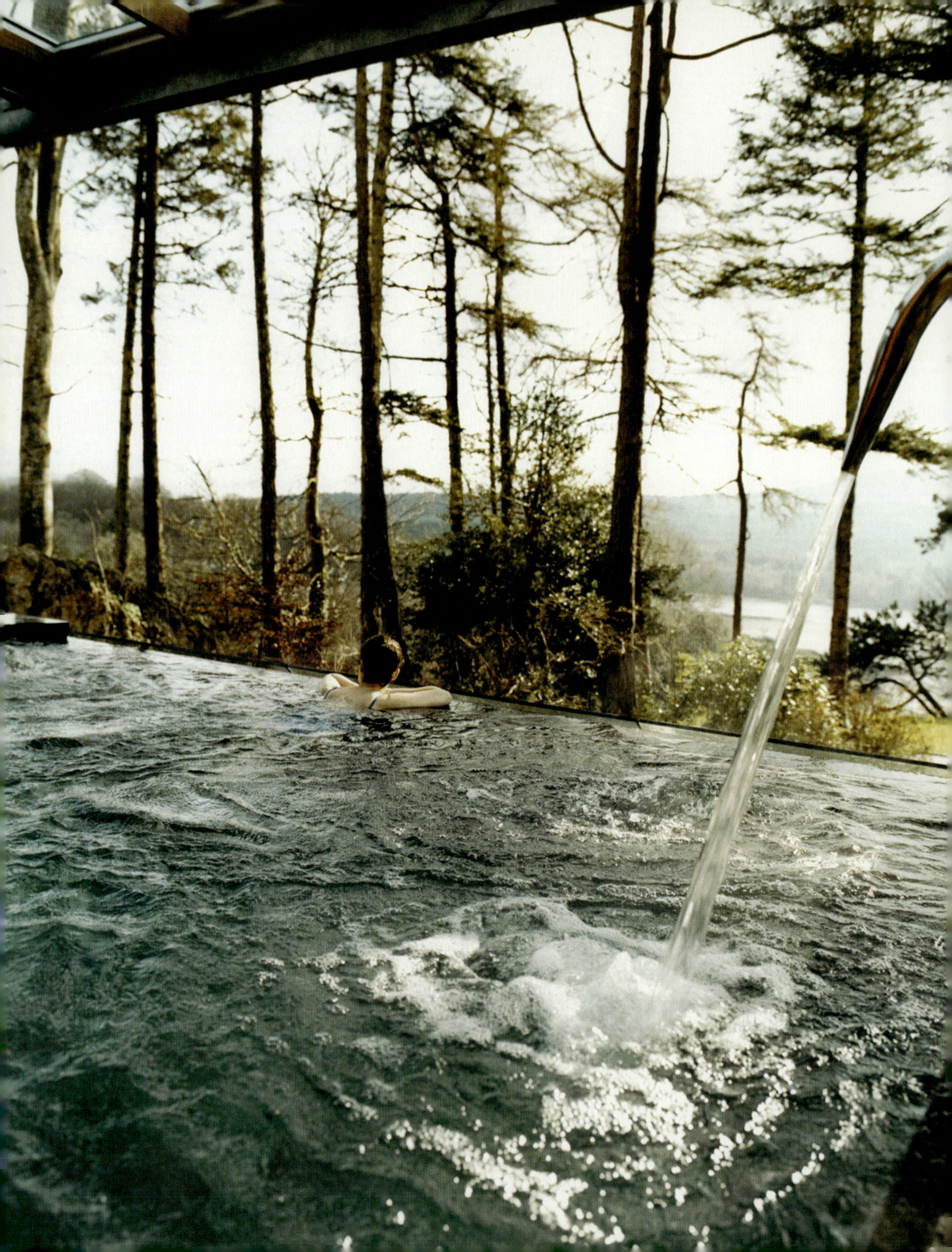

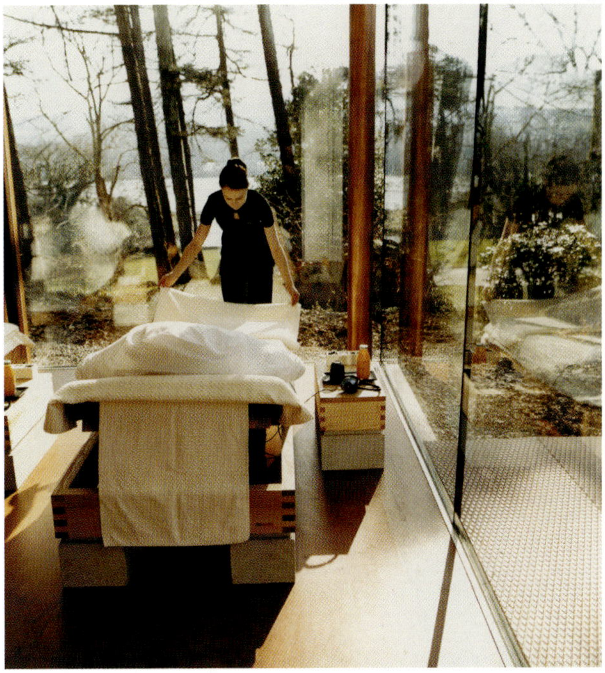

Der Gang durch alle Behandlungsräume, Sauna, Entspannungsbereich und Swimming Pool nimmt etwa drei Stunden in Anspruch.

The route through all the treatment rooms, the sauna, the relaxation area and the swimming pool lasts about three hours.

Le programme complet des traitements, intégrant sauna, piscine et relaxation, dure environ trois heures.

Het traject door behandelkamers, sauna, ontspanningsruimte en zwembad neemt een uur of drie in beslag.

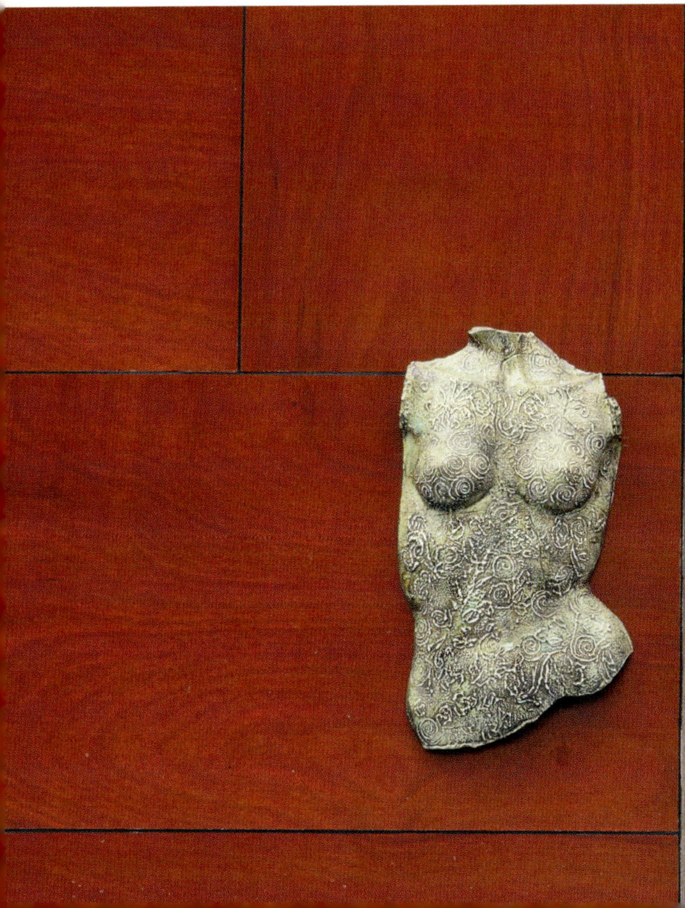

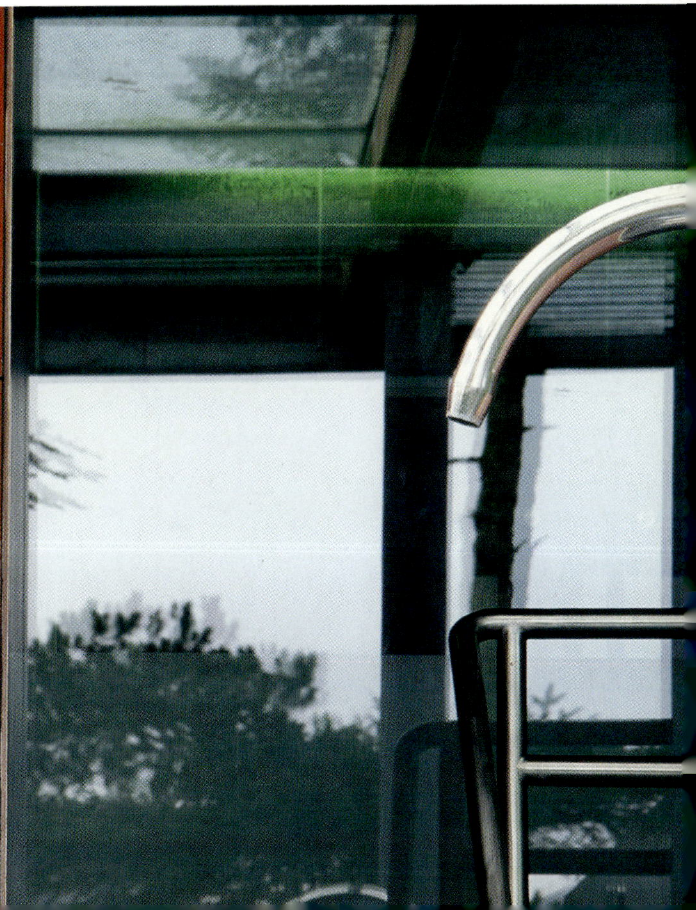

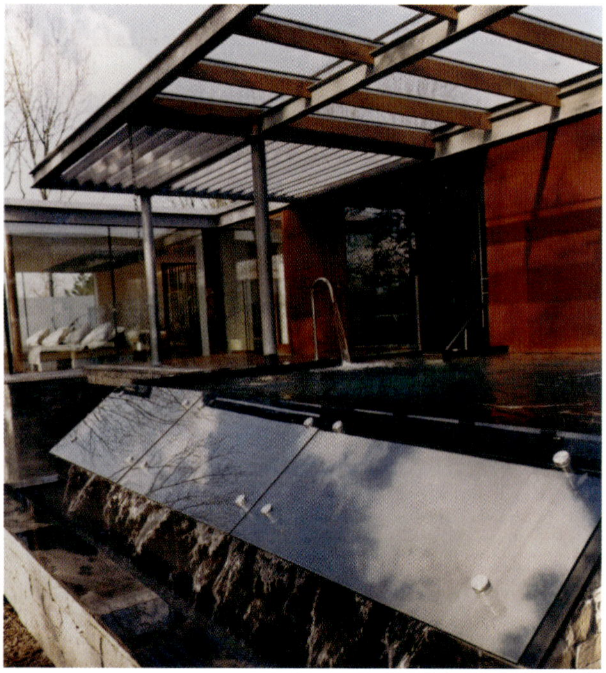

Das Spa-Programm wird durch Aktivitäten wie Bergwandern und Mondscheinmeditation abgerundet.

The spa program is completed with activities such as hikes in the mountains and meditation lessons by moonlight.

Outre les prestations du spa, d'autres activités sont proposées, comme des excursions dans les proches montagnes ou des séances de méditation au clair de lune.

Het kuurprogramma wordt aangevuld met activiteiten zoals bergwandelen en meditatielessen bij maanlicht.

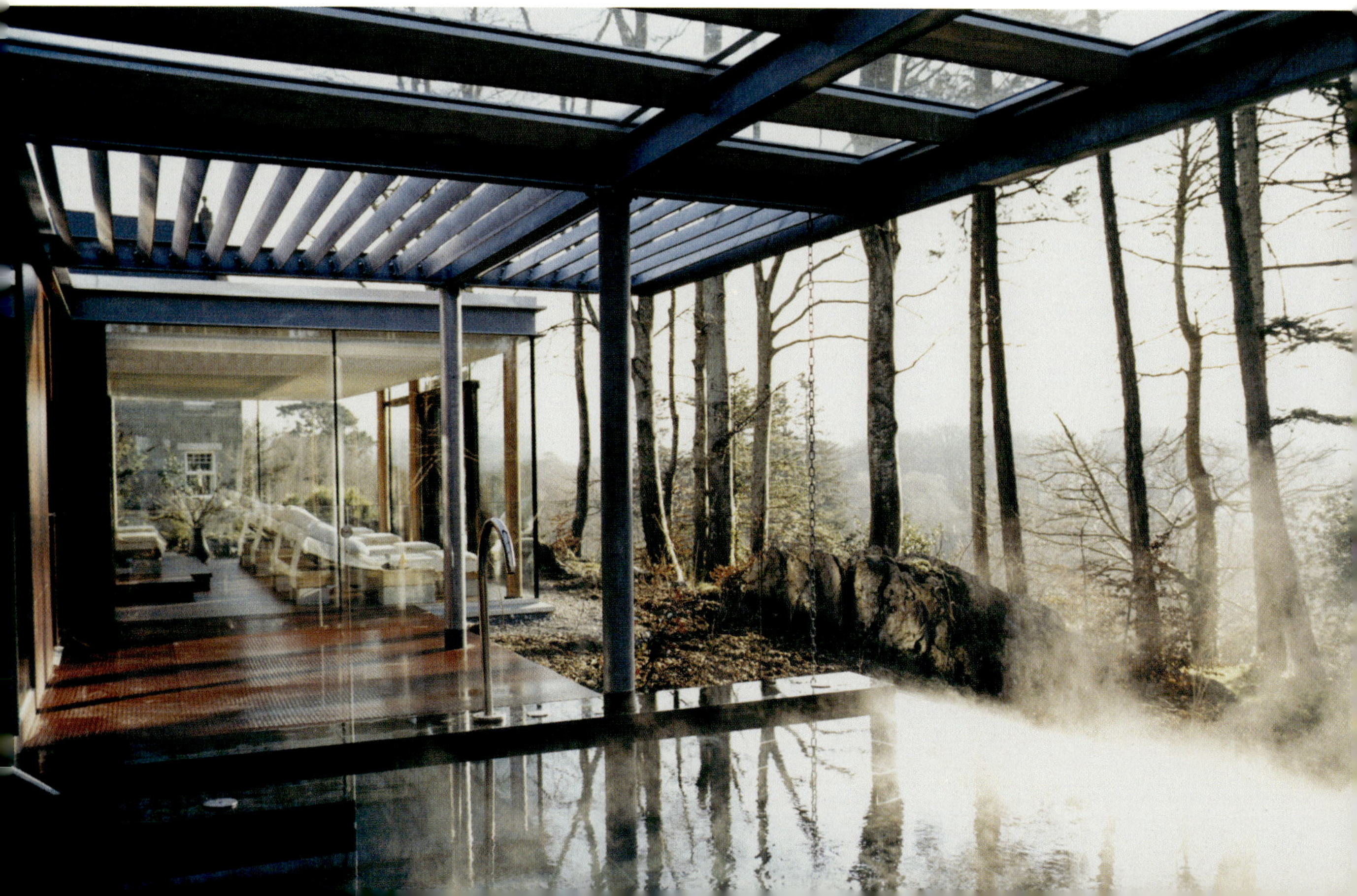

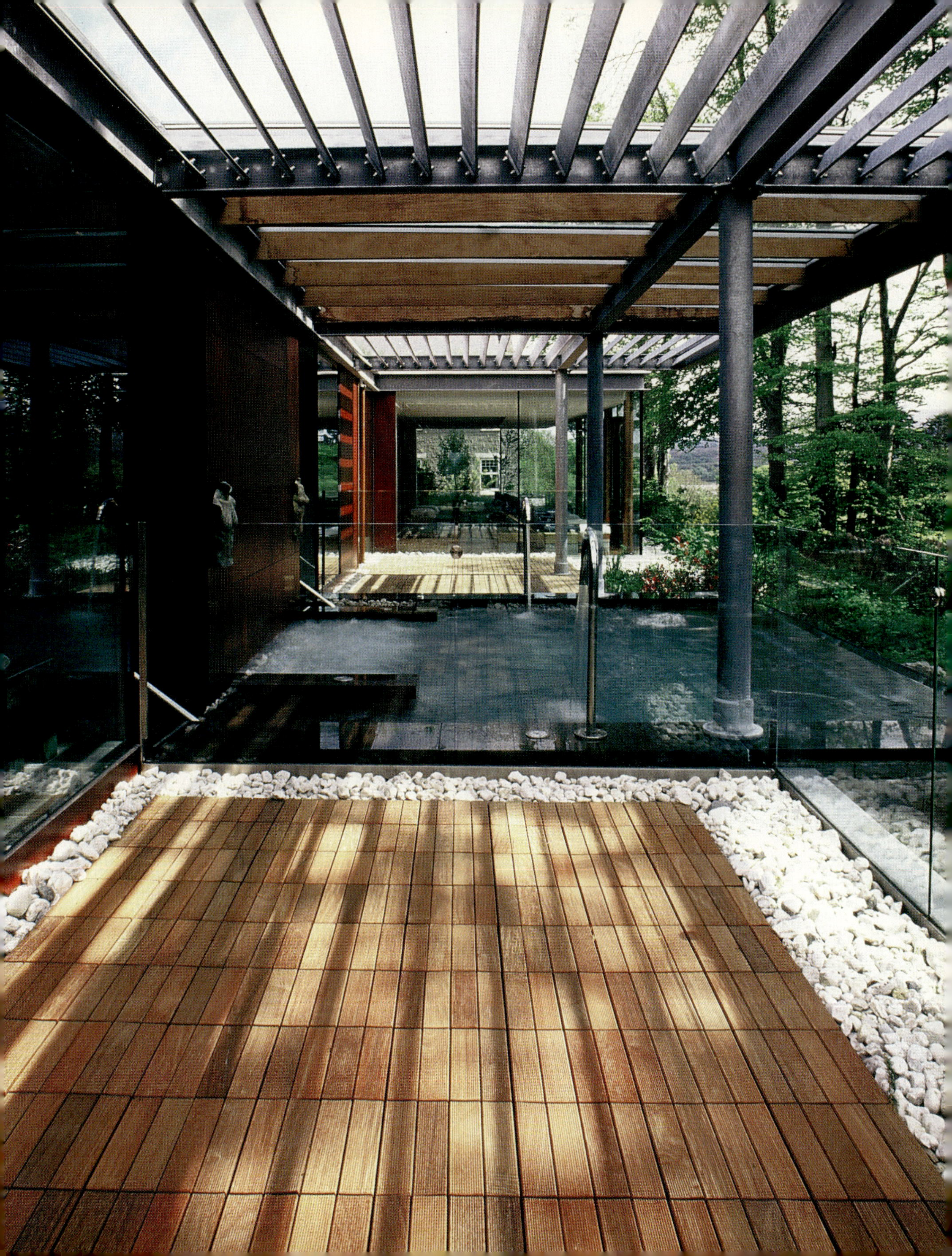

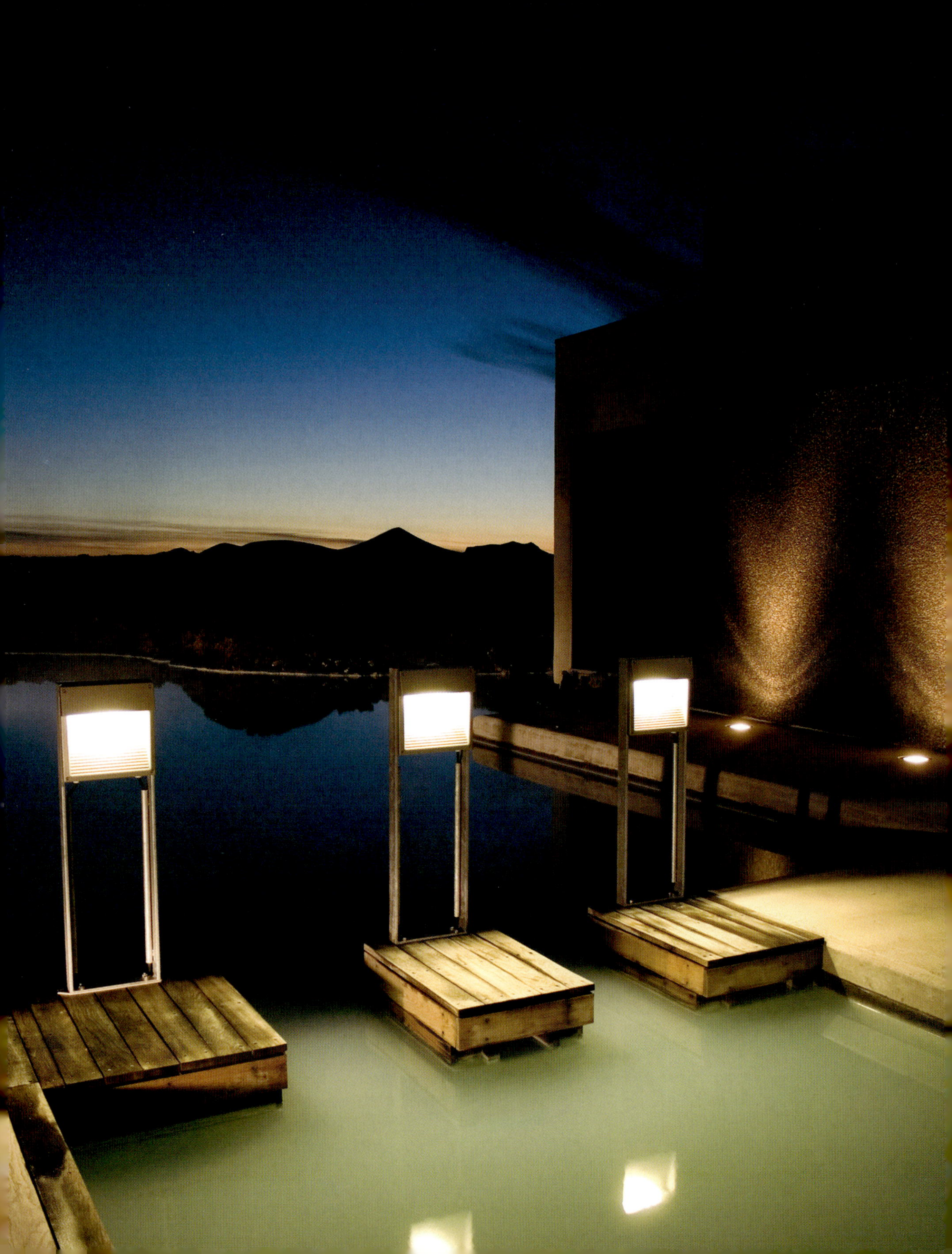

Blue Lagoon

Die 5.000 qm große Badezone umsäumt den Gebäudekomplex mit Spa, Klinik und Hotel. Die Anlage grenzt an einen Krater und einen Lavafelsen, der sich innerhalb des Areals durch den Hauptgang fortsetzt, an Restaurant und Terrasse vorbeiführt und schließlich in der Badelandschaft endet. Design und eingesetzte Materialien vermitteln ein angenehmes Gefühl von behaglicher Wärme in Harmonie mit der einzigartigen Landschaft.

The 54,000 square feet of the bath zone surrounds a building that holds the spa, the clinic and a hotel. The construction is on the edge of a crater and a precipice of lava, that continues inside the precincts through the hallway, passing by the restaurant on its way to the terrace and ending in the bath zone. The warm sensation that predominates in the facilities responds to the design and the materials selected to capture the energy of the atmosphere.

Les 5.000 m² de la zone de baignade entourent un bâtiment qui comporte le spa, l'institut et un hôtel. La construction est implantée sur le bord d'un cratère et d'une coulée de lave, laquelle se prolonge à l'intérieur par le vestibule, passant par le restaurant jusqu'à la terrasse et l'extrémité de la zone de bain. L'impression de chaleur qui prédomine dans les équipements répond à la conception et aux matériaux choisis pour capter l'énergie de l'atmosphère.

Het 5000 m² tellende oppervlak van dit badcomplex ligt rond een gebouw met bronnenbad, thermale kliniek en hotel. Het gebouw grenst aan een krater en een steile lavahelling, die het complex binnenkomt via de hal, doorloopt langs het restaurant en via het terras uitkomt in de badenzone. Zijn warme uitstraling dankt dit complex aan de inrichting en de materiaalkeuze, die gericht is op het vasthouden van de sfeer van energie die er hangt.

Svartsengi, Iceland

VA ARKITEKTAR

Photos © Ragnar Th. Sigurdsson, Rafn Sigurdsson, Oddgeir Karlsson

www.bluelagoon.com

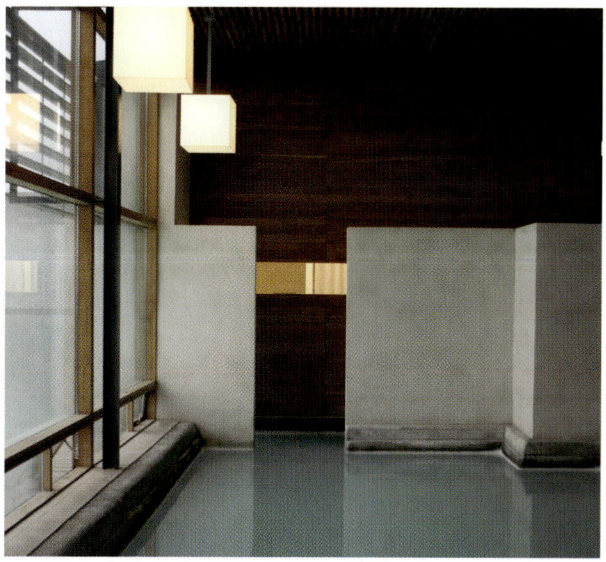

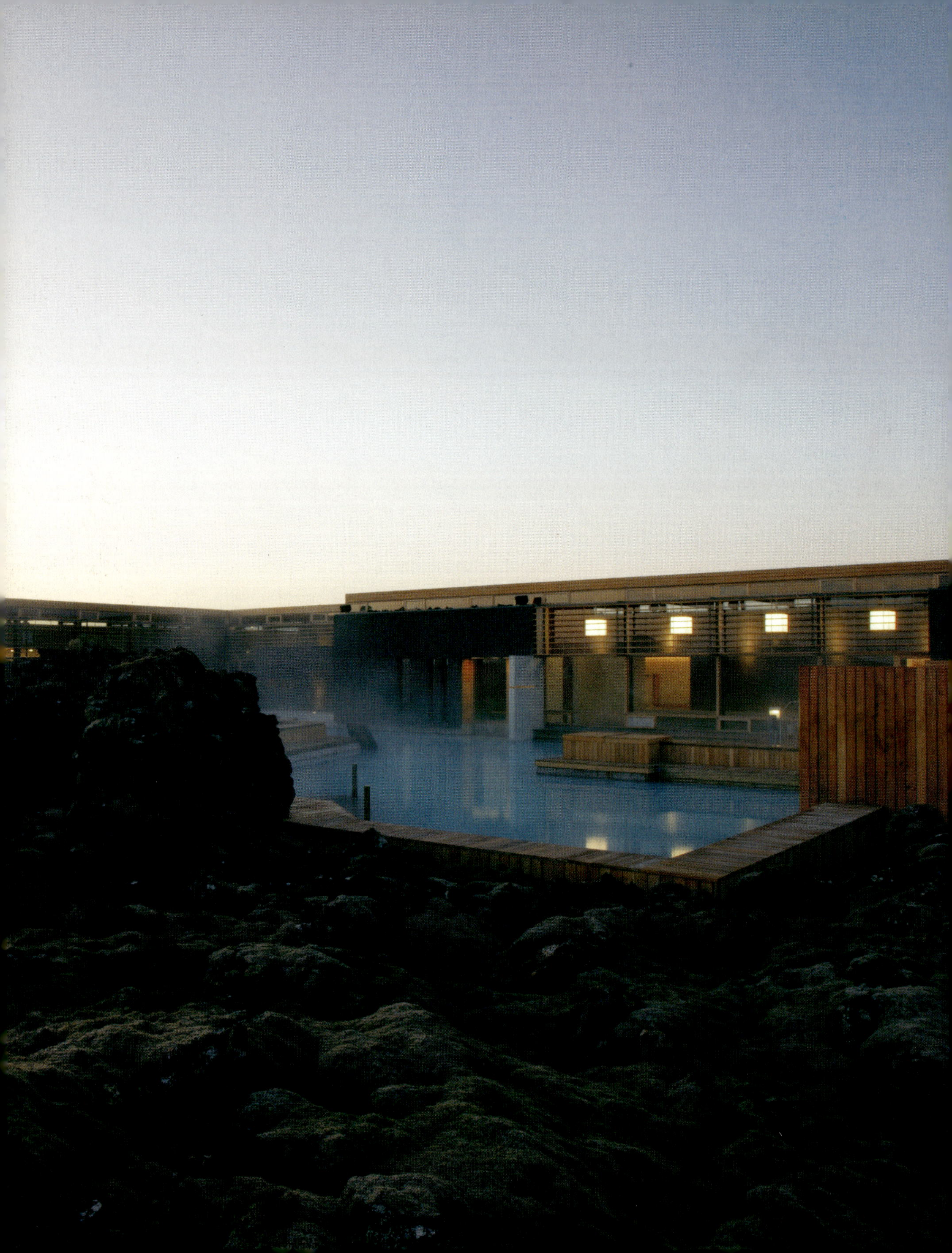

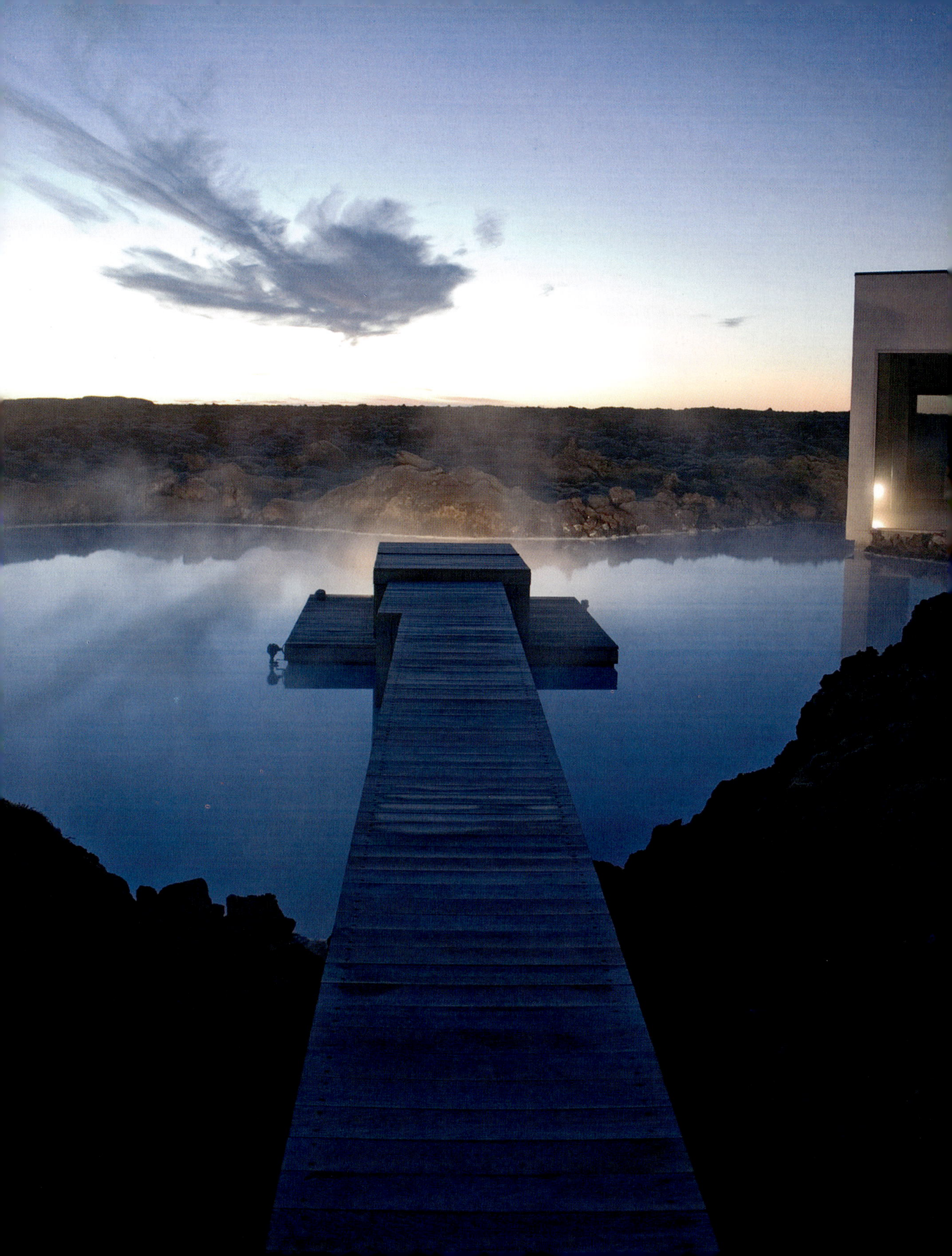

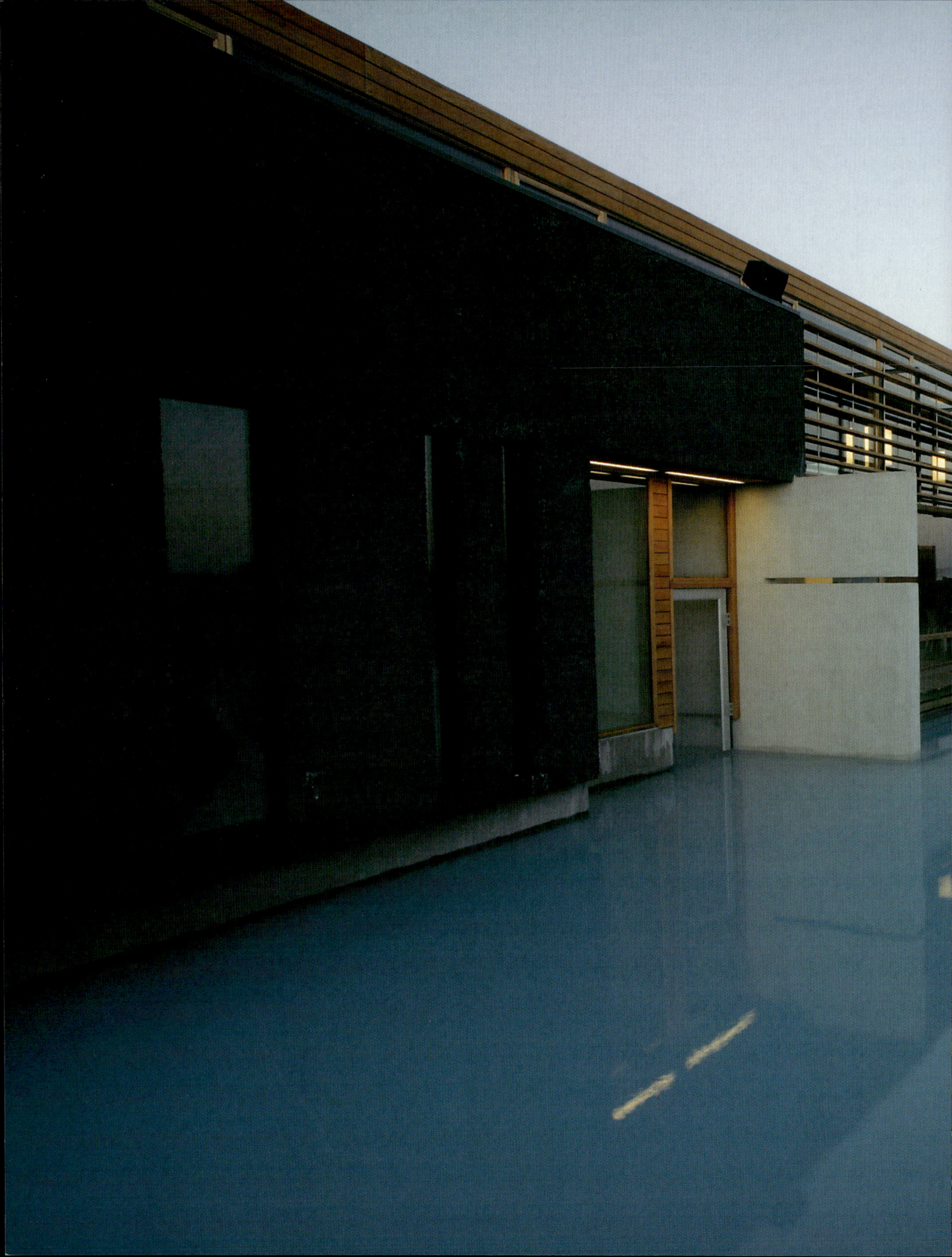

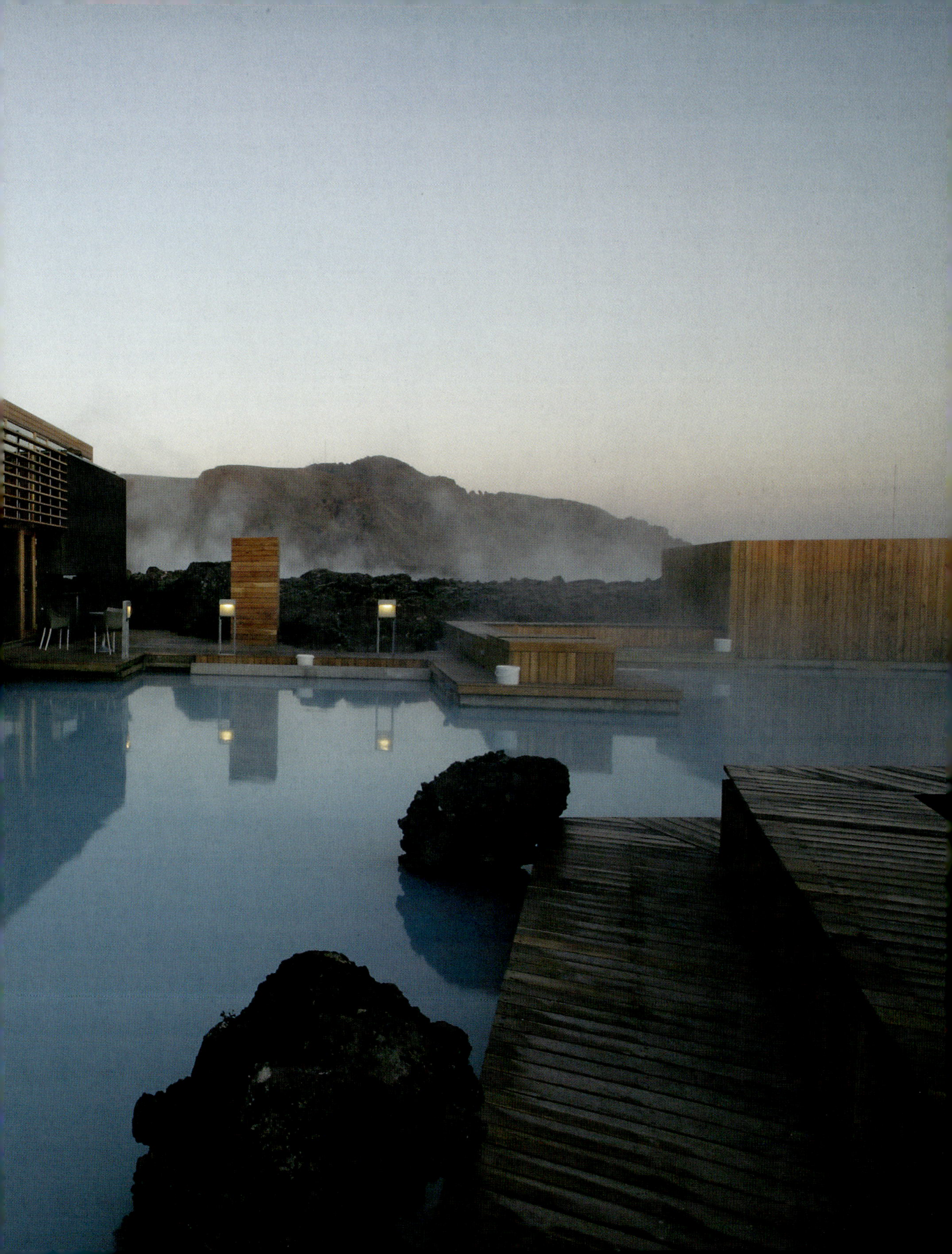

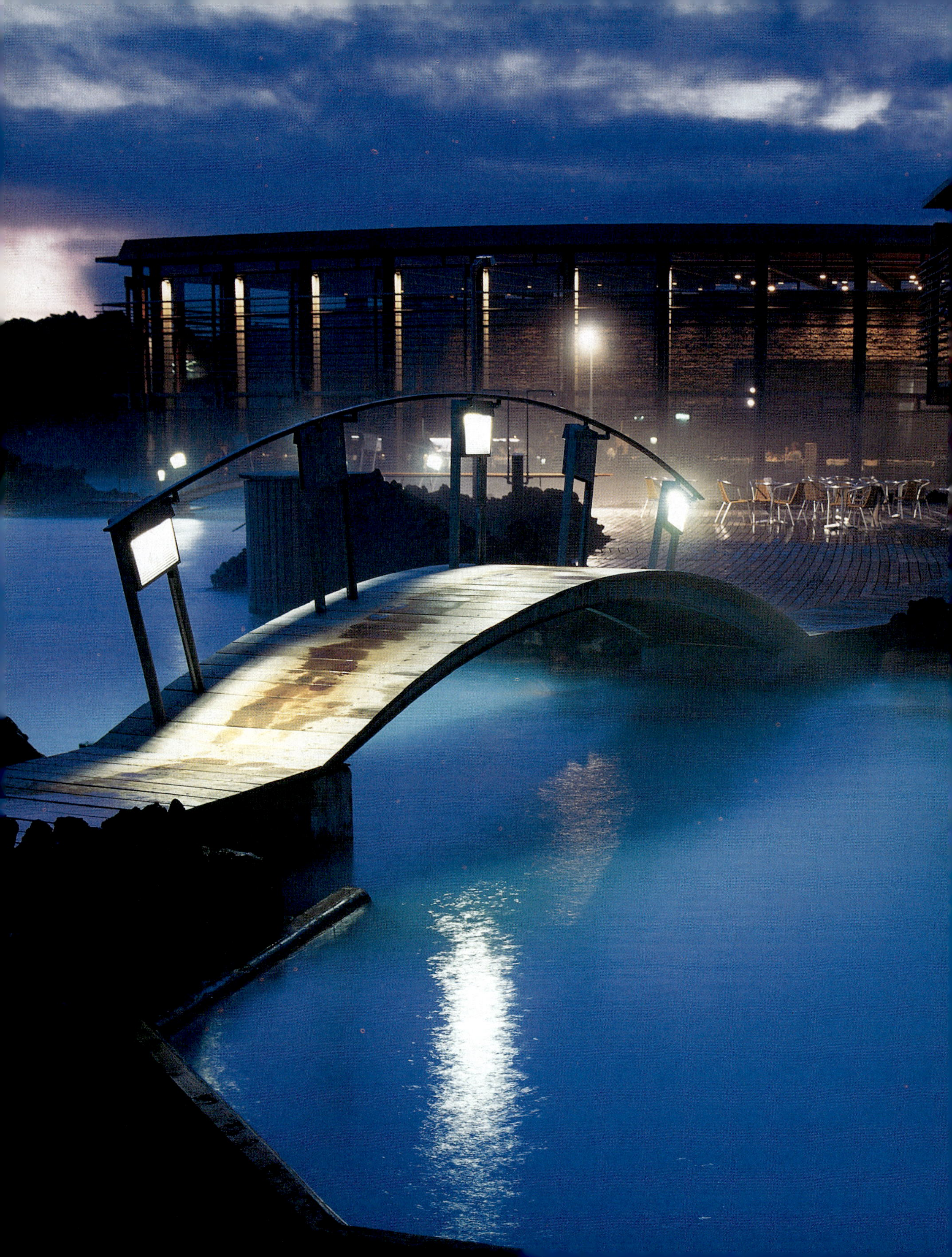

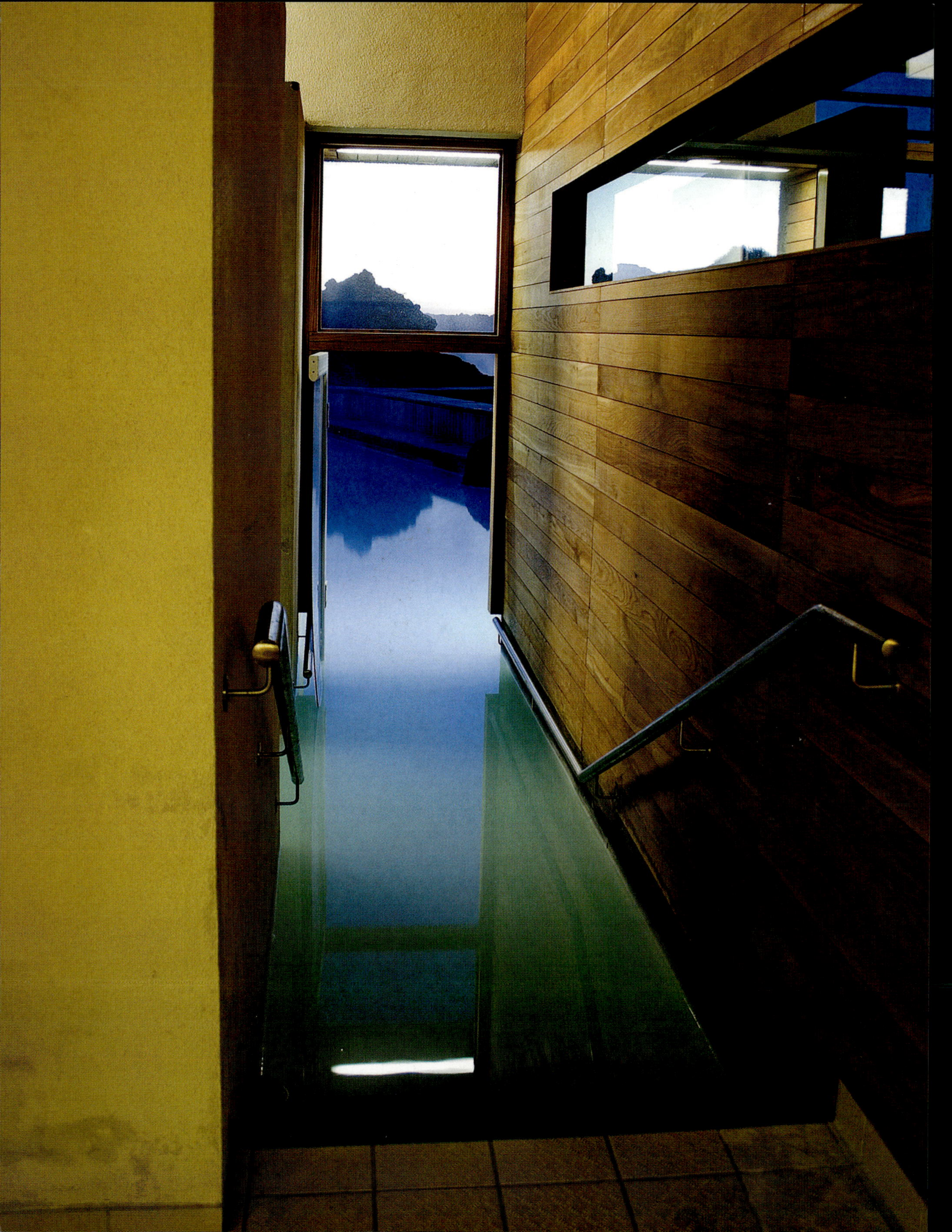

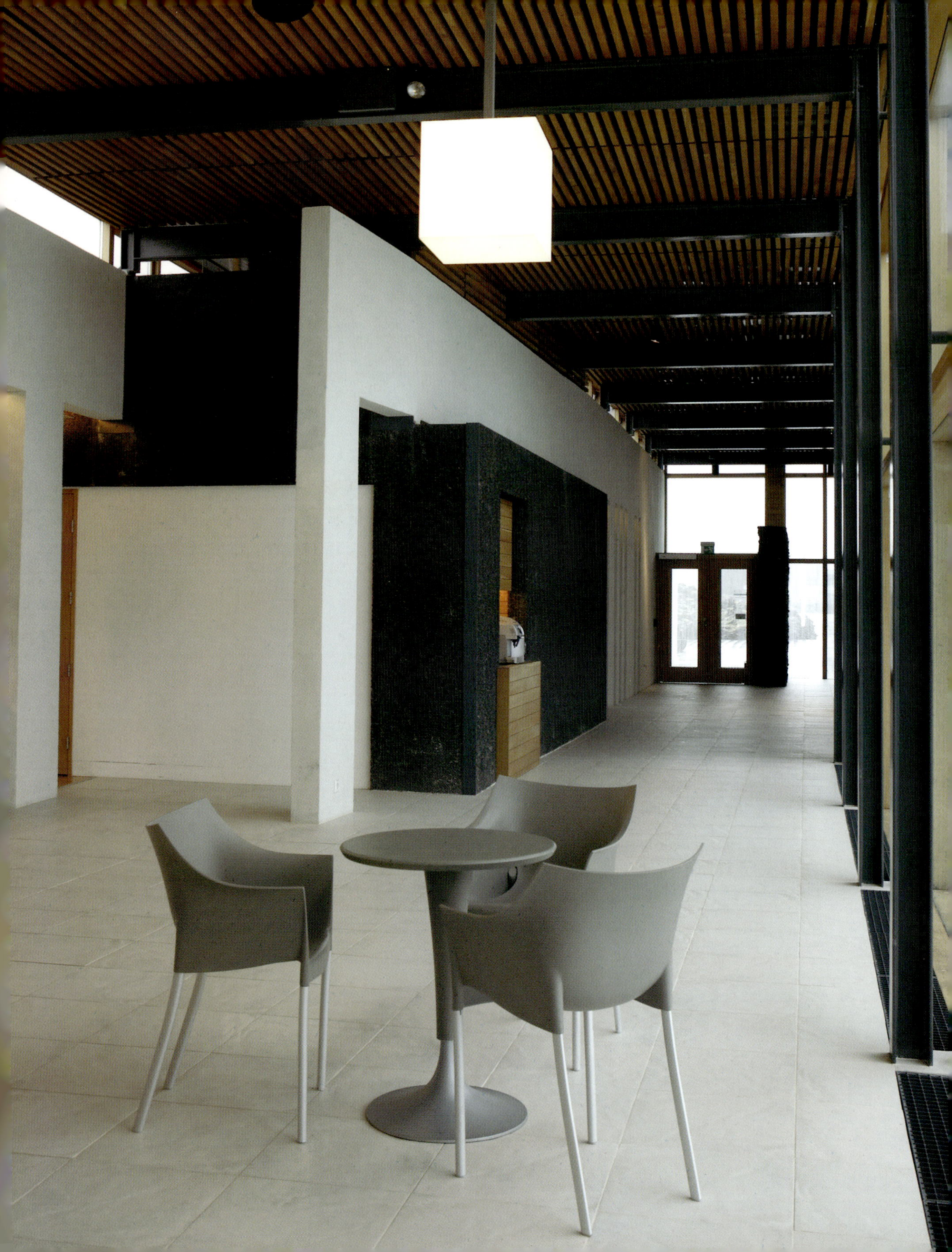

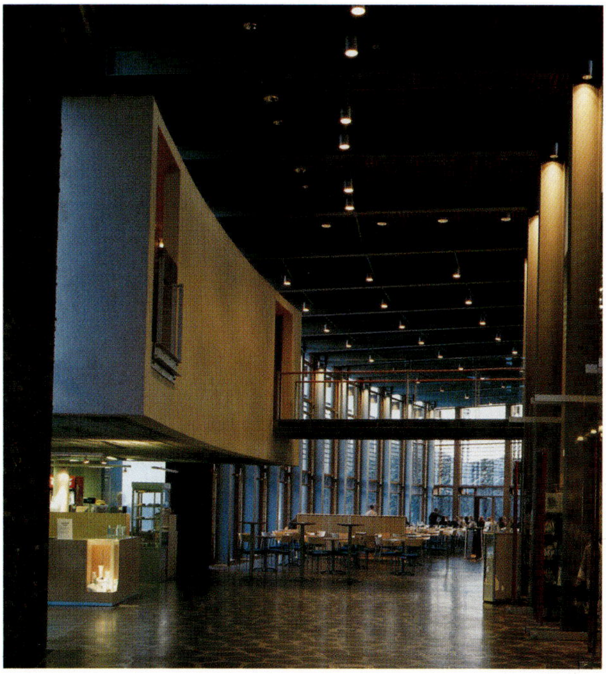

Die 6 Millionen Liter Wasser der Blue Lagoon werden innerhalb von 40 Stunden ausgetauscht.

The 6 million liters of water of the Blue Lagoon are renewed every 40 hours.

Les 6 millions de litres d'eau du Blue Lagoon sont renouvelés toutes les 40 heures.

De 6 miljoen liter water van de Blue Lagoon wordt om de 40 uur ververst.

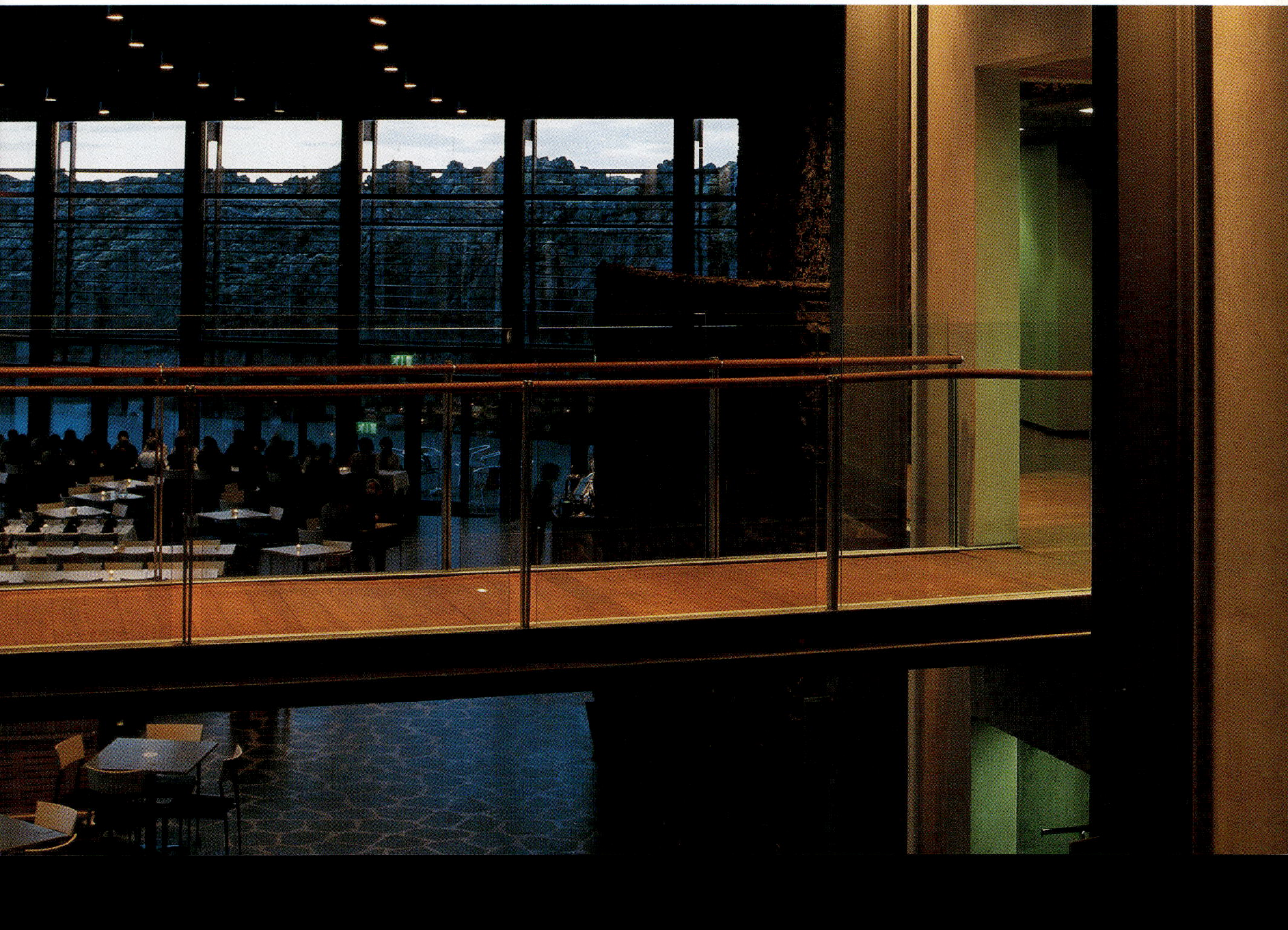

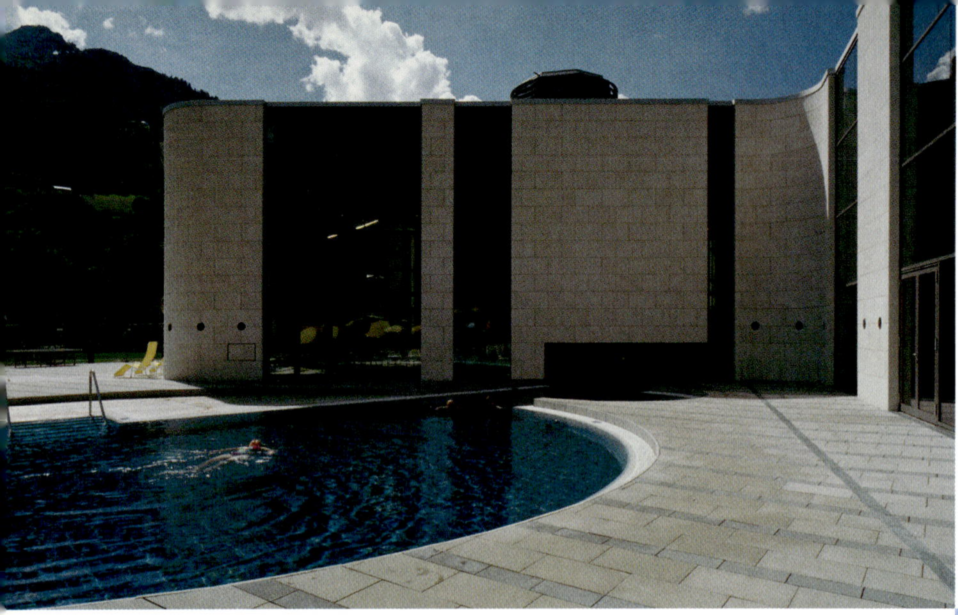

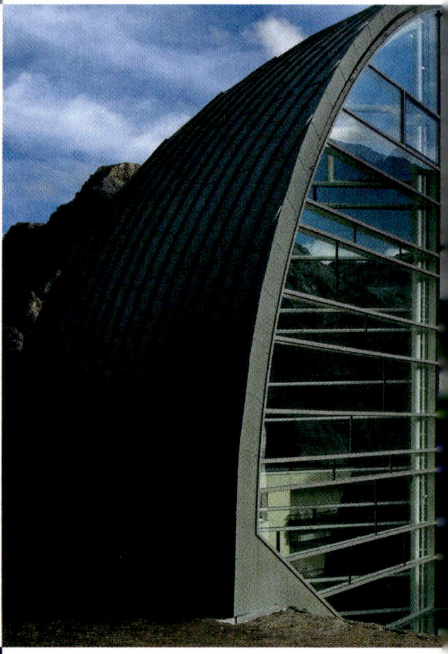

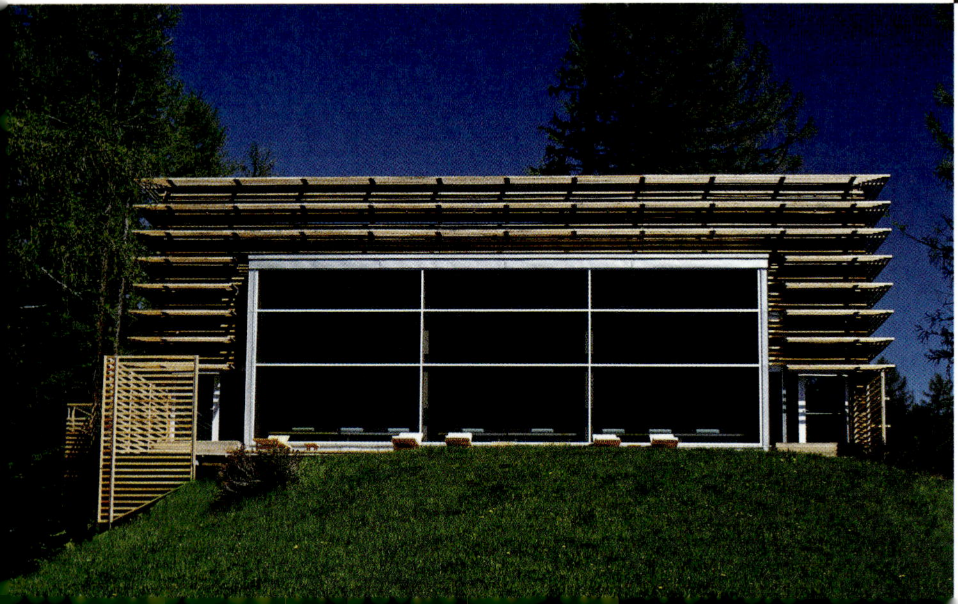

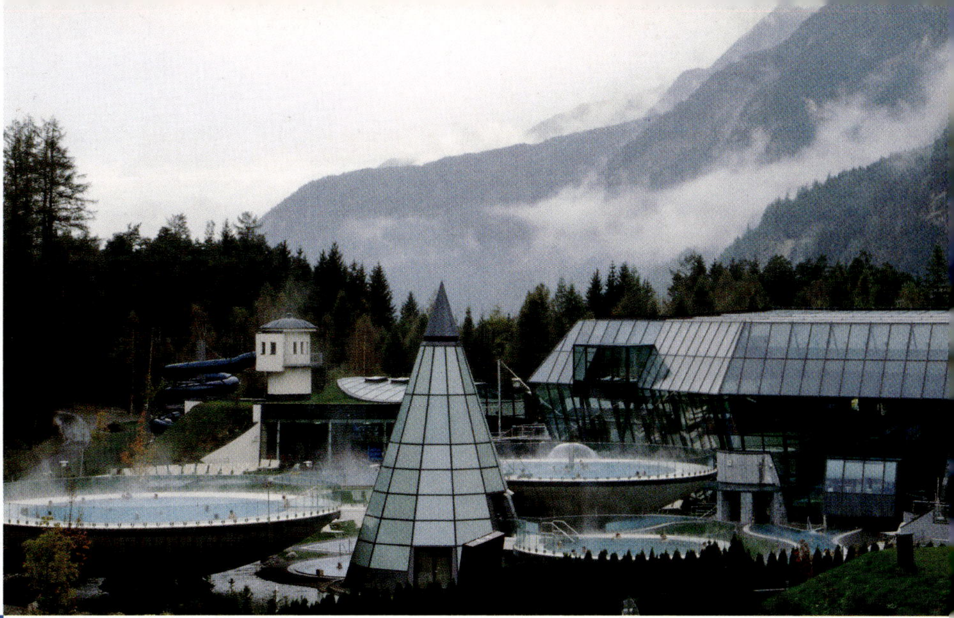

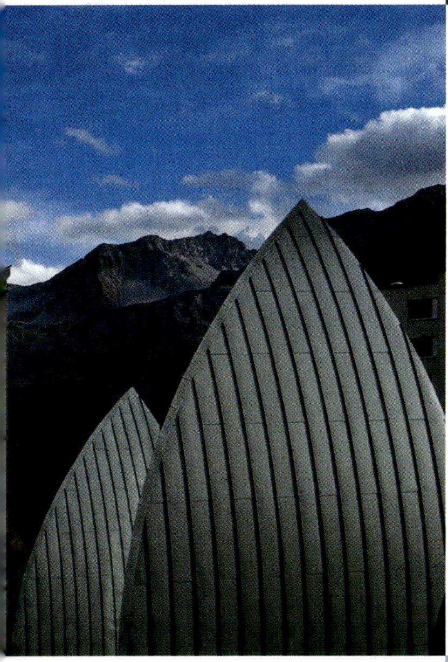

Mountain & Seaside Spas

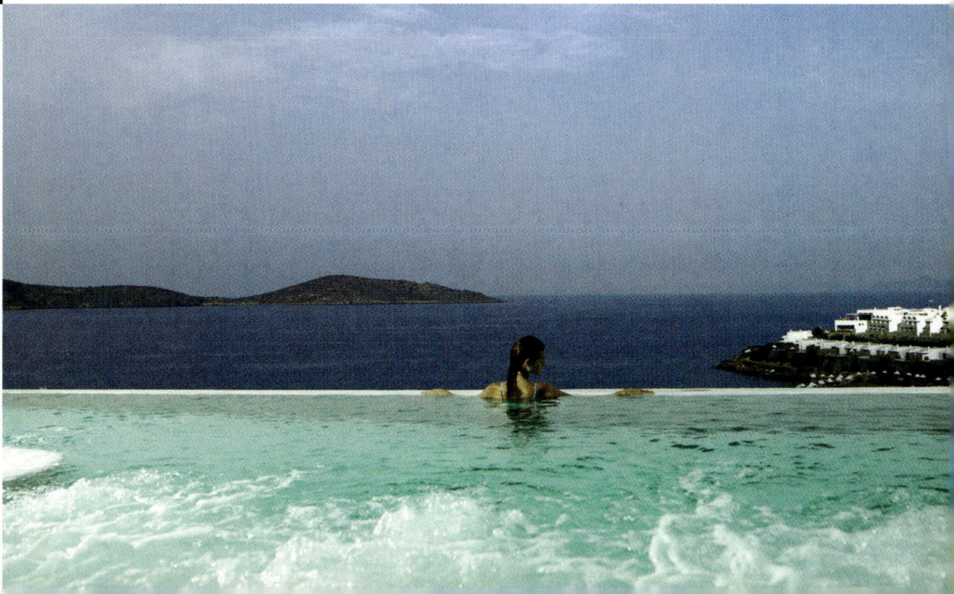

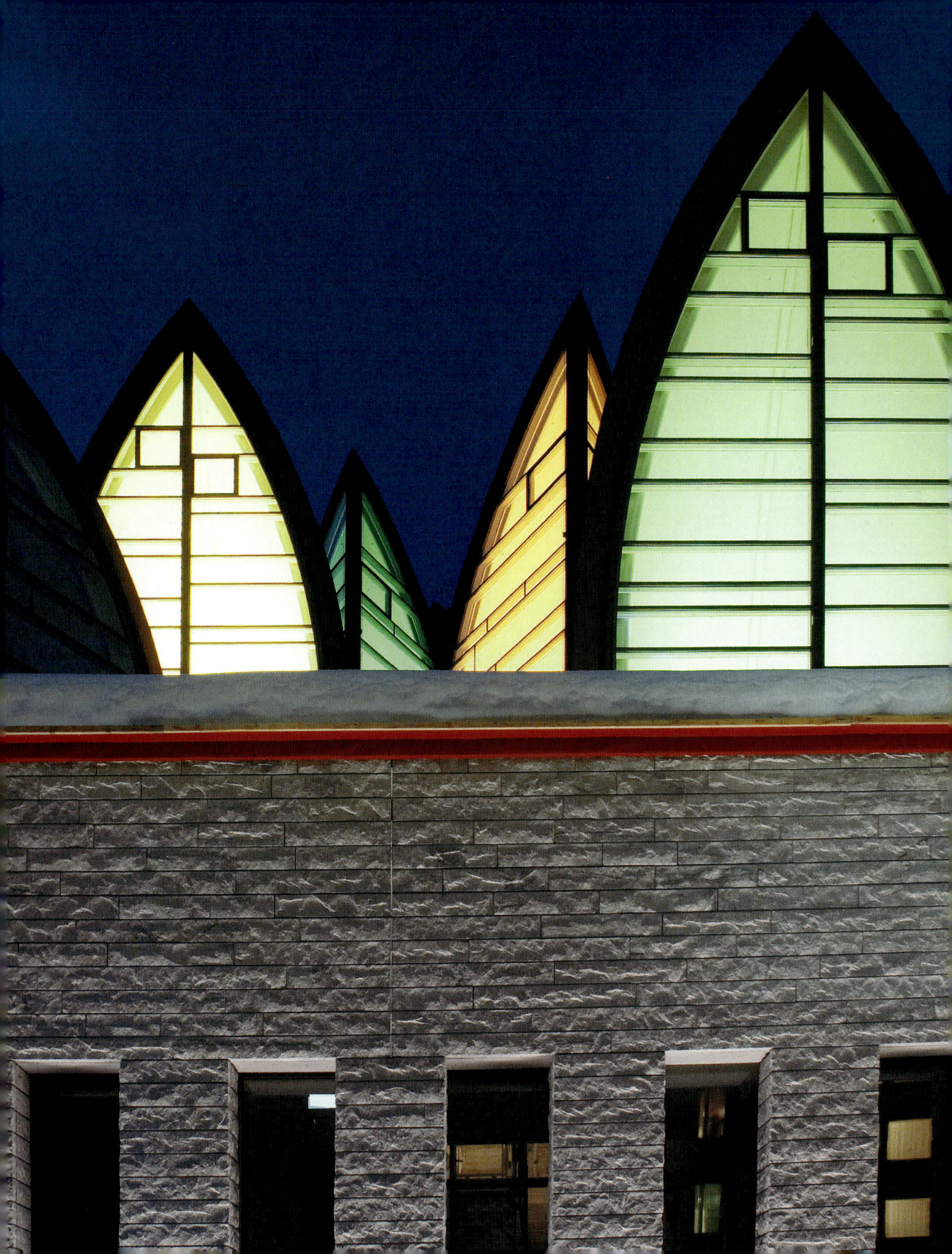

Wellness Centre Tschuggen Bergoase

Stararchitekt Mario Botta gestaltete dieses zum Hotel Tschuggen gehörende Spa wie eine futuristische Baumlandschaft im Herzen der Schweizer Alpen. Die Innenräume des Spas sind als durchgängige Terrasse angeordnet, die der Form des Berghügels folgt und durch zwei Brücken mit dem Hotelgebäude verbunden ist. Innen- und Außenpools, Sonnenterrassen und Fitnessräume laden zu sportlichen Aktivitäten oder zum entspannten Blick auf die grandiose Gebirgsnatur ein.

Architect Mario Botta, famous for his museums and temples, has designed this building that stands next to hotel Tschuggen like woods of futuristic trees in the middle of nature. The inside spaces of the spa are distributed like a continuous terrace that follows the shape of the hill and two bridges connect them to the hotel building. Outside areas include an open-air pool and esplanades with solariums, some of which are equipped to do exercise and others to enjoy the snow.

L'architecte Mario Botta, célèbre pour ses musées et ses temples, a conçu cette construction qui se dresse en pleine nature à côté de l'hôtel Tschuggen comme des arbres futuristes. Les espaces intérieurs du spa sont distribués comme une terrasse continue qui suit les courbes de la montagne et reliés au bâtiment de l'hôtel par deux passerelles. À l'extérieur, différentes zones comprennent une piscine et des solariums, dont certains sont équipés pour faire de la remise en forme et d'autres pour profiter de la neige.

Mario Botta, architect van musea en tempels, ontwierp dit gebouw dat naast hotel Tschuggen staat als een bos futuristische bomen midden in de natuur. De binnenruimten van de kuurinrichting zijn geconstrueerd als een doorlopend terras dat de vorm van de heuvel volgt. Twee bruggen verbinden het met het hotel. De buitenruimten hebben een buitenbad en promenades met zonnebanken. In sommige ruimten staan fitnessapparaten, in andere kun je van de sneeuw genieten.

Arosa, Switzerland

MARIO BOTTA

Photos © Enrico Cano, Pino Musi

www.tschuggen.ch

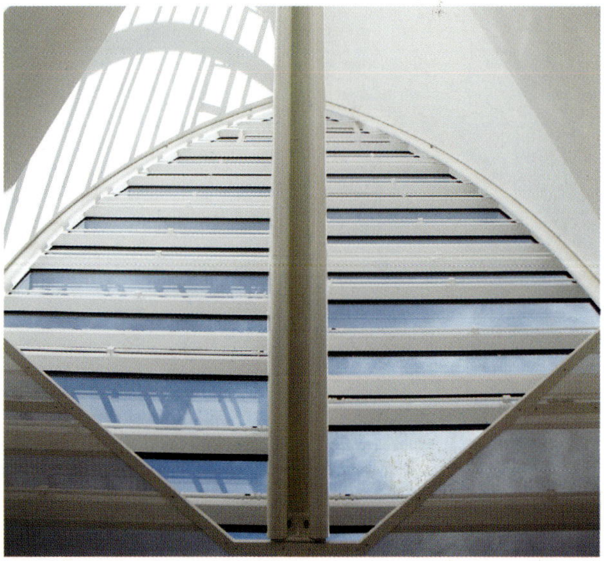

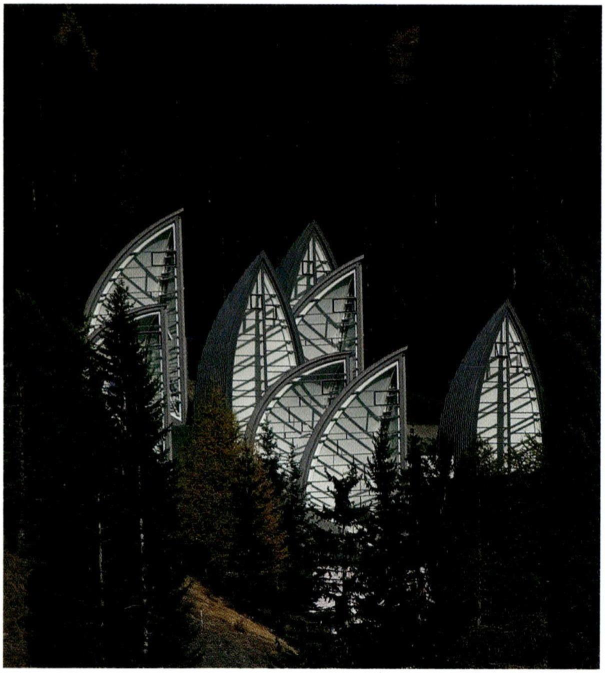

Die Bergoase, ein Spa im Stil des 21. Jahrhunderts, bietet Erholung für Geist und Körper.

The Bergoase was built as a 21st century spa in which the regeneration of the body and the spirit are equally important.

Le Bergoase a été construit comme une station thermale du XXIe siècle dans laquelle la notion de revitalisation du corps et de l'esprit prend toute sa signification.

De Bergoase is gebouwd als een kuuroord voor de 21e eeuw, waarin regeneratie van het lichaam centraal staat.

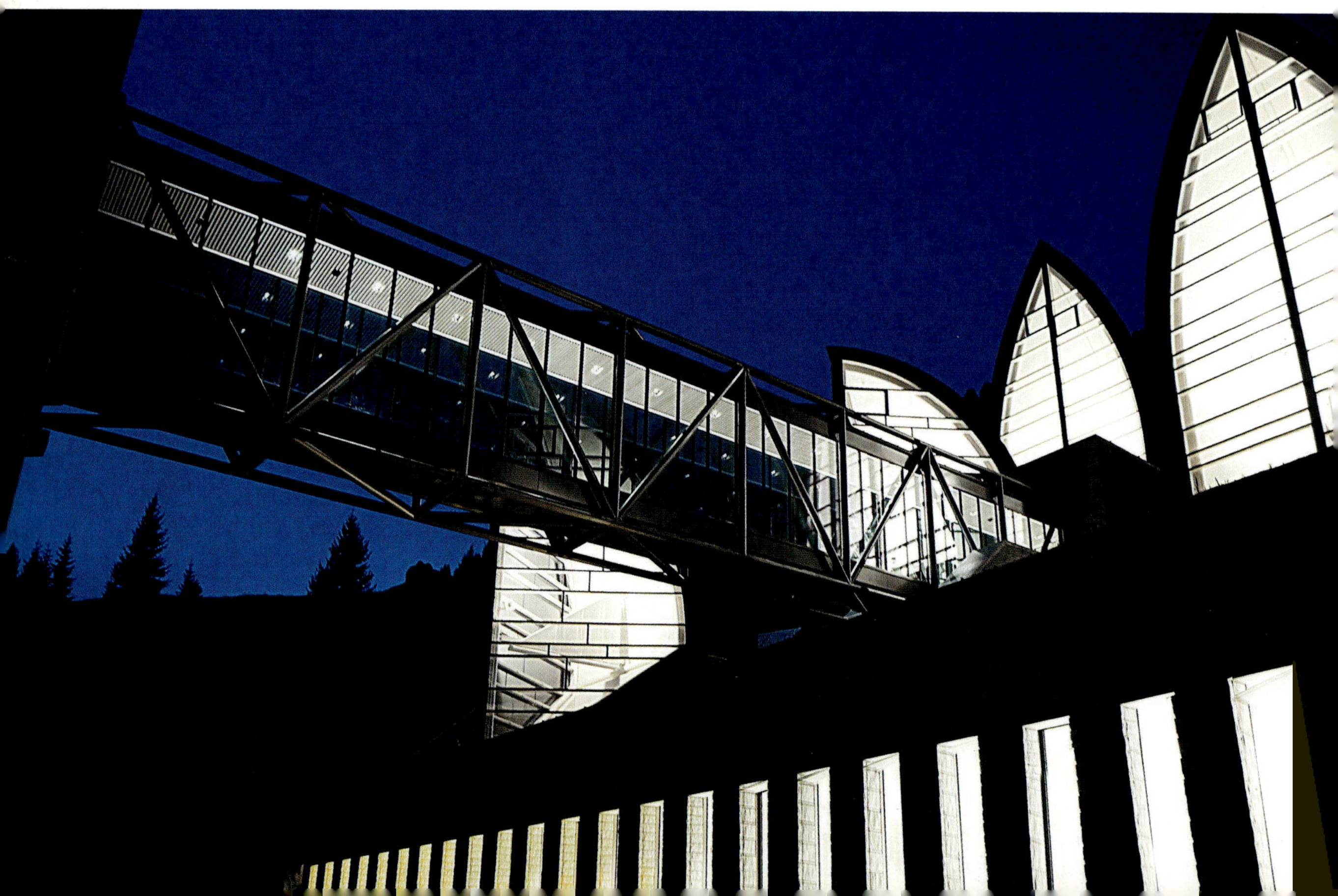

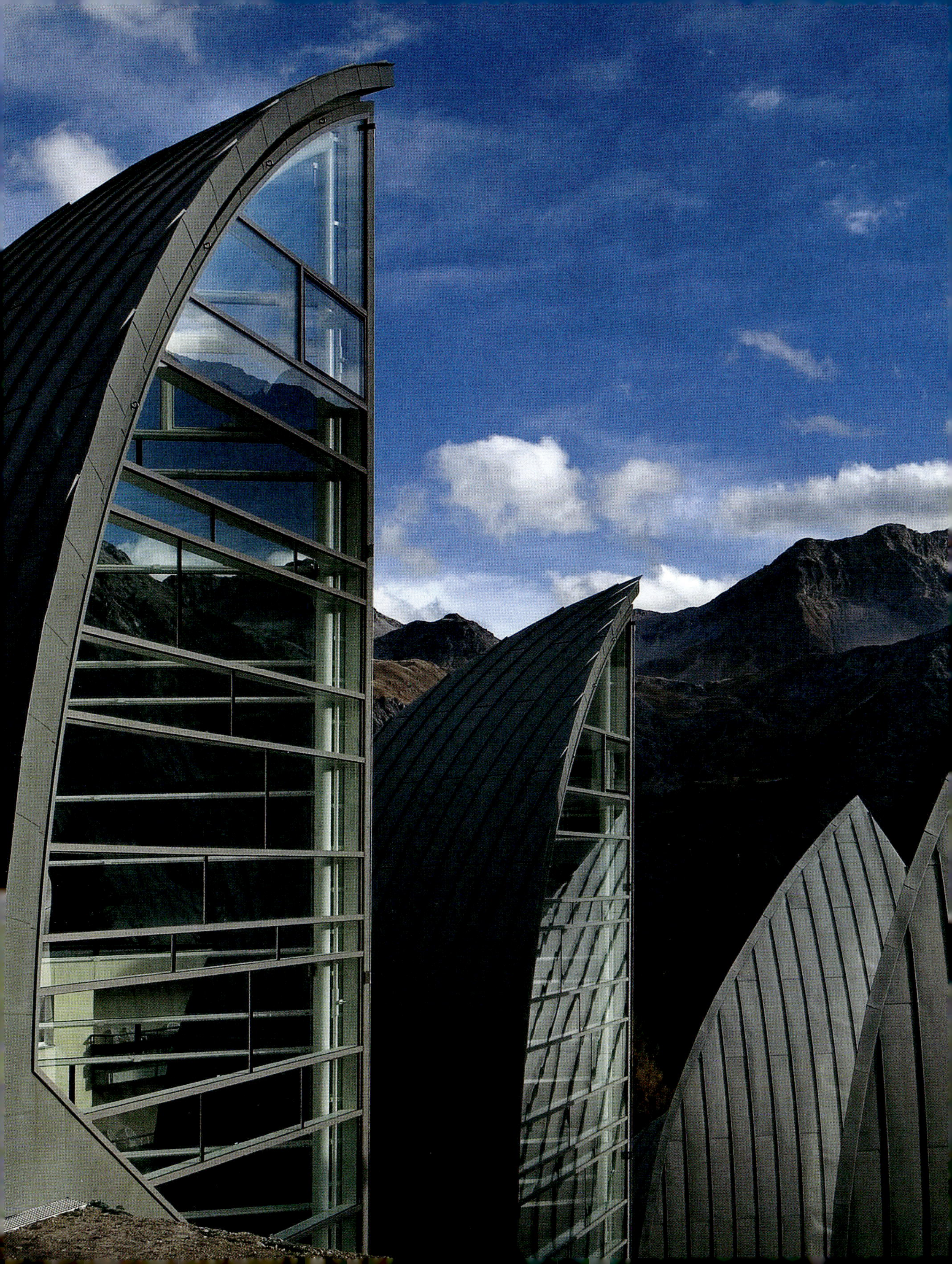

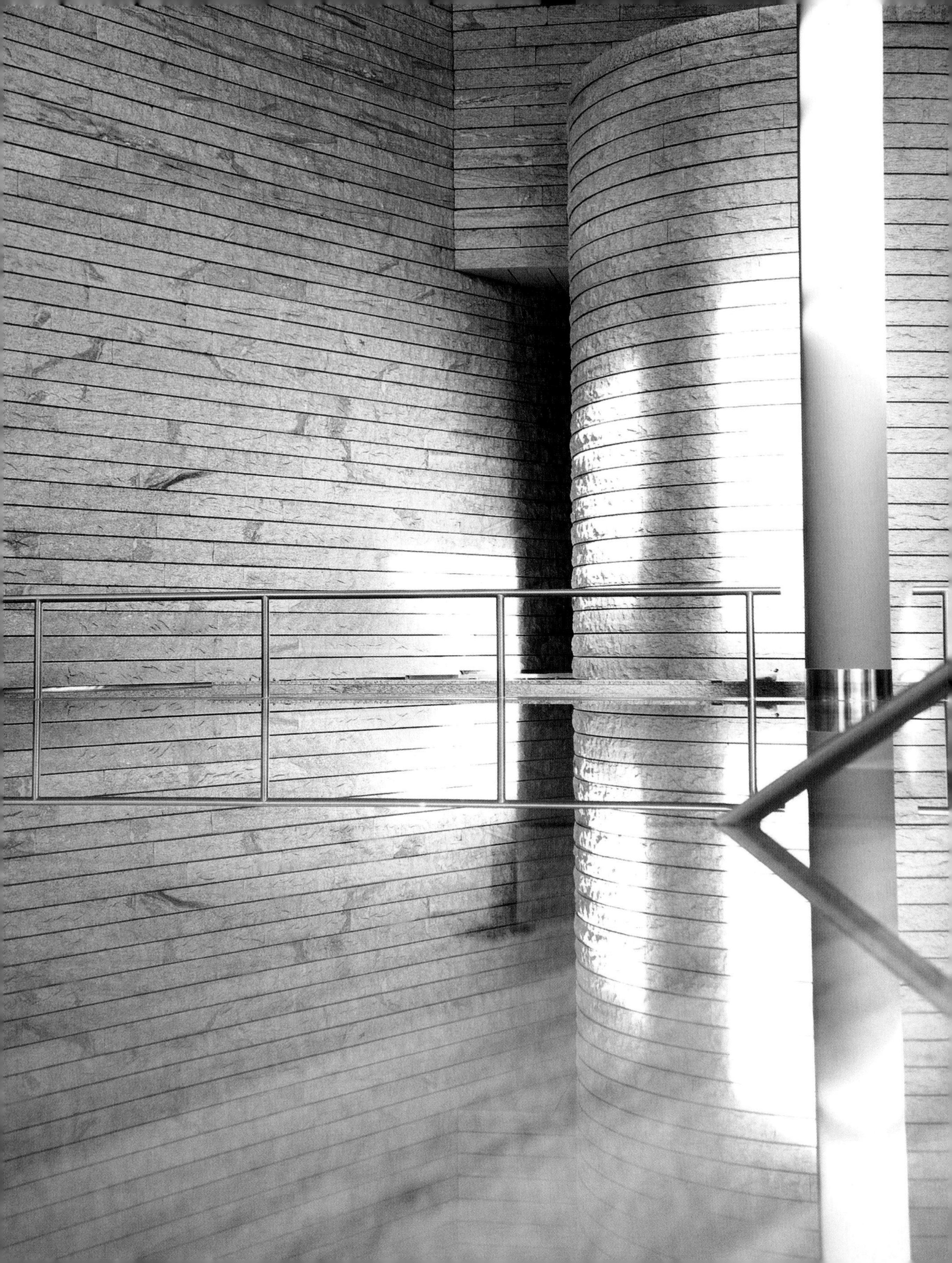

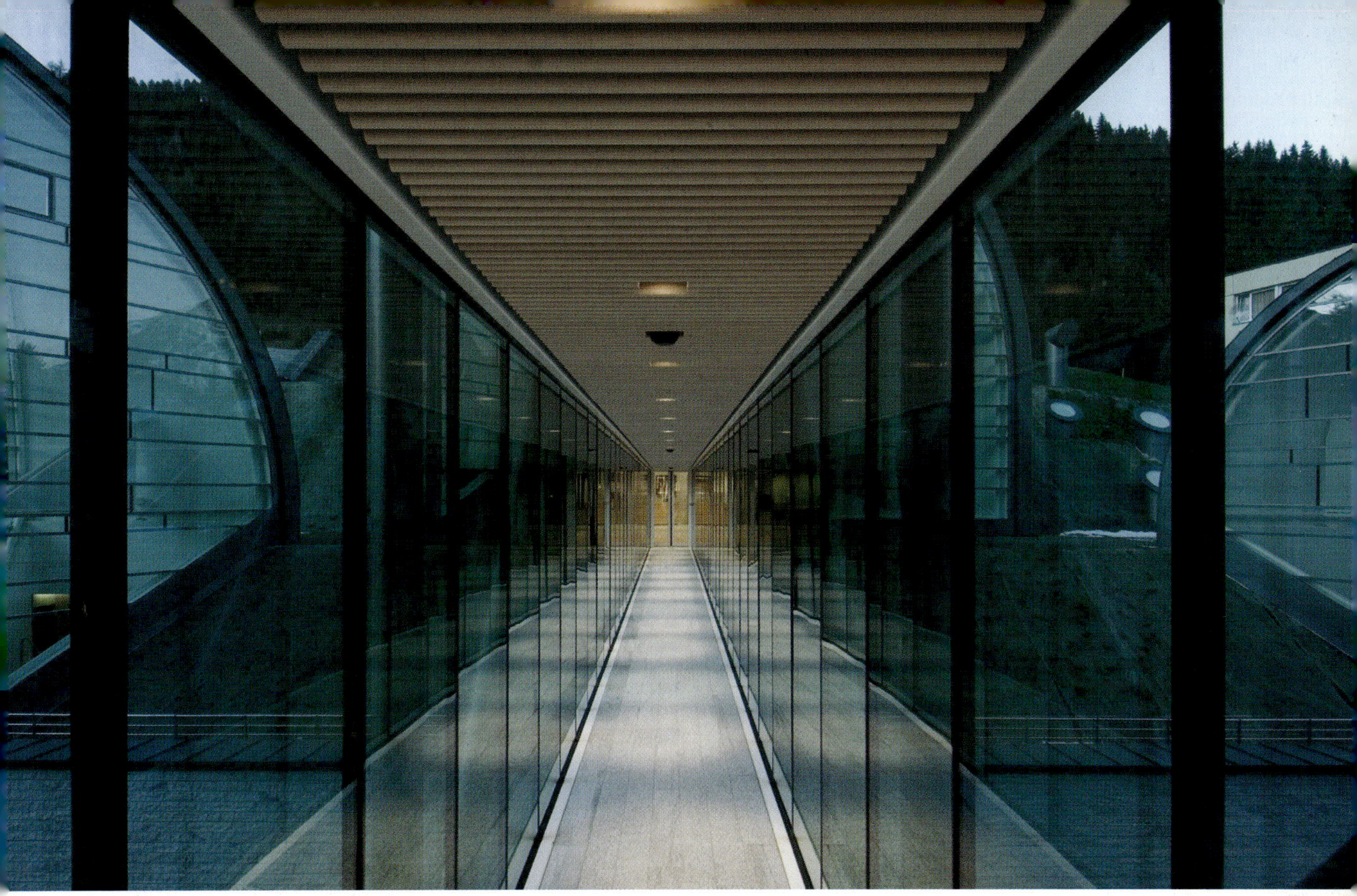

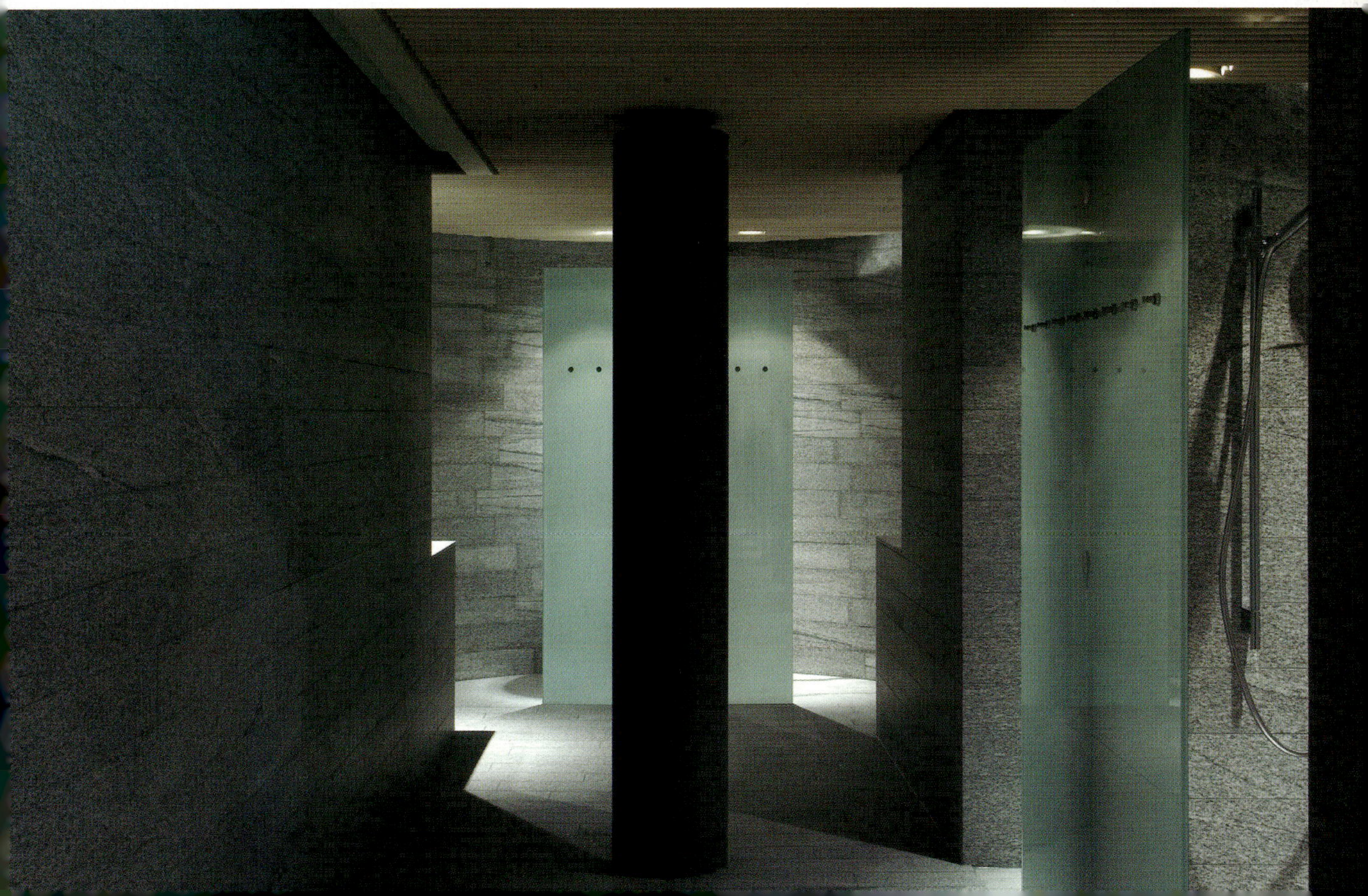

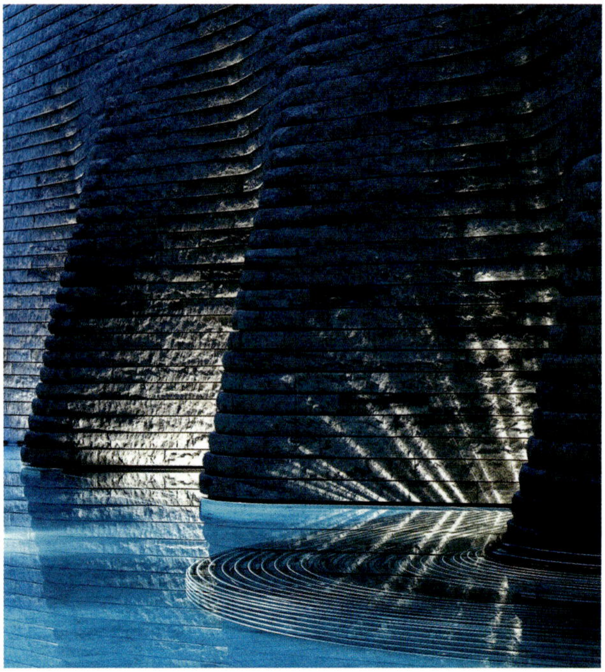

Die Granitwand des Pools erinnert mit ihren gewölbten Einbuchtungen an das Innere einer Höhle.

The texturized granite wall in the pool, with all its curves, looks like the inside of a cave.

Avec toutes ses courbes, le mur de granit plongeant dans la piscine ressemble à l'intérieur d'une caverne.

De ongelijkmatige, ruwgranieten muur in het zwembad ziet eruit als de binnenkant van een grot.

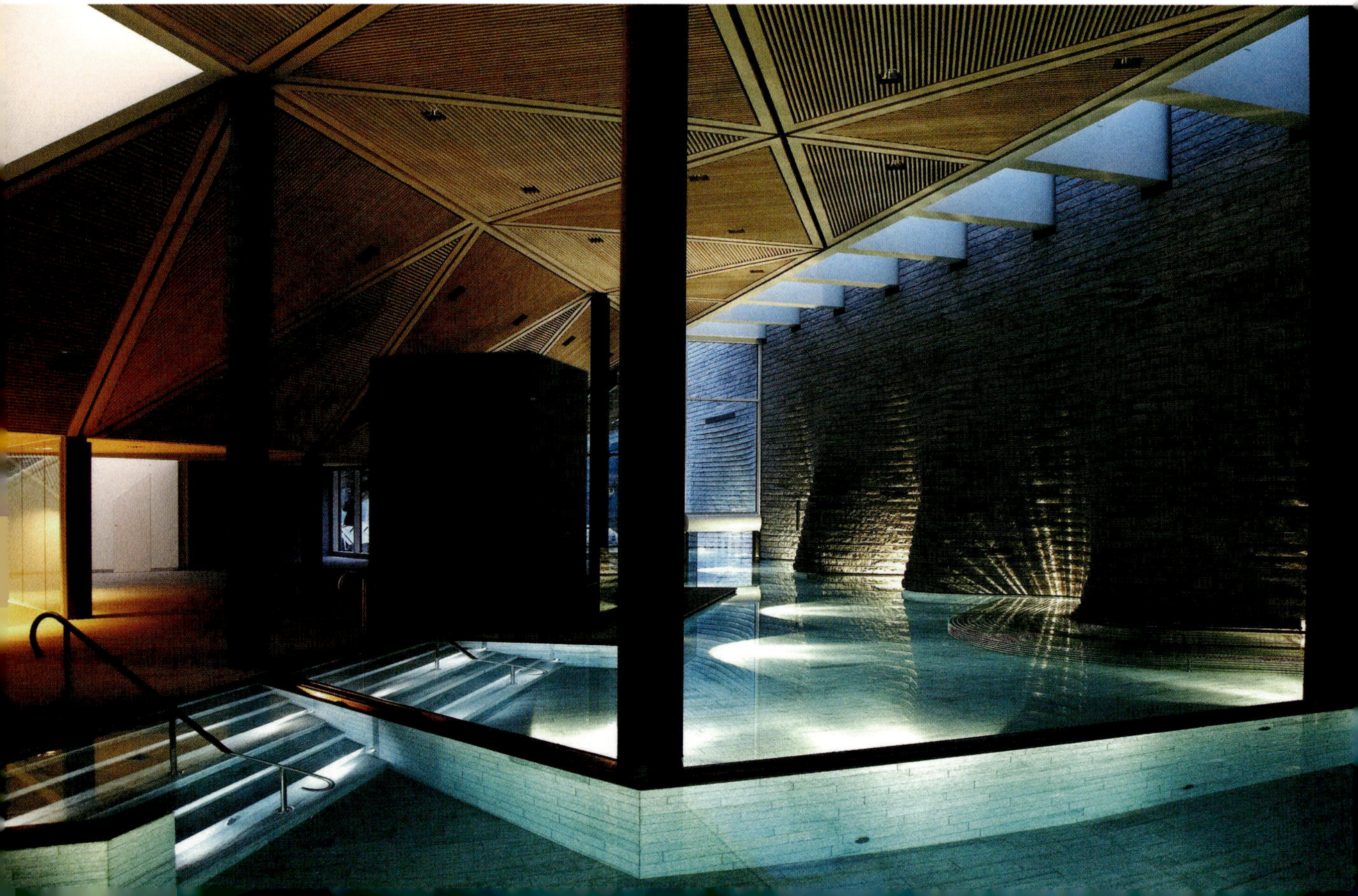

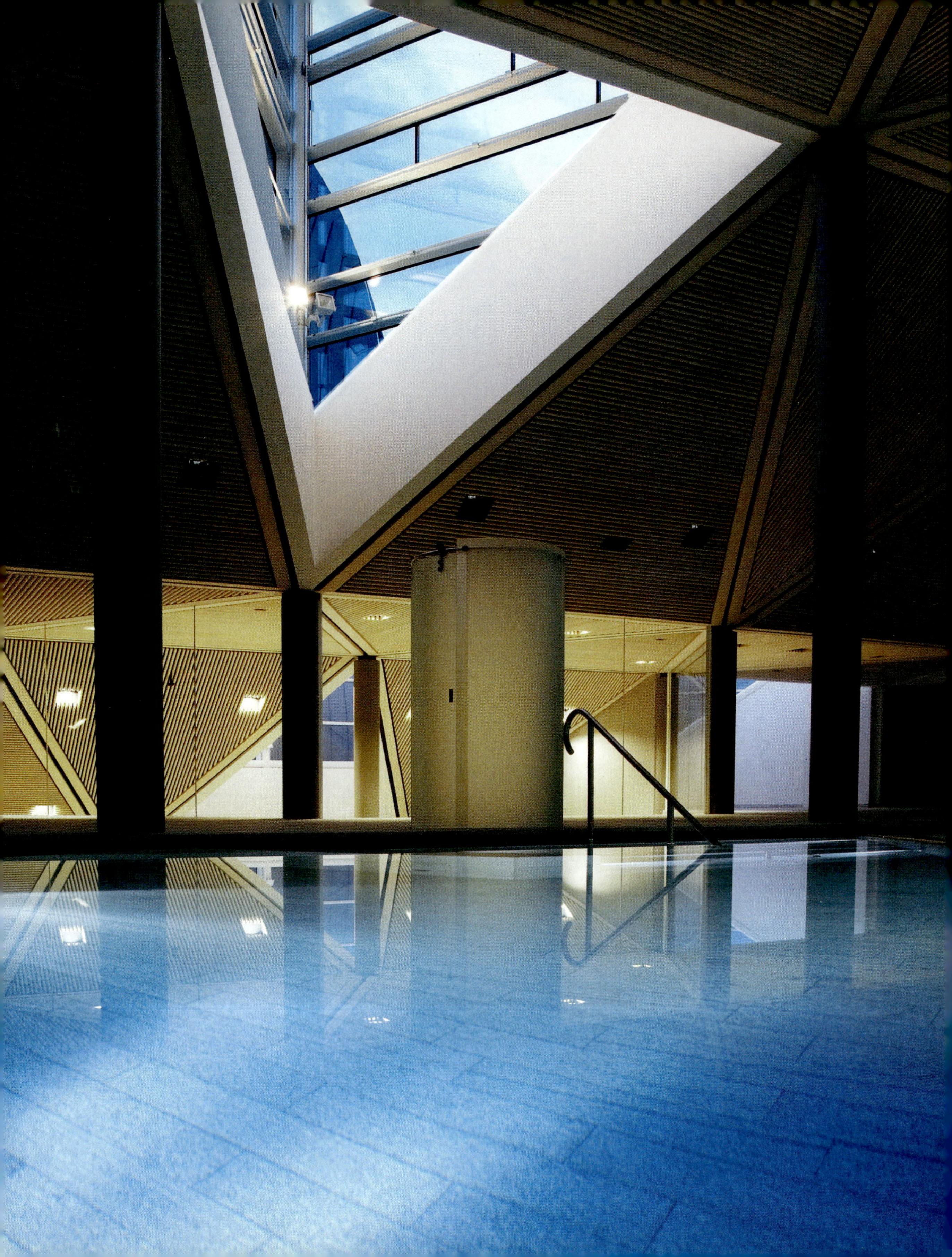

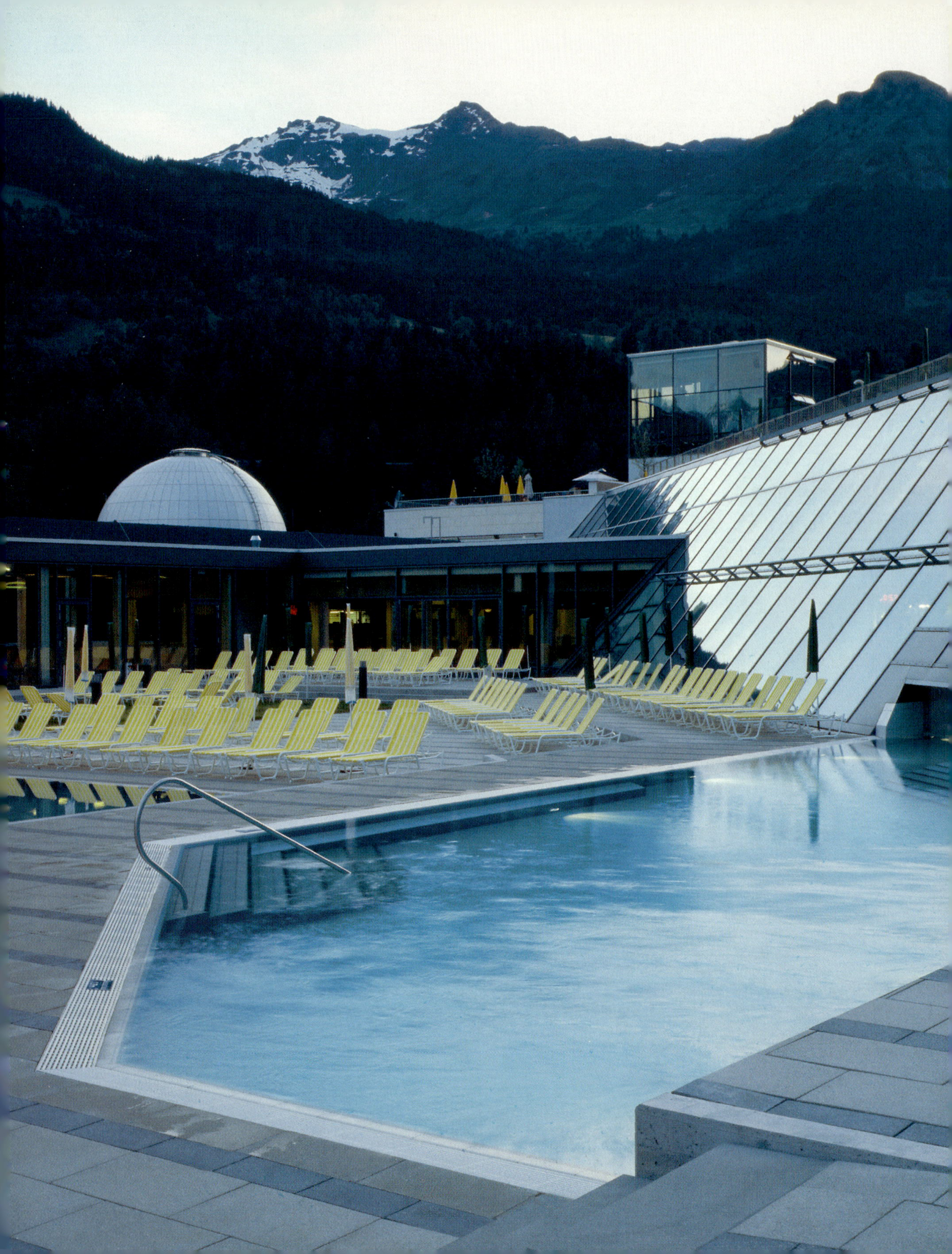

Alpen Therme Gastein Spa

Dieses Spa präsentiert sich als komplexer plastischer Bau. Kubusförmige Strukturen, die eine Sauna bergen, stehen in harmonischem Einklang mit langen Wasserrutschen und der Metallkuppel, unter der sich ein Multimedia Erlebnisdom befindet. Die Einrichtungen verteilen sich auf ein Areal von insgesamt 36.000 qm. Von dieser Fläche, die doppelt so groß ist wie die der ursprünglichen Thermalbäder, entfallen 1.500 qm auf die Wasserbecken der Entspannungs- und Erholungszonen.

This Spa is a sculptural, complex building, where structures in the shape of a cube holding saunas are assembled harmonically with long water slides, and with the metal covered dome holding a multimedia space. The facilities occupy a total of 387,000 square feet –twice as much as the original thermal baths-, of which 16,200 correspond to water surfaces divided into relaxation and recreation areas.

Ce spa est une construction sculpturale, complexe, où les structures en forme de cube intégrant des saunas répondent harmonieusement aux longues bandes d'eau et au métal du dôme accueillant un espace multimédia. Les équipements occupent un total de près de 32.000 m² – deux fois plus que la station thermale d'origine – , dont la moitié correspond aux surfaces d'eau dédiées aux espaces ludiques et de relaxation.

Dit kuuroord is een plastisch aandoend, complex gebouw, waar kubusvormige sauna's harmonieus samengaan met lange waterglijbanen en een metalen koepeldak, waaronder een multimediaruimte zit. De faciliteiten beslaan in totaal zo'n 40.000 m² – twee keer zoveel als het oorspronkelijke bronnenbad – waarvan zo'n 1500 m² bestaat uit waterpartijen, sommige voor ontspanning, andere voor recreatie.

Bad Hofgastein, Austria

MARTIN KOHLBAUER ZT

Photos © Rupert Steiner

www.alpentherme.com

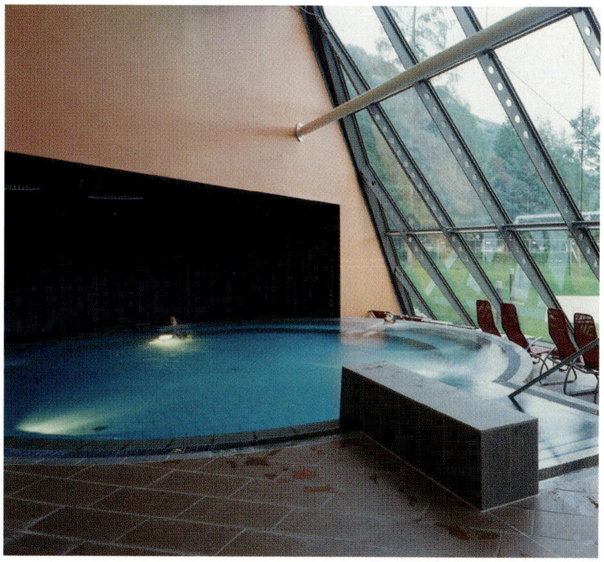

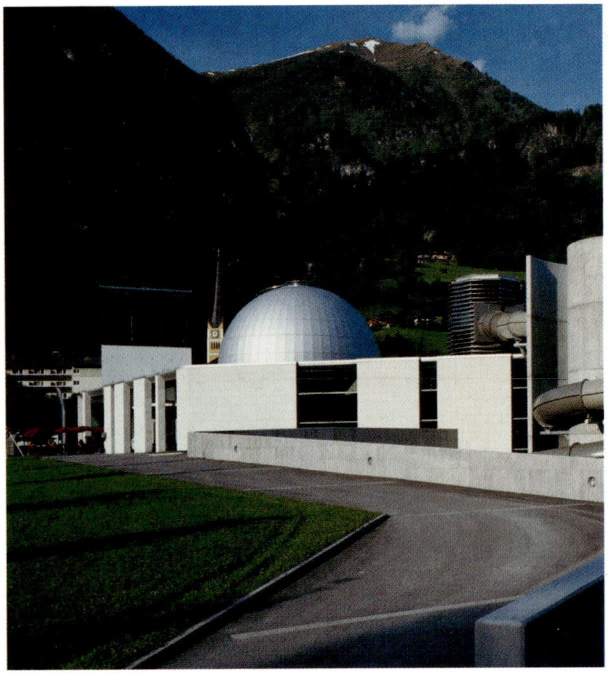

Das Gasteinertal, in dem die Alpen Therme liegt, ist für die heilenden Kräfte seiner Mineralquellen berühmt.

The Gastein valley, where Alpen Therme is located, is famous for the curative properties of its mineral waters.

La vallée de Gastein, où l'Alpen Therme est situé, est célèbre pour ses eaux minérales aux nombreuses propriétés curatives.

Het dal van Gastein, waar de Alpen Therme ligt, is beroemd om de heilzame eigenschappen van het lokale mineraalwater.

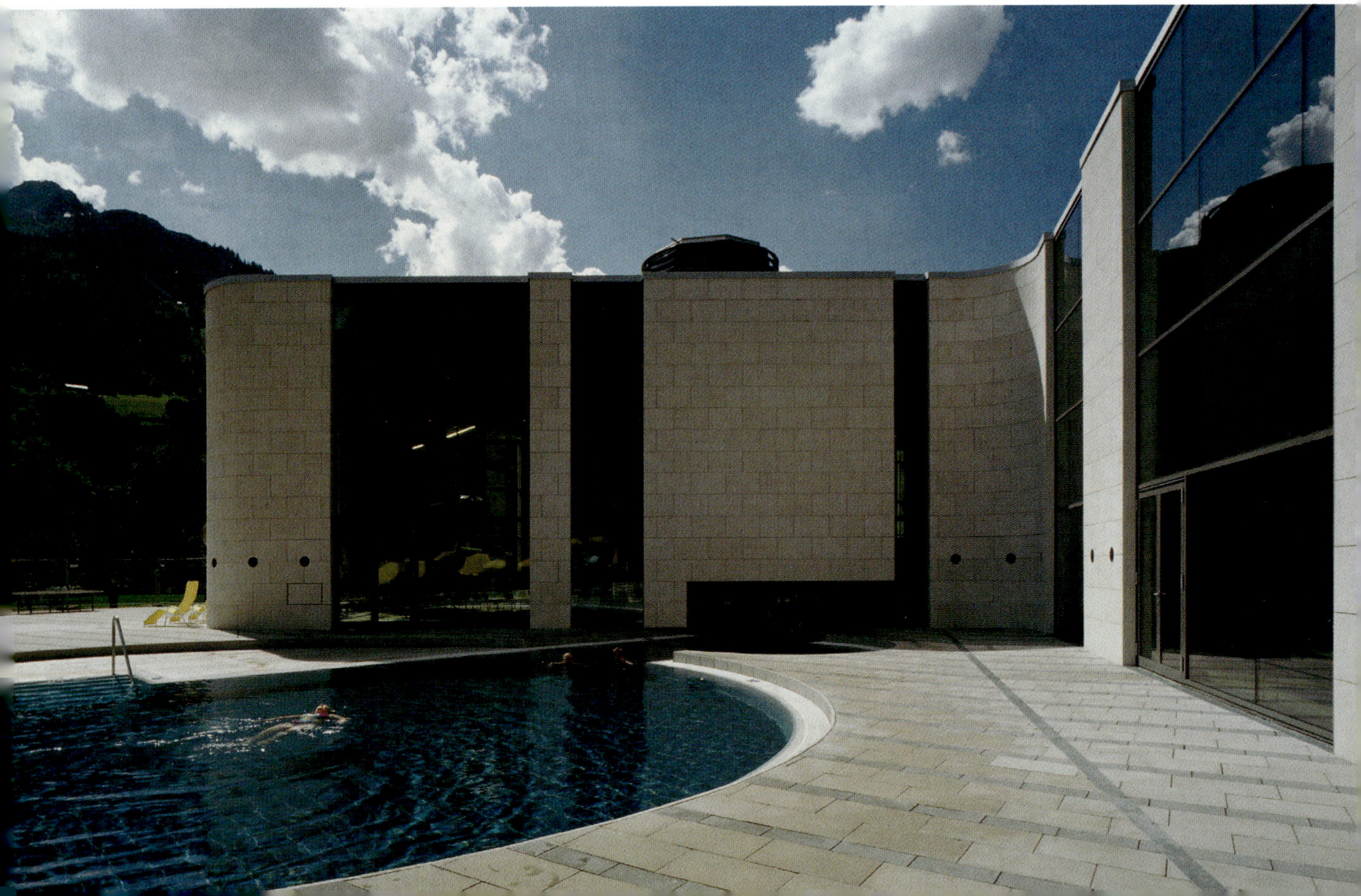

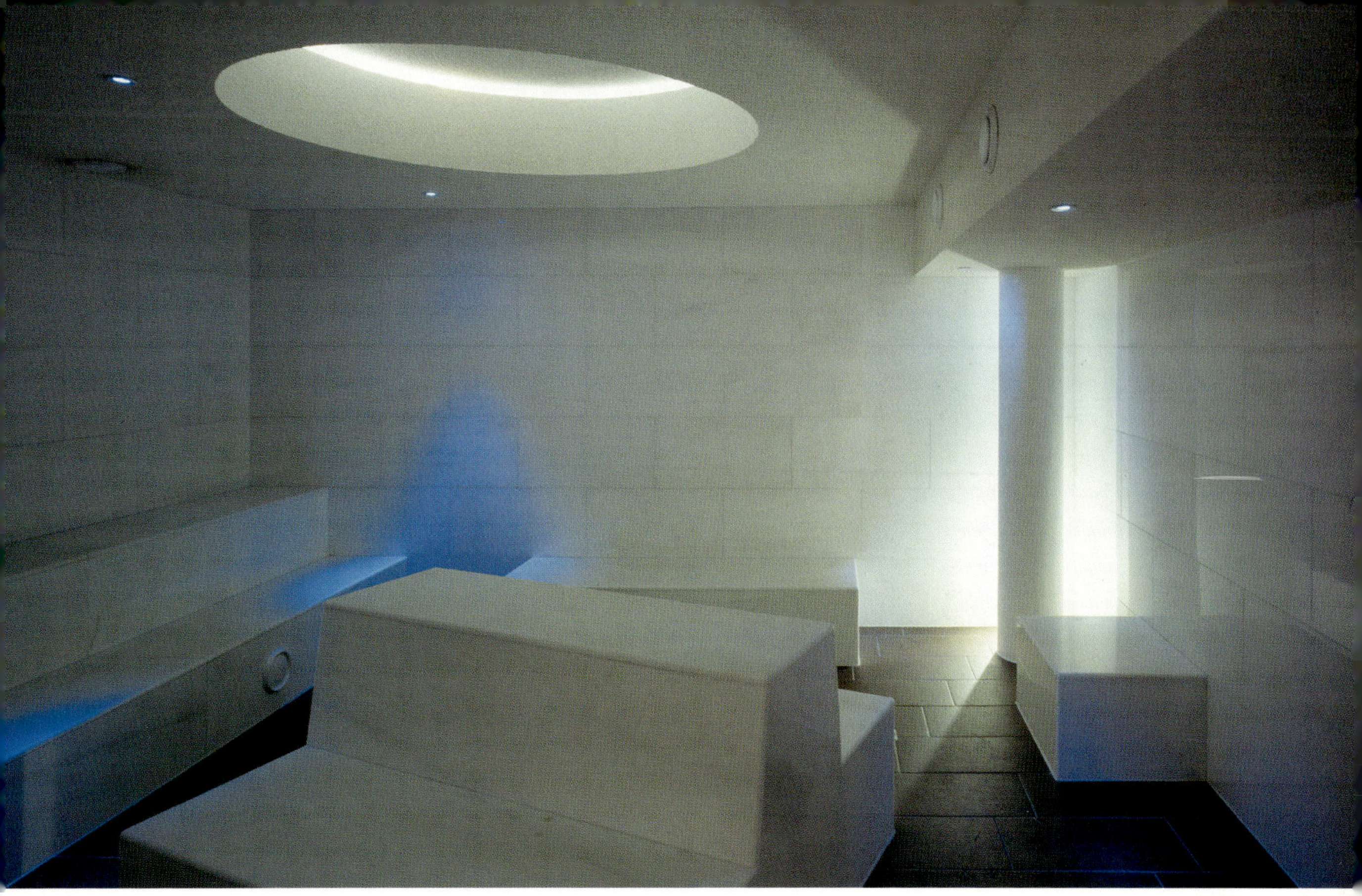

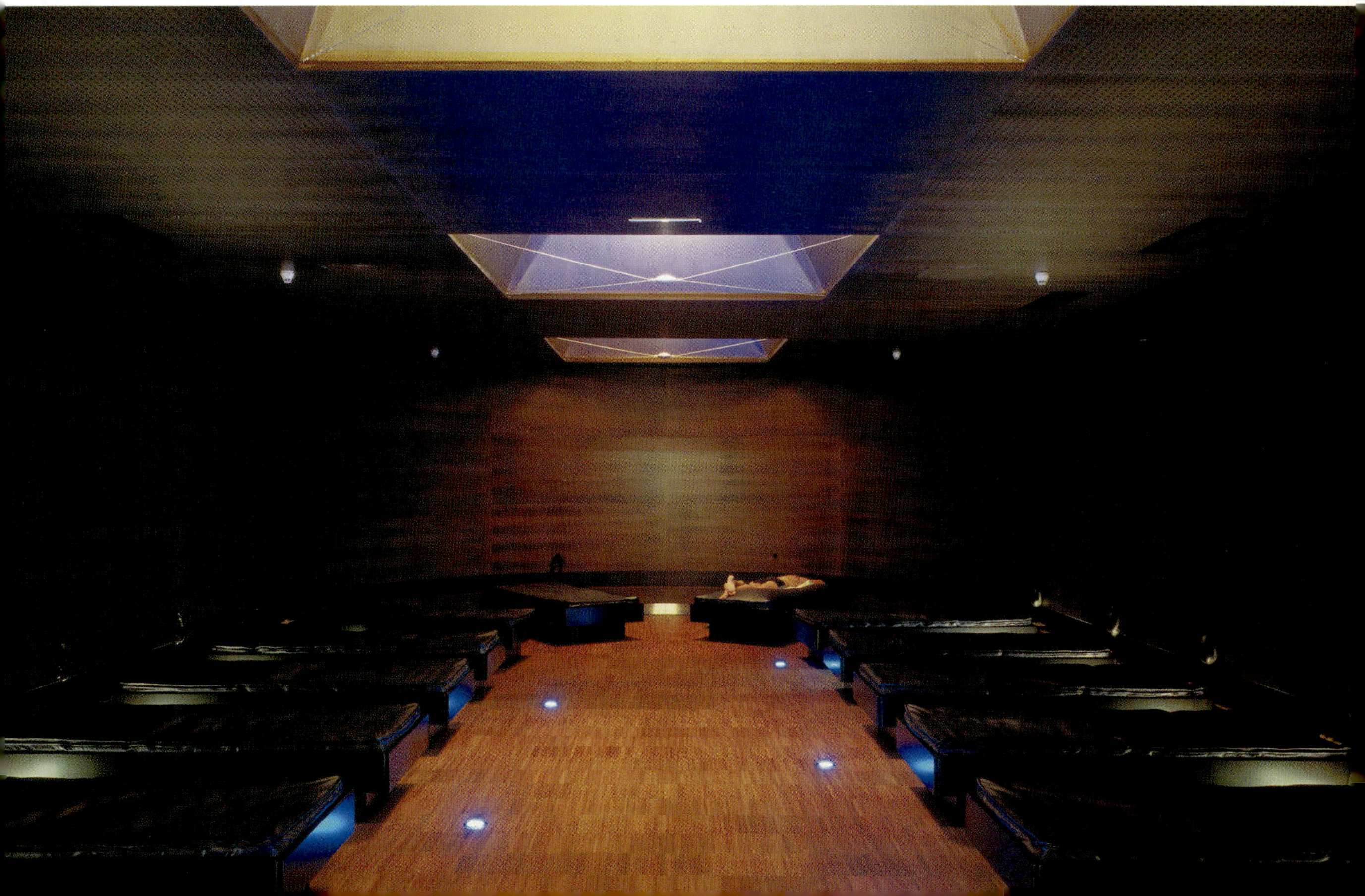

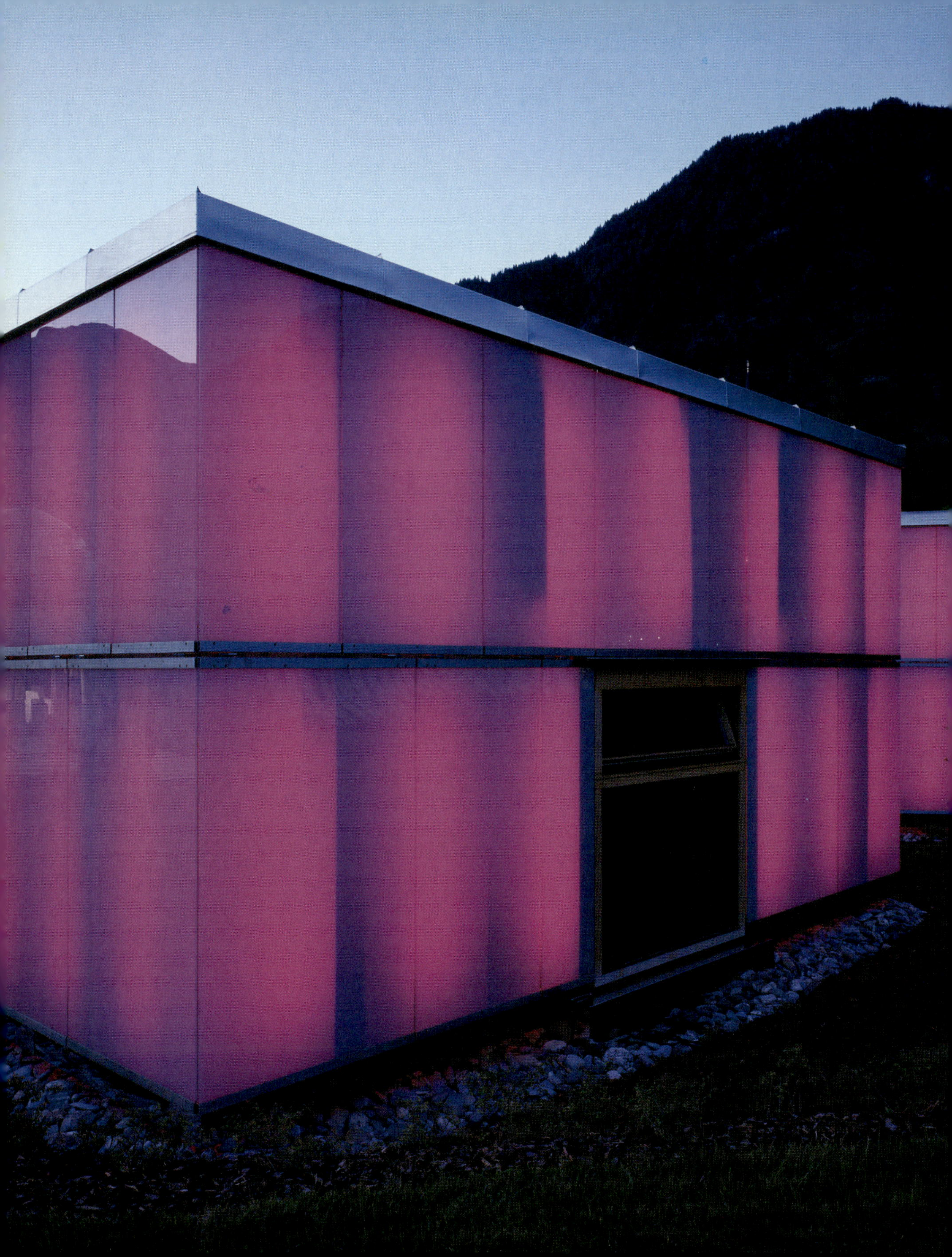

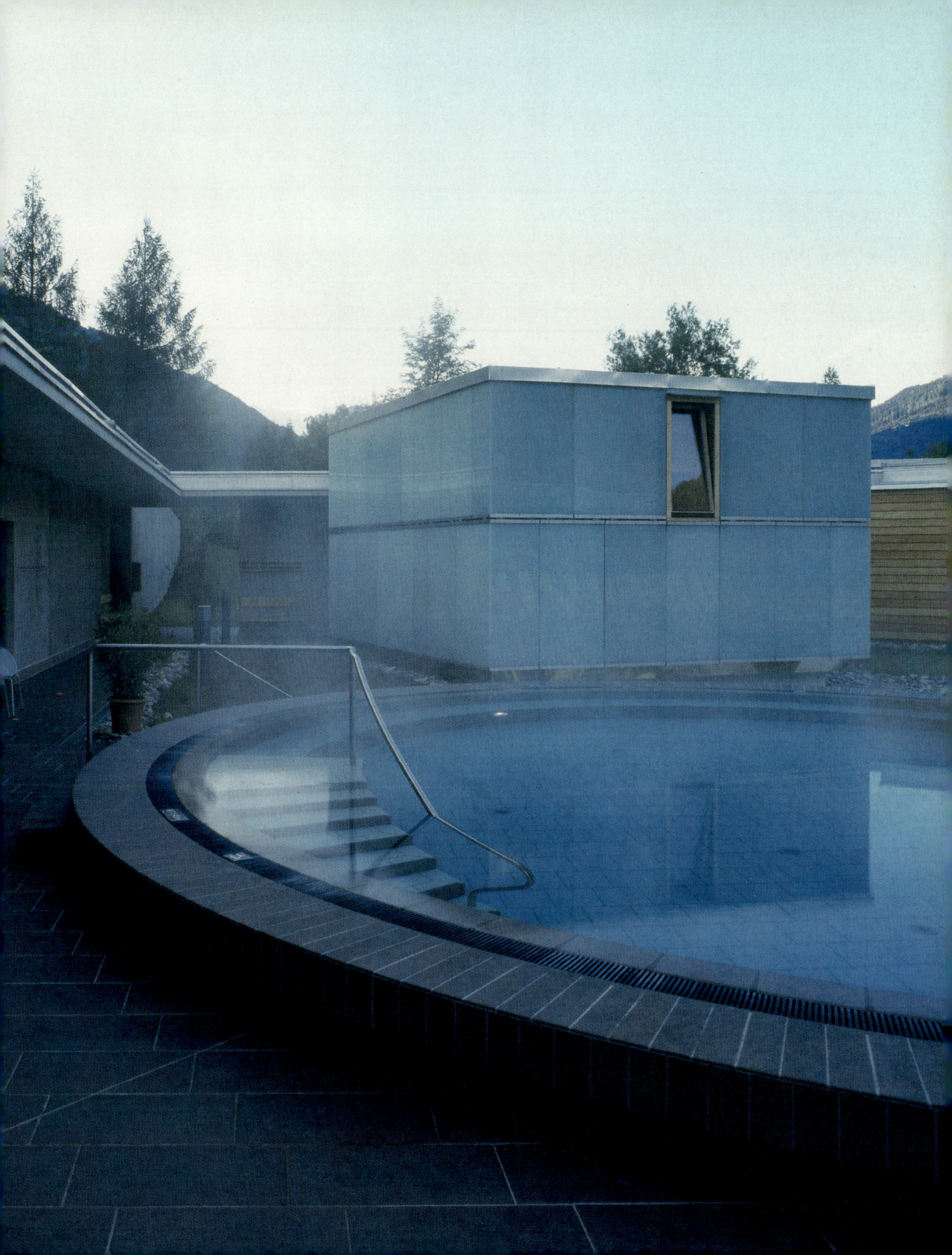

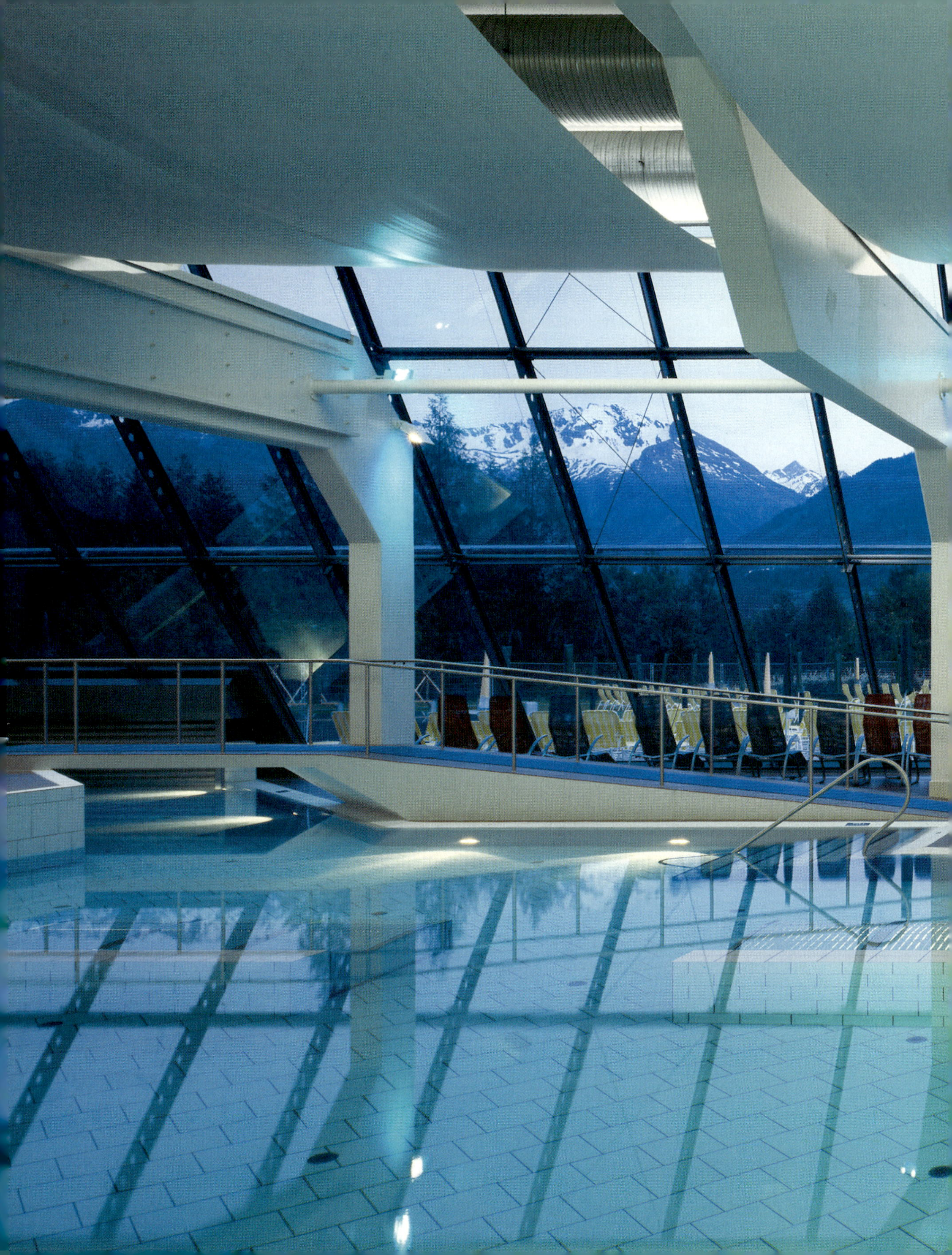

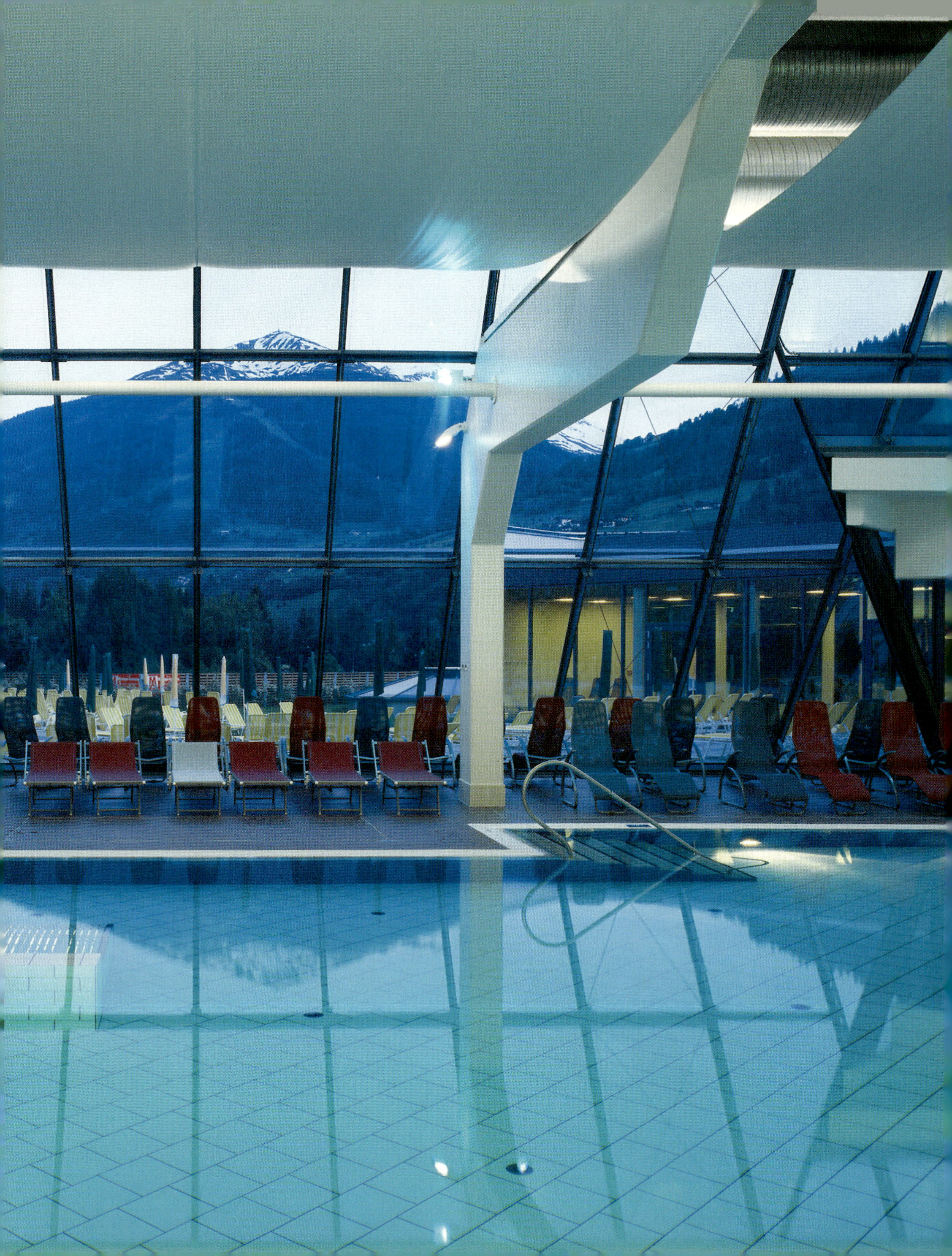

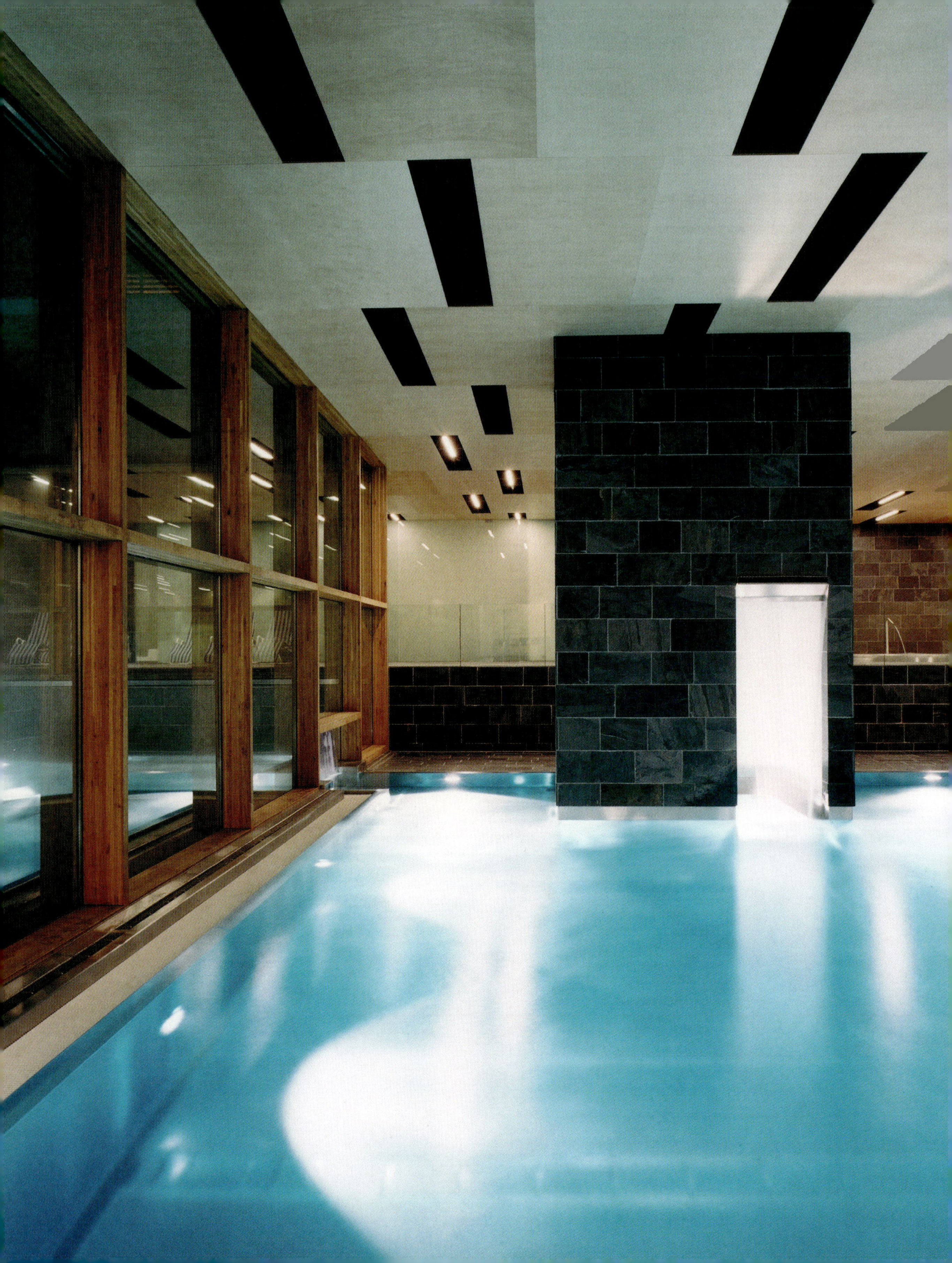

Arlberg-well.com

Diese Wellnessoase lockt mit Indoorpools, beheizten Außenpools, Gegenstromschwimmbahn, Wasserfall und speziellem Kinderbereich mit Wasserrutschen und Düsenstrahlen. Der Bau ist in eine Landschaft eingebettet, die zu jeder Jahreszeit beeindruckt. Im Sommer leuchten die ausgedehnten Wiesen sattgrün, dazwischen glitzern Seen. Im Winter liegt der Park unter einer strahlend weißen Scheedecke, während das Licht- und Schattenspiel der Bäume auf dem Eis reflektiert.

This is the fancy wet zone of Arlberg-well.com, composed of indoor pools, and open-air, heated pools; a lane to swim against the current, a cascade, and an area especially for children with water slides and jets. The landscape that surrounds the location is spectacular all year long. In summer, the vast meadows are deep green and one can see lakes here and there. In winter, the park is covered in snow, and the trees are decorated with colored lights that reflect upon the ice.

Voici l'original espace aquatique d'Arlberg-well.com, composé de piscines chauffées d'intérieur et de plein air : un couloir d'eau pour nager contre le courant, une cascade et une zone réservée aux enfants avec toboggan et jets d'eau.
Le paysage environnant est spectaculaire toute l'année. En été, les prés sont d'un vert profond et l'on peut voir des lacs ici et là. En hiver, le parc est recouvert de neige et les arbres sont décorés de lumières de toutes les couleurs qui se reflètent sur la glace.

Dit is een luxueuze badinrichting met binnenbaden en warme buitenbaden, een watertraject om tegen de stroom in te zwemmen, een waterval en een kinderafdeling met waterglijbanen en fonteinen. Het omringende landschap is het hele jaar door spectaculair. Zomers's zijn de alpenweiden diepgroen van kleur en zijn hier en daar bergmeertjes te zien. Winters's is het park overdekt met sneeuw en worden de gekleurde lampjes in de bomen weerspiegeld door het ijs.

Arlberg, Austria

DIETRICH UNTERTRIFALLER ARCHITEKTEN

Photos © Bruno Klomfar/
Tourism office of St. Anton am Arlberg

www.arlberg-well.com

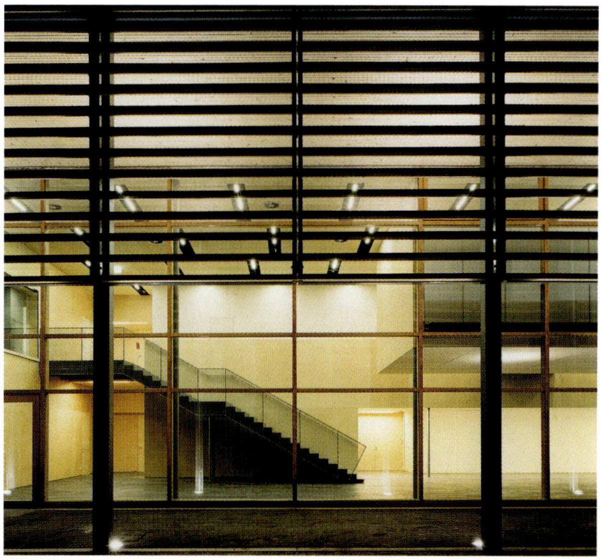

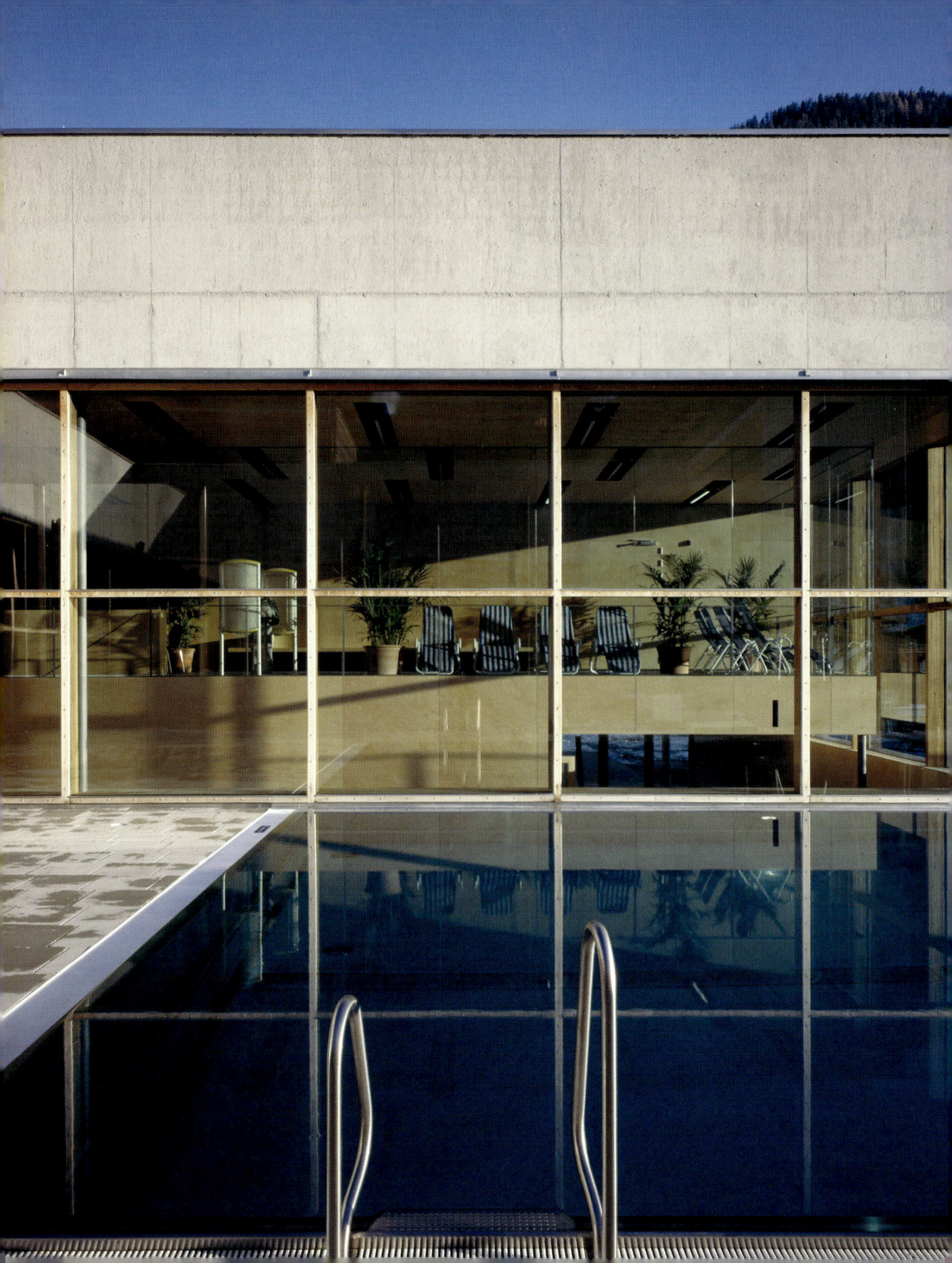

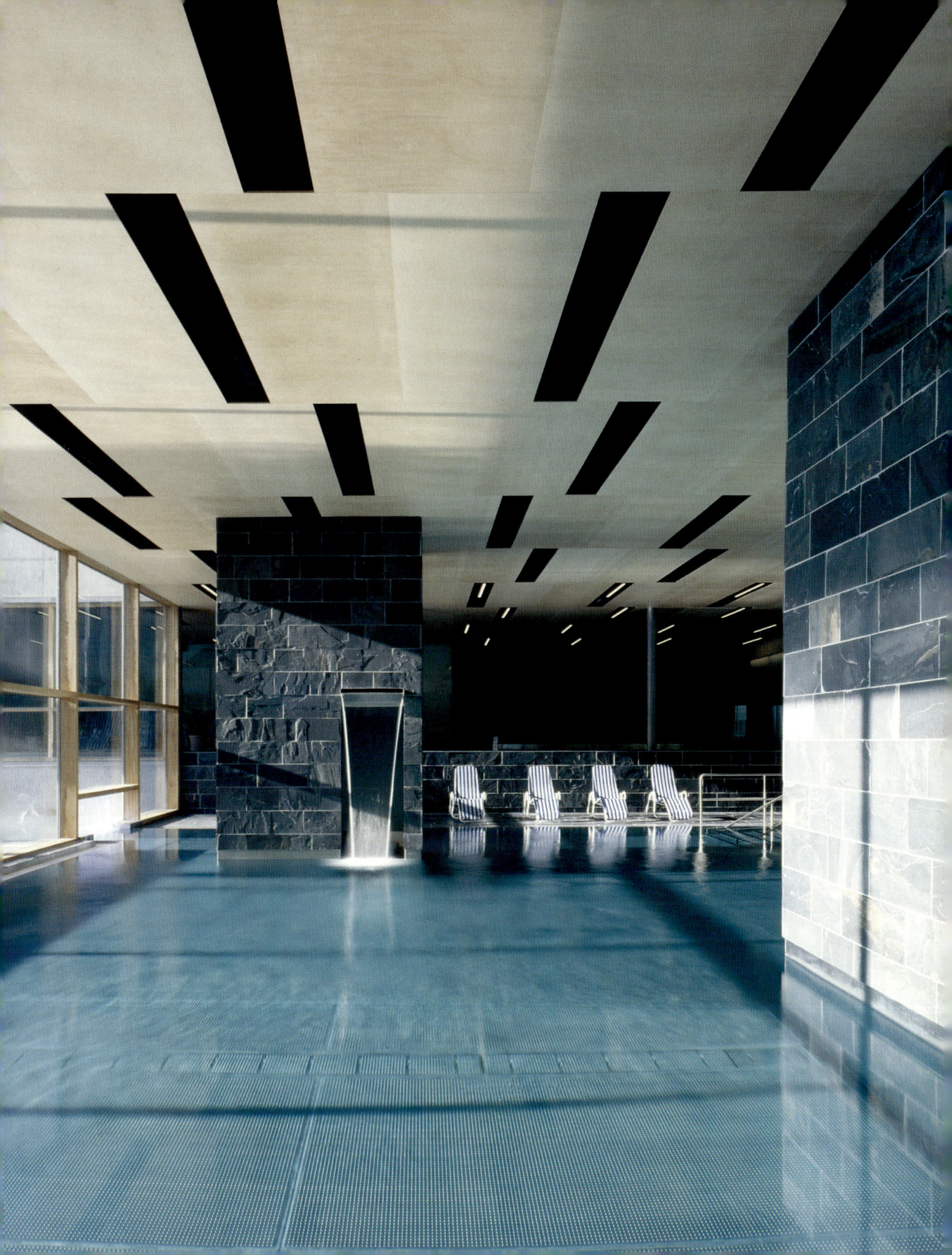

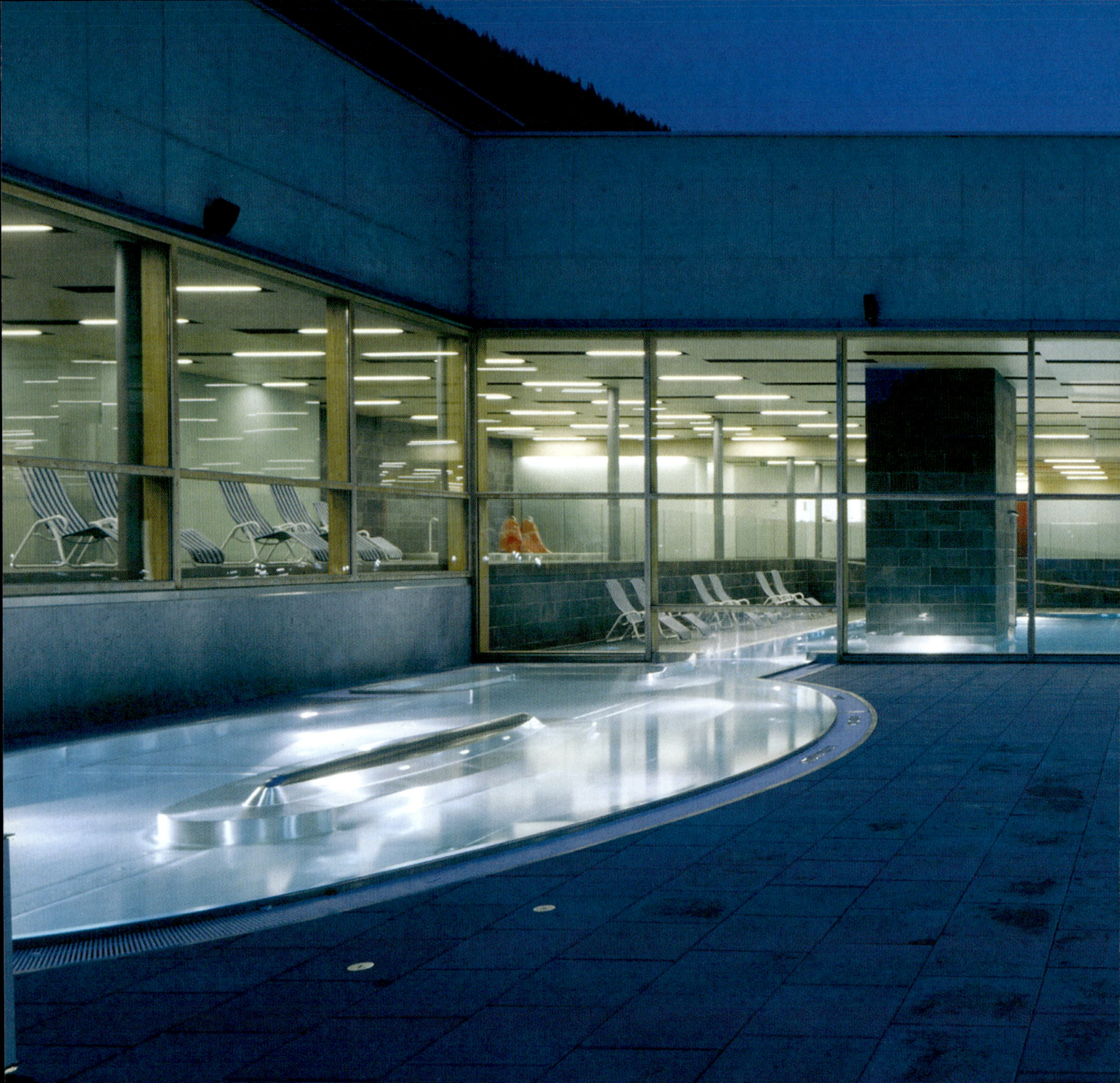

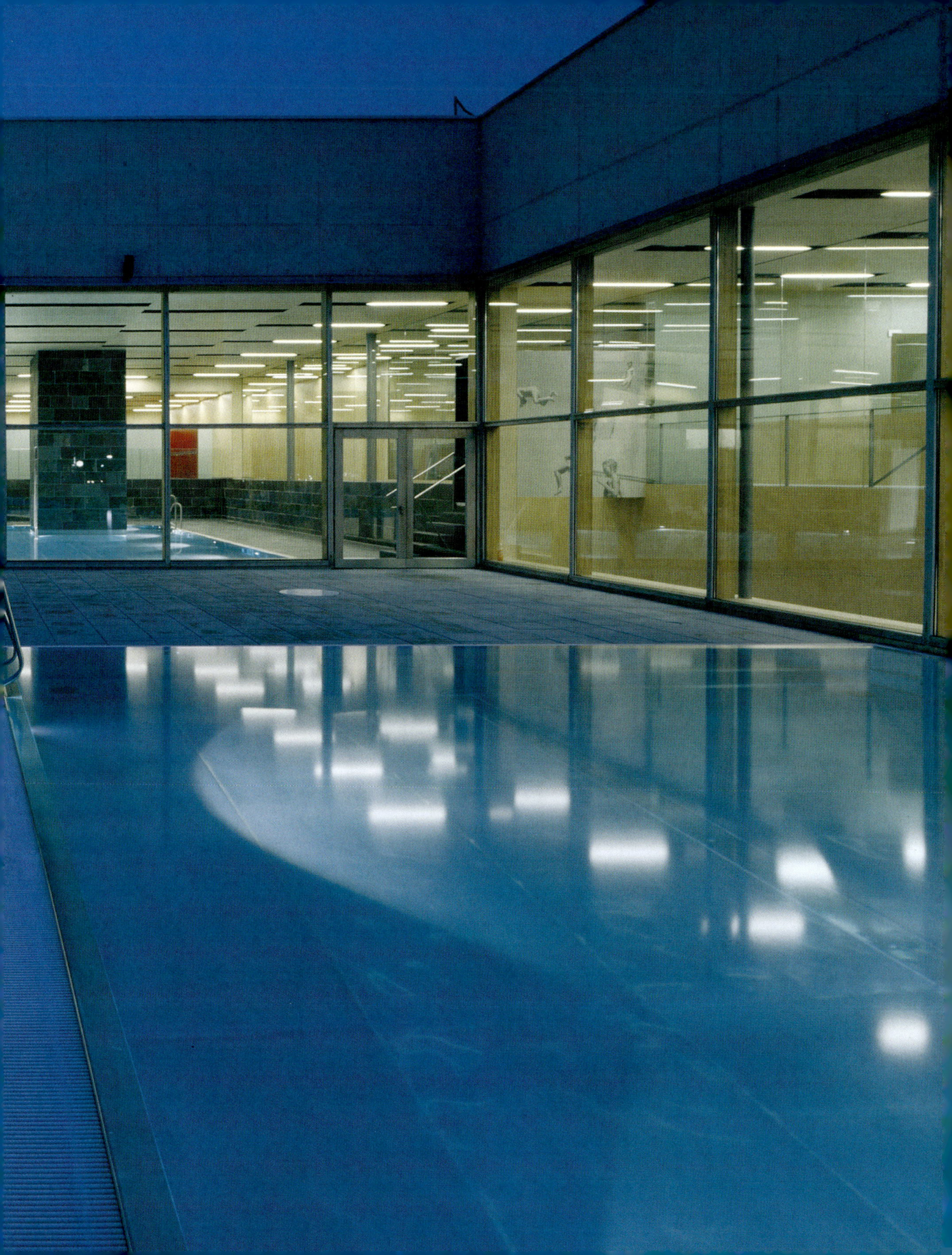

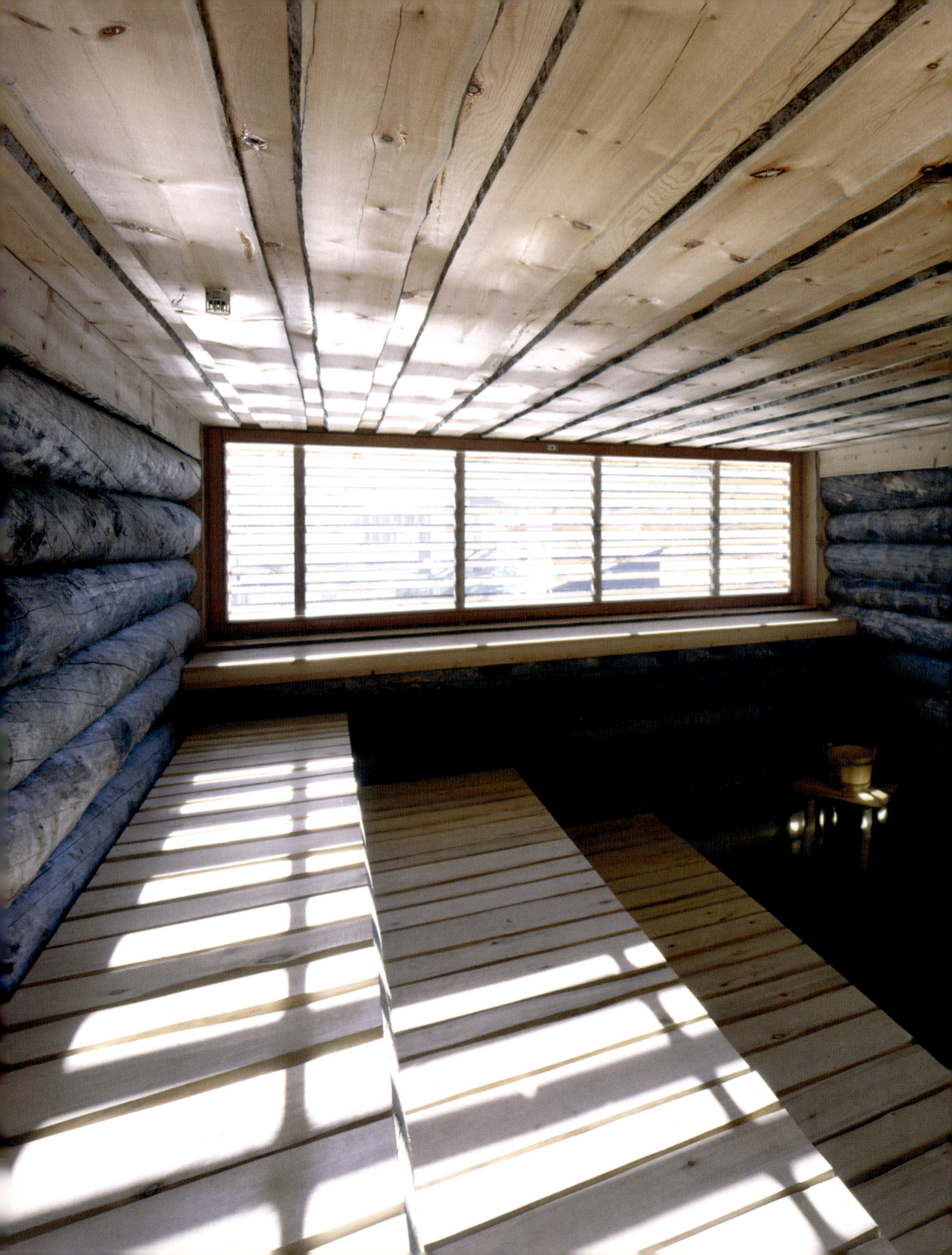

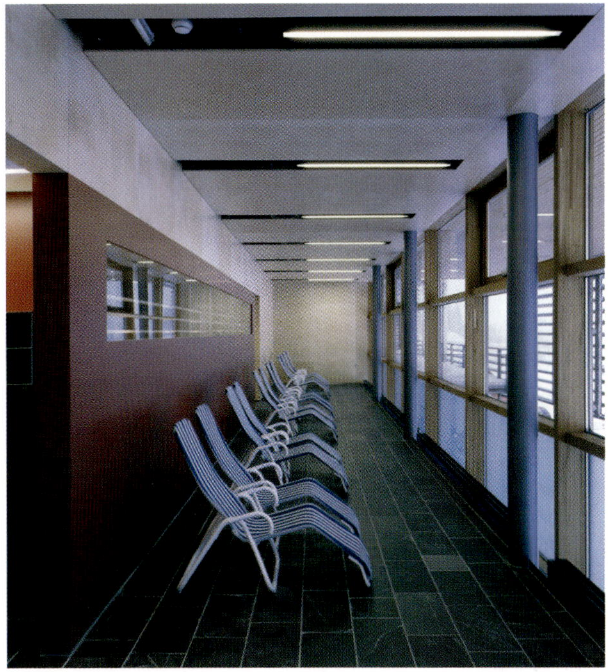

Die Einrichtung umfasst mehrere Dampfbäder, eine finnische Sauna, eine Kelo-Sauna und Sanarien.

The facilities include a variety of steam baths, a Finnish sauna, a kelo-sauna and sanariums.

Les équipements, d'une grande diversité, incluent bains à vapeur, sauna finlandais, kelo-sauna et autres sanariums.

Het complex bevat allerlei soorten stoombaden, een Finse sauna, een kelosauna en sanaria.

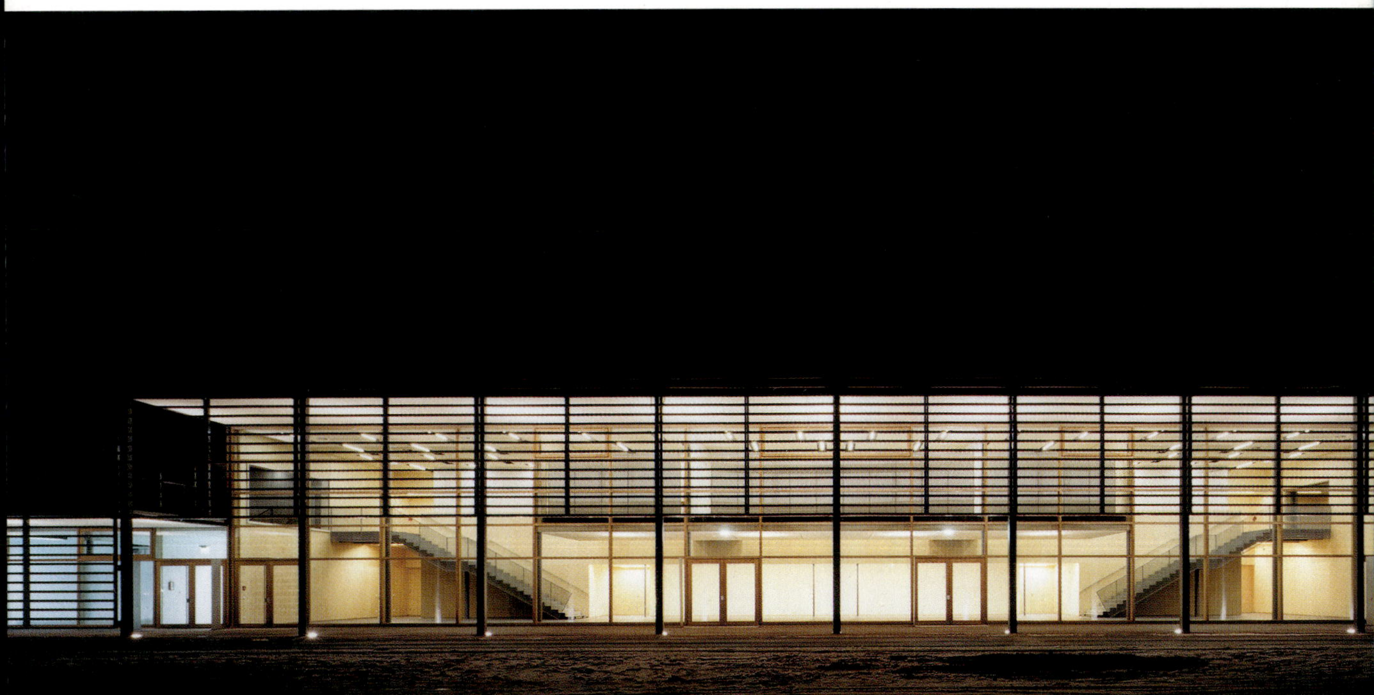

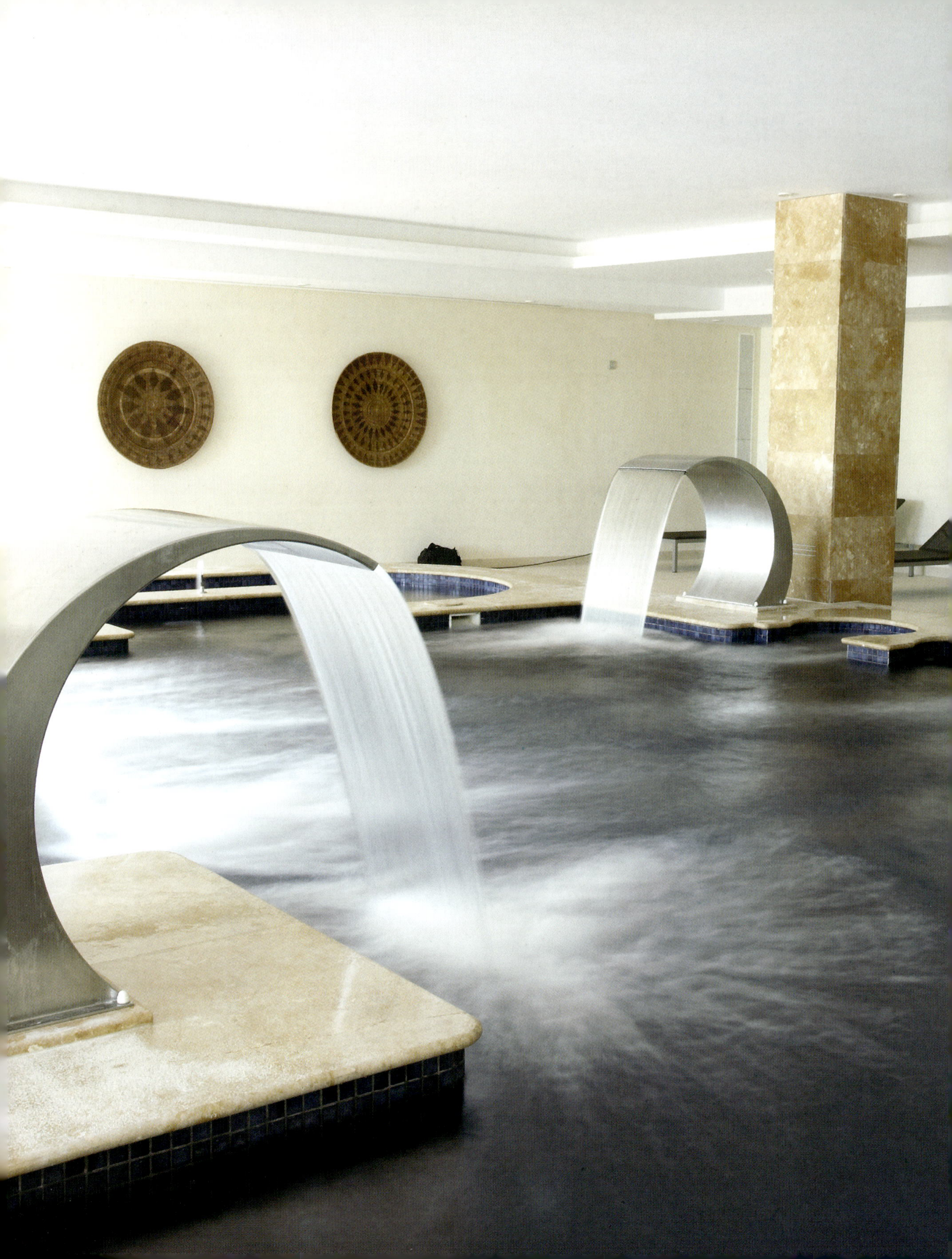

Thalasso Spa Fenicia

Bei diesem Spa steht die Thalassotherapie im Mittelpunkt, bei der Meerwasser und Meerwasserprodukte für die Schönheits- und Gesundheitspflege zum Einsatz kommen. Die Einrichtungen umfassen Sprudelmatten, Gegenstromdüsen, türkische Bäder, Sauna, Whirlpool, beheizte Liegestühle, Erlebnisduschen sowie Entspannungszonen im Innen- und Außenbereich. Zudem verfügt dieses Spa über einen VIP-Bereich samt Terrasse mit Panoramablick auf die Küste.

Thalassotherapy is based on the use of sea water and products that come from this medium. Their benefits for health and beauty constitute the axis of this spa. Bubble beds, counter current jets, Turkish baths, sauna, Jacuzzi, thermal deck chairs, sensation showers, inside and outside relaxation areas are all part of the central facilities of the thermal club. This center also has a VIP area with a terrace offering a panoramic view of the coast.

La thalassothérapie est basée sur l'utilisation de l'eau de mer et des produits qui en sont issus. Leurs bienfaits pour la santé et la beauté constituent l'essence même de ce spa. Les lits à bulles, les jets à contre-courant, le hammam, le sauna, le jacuzzi, les lits de soins, les douches de sensations, ainsi que les espaces de relaxation à l'intérieur et à l'extérieur constituent autant d'équipements majeurs de ce club thermal. Ce centre dispose également d'une zone VIP, dont la terrasse offre une vue panoramique sur la côte.

Thalassotherapie is gebaseerd op zeewater en derivaten daarvan. De heilzame werking hiervan op gezondheid en uiterlijk staan centraal in deze kuurinrichting. Bubbelbedden, waterstralen, Turkse baden, sauna's, jacuzzi, thermale ligstoelen, massagedouches en rustruimten – zowel binnen als in de buitenlucht – behoren tot de centrale faciliteiten. Dit centrum heeft ook een vip-gedeelte met een terras met een schitterend uitzicht op de kust.

Ibiza, Spain

MIREIA VILA MERINO

Photos © Jordi Escandell

www.tesal.com

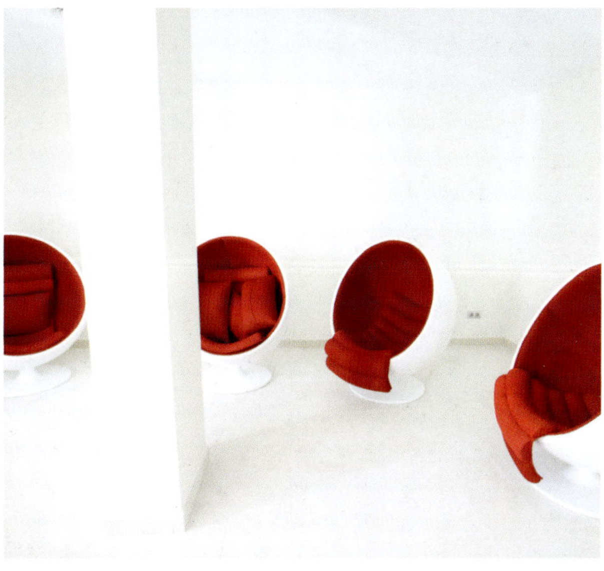

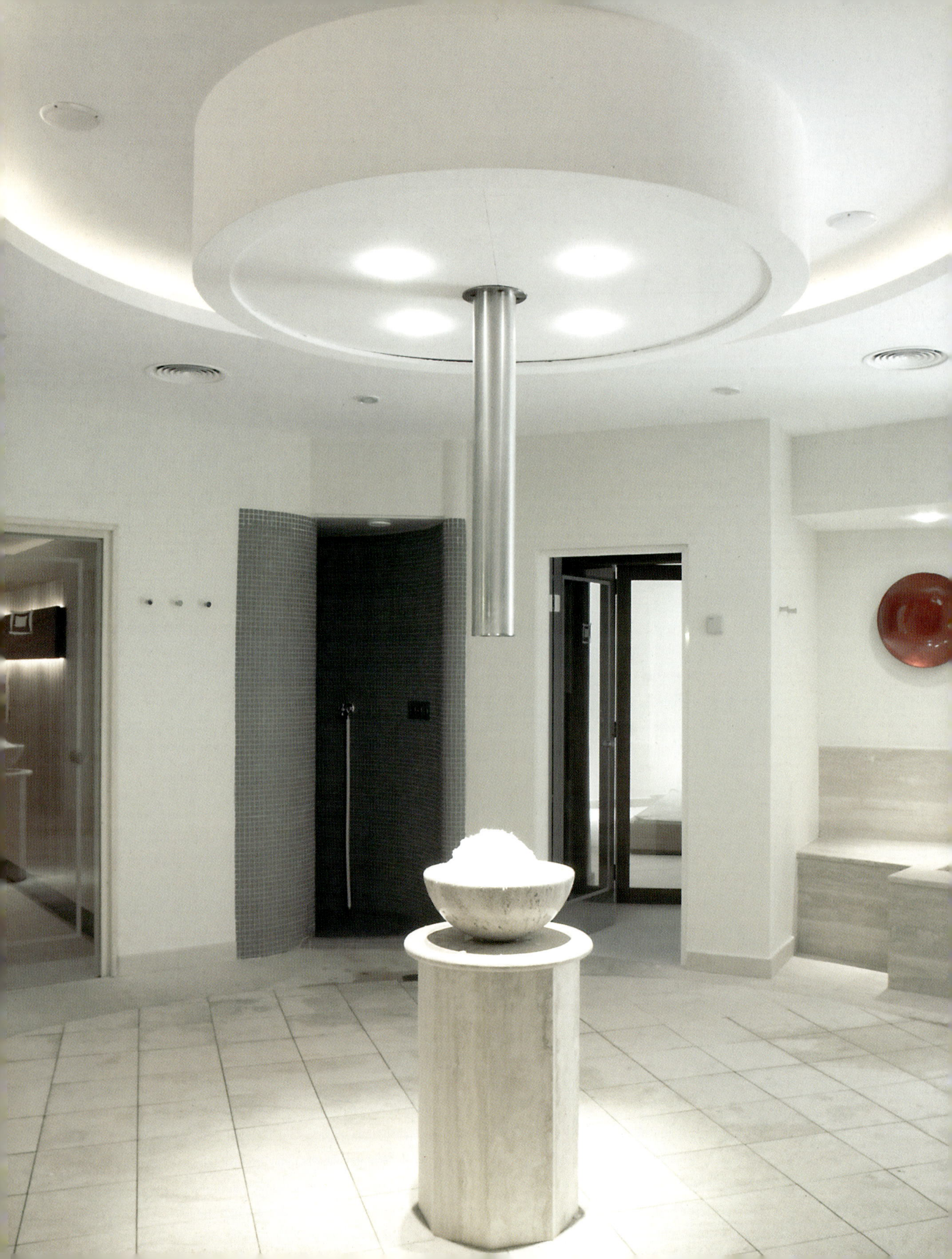

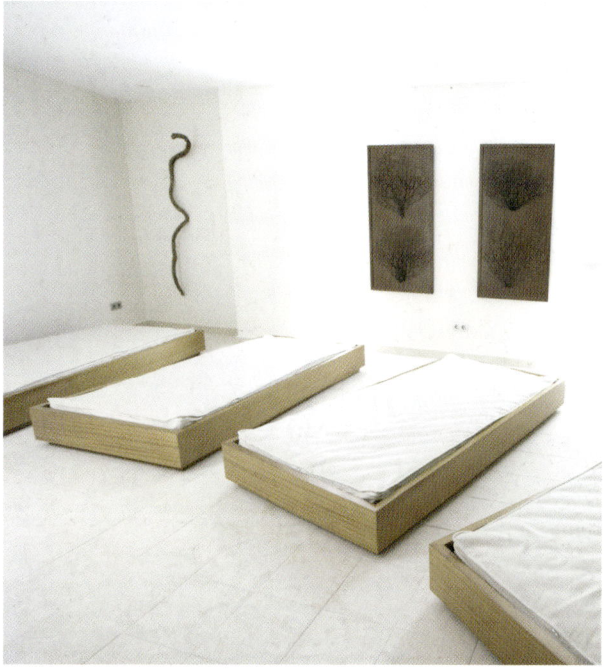

Neutrale Farben und minimalistische Formen prägen die erholsame Atmosphäre des Thalasso Spa Fenicia.

Neutral colors and minimalist shapes: the Thalasso Spa Fenicia calls for calm.

Couleurs neutres et formes épurées : le Thalasso Spa Fenicia invite à la sérénité.

Neutrale kleuren en minimalistische vormgeving: de Thalasso Spa Fenicia is gericht op rust.

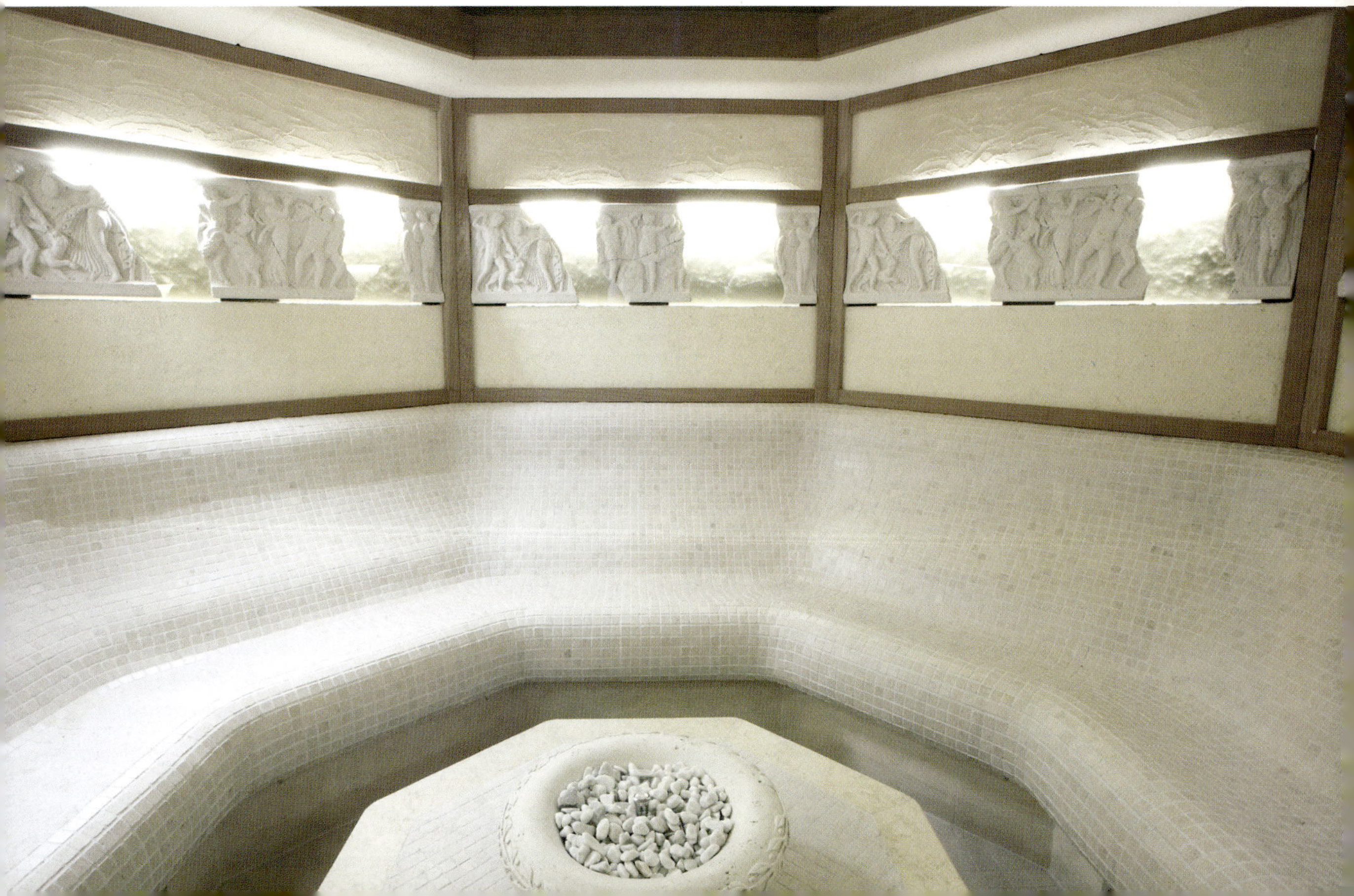

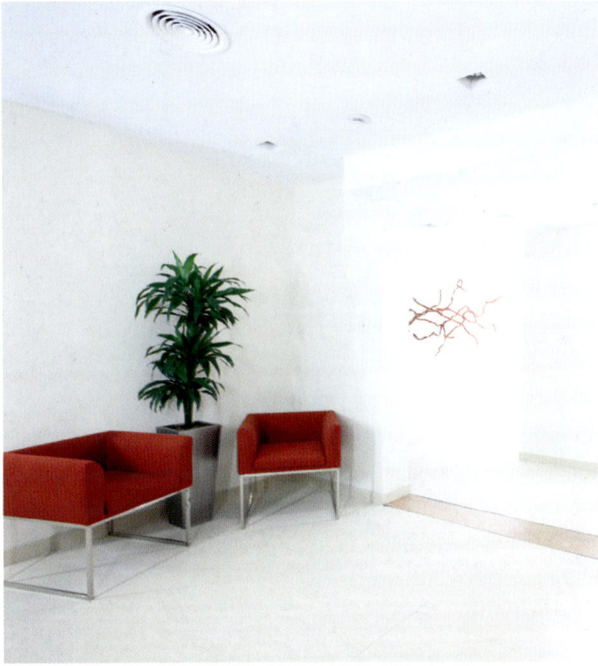

Die Terrasse des Spa bietet einen herrlichen Panoramablick auf die ibizenkische Küste.

From the spa terrace there is a privileged panoramic view of Ibiza's coastline.

Depuis la terrasse du spa, on jouit d'une vue panoramique privilégiée sur la côte d'Ibiza.

Het terras biedt een exclusief uitzicht op de kustlijn van Ibiza.

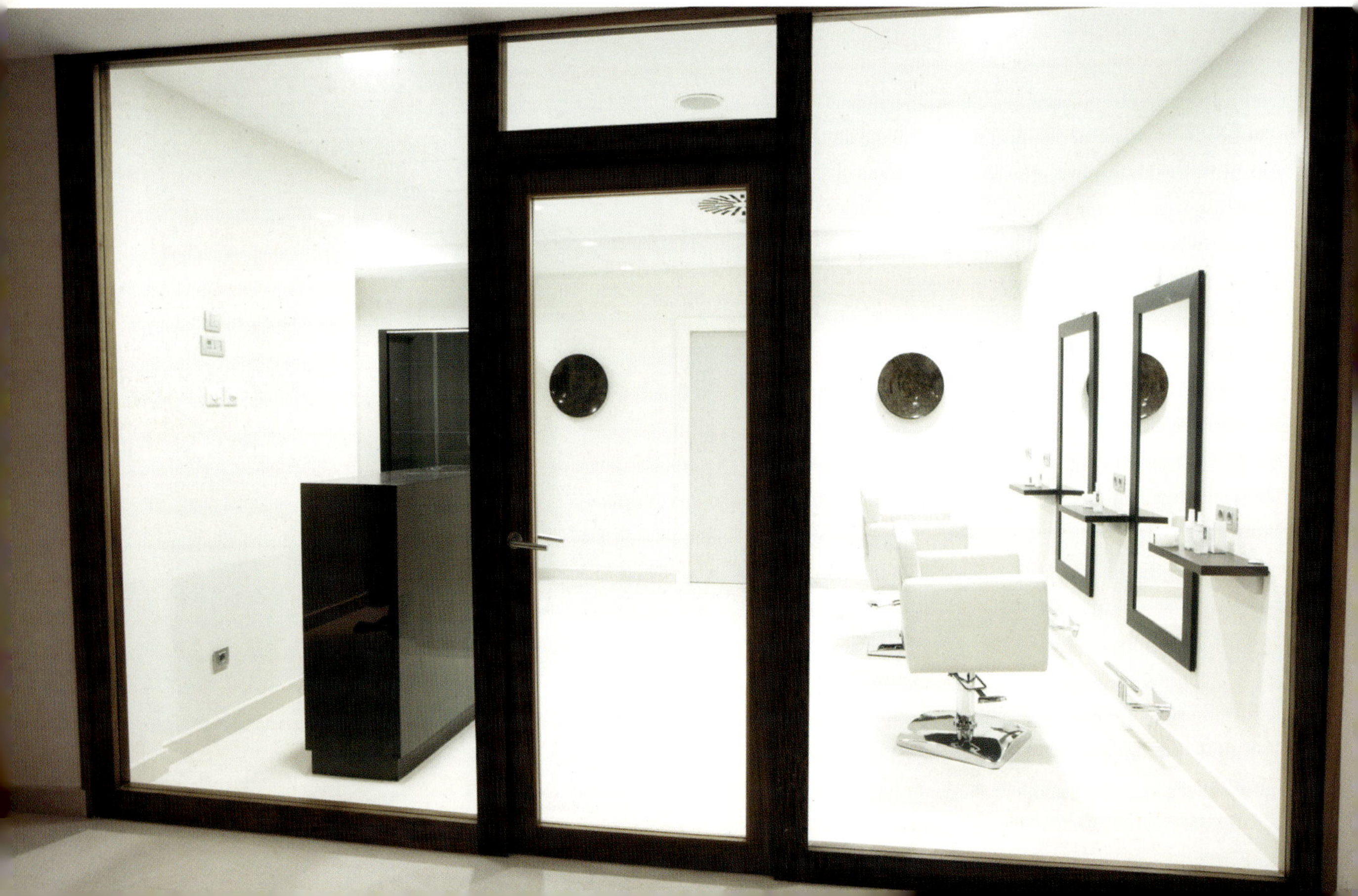

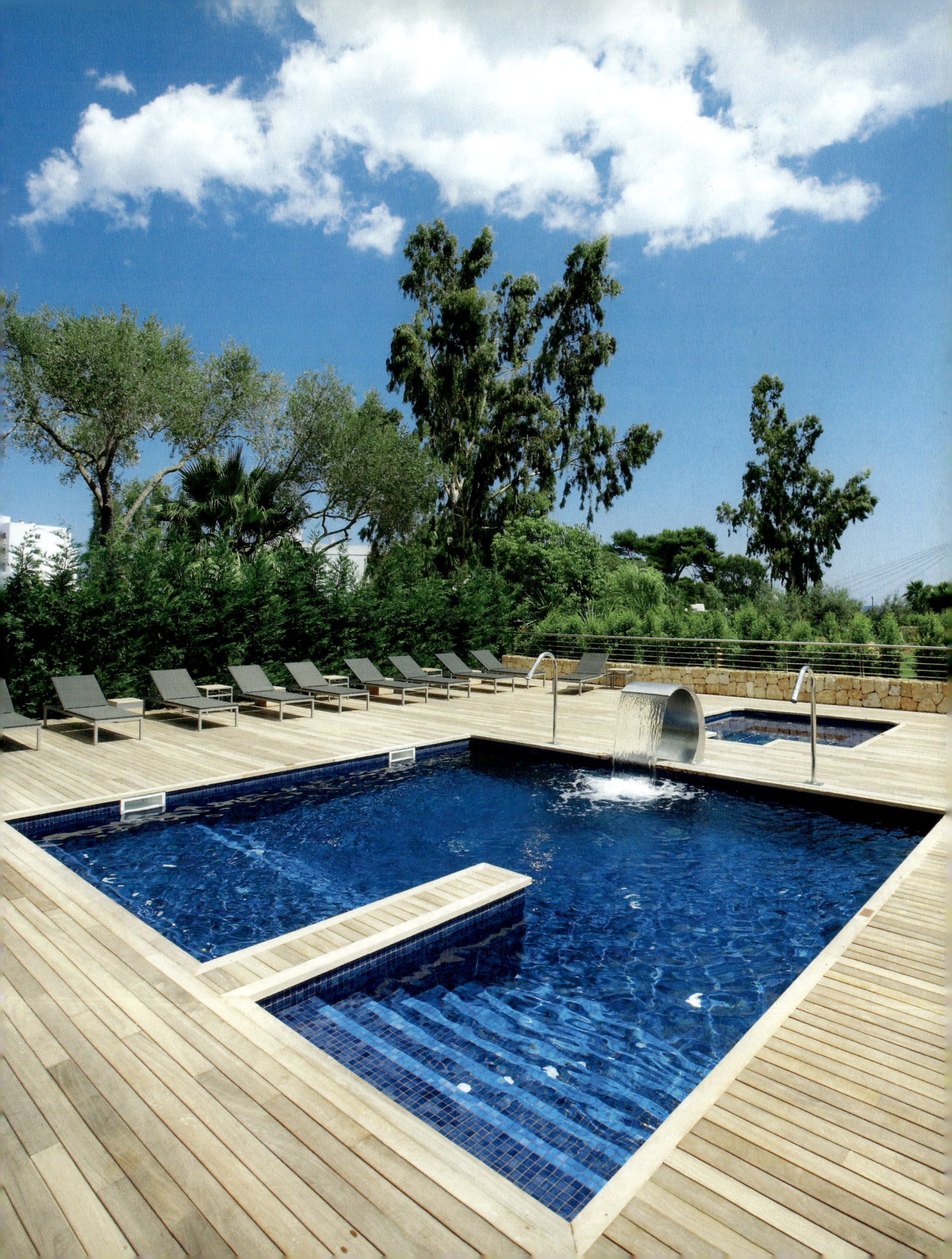

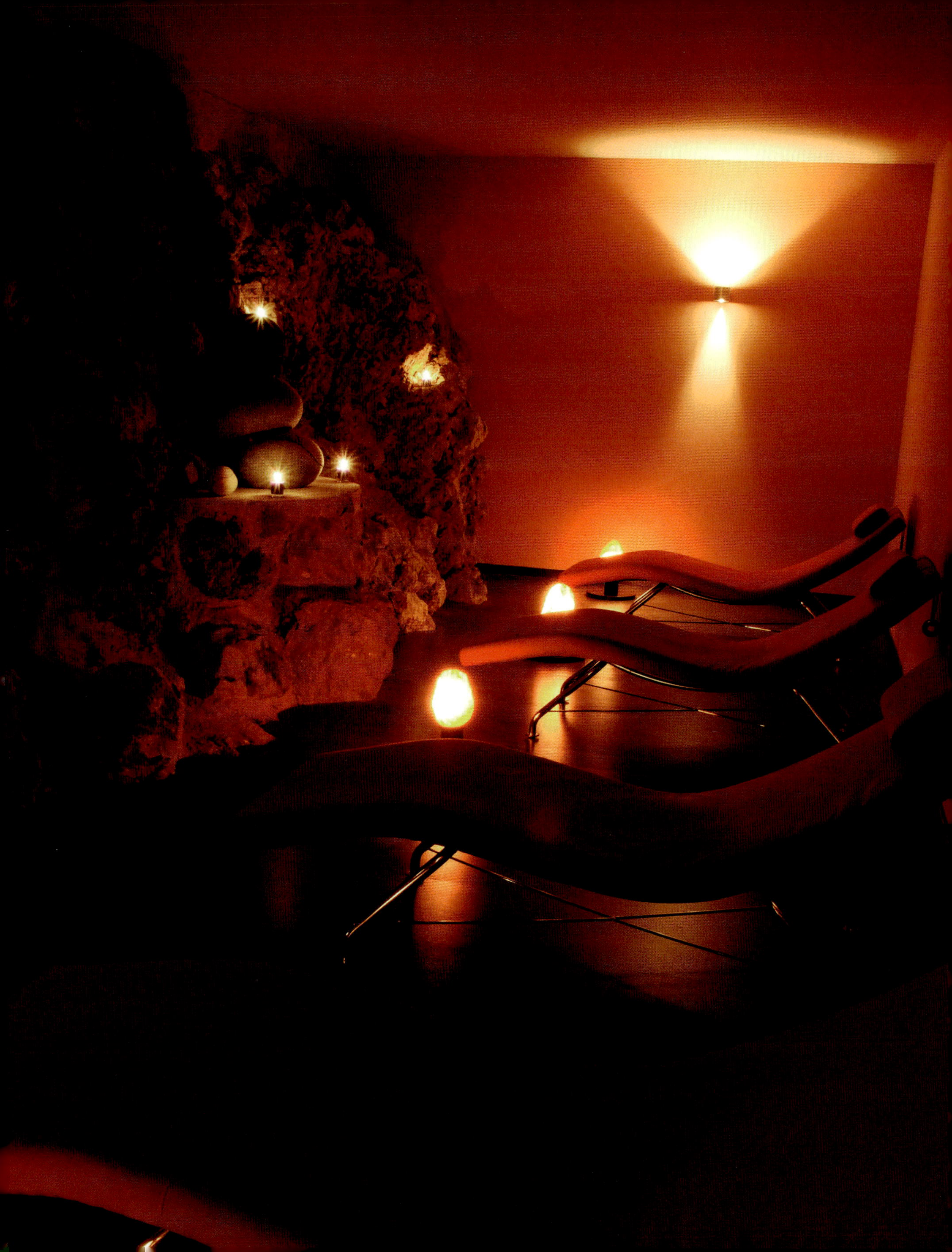

Spa Néocéa

Das 750 qm große Gelände des Spas beherbergt 11 innovative Räume für Schönheitsrituale wie „Grand Soin Aquananda“ mit rosafarbenen Himalayasalzen oder „Grand Soin Aquadream“ mit magnesiumhaltigem Meerwasser zur Remineraliserung des Körpers. Die Steinblöcke am Rande des Pools, entworfen von Stéphanie Marin, scheinen frei zu schweben und bilden ein surrealistisches Szenario, das die Balance zwischen Körper und Geist neu definiert.

The 8,000 square feet of the spa holds 11 innovative areas that have been designed for the beauty rituals such as the "Grand Soin Aquananda," with pink Himalayan salts, or the "Grand Soin Aquadream," with sea-water rich in magnesium to recharge the body with minerals. Designed by Stèphanie Marin, the large boulders that surround the pool seem to be levitating, and offer a surrealistic scenario in which the balance between mind and body is redefined.

Les 750 m² du spa comportent 11 cabines, conçues pour des rituels de beauté comme le « Grand Soin Aquananda » , à base de sel rose de l'Himalaya, ou le « Grand Soin Aquadream » , à base d'eau de mer riche en magnésium, un soin idéal pour recharger le corps en minéraux. Conçues par Stéphanie Marin, les imposantes pierres qui entourent la piscine semblent être en lévitation et offrent un décor surréaliste dans lequel l'équilibre entre l'esprit et le corps est redéfini.

Op een terrein van 750 m² liggen elf innovatieve ruimten die zijn ontworpen voor schoonheidsbehandelingen als de 'Grand Soin Aquananda', met roze Himalayazout, en de 'Grand Soin Aquadream', met magnesiumrijk zeewater, om het lichaam van mineralen te voorzien. Dit is een ontwerp van Stéphanie Marin, met grote zwerfkeien die rond het zwembad lijken te zweven en voor een surrealistisch decor zorgen, waarin de balans tussen geest en lichaam hernieuwd wordt.

Saint Paul de Vence, France

DANIEL JOUVANCE

Photos © Gilles Bailleux

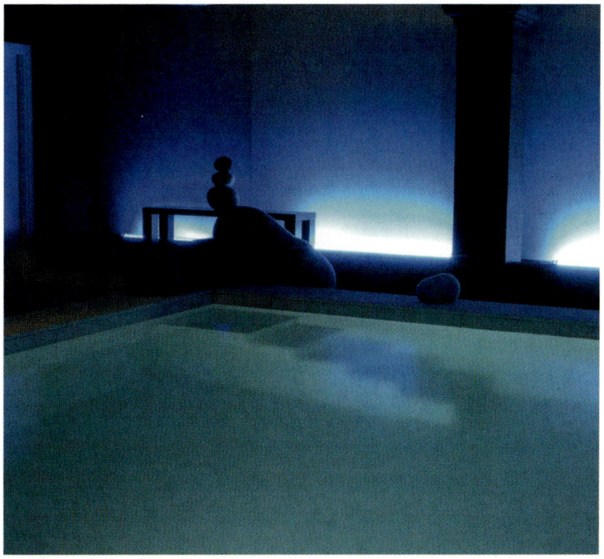

www.mas-artigny.com

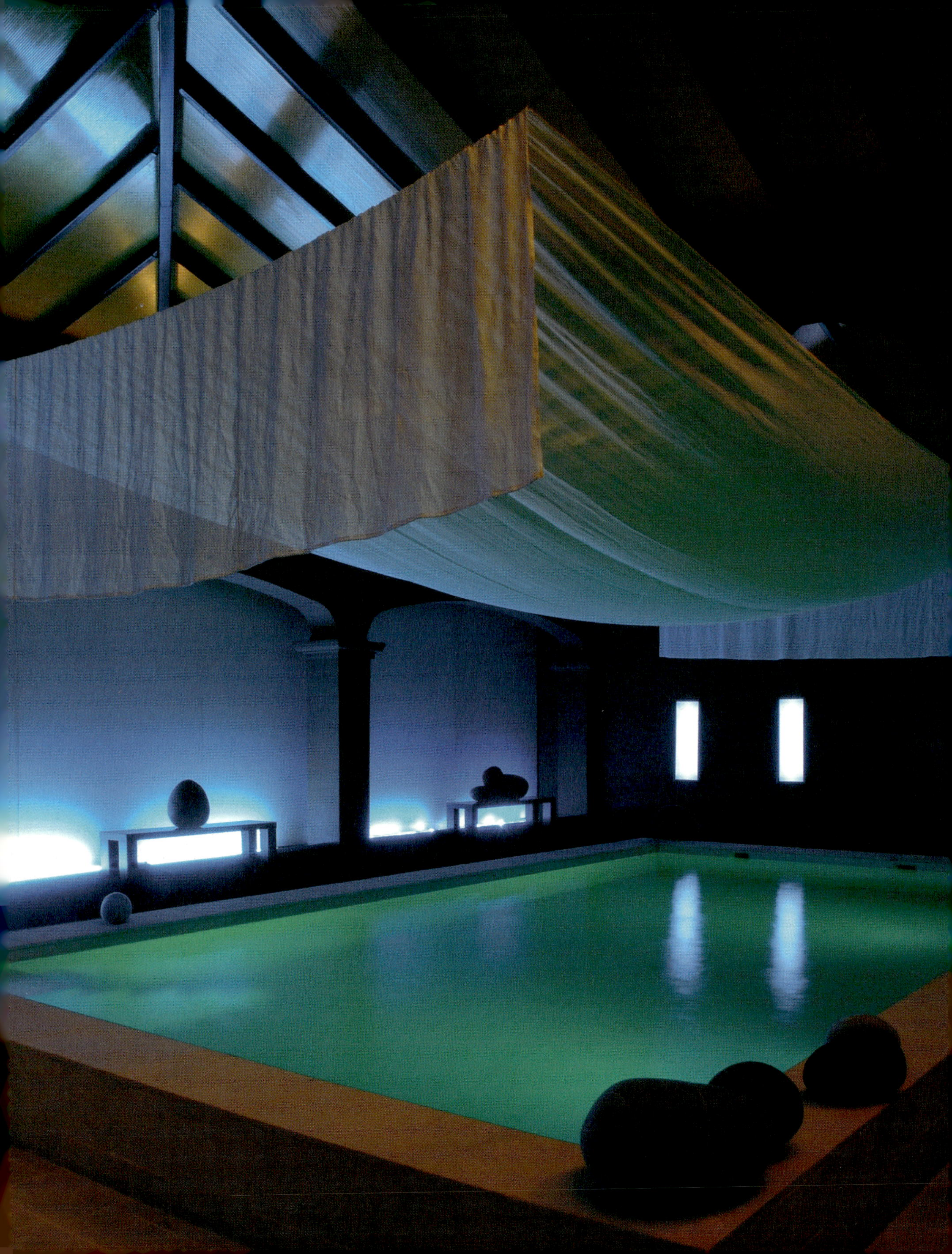

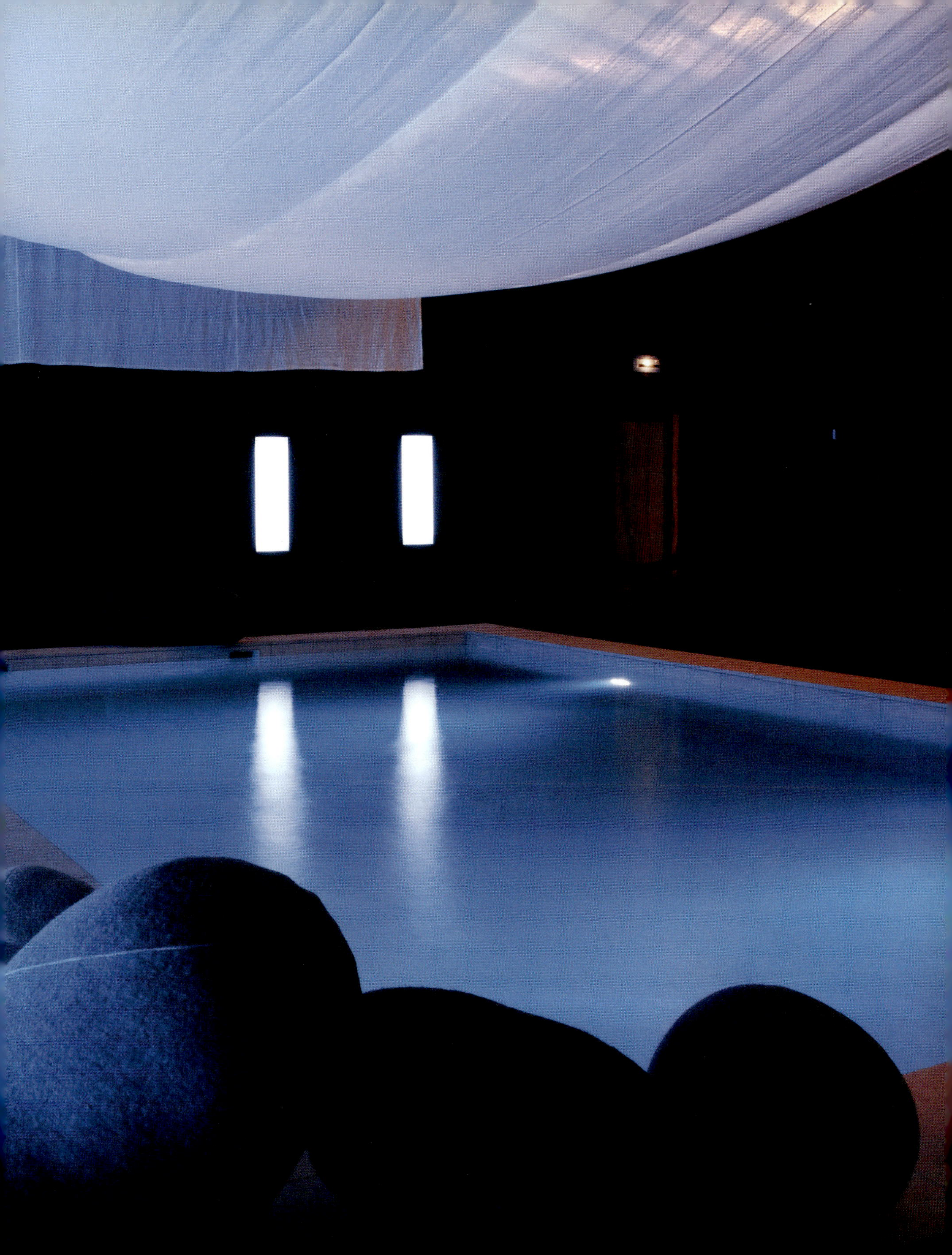

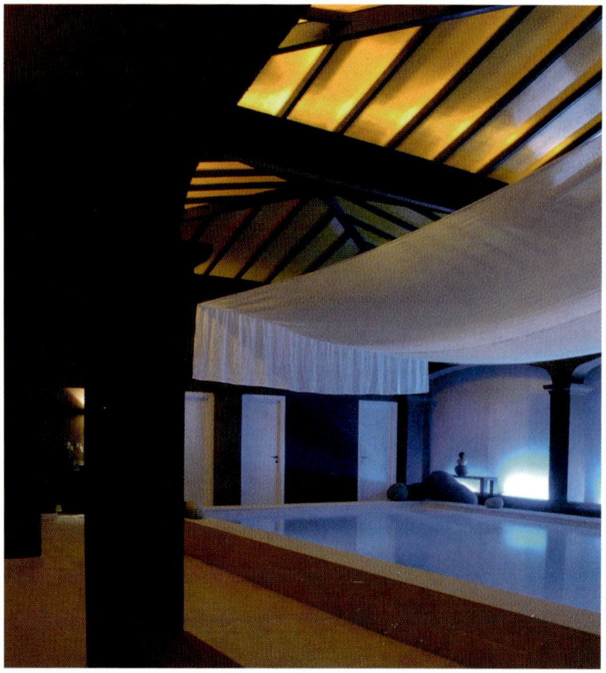

Das Zusammenspiel von Licht, Farben und Steinen verleiht dem Swimming Pool ein surrealistisches Ambiente.

The variations in the light and the boulders offer a surrealist image of the main swimming pool.

Les variations de lumière et les rochers confèrent à la piscine principale une ambiance onirique.

De belichting en de zwerfkeien geven het grote zwembad iets surrealistisch.

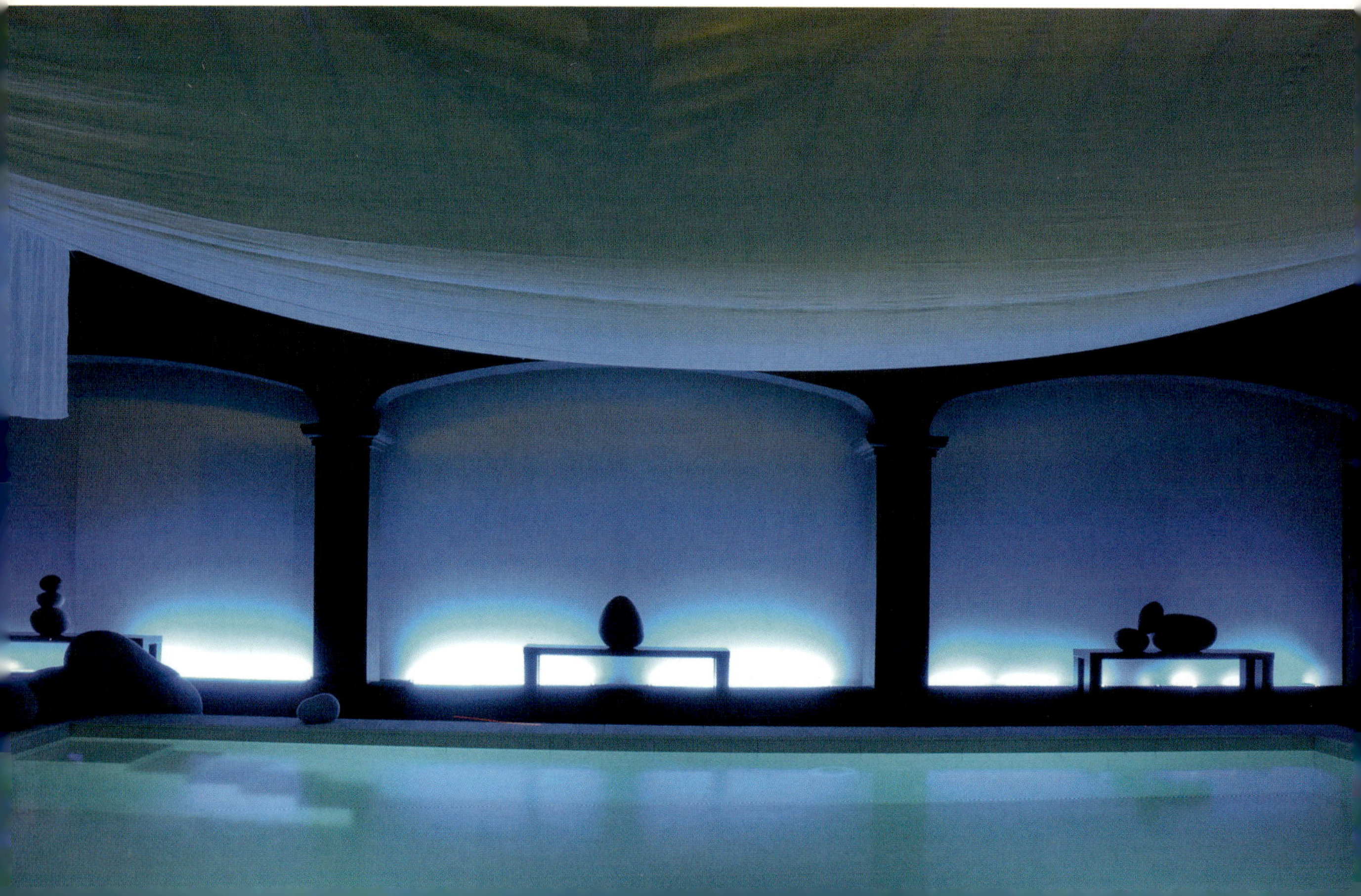

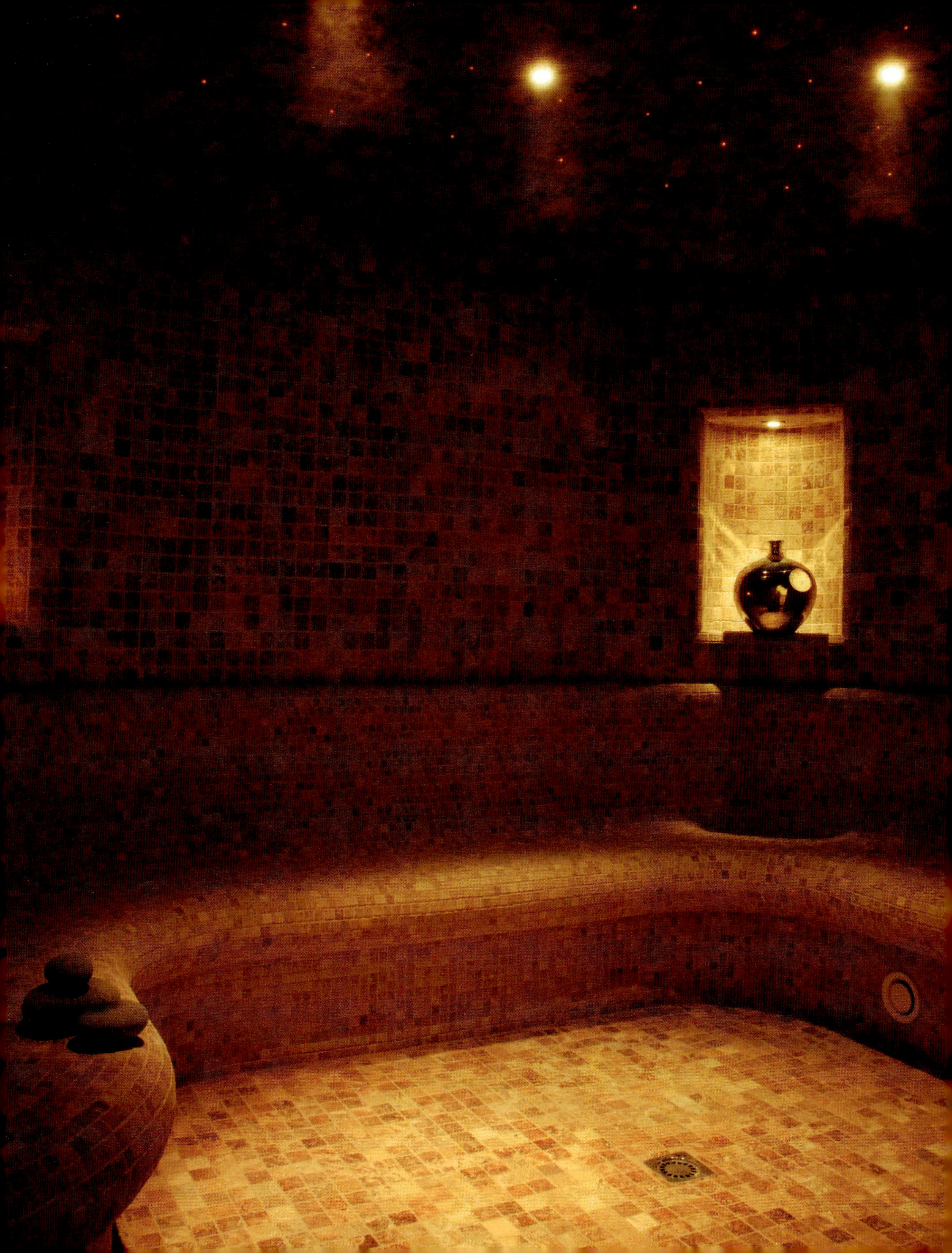

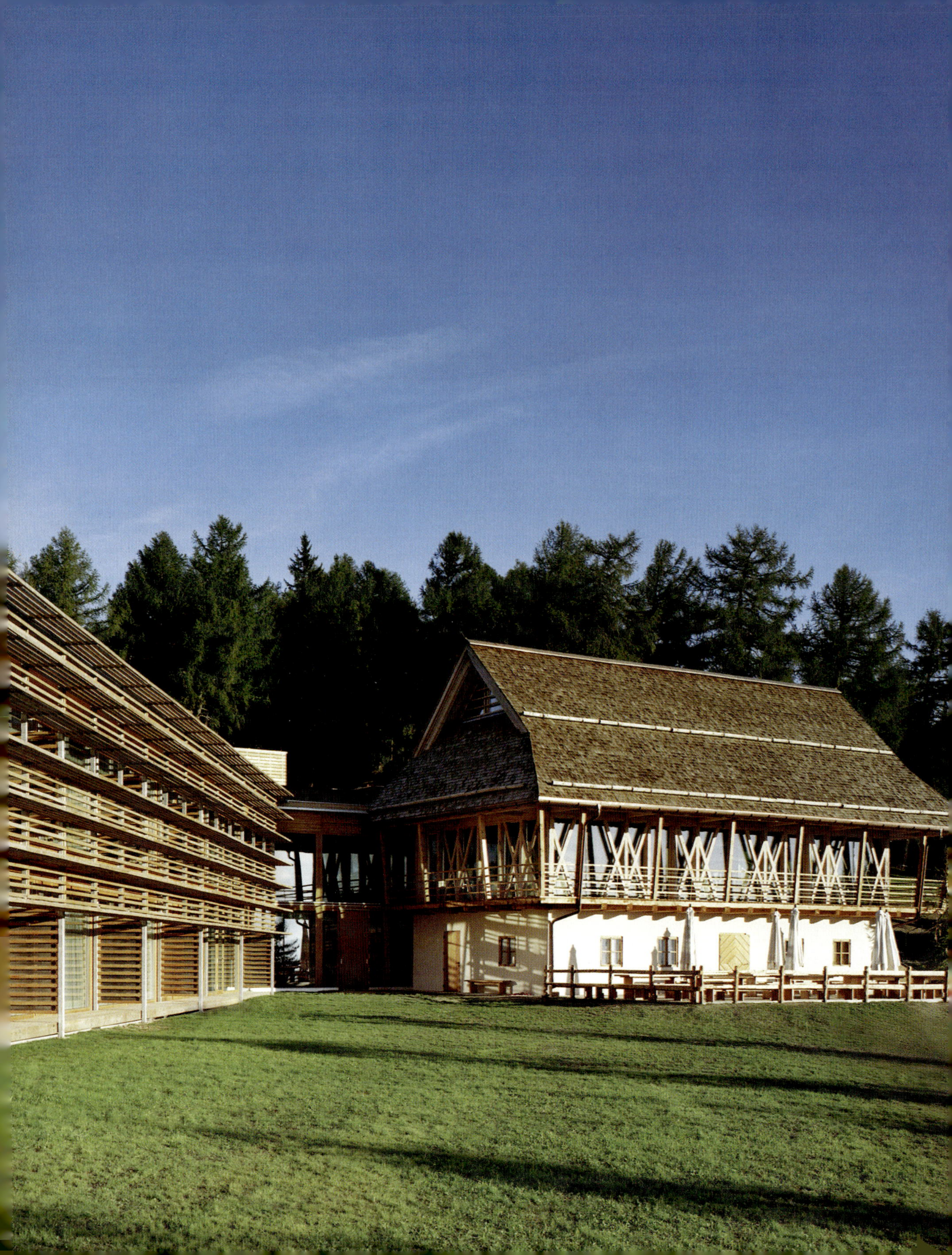

Vigilius Mountain Resort

Dieses in 1.500 Meter Höhe gelegene Resort scheint gleichsam mit der umliegenden Natur zu verschmelzen. Die Fassade mit den parallel angeordneten Holzplanken unterstreicht den Horizontalcharakter des Gebäudes und lenkt zudem den Blick auf das herrliche Waldpanorama. Gedeckte Farben, Holz und heller Naturstein vermitteln eine luxuriöse und zugleich behagliche Atmosphäre, die den geeigneten Rahmen für unterschiedlichste Anwendungen und Massagen bietet.

At 4,900 feet above sea level, the Vigilius Mountain Resort is able to blend with the nature that surrounds it. In the façade, the wooden planks placed parallel to each other highlight the horizontal characteristic of the construction without renouncing the amazing views over the woods. The neutral colors, the wood and the stone in light tones achieve luxurious and cozy aesthetics, which create an atmosphere that is suitable for receiving all sorts of treatments and massages.

À 1.500 m d'altitude, le Vigilius Mountain Resort semble se fondre dans la nature qui l'environne. Les lattes de bois parallèles sur la façade soulignent le caractère horizontal de la construction sans pour autant obturer le panorama étonnant sur les bois. Les couleurs douces et les tons légers du bois et de la pierre confèrent une esthétique luxueuse et confortable, créant une atmosphère propice à toutes sortes de soins et massages.

Het Vigilius Mountain Resort, dat 1500 meter boven zeeniveau ligt, voegt zich naadloos in de omringende natuur. De parallel aangebrachte planken op de gevel benadrukken het horizontale karakter van het gebouw zonder afbreuk te doen aan het verbluffende uitzicht op de bossen. De neutrale kleuren en de lichte tinten van hout en steen leveren een stijlvolle gezelligheid op en een sfeer die bij uitstek geschikt is voor allerlei kuurbehandelingen en massages.

Monte San Vigilio, Italy

MATTEO THUN

Photos © Design Hotels

www.vigilius.it

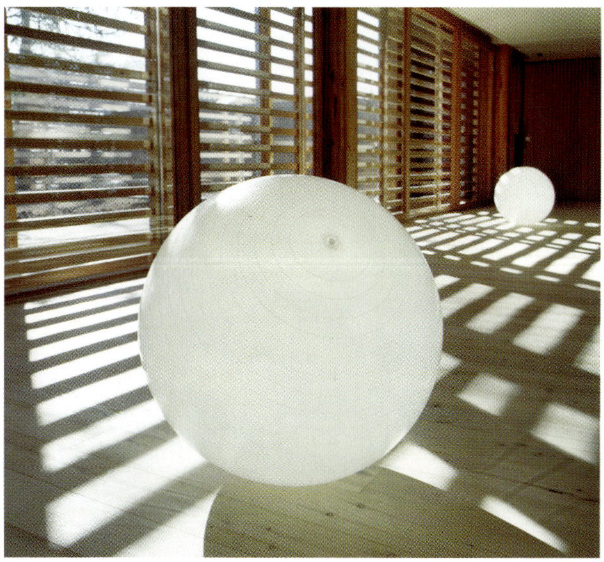

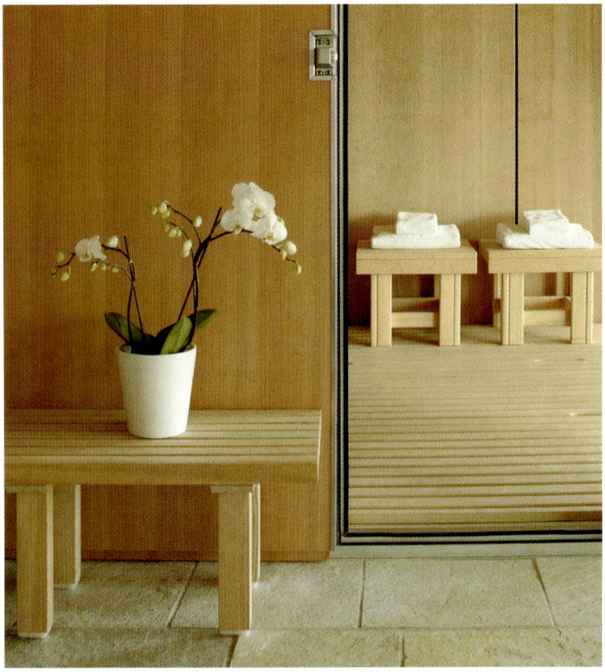

Außergewöhnliche Interieurs, exquisite italienische Küche und ein extravagantes Spa zeichnen dieses Luxusrefugium aus.

The exceptional interiors, exquisite Italian food, and the hedonistic spa represent the future of luxurious retreats.

Les intérieurs exceptionnels, l'incomparable cuisine italienne et le spa hédoniste symbolisent l'avenir des retraites voluptueuses.

De inrichting, het verfijnde eten en de hedonistische baden vertegenwoordigen de toekomst van het luxe ontspanningsoord.

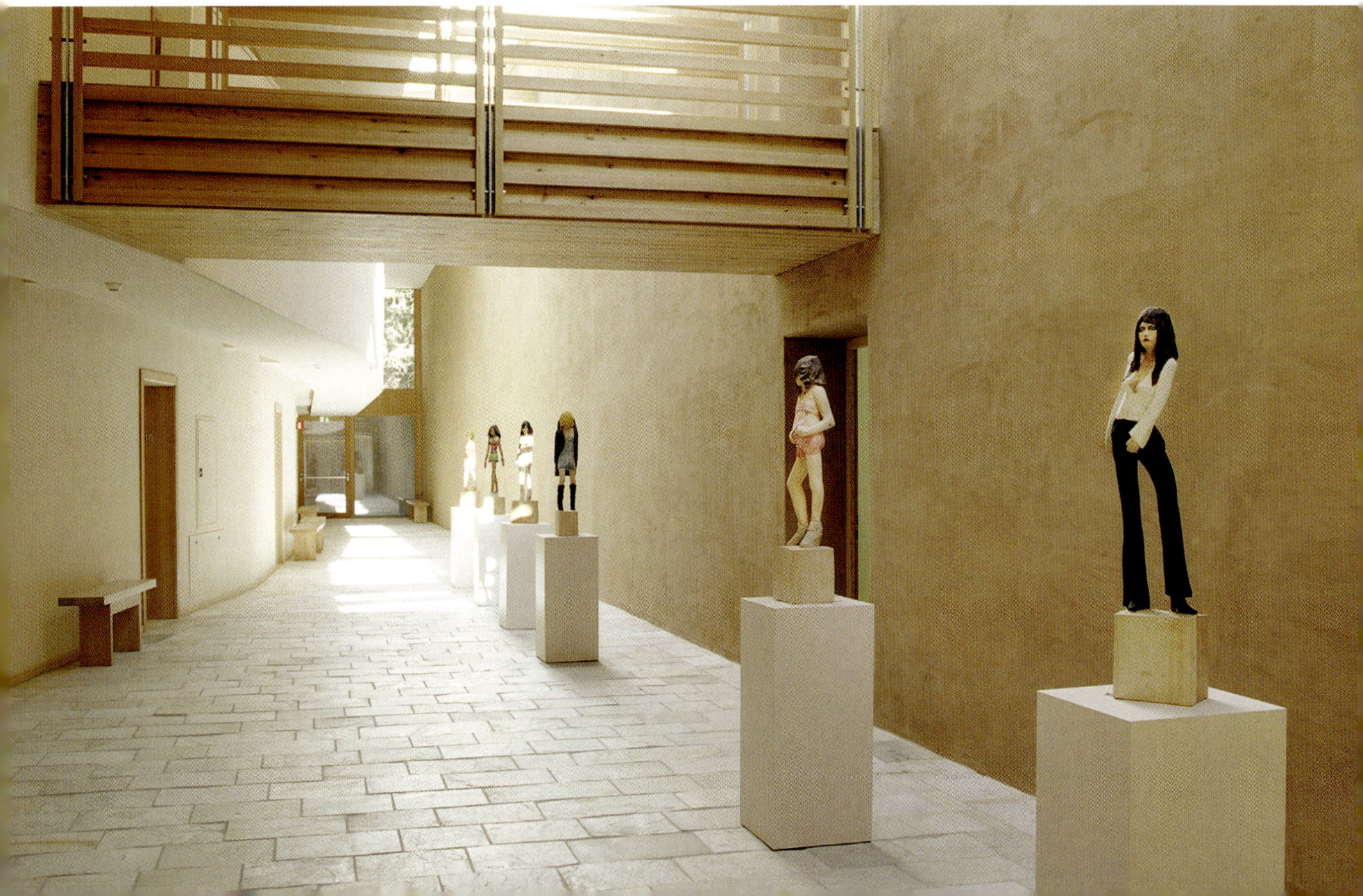

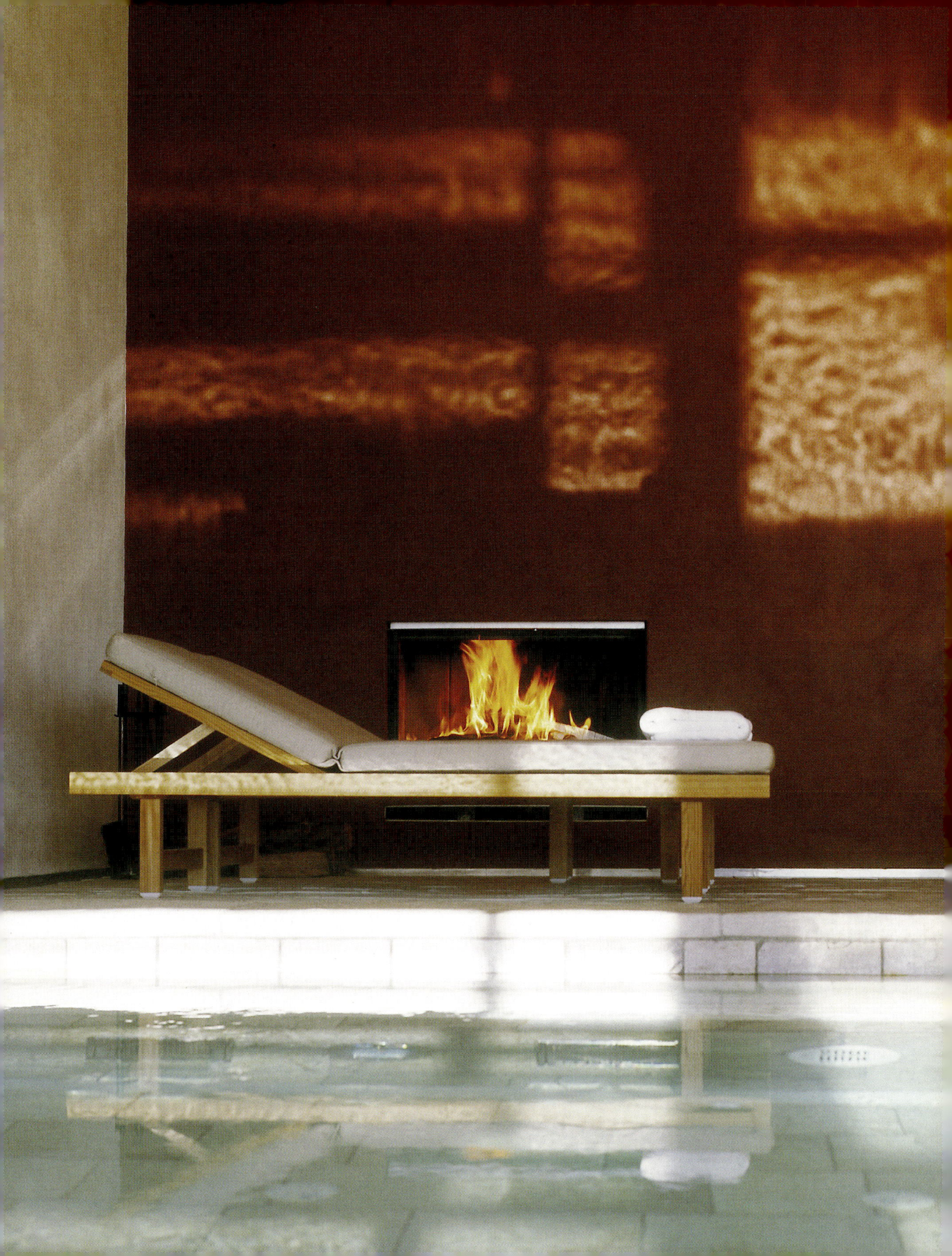

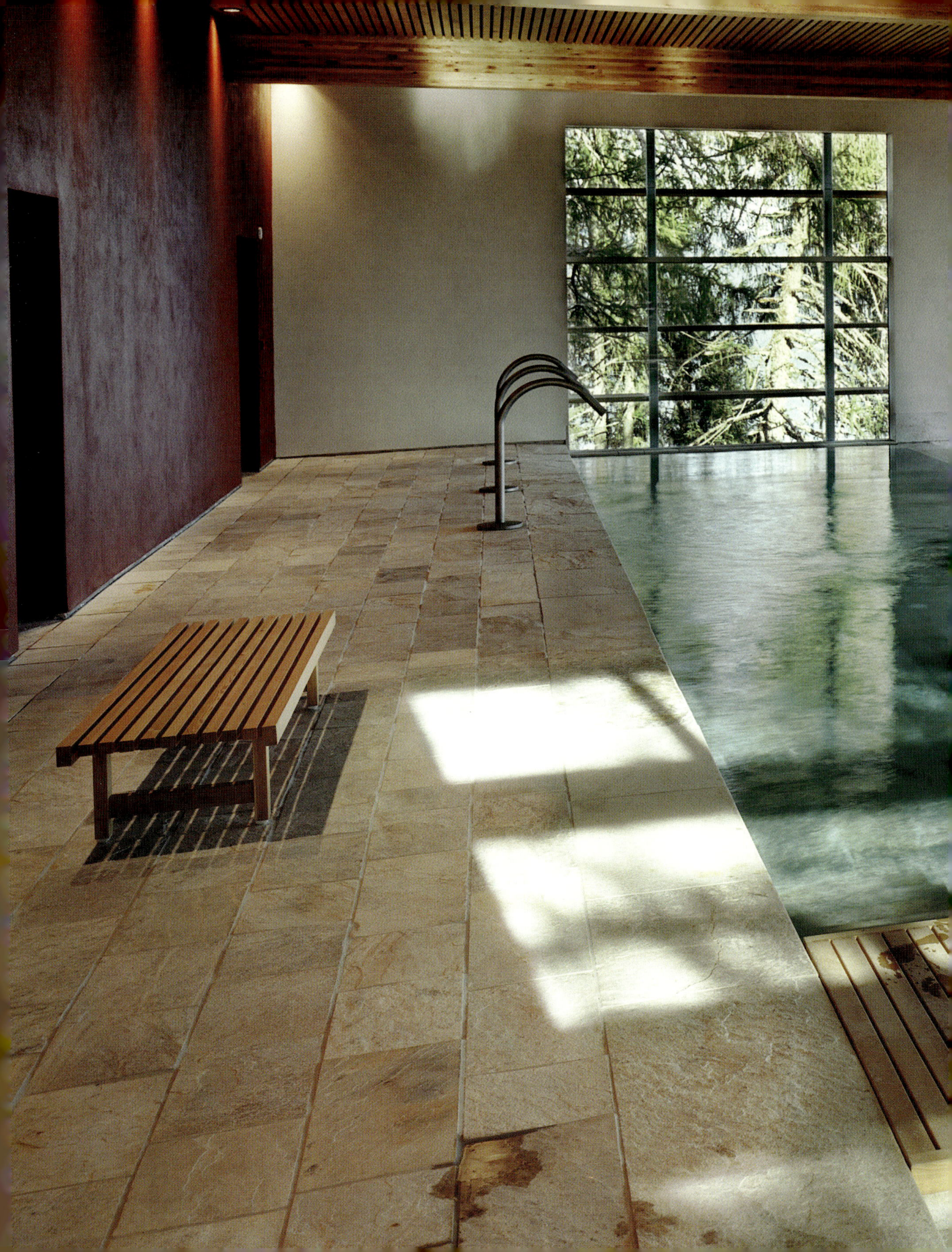

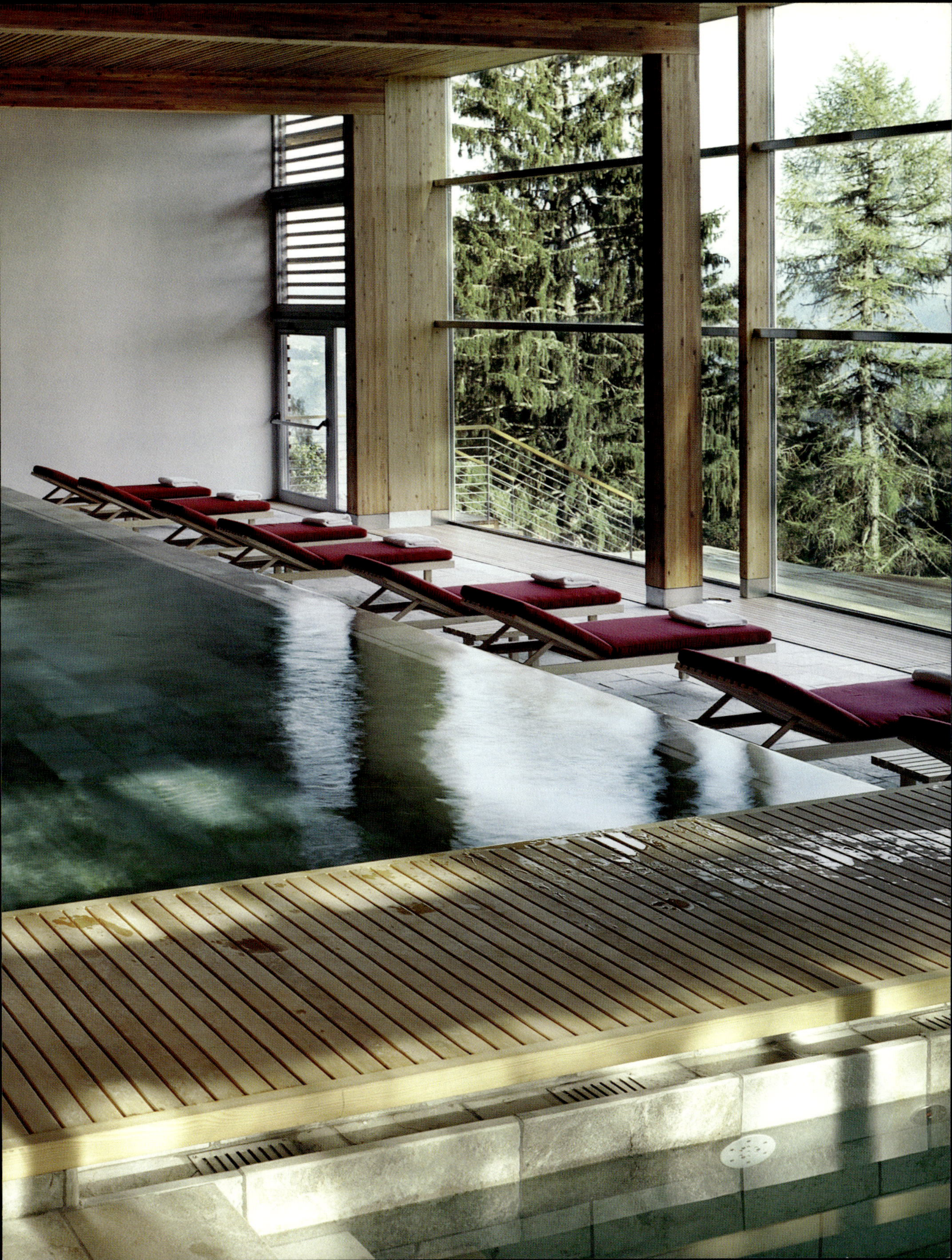

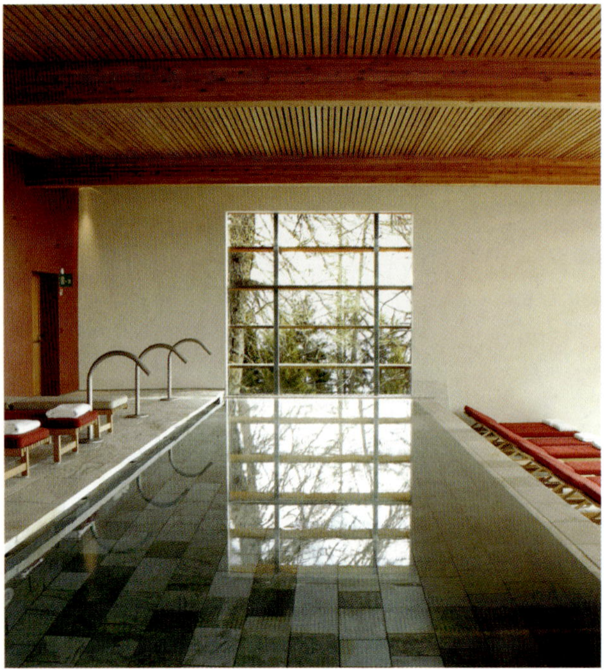

Vom überdachten Pool aus bieten große Fassadenfenster einen herrlichen Blick auf die Gebirgslandschaft.

The great windows that cover the façade offer views of the mountainous landscape from the covered pool.

Les grandes baies vitrées de la façade de la piscine couverte offrent une superbe vue sur le paysage montagneux.

De grote vensters bieden vanuit het binnenbad uitzicht op het berglandschap.

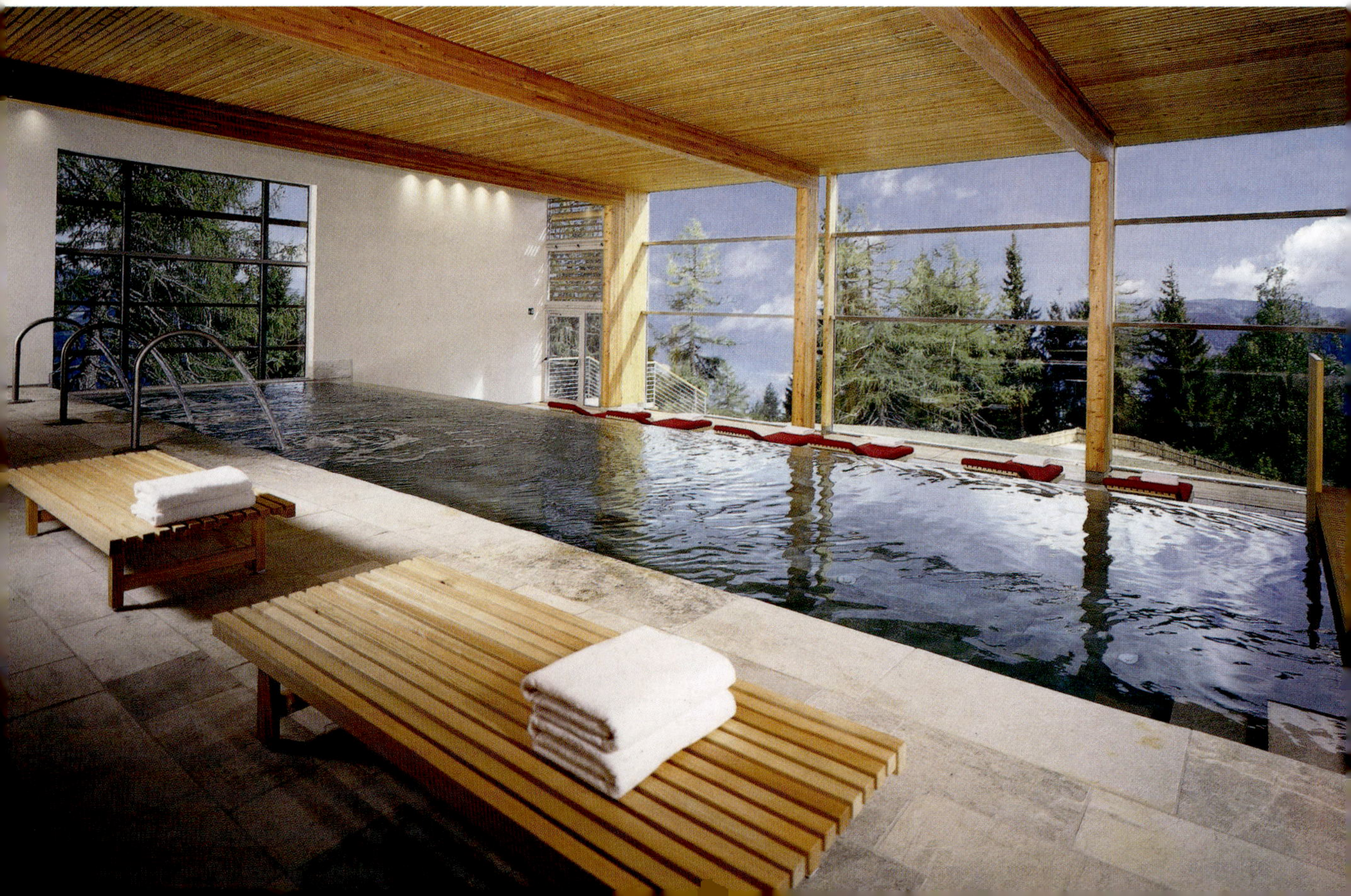

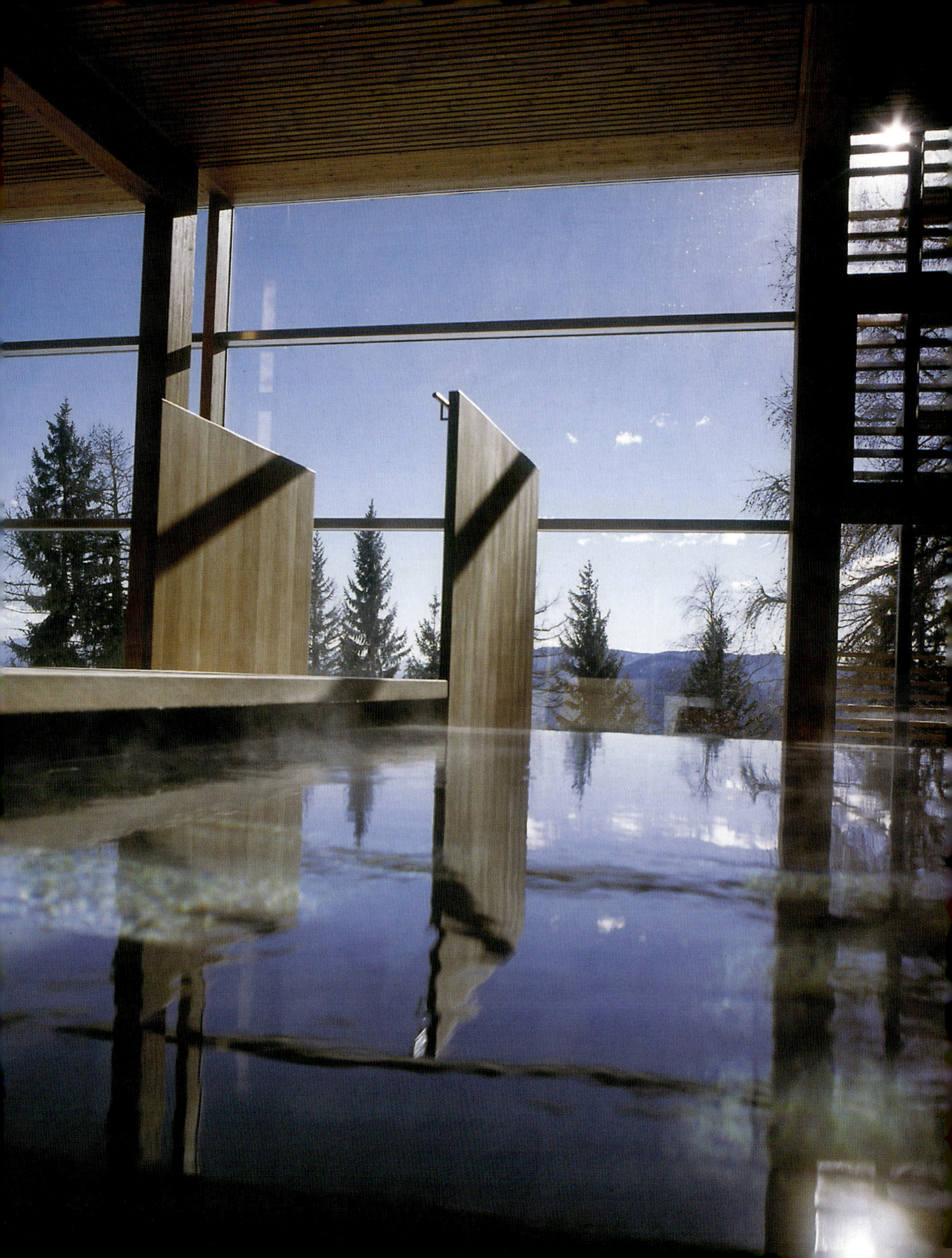

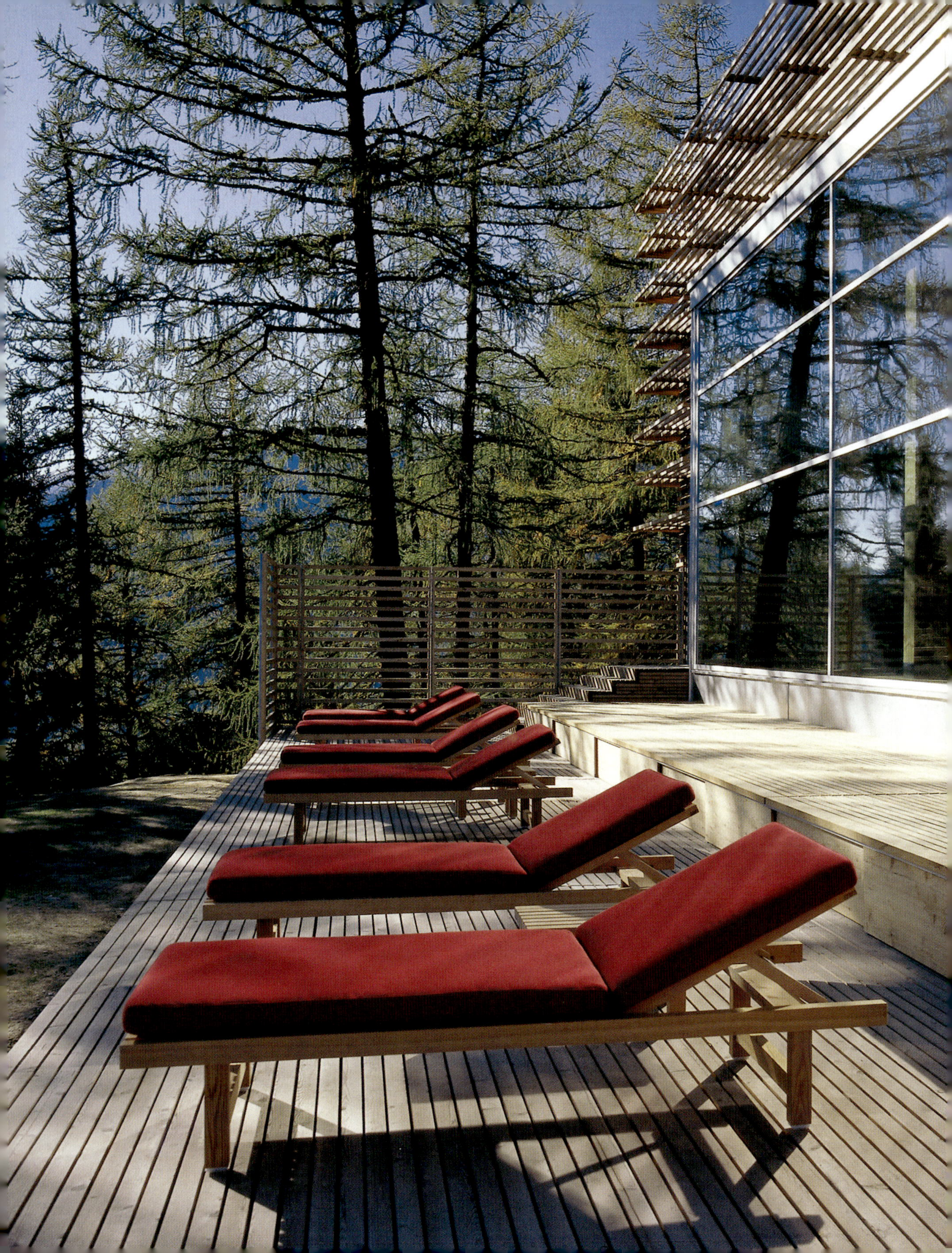

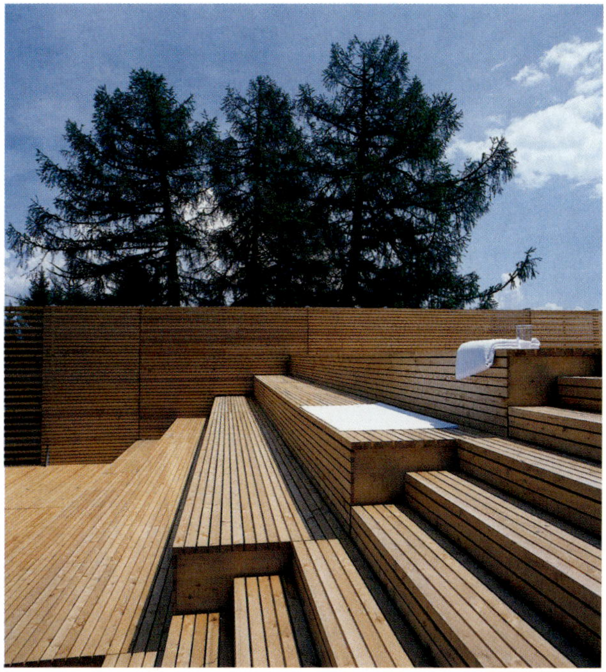

Im gesamten Spa vermitteln Holz und andere Naturmaterialien eine warme und entspannte Atmosphäre.

Throughout the spa one gets a feeling of warmth and serenity thanks to the predominance of wood and natural materials.

L'impression de chaleur et de sérénité prédomine partout dans le spa grâce à l'emploi du bois et de matériaux naturels.

Het complex ademt een sfeer van warmte en rust, dankzij het gebruik van hout en andere natuurlijke materialen.

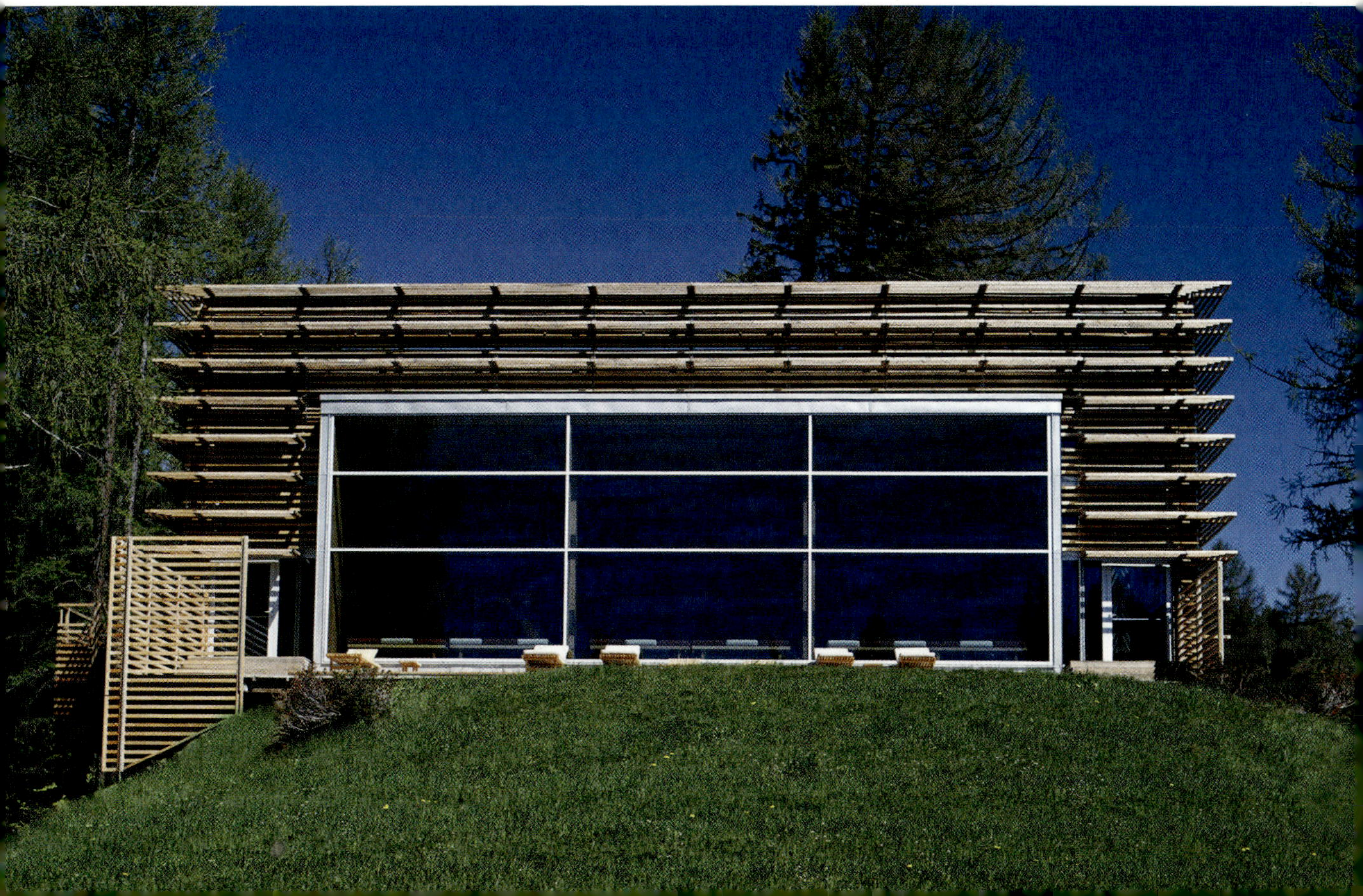

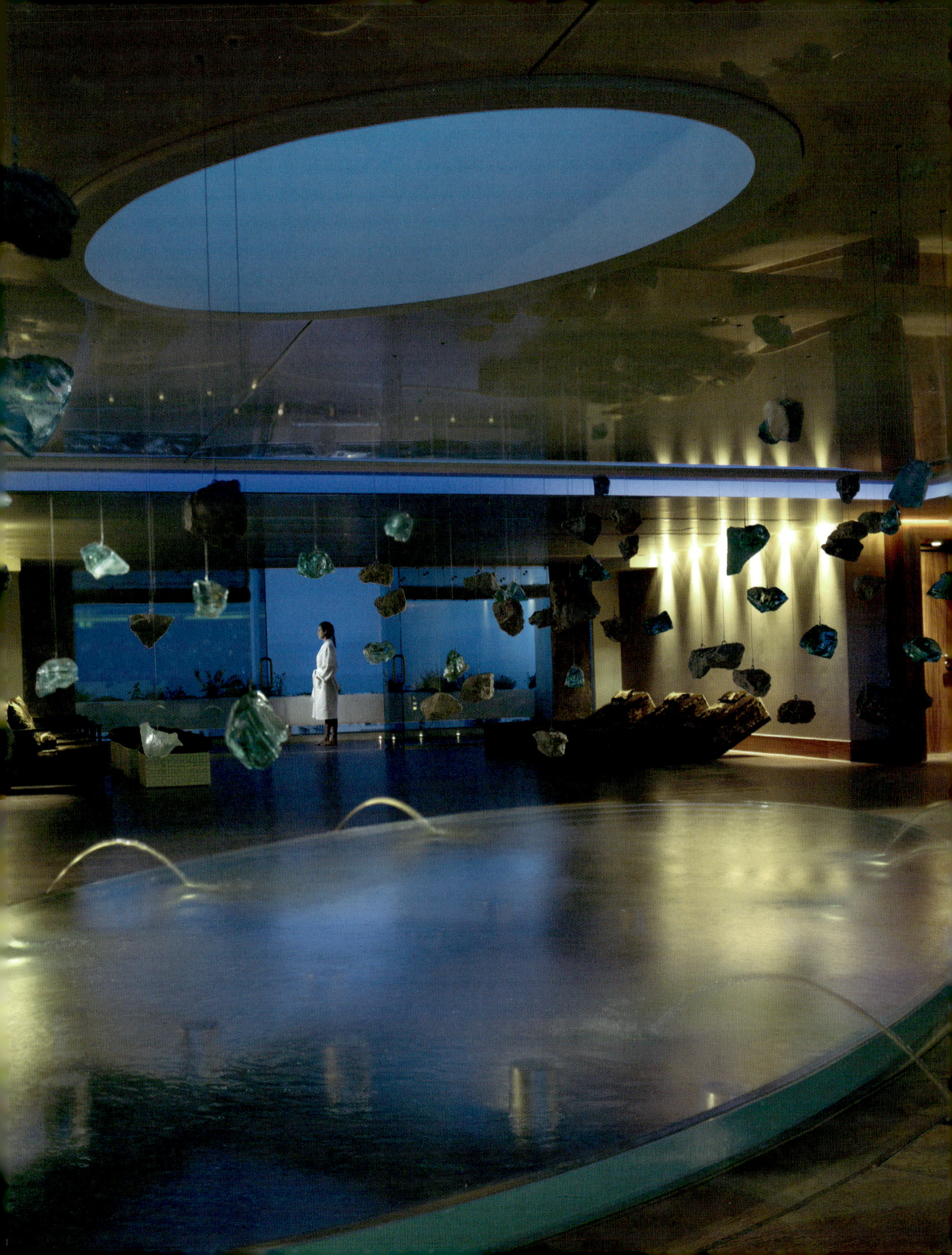

Porto Elounda De Luxe Resort

Dieses in der Mirabello Bucht gelegene Spa lockt mit Sprudelbädern auf der Terrasse und einem Thalassopool mit herrlichem Blick auf die griechischen Inseln. Als gleichfalls spektakuläre Kulisse erweist sich der Hauptbereich des Spas, das Tepidarium, wo Wasser als eines der Grundelemente der Natur sehr eindrucksvoll in Szene gesetzt wird: Es stürzt kaskadenartig in die Tiefe, sprudelt in Glasbecken und leuchtet in Kristallteichen.

Taking a bubble bath on the terrace or diving into the thalassotherapy pool with views of the Greek islands is a pleasure available at the Elounda, located on the Mirabello bay. As a fantastic stage, the main precinct, called tepidarium, holds outstanding facilities that appeal to the basic elements of nature. Water is the protagonist here, transparent in the great waterfall, bubbling in the glass pools and bright in the elevated crystal ponds.

Prendre un bain bouillonnant sur la terrasse ou plonger dans la piscine dédiée à la thalassothérapie en profitant d'une vue imprenable sur les îles grecques est un plaisir à votre portée à Elounda, situé sur la baie de Mirabello. Comme une scène fantastique, l'enceinte principale, ou tepidarium, propose des équipements fantastiques basés sur les éléments naturels. L'eau est ici au centre de tout, transparente dans la grande chute d'eau, bouillonnante dans les piscines de verre et lumineuse dans le bassin translucide du plafond.

Een bubbelbad op het terras of een duik in het thalassotherapiebad met uitzicht op de Griekse eilanden – het kan in het Elounda, gelegen aan de baai van Mirabello. Het zogenaamde tepidarium ziet eruit als een fantastisch podium voor allerlei faciliteiten die teruggrijpen op de basiselementen van de natuur. Water speelt de hoofdrol: het valt transparant neer in de grote waterval, borrelt in de glazen baden en schittert in de verhoogde, kristalheldere vijvers.

Crete, Greece

THE SYNTAX GROUP

Photos © Dimitris Poupalos

www.portoelounda.com

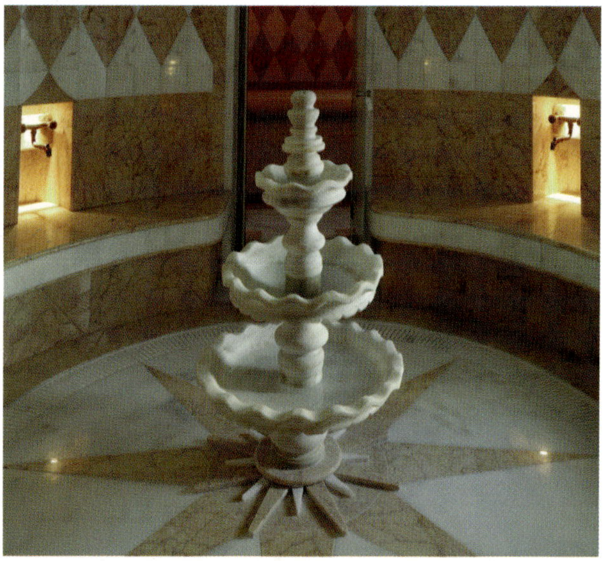

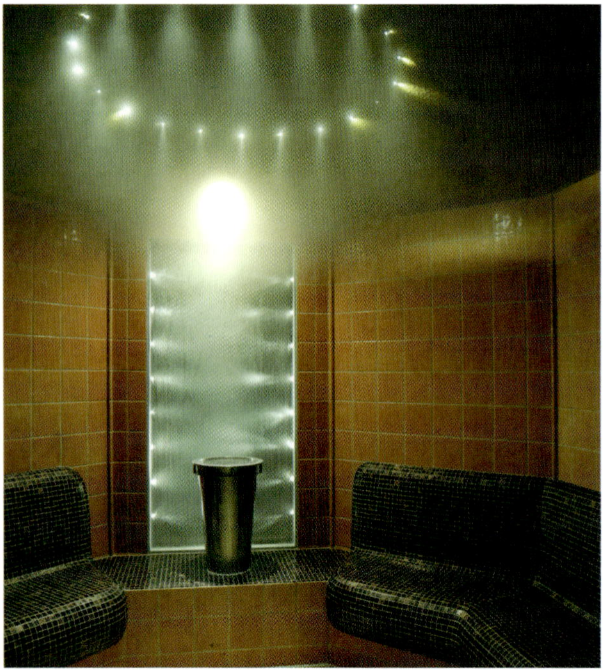

Im Tepidarium, dessen Name auf römische Badehäuser zurückgeht, ist Wasser das gemeinsame Element aller Therapien.

At the tepidarium, which takes its name from Roman baths, water is the main thread connecting all therapies.

Dans le tepidarium, qui tient son nom des bains romains, l'eau est le fil conducteur reliant toutes les zones de soins.

In het tepidarium, een naam die komt uit de oude Romeinse baden, is water het verbindende motief tussen de therapieën.

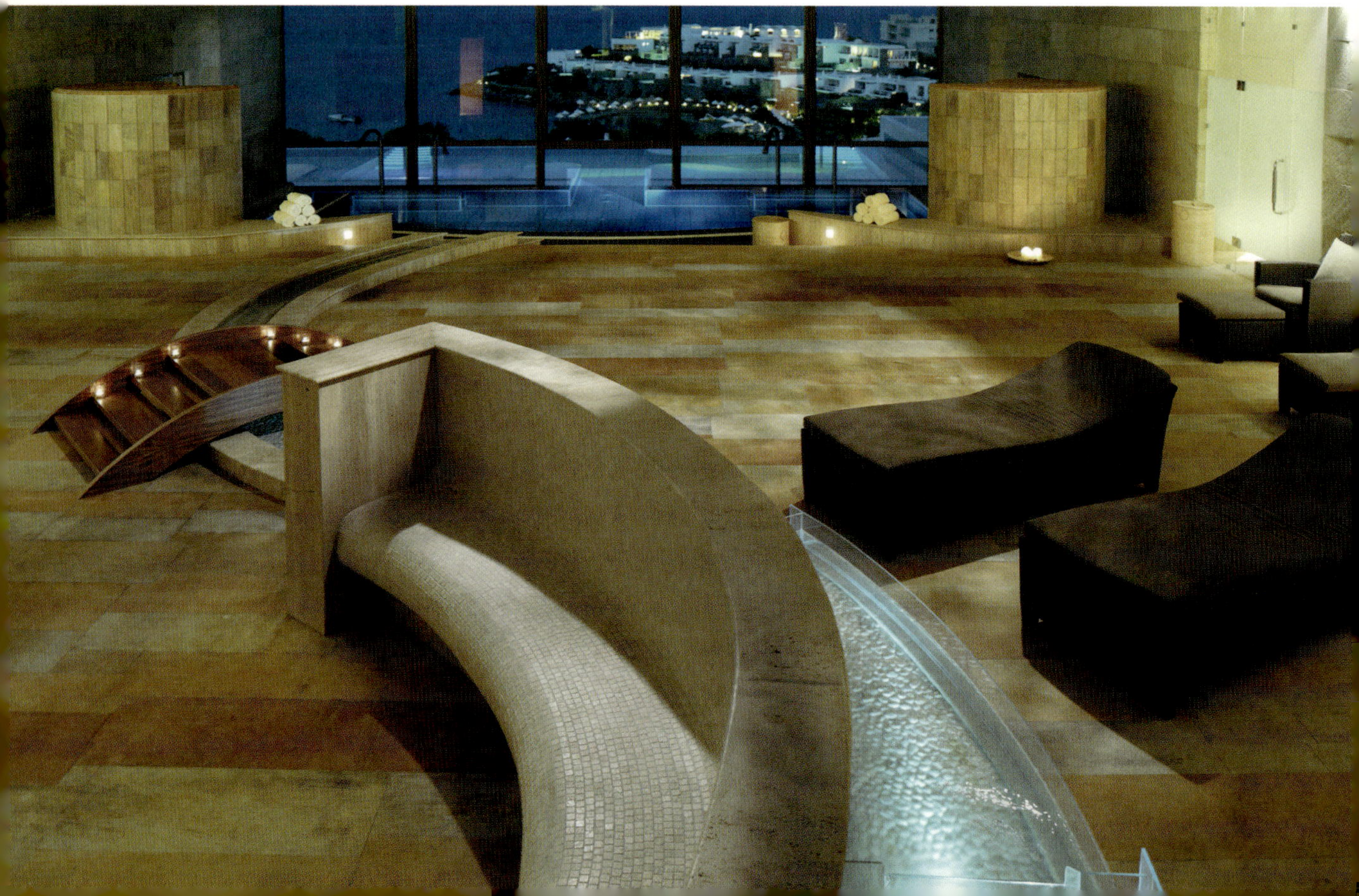

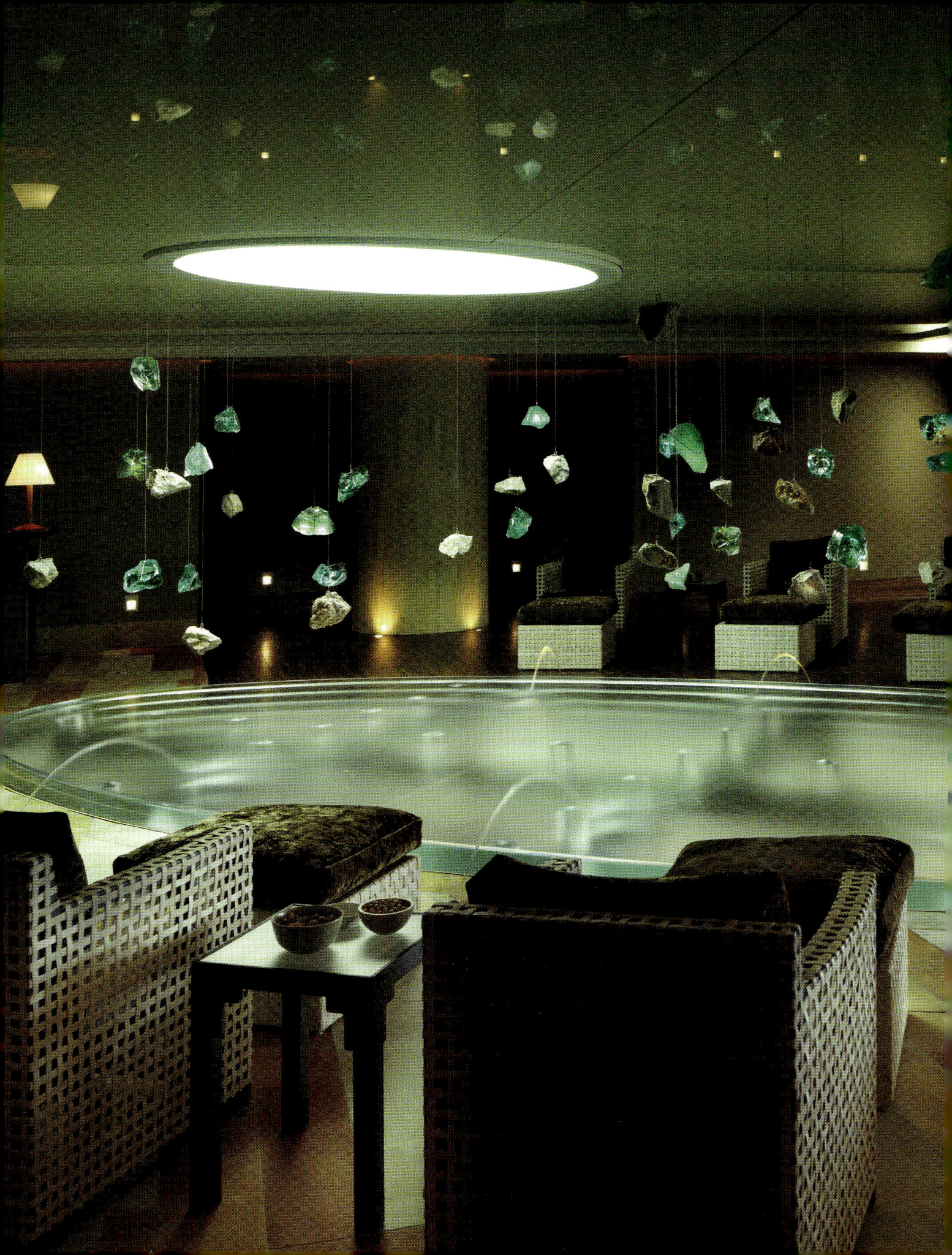

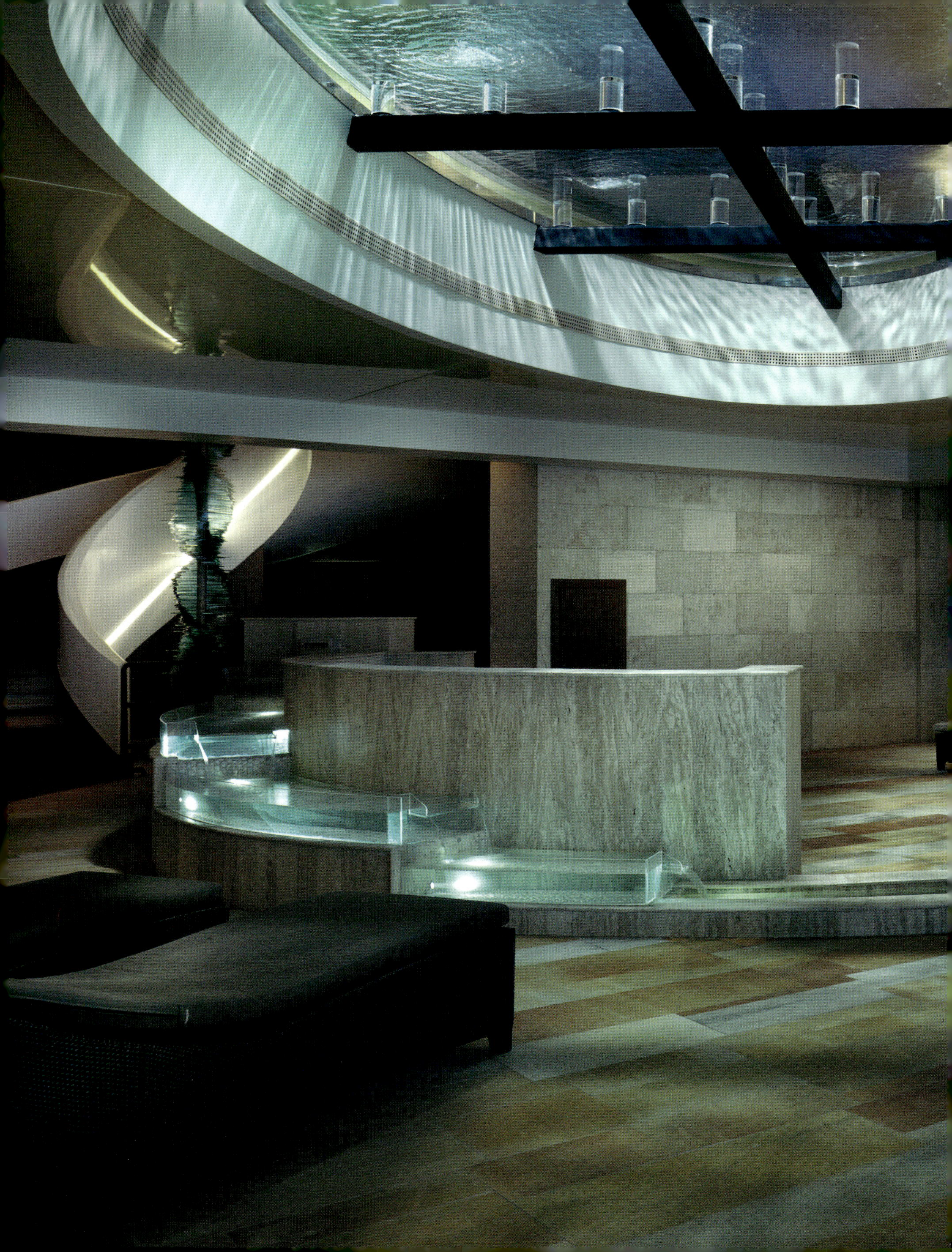

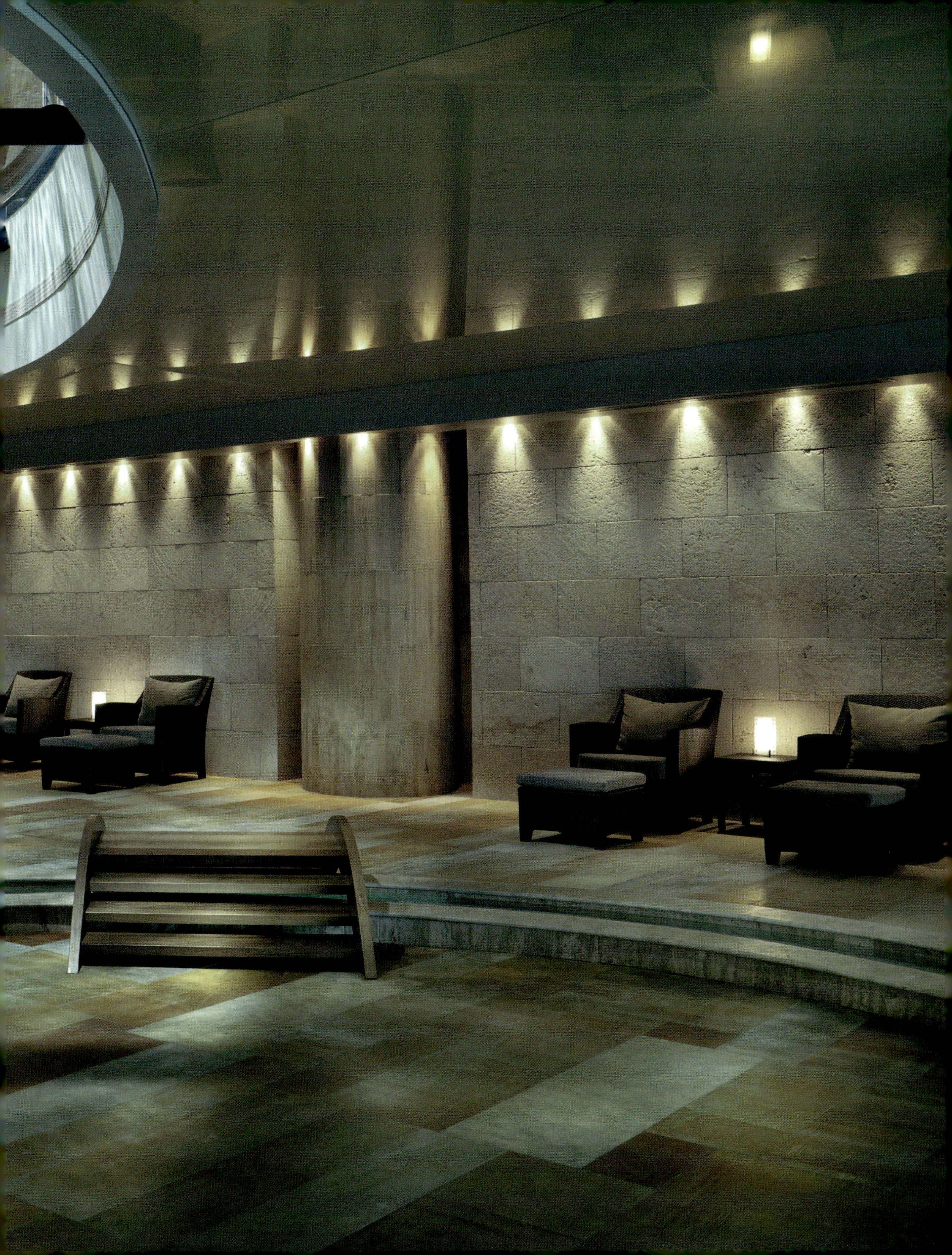

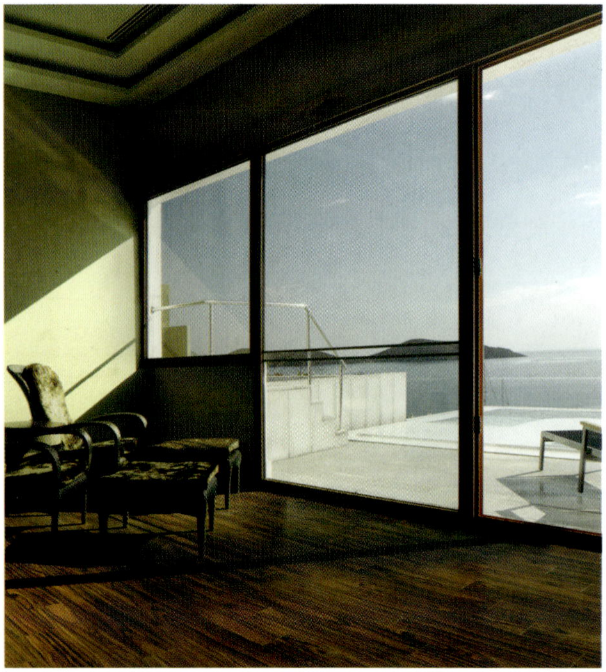

Der Whirlpool mit Innen- und Außenbereich bietet einen herrlichen Meerblick.

The whirlpool has an inside section and an outside one from which it is possible to see the marine landscape.

Intérieur et extérieur communiquent par la piscine à bulles, d'où l'on peut contempler le paysage marin.

De whirlpool heeft een binnengebied en een openluchtafdeling met uitzicht op zee.

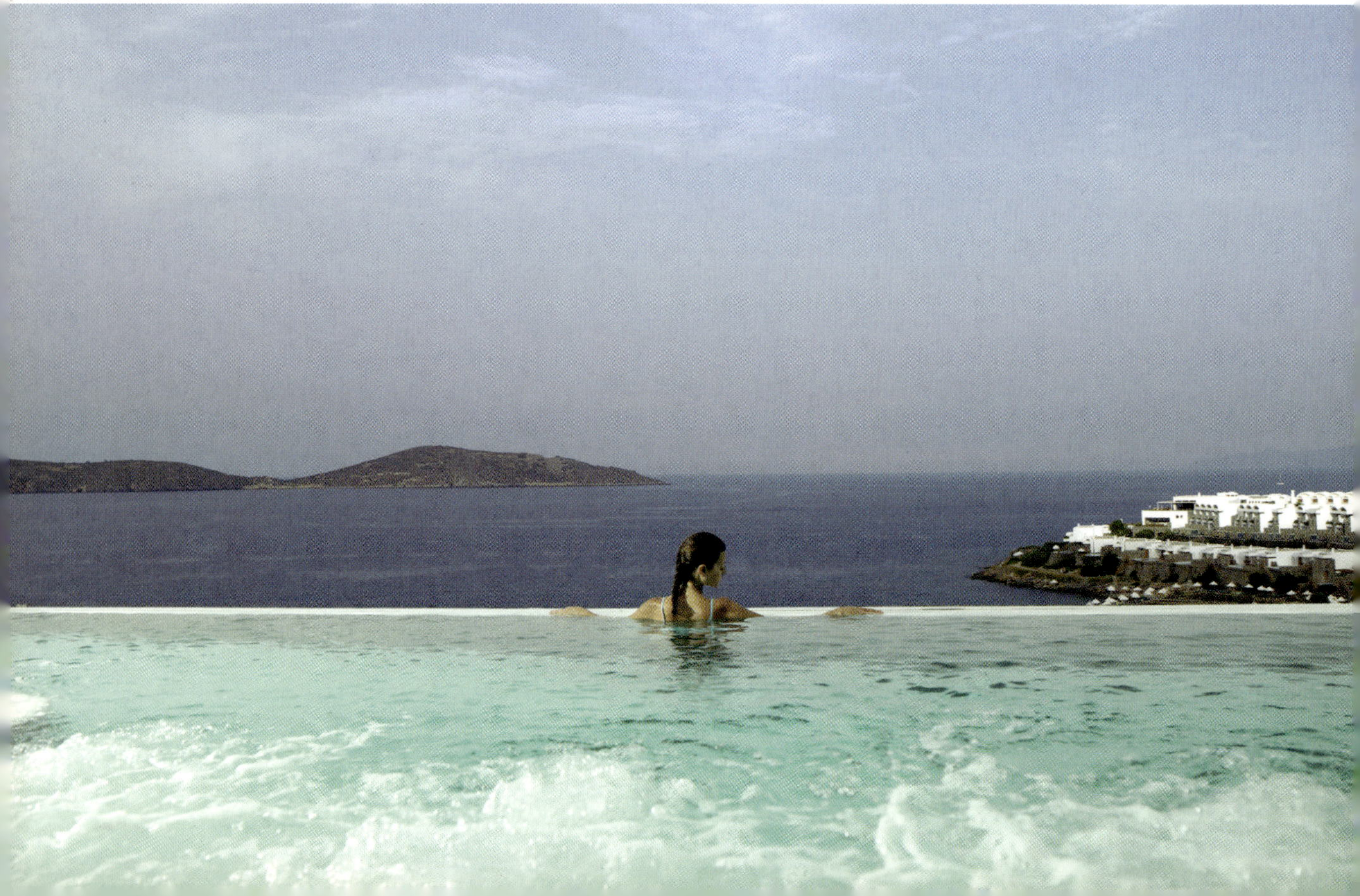

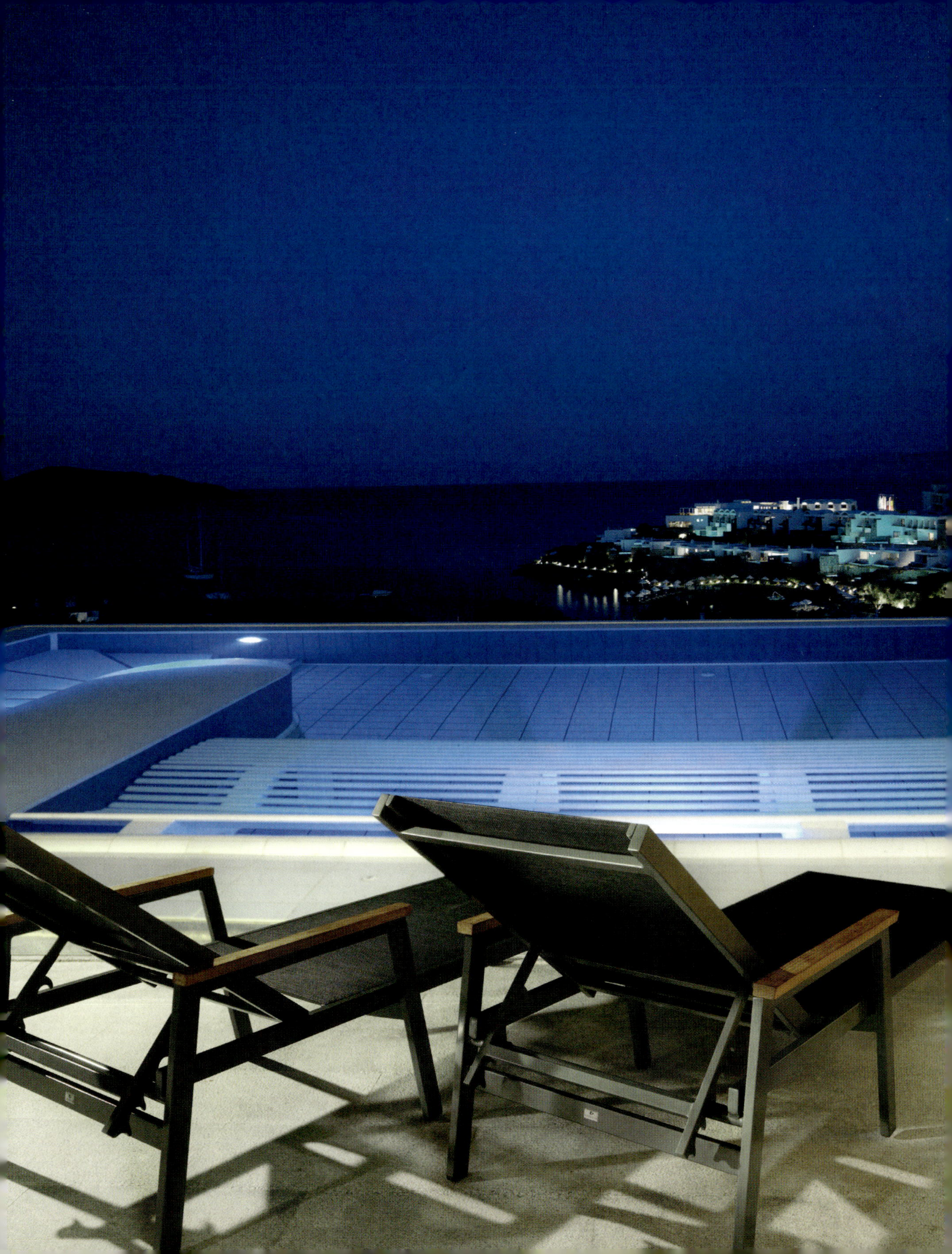

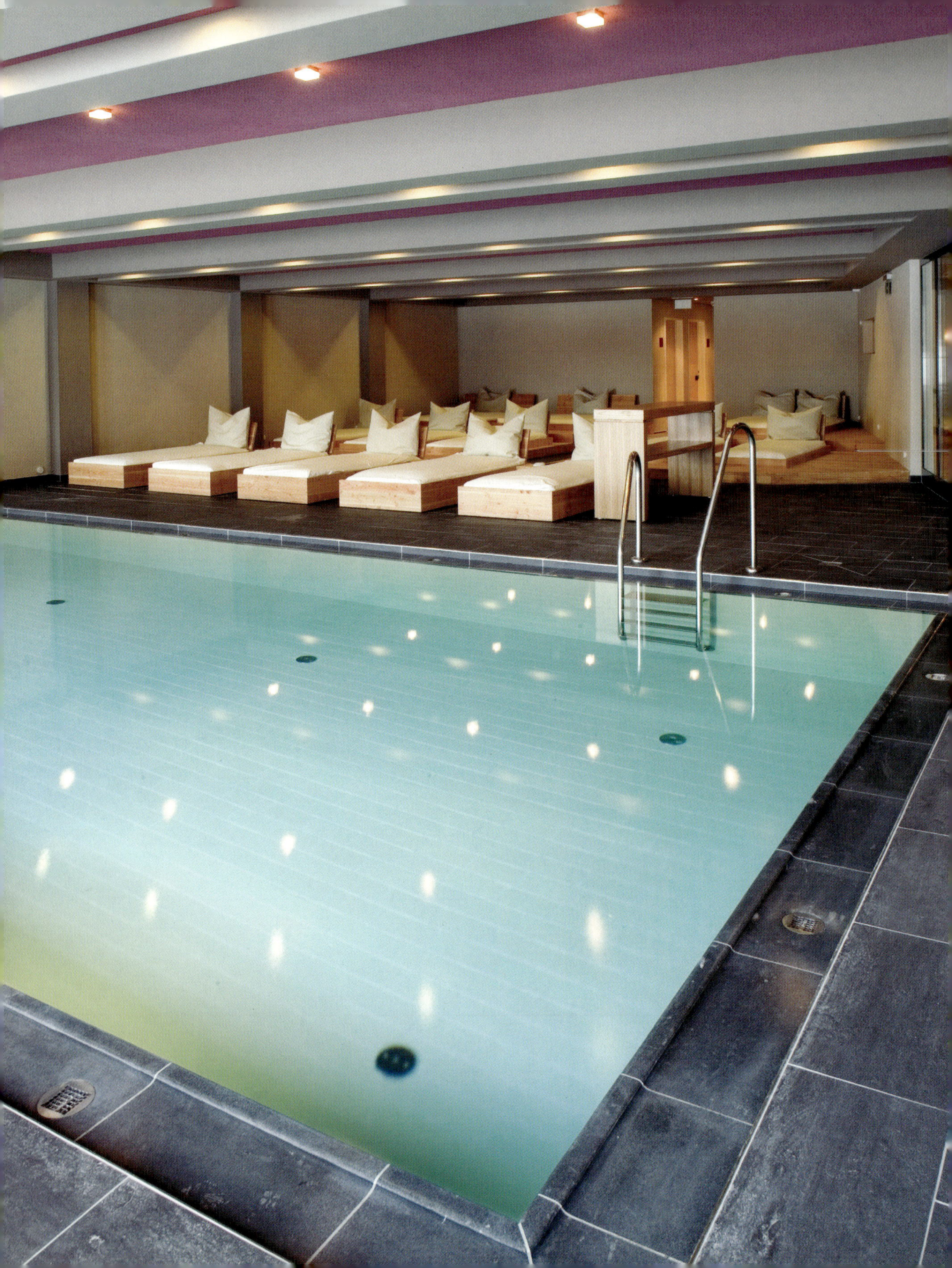

Balance Center & Spa

Dieses zu einem Hotel gehörende Spa ist ein wahres Refugium. Polierter Stein, kunsthandwerklich gefertigte Möbel und Schiefer prägen das Design. Neutrale Farben wie Beige, Braun, Sand und Schwarz vermitteln eine Atmosphäre, die Ruhe und Entspannung ausstrahlt. Licht ist das Hauptwerkzeug des „Mentaltrainers", der sich unterschiedlicher Methoden wie Entspannung, Meditation und Hypnose bedient, um Harmonie zwischen Körper und Geist herzustellen.

Behind the comfortable hotel there is a real sanctuary, the Balance Center & Spa. Polished stone, artisan furniture and slate stone stand out in the design. The colors of beige, brown, sand and black manage a neutral atmosphere that radiates calm and relaxation. Light is the main tool with which the "mental trainer" works, using different methods such as relaxation, meditation and hypnosis to acquire harmony between the body and the mind.

Derrière l'hôtel confortable se cache un véritable sanctuaire, le Balance Center & Spa. La pierre polie, les meubles artisanaux et l'ardoise se distinguent tout particulièrement dans sa conception. Les couleurs beige, brun, sable et noir créent une atmosphère douce qui invite à la sérénité et à la relaxation. La lumière est l'élément principal utilisé lors des traitements, que ce soit pour la relaxation, la méditation ou l'hypnose, afin de renforcer l'harmonie entre le corps et l'esprit.

Achter het comfortabele hotel ligt een waar reservaat voor ontspanning. Gepolijste stenen, handgemaakt meubilair en leisteen zijn opvallende kenmerken van de inrichting. Verschillende tinten beige, bruin, zandgeel en zwart creëren een neutrale sfeer die rust en ontspanning uitstraalt. Licht is een belangrijk werktuig voor de 'mentale trainers', die verschillende technieken toepassen om lichaam en geest weer in balans te brengen, zoals ontspanning, meditatie en hypnose.

Salzburg, Austria

NIKI SZILAGYI

Photos © Design Hotels

www.mavida.at

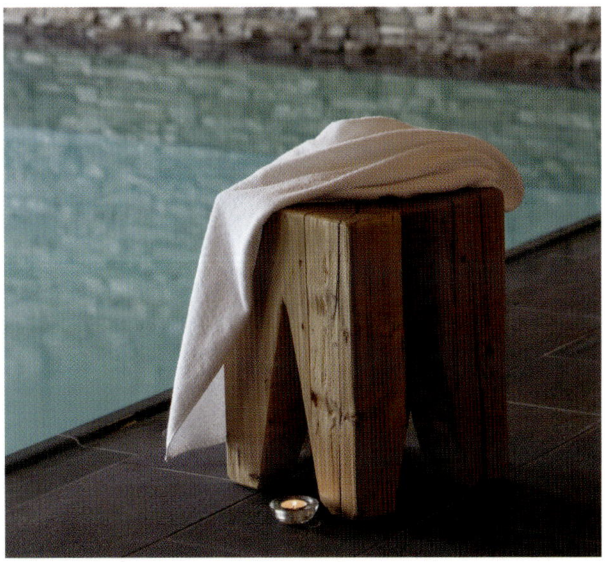

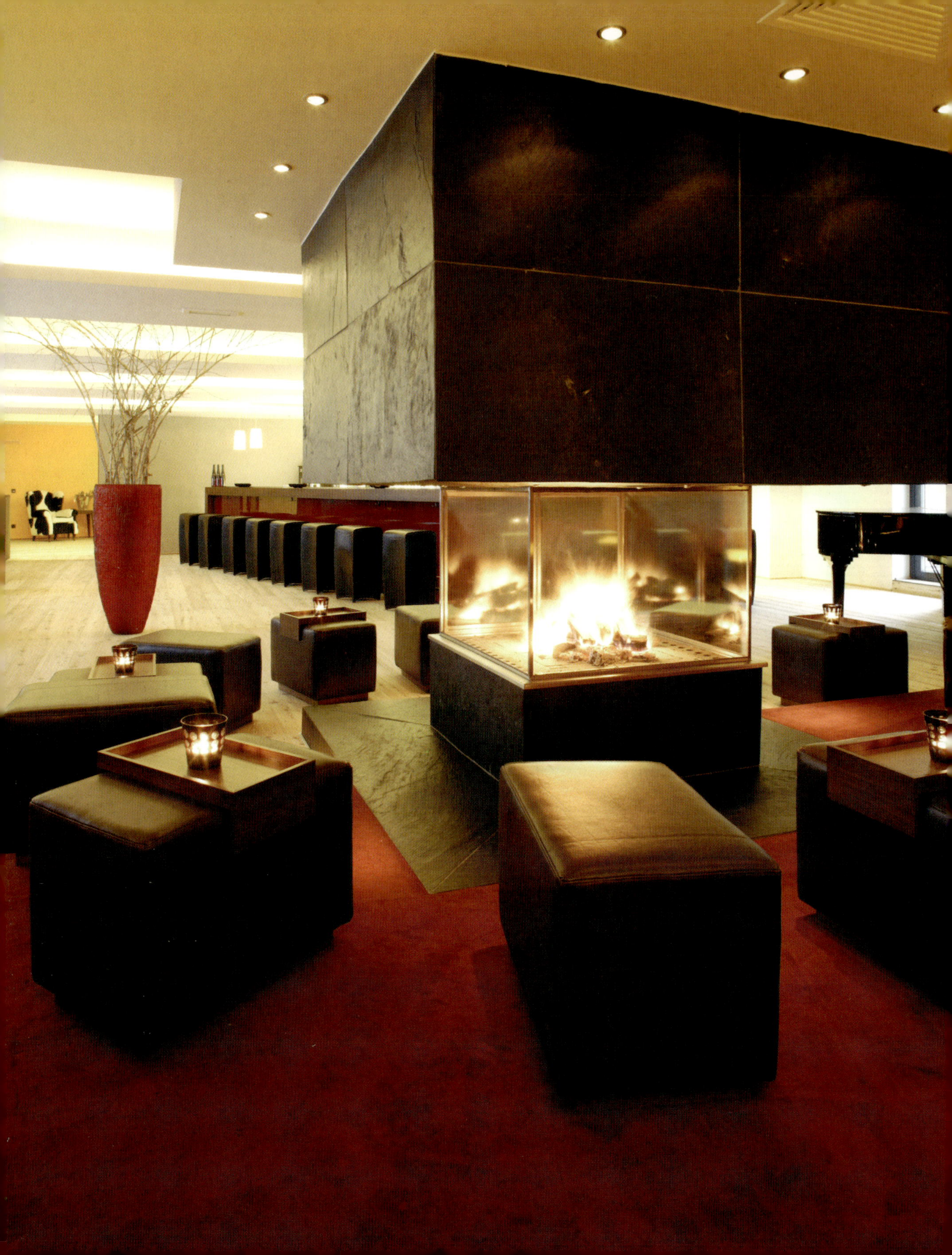

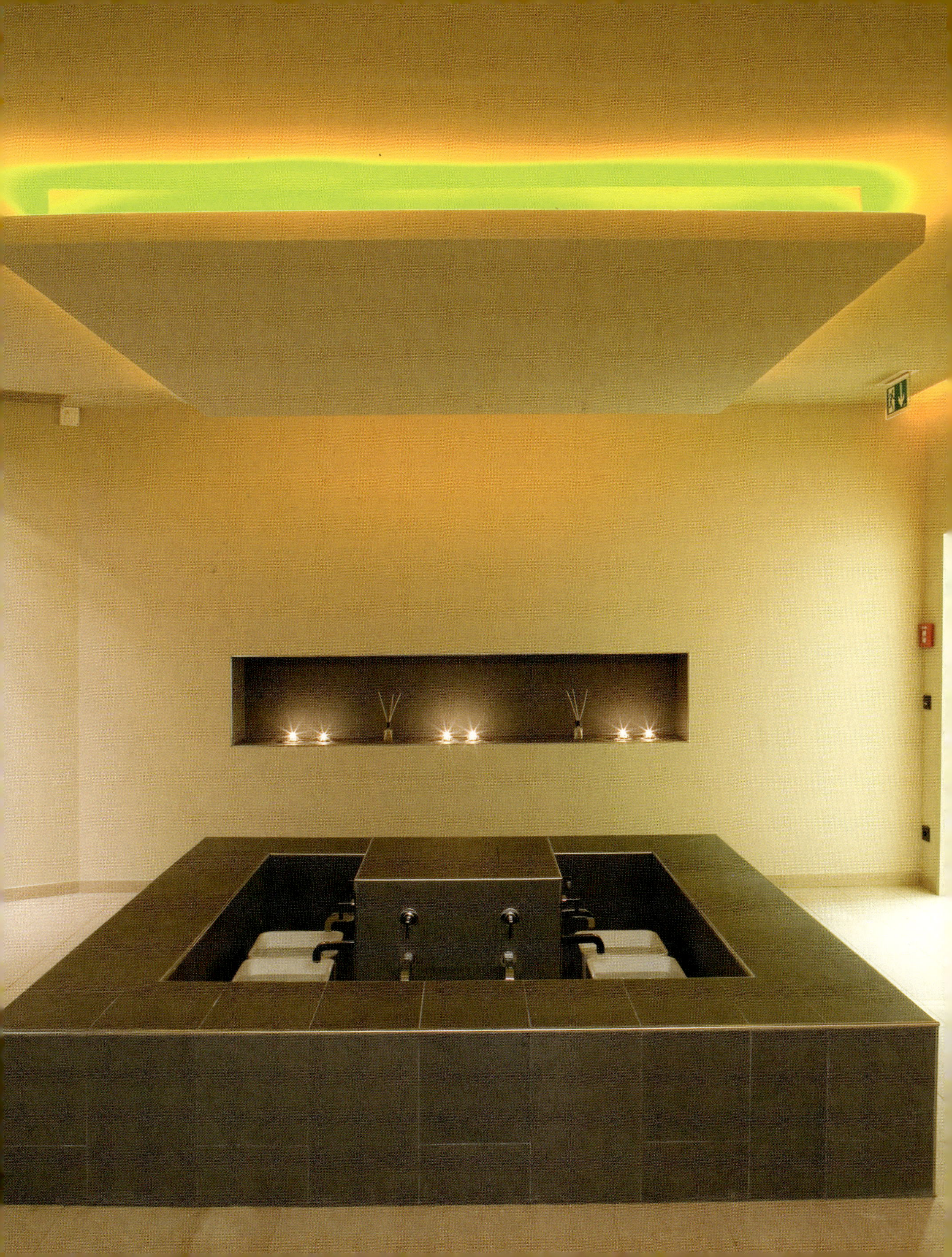

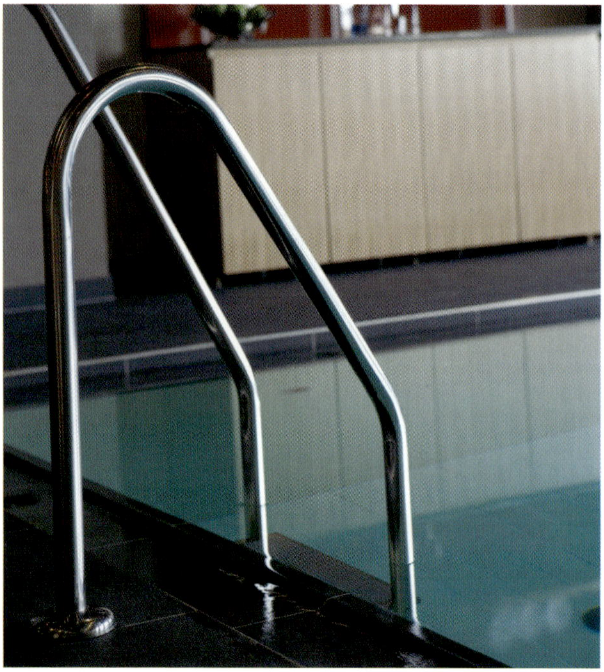

Neben dem Pool laden große Holzliegen zum Entspannen und zum Genuß der aromatischen Düfte ein, die die Luft erfüllen.

Next to the pool is the lounge where large wooden beds invite you to relax, enjoying the sweet aromas in the air.

À côté de la piscine se trouve le salon, où de grands lits en bois invitent à la détente et à savourer les doux parfums qui flottent dans l'air.

De lounge is naast het zwembad. Hier kunnen gasten uitrusten op grote houten bedden en zoete geuren opsnuiven.

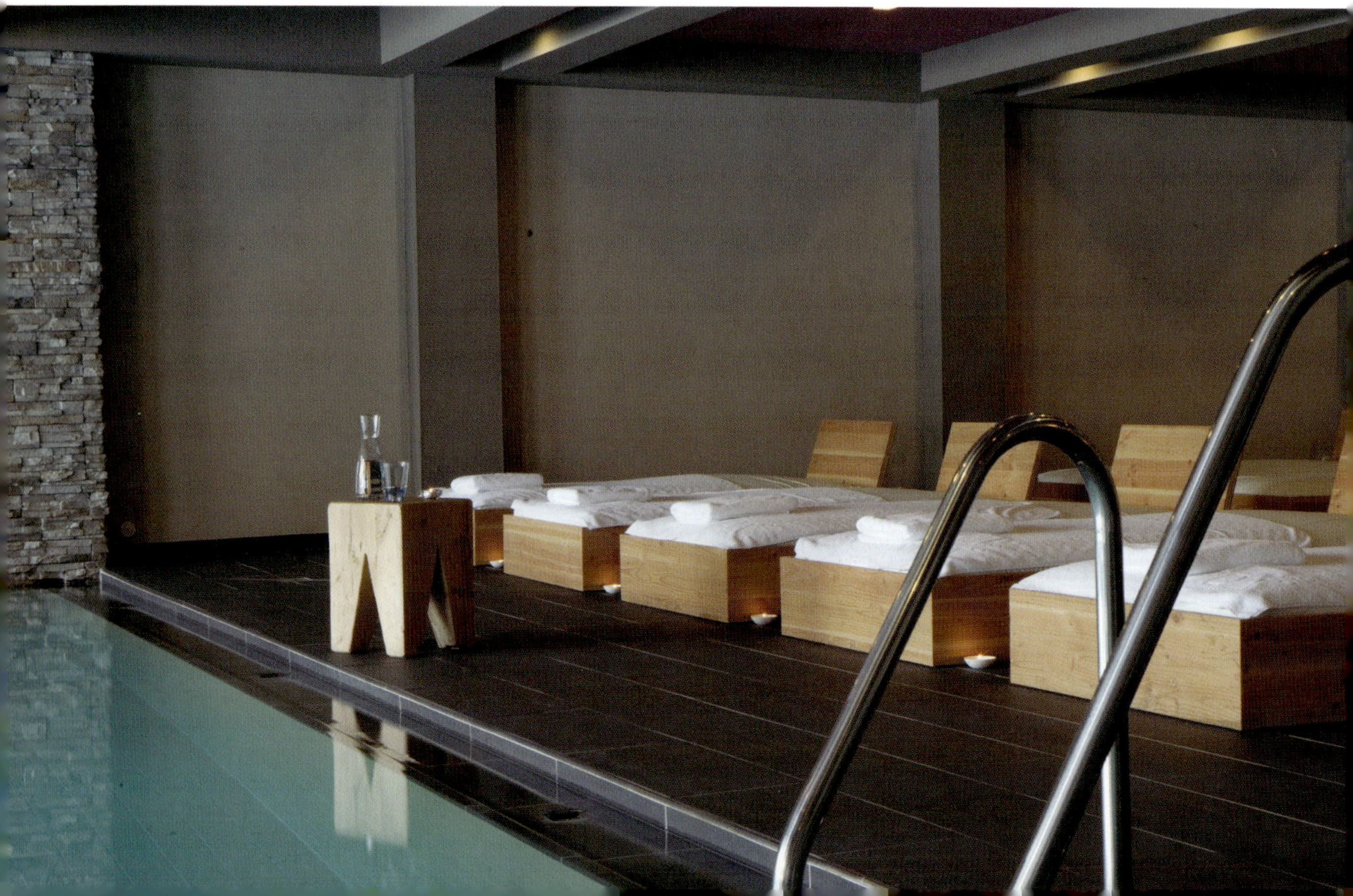

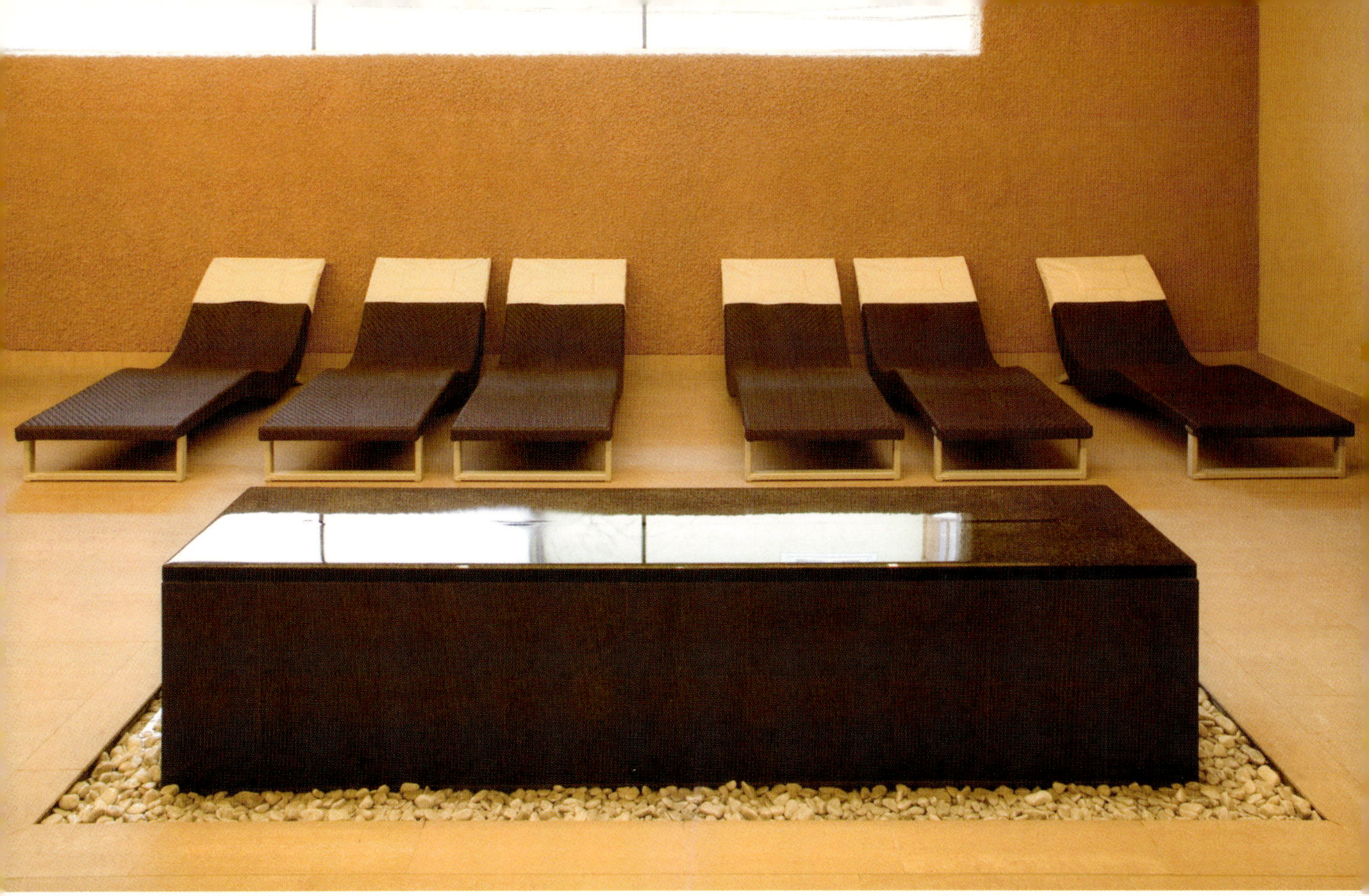
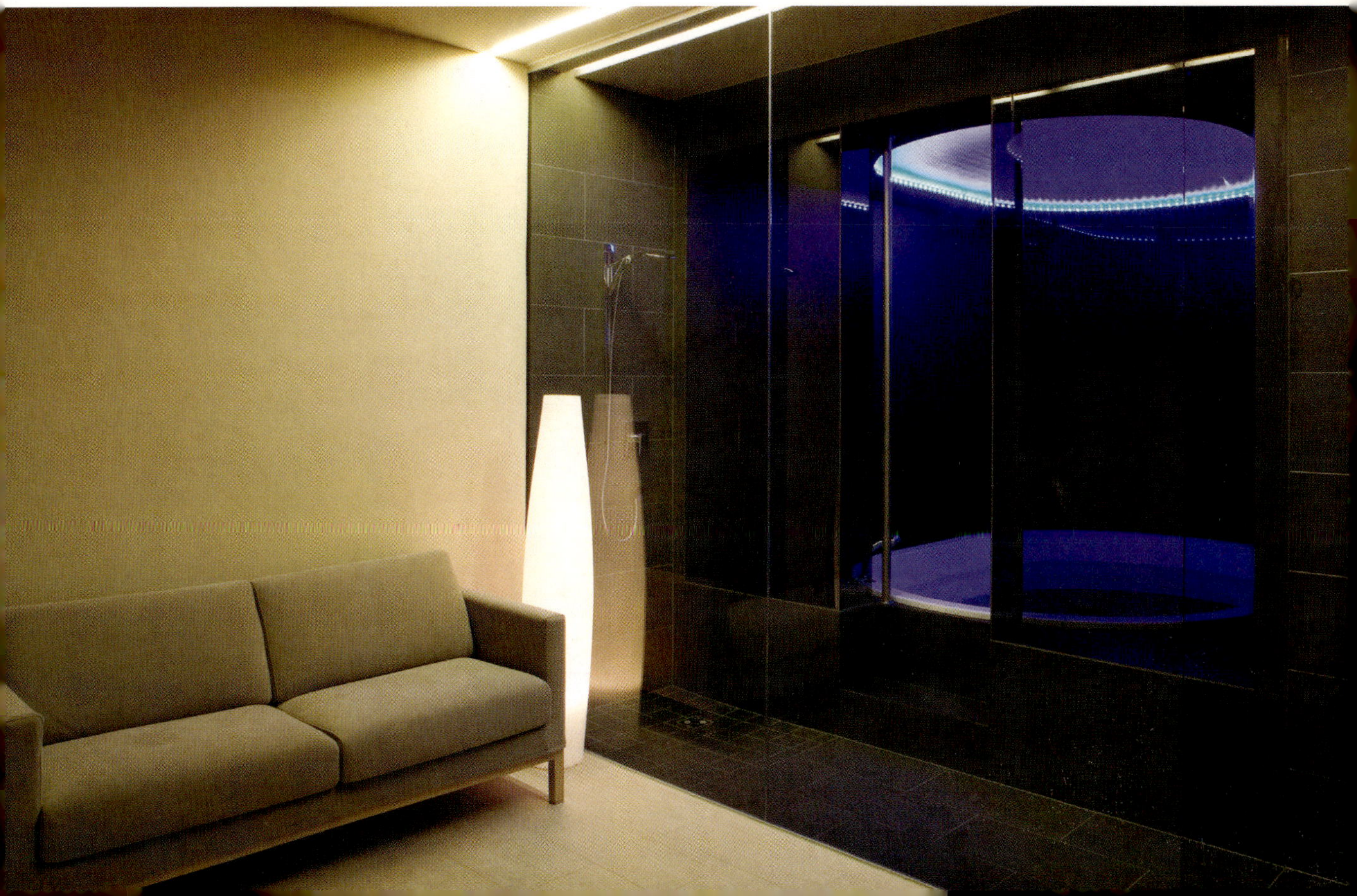

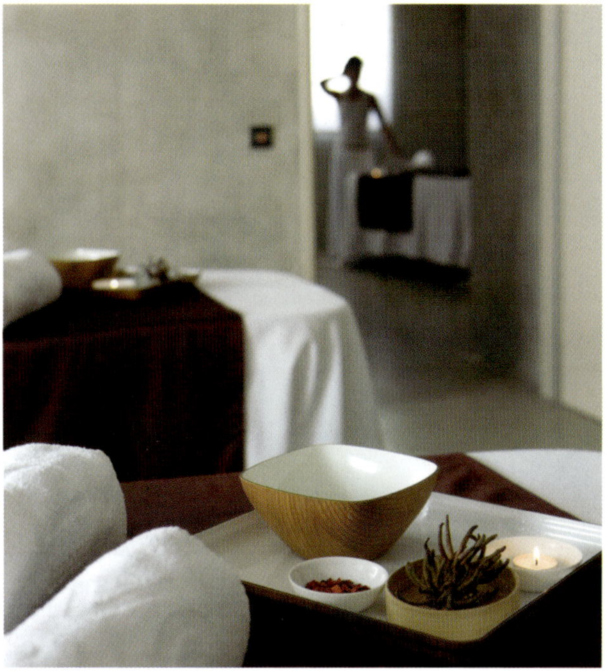

Riesige Schieferblöcke fungieren als eindrucksvolle Kulisse des von Holz und Erdtönen dominierten Spas.

Huge slate blocks create the spectacular backdrop of the spa, in which wood and a palette of earth colors predominate.

D'immenses dalles d'ardoise créent l'impressionnante toile de fond de ce spa, dans lequel le bois et les couleurs naturelles prédominent.

Enorme blokken leisteen vormen de spectaculaire achtergrond van het complex, waarin hout en aardse kleuren domineren.

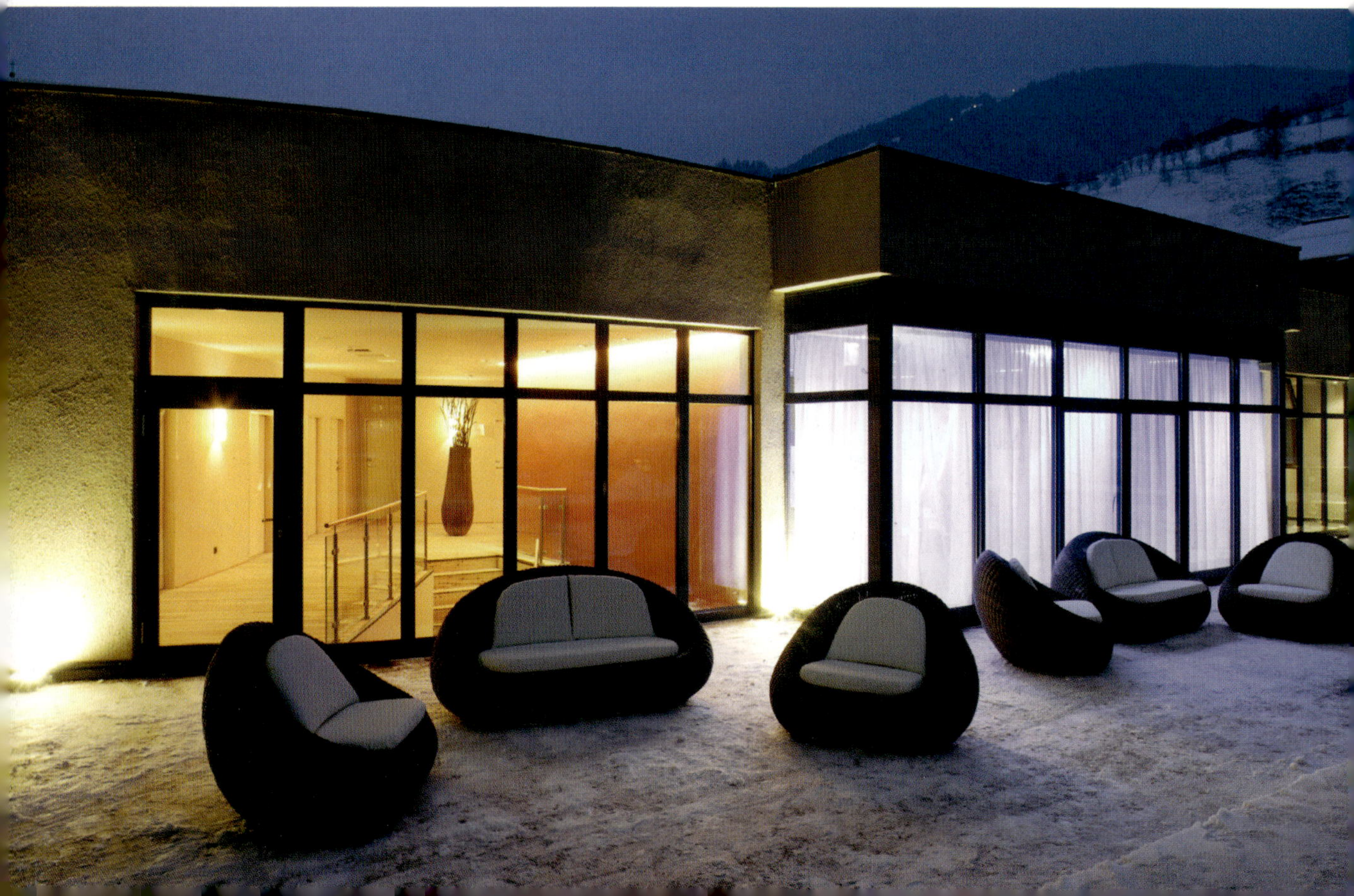

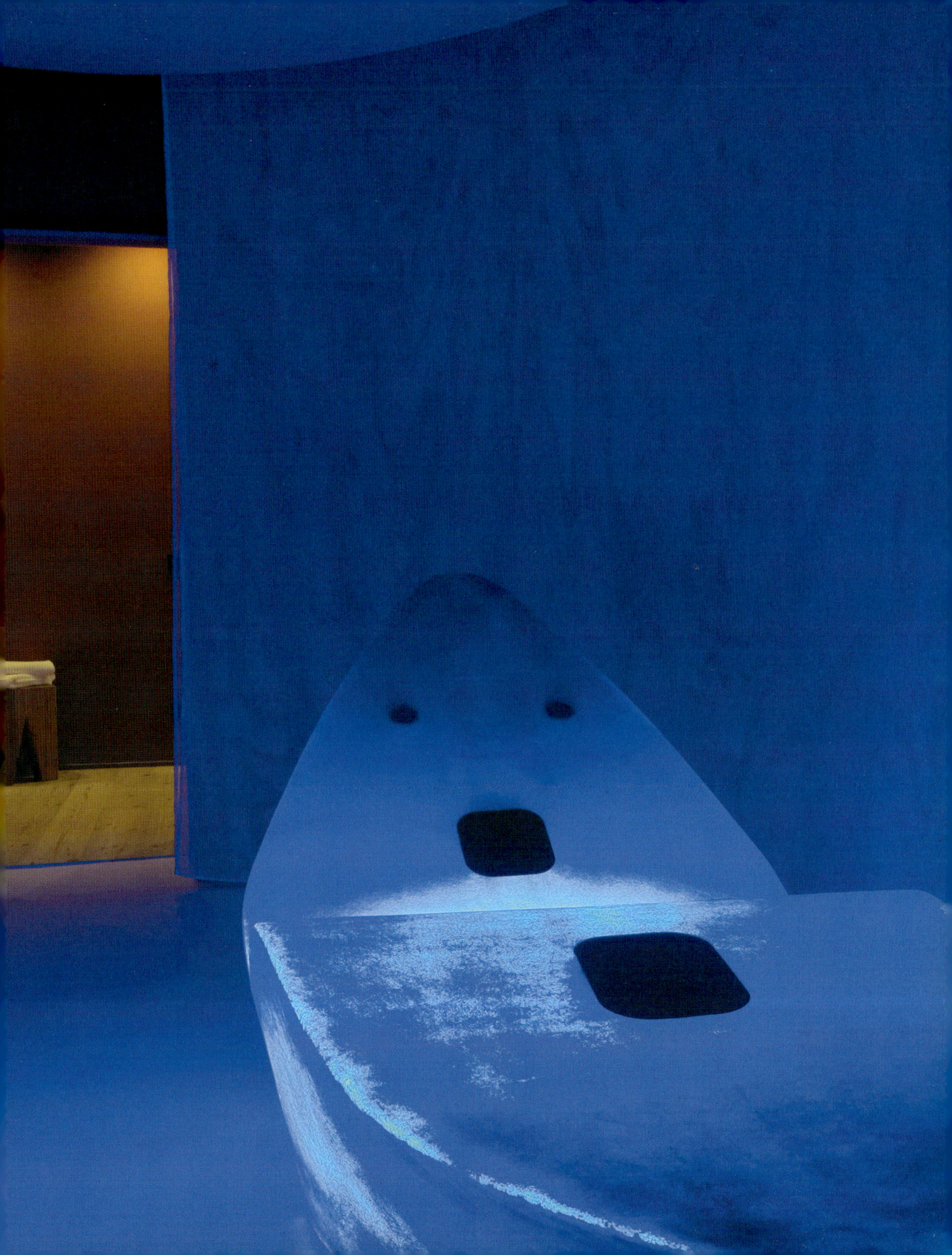

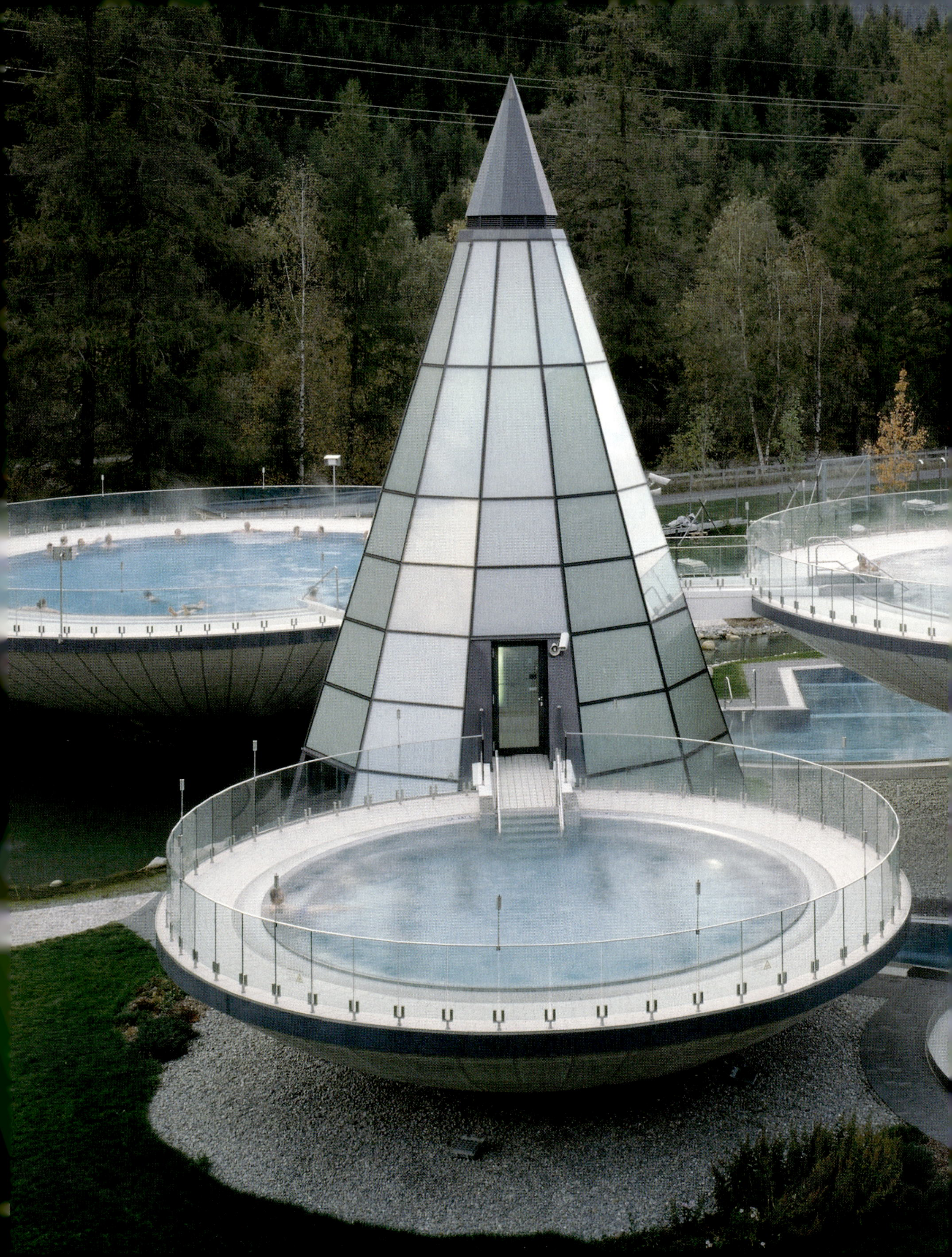

Therme Aqua Dome

Trotz seiner futuristischen Formen fügt sich dieser Bau harmonisch in die Natur ein, denn Landschaft und Wasser spiegeln sich in seiner gläsernen Fassade. Der Komplex beherbergt ein Hotel, innere und äußere Thermalzonen, Saunabereich, Fitnessbereich, Health Club und Spa. Die wie Scheiben geformten Außenpools scheinen frei zu schweben. Zu ihnen zählen ein Salzwasserbecken, ein Whirlpool sowie ein Entspannungs- und Massagebecken.

Despite its futuristic shape, the complex fits harmoniously with the surroundings because of the reflections of the landscape and the water on its crystal skin. The complex includes a hotel, inside and outside thermal zones, sauna area, fitness area, health clinic and spa. The outside pools are shaped as discs and seem to be floating in the air. They all have different characteristics: salt water, a whirlpool bath, and the third, dedicated to massages and relaxation.

En dépit de sa forme futuriste, le complexe s'accorde harmonieusement avec le cadre naturel, grâce à sa construction où se reflètent le paysage et l'eau. L'Aqua Dome comprend un hôtel, des zones thermales en intérieur et en extérieur, un espace sauna, une salle de remise en forme, une clinique et un spa. Trois des piscines extérieures, en forme de disque, semblent flotter dans l'air. Chacune possède ses spécificités : eau salée pour la première, bain bouillonnant pour la deuxième, massages et relaxation pour la troisième.

Ondanks de futuristische buitenkant harmonieert dit complex goed met de omgeving, dankzij de weerkaatsing van landschap en water op de muren. Het complex bevat een hotel, een thermaal gedeelte met binnen- en buitenafdelingen, sauna's, een fitnessruimte, een thermale kliniek en een bronnenbad. De buitenbaden zijn rond en lijken wel te zweven. Ze hebben allemaal hun eigen kenmerken: een zoutwaterbad, een whirlpool en een bad voor massage en ontspanning.

Längenfeld, Austria

SCHNÖGASS & PARTNER ZIVILTECHNIKER

Photos © Angelo Kaunat

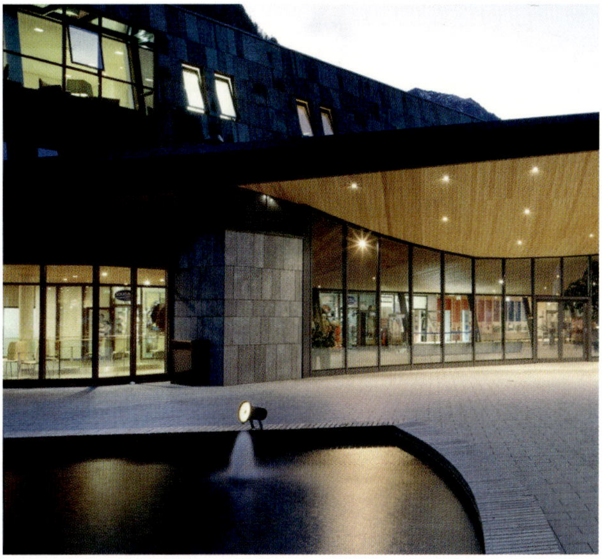

www.aqua-dome.at

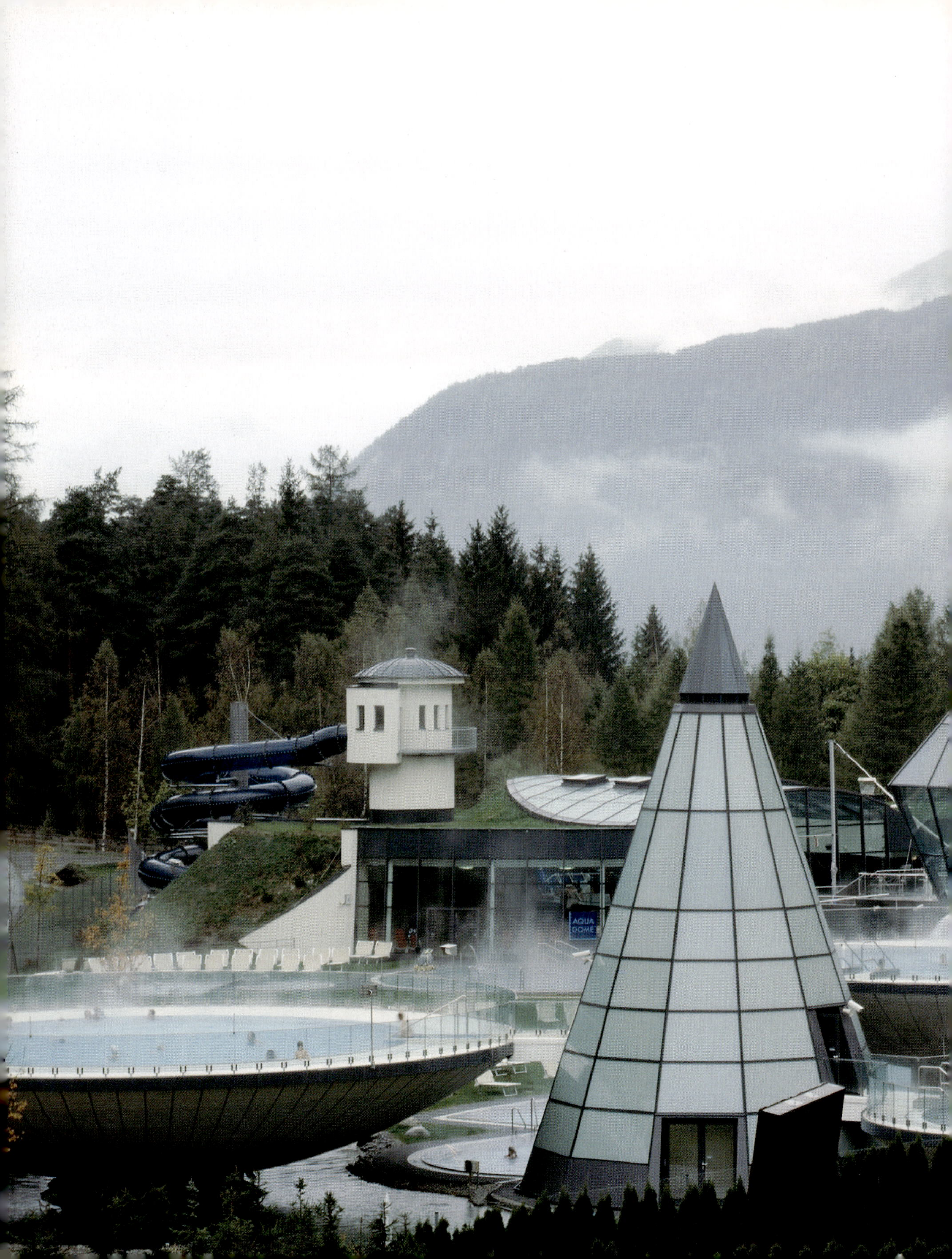
AQUA
DOME

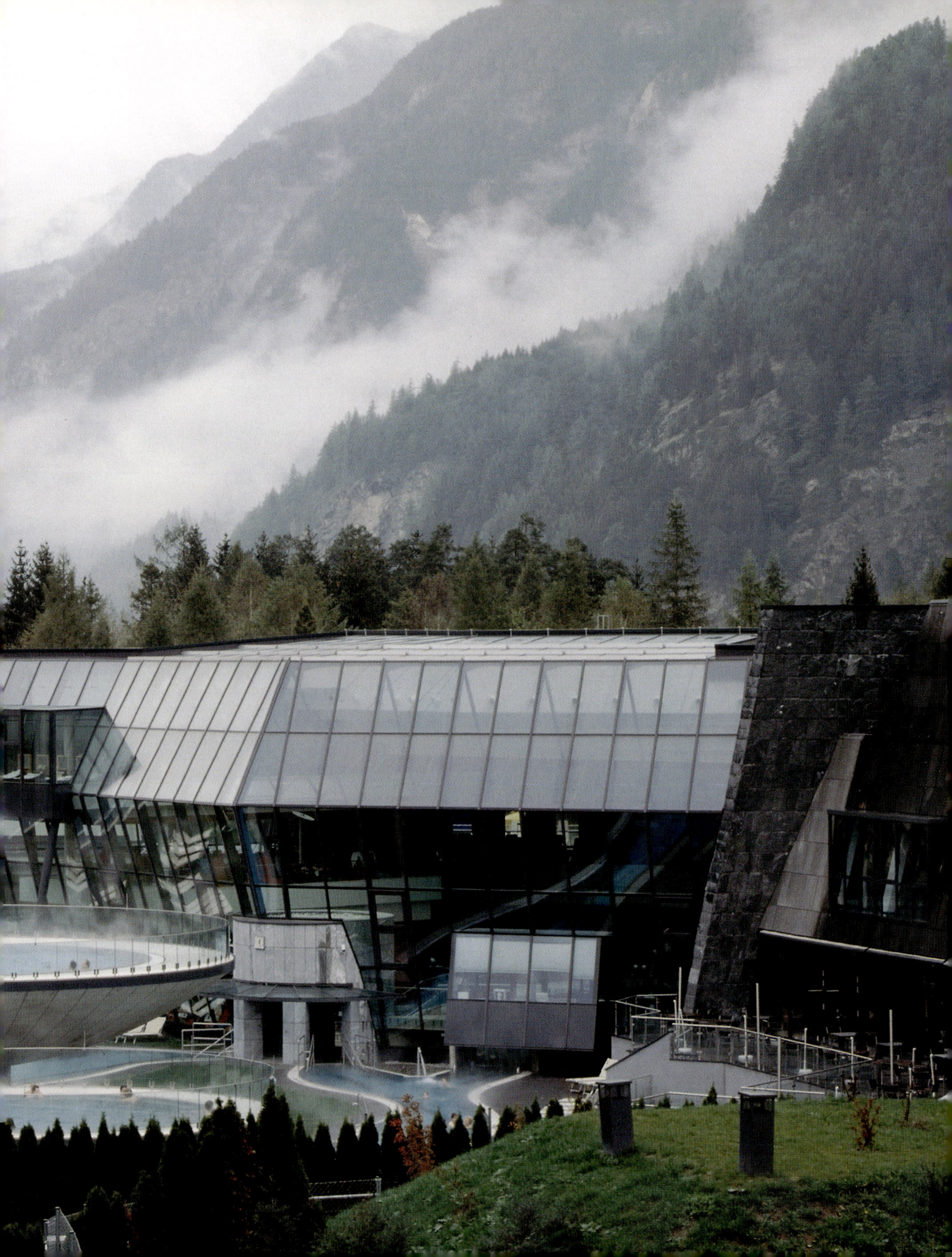

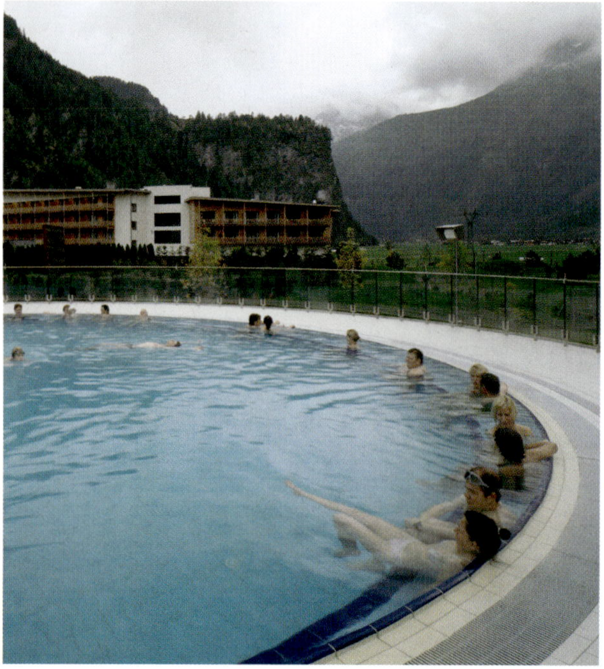

Die Landschaft Tirols ist durch die Glasfassaden in allen Gebäudeteilen präsent.

The Tyrolese landscape penetrates the complex through the glass facades of all its buildings.

Grâce aux façades vitrées de tous les bâtiments, le paysage tyrolien est ici véritablement « invité » au cœur du complexe.

Het landschap van Tirol dringt via de glazen wanden door tot in het gebouw.

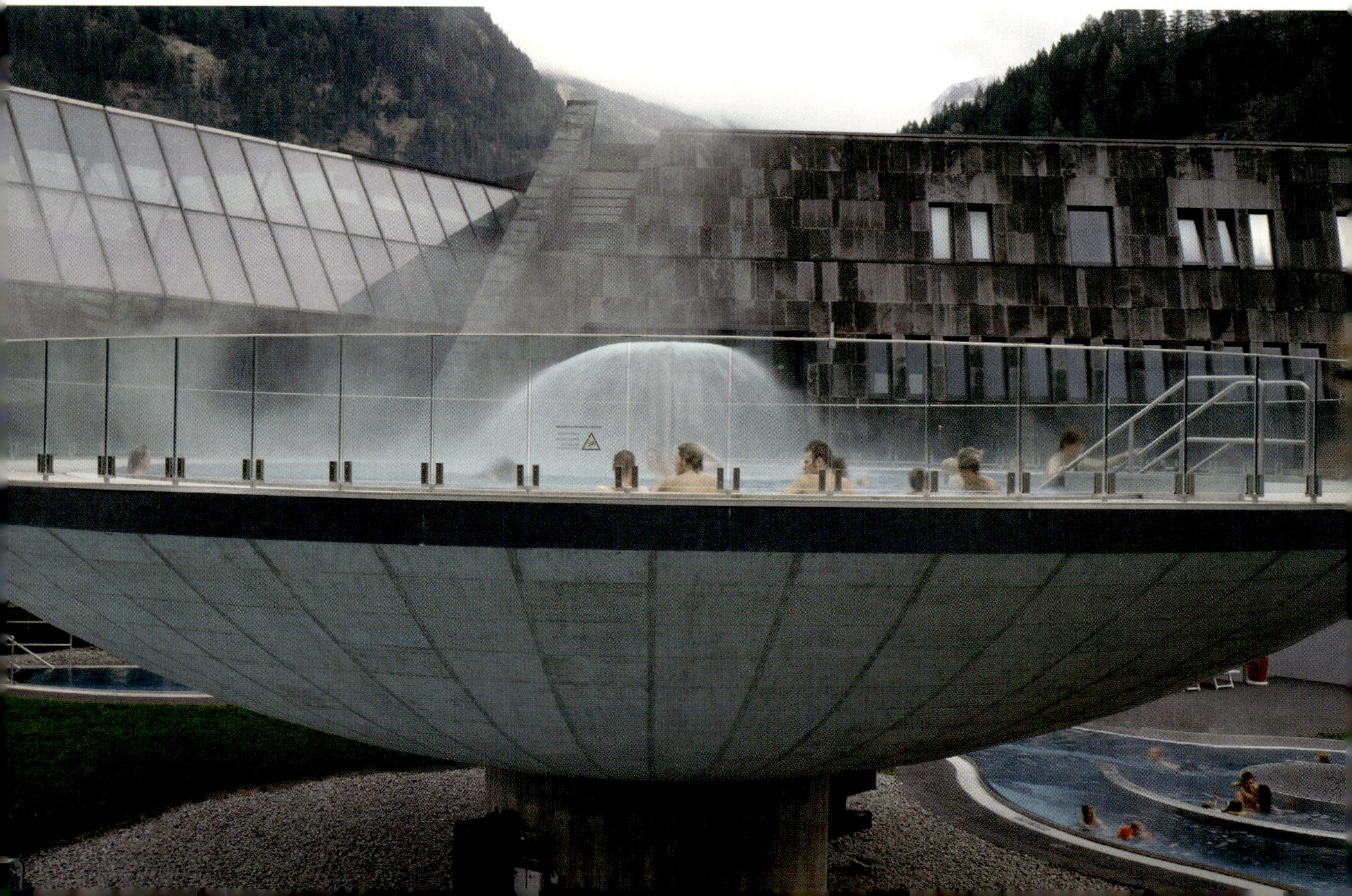

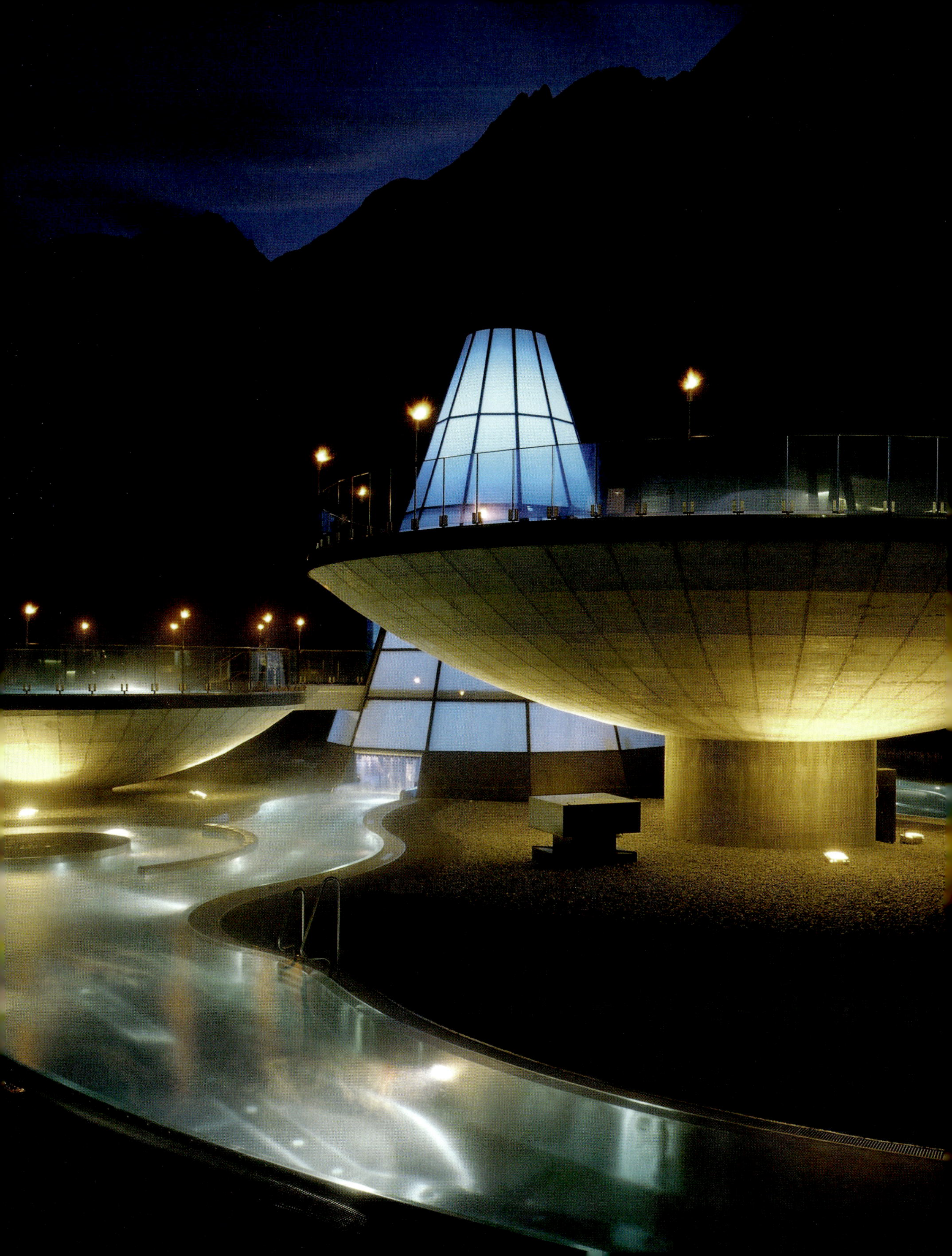

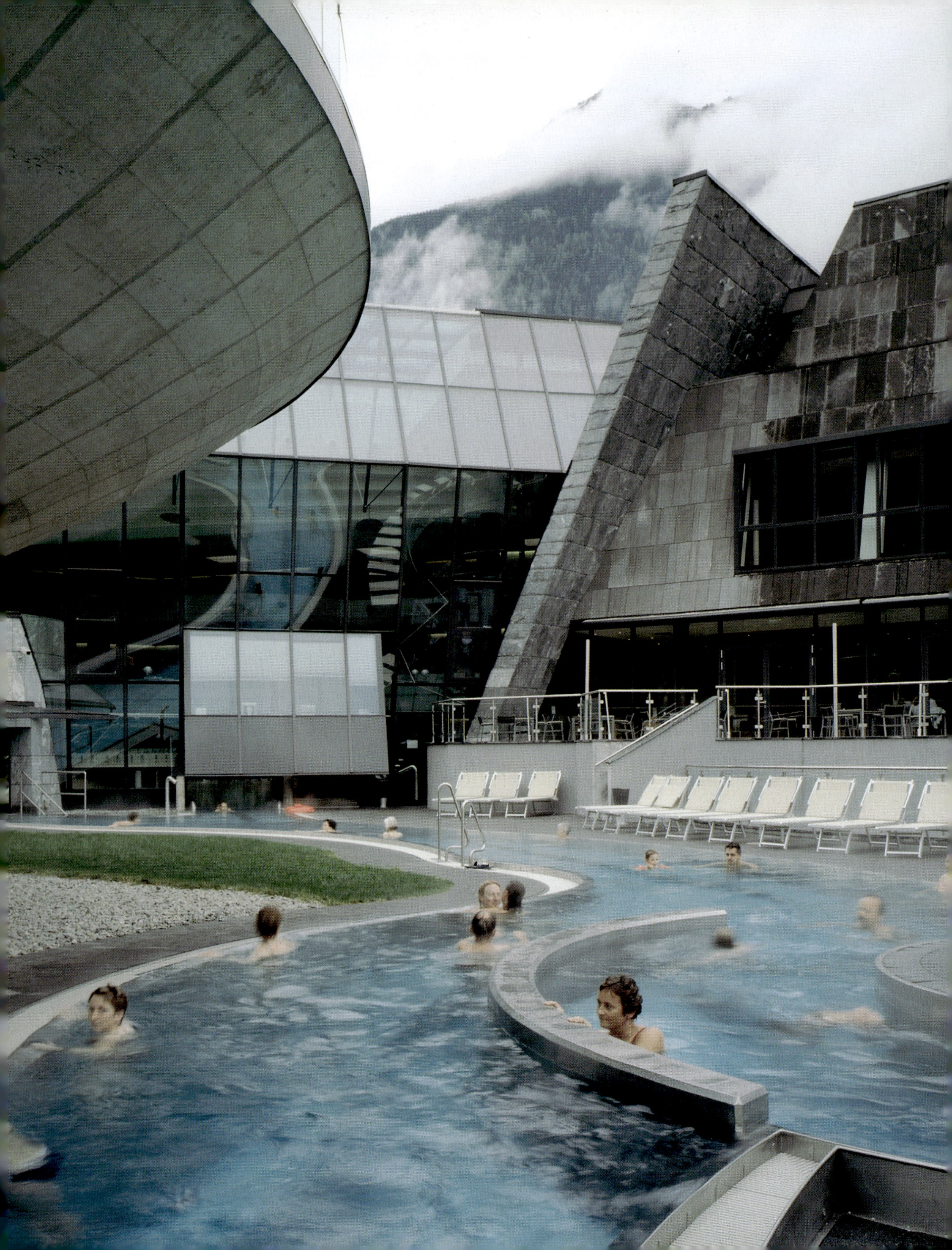

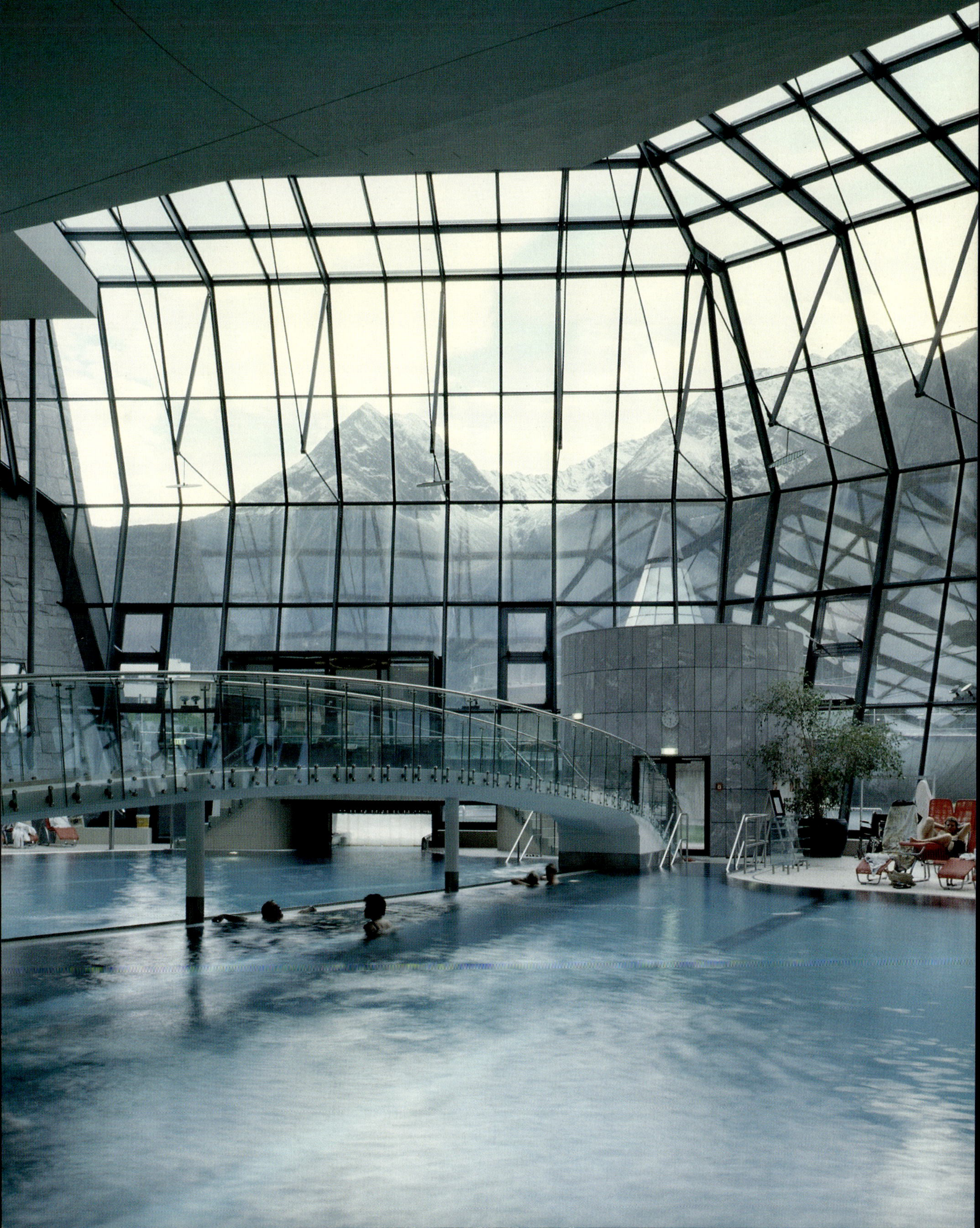

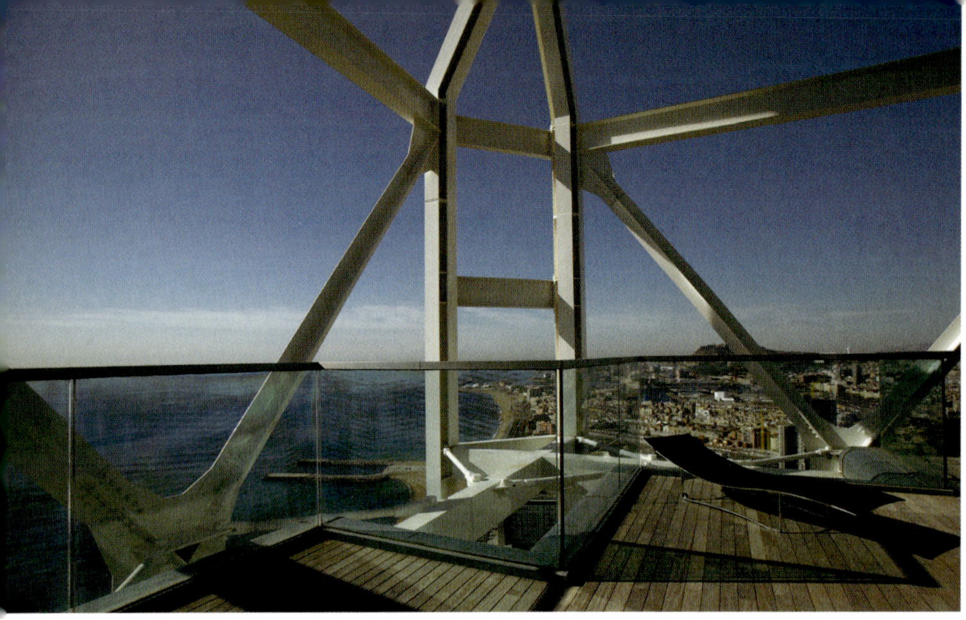

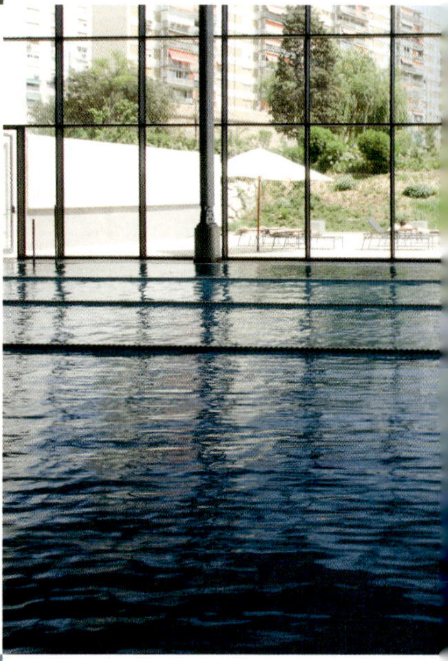

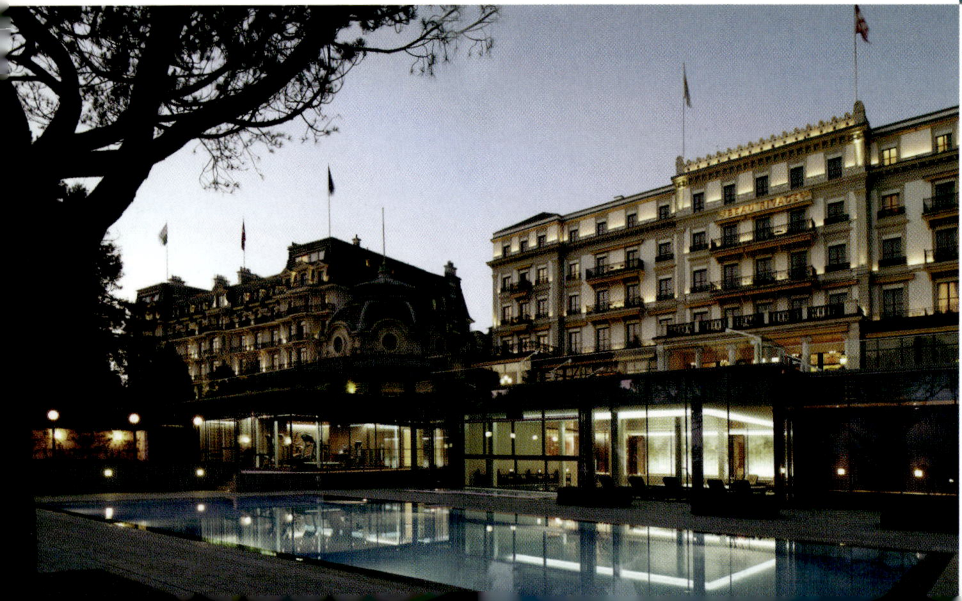

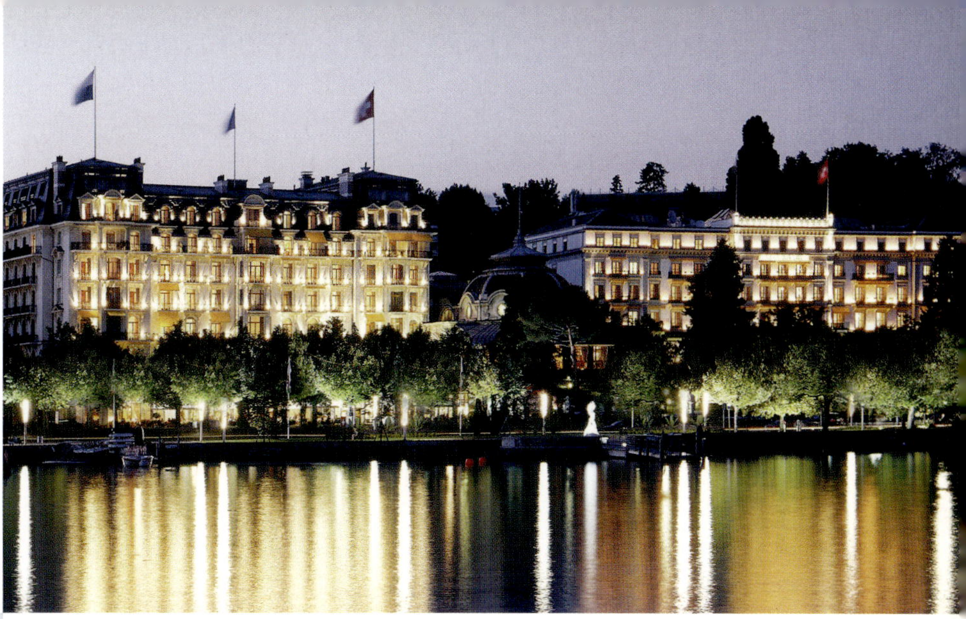

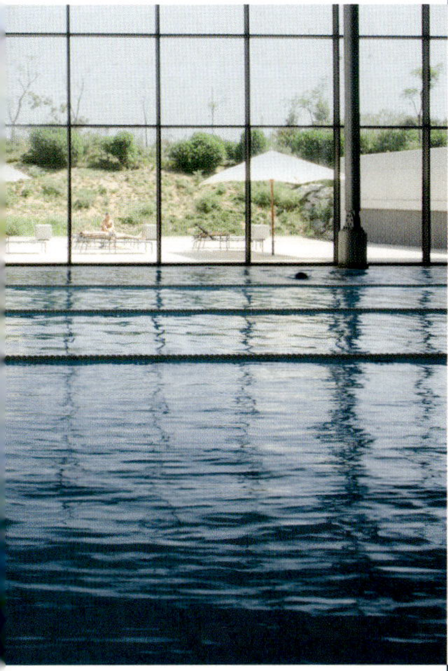

Urban Spas

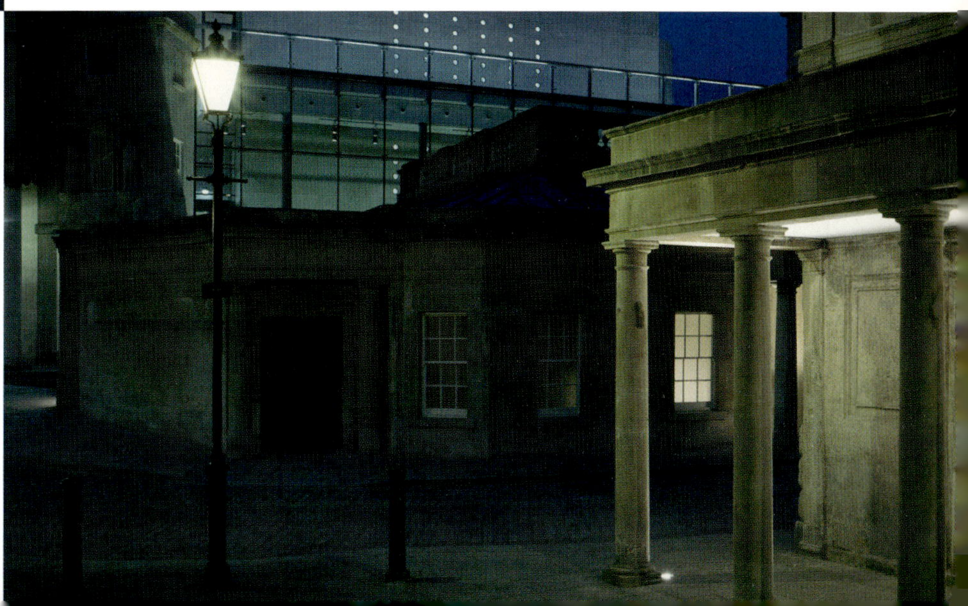

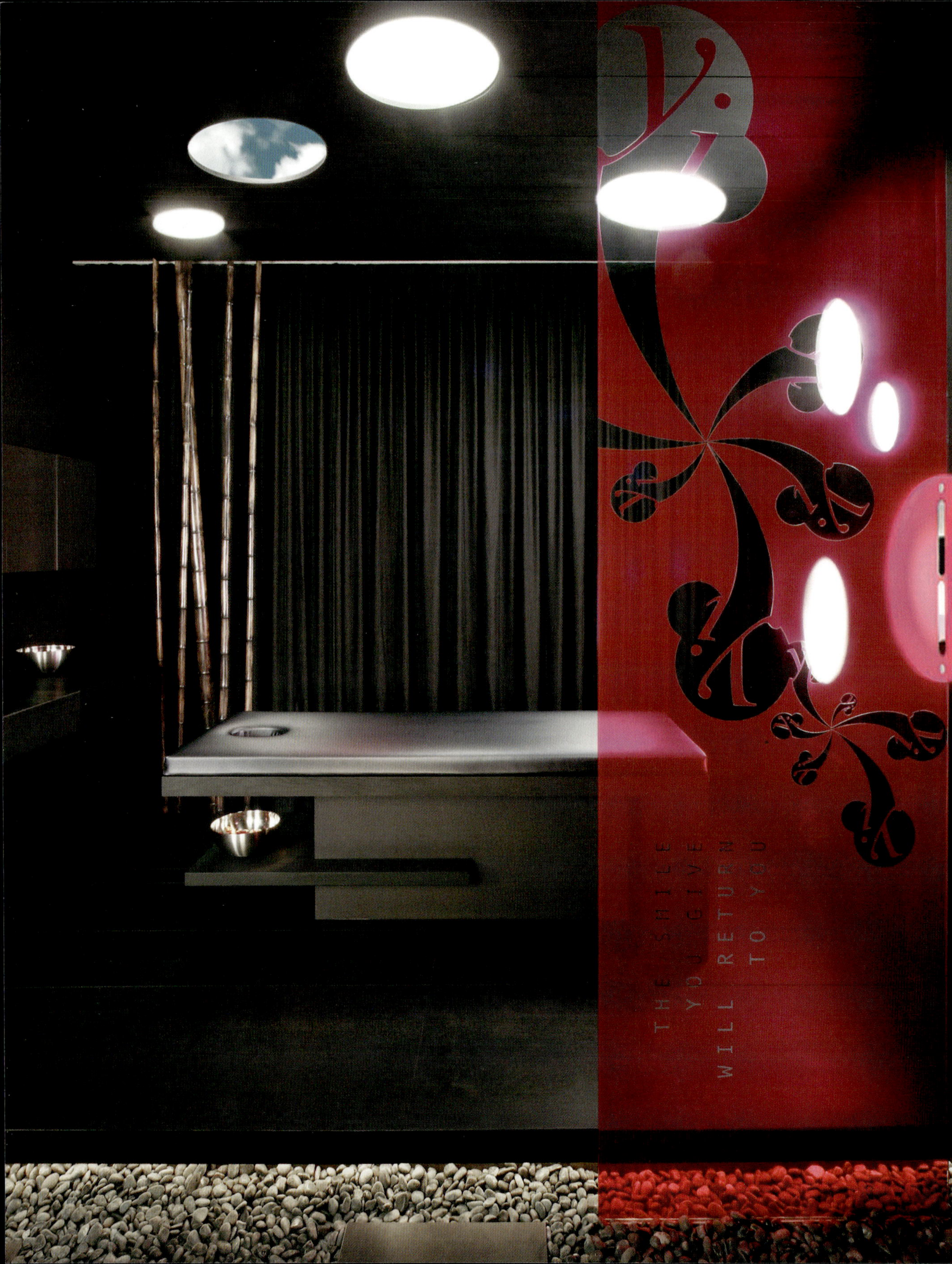
THE SMILE
YOU GIVE
WILL RETURN
TO YOU

Yi-Spa

Im Zentrum Berlins wurde dieses asiatisch inspirierte Spa als Oase der Ruhe für Körper, Geist und Seele konzipiert. Die Behandlungen werden in drei Räumen durchgeführt, die in unterschiedlichen Farbtönen gestaltet sind, doch zugleich alle durch beleuchtete Glastrennwände in rosafarbenes Licht getaucht werden. Eine große in das Dach eingelassene Scheibe gewährt einen Blick in den Himmel.
Alle Anwendungen werden durch asiatische Meister ihres Fachs durchgeführt.

Located in downtown Berlin, this spa-boutique of Asian inspiration was designed as a refuge of serenity for body, mind and spirit. Treatments are done in three rooms that, although differentiated by the color that predominates in each of them, are all bathed in a pink light that comes from the glass separations. A large screen placed on the roof lets the sky be seen. All the treatments are in the hands of professional Asians, experts in their task.

Situé dans le centre-ville de Berlin, cette boutique-spa d'inspiration asiatique a été conçue comme un havre de paix pour le corps et l'esprit. Les soins, laissés au savoir-faire de professionnels asiatiques, sont prodigués dans trois cabines, chacune de couleur différente, toutes baignées d'une lumière rose provenant de claustras en verre. À noter : une ouverture dans le toit permet de voir le ciel.

Deze op Azië geïnspireerde design-spa in het centrum van Berlijn is ontworpen als een sereen toevluchtsoord waar rust voor lichaam en geest centraal staat. De behandelingen vinden plaats in drie ruimten die weliswaar verschillende kleurstellingen hebben, maar allemaal baden in een rozig licht dat door de glazen scheidingsmuren valt. Door een groot scherm op het dak is de lucht te zien. Alle behandelingen worden uitgevoerd door professionele experts uit Azië.

Berlin, Germany

MARCO THIELE, PLAJER & FRANZ STUDIO

Photos © Die Photodesigner.de

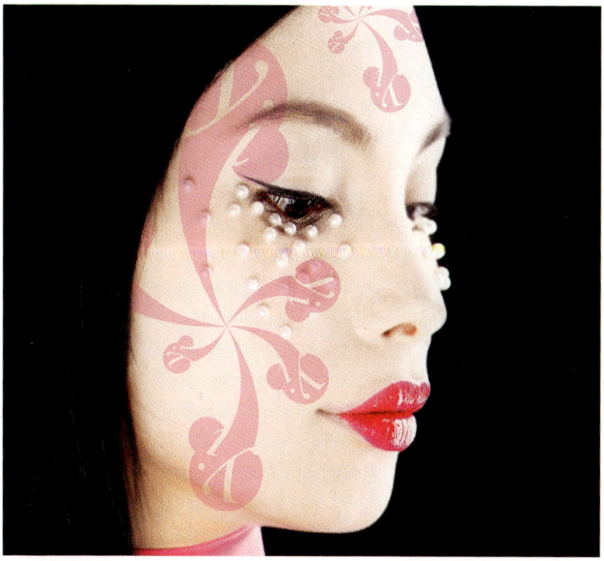

www.yi-spa.com

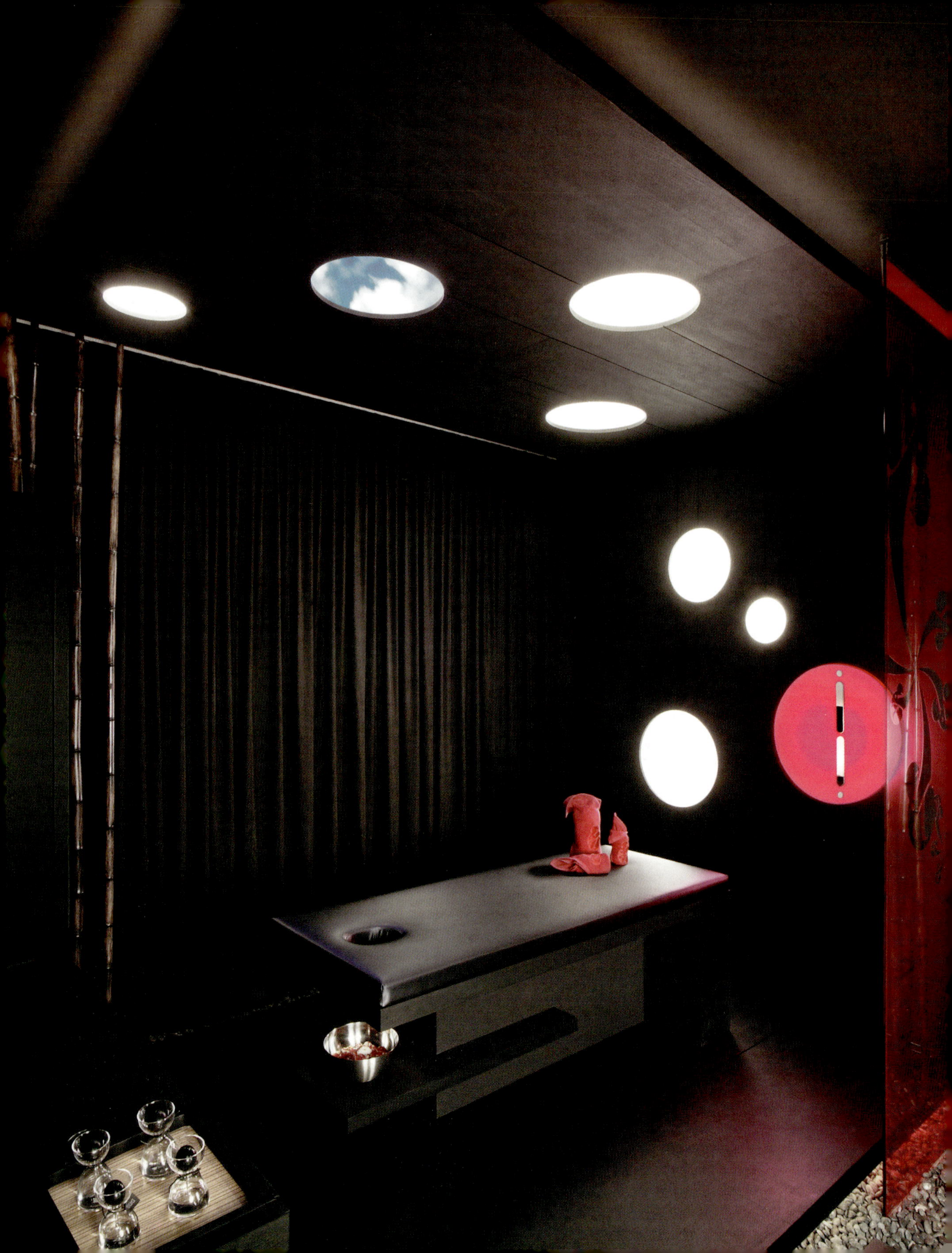

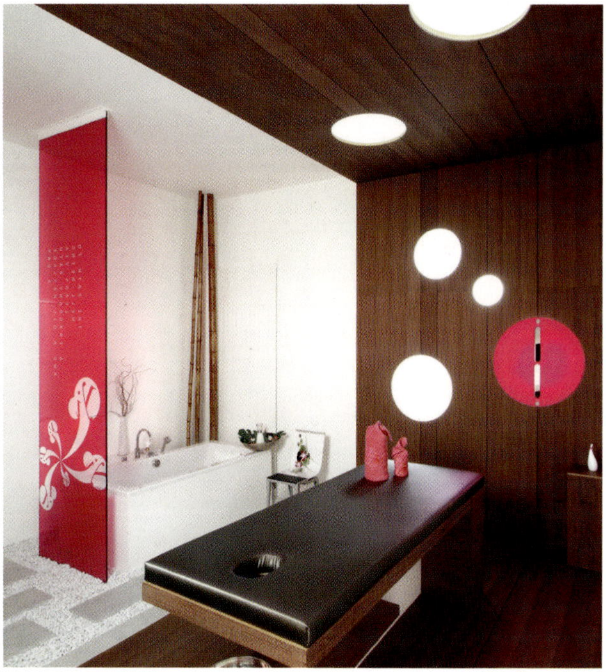

Oberflächen und Accessoires harmonieren mit der Farbe Schwarz, die in einem der Behandlungsräume dominiert.

Surfaces and accessories are combined with the color black that predominates in one of the three treatment rooms.

Les surfaces et les accessoires s'harmonisent avec la couleur noire, prédominante dans l'une des trois cabines.

Werkbladen en benodigdheden zijn gecombineerd met de kleur zwart, die in een van de drie behandelruimten overheerst.

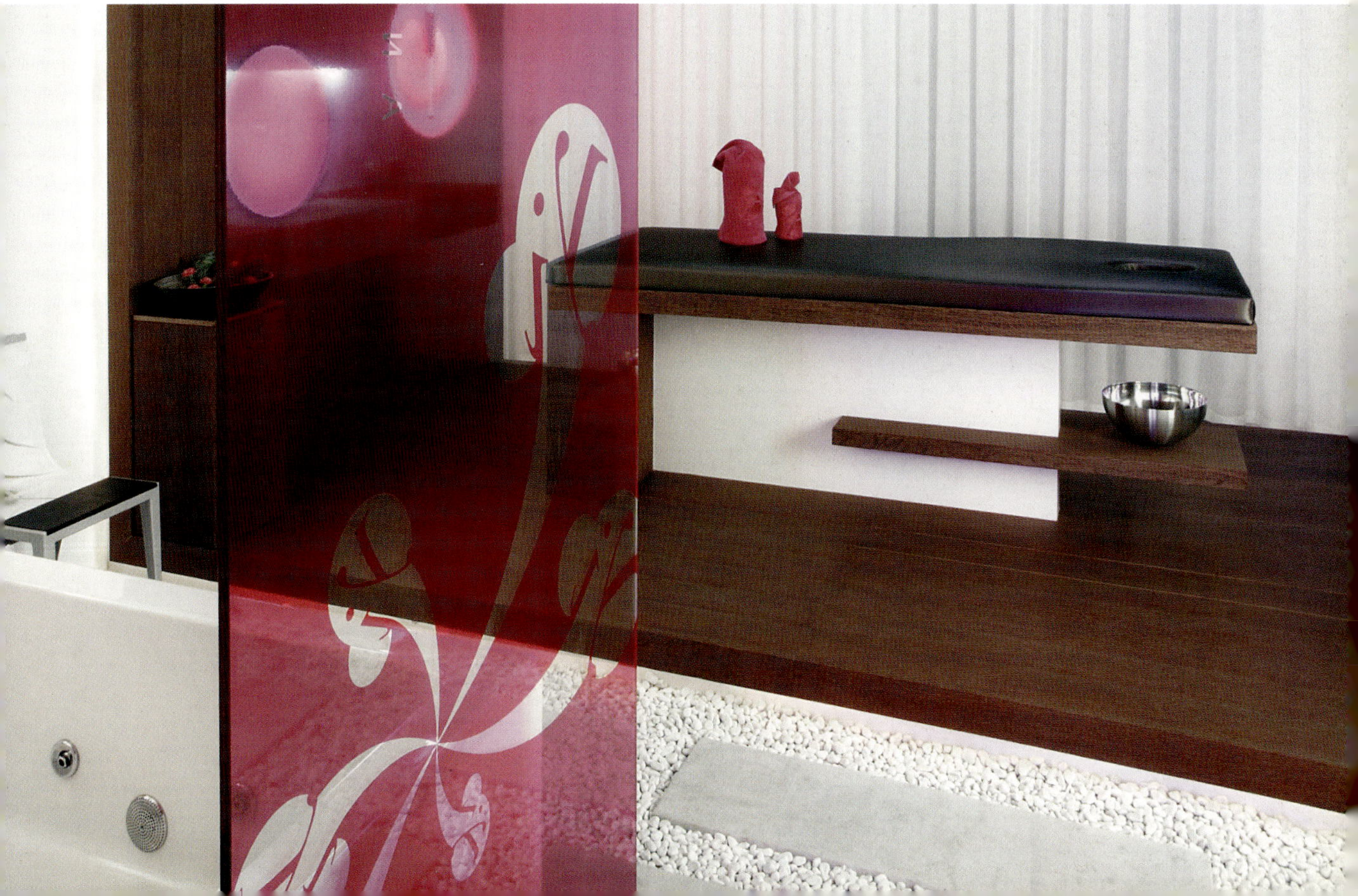

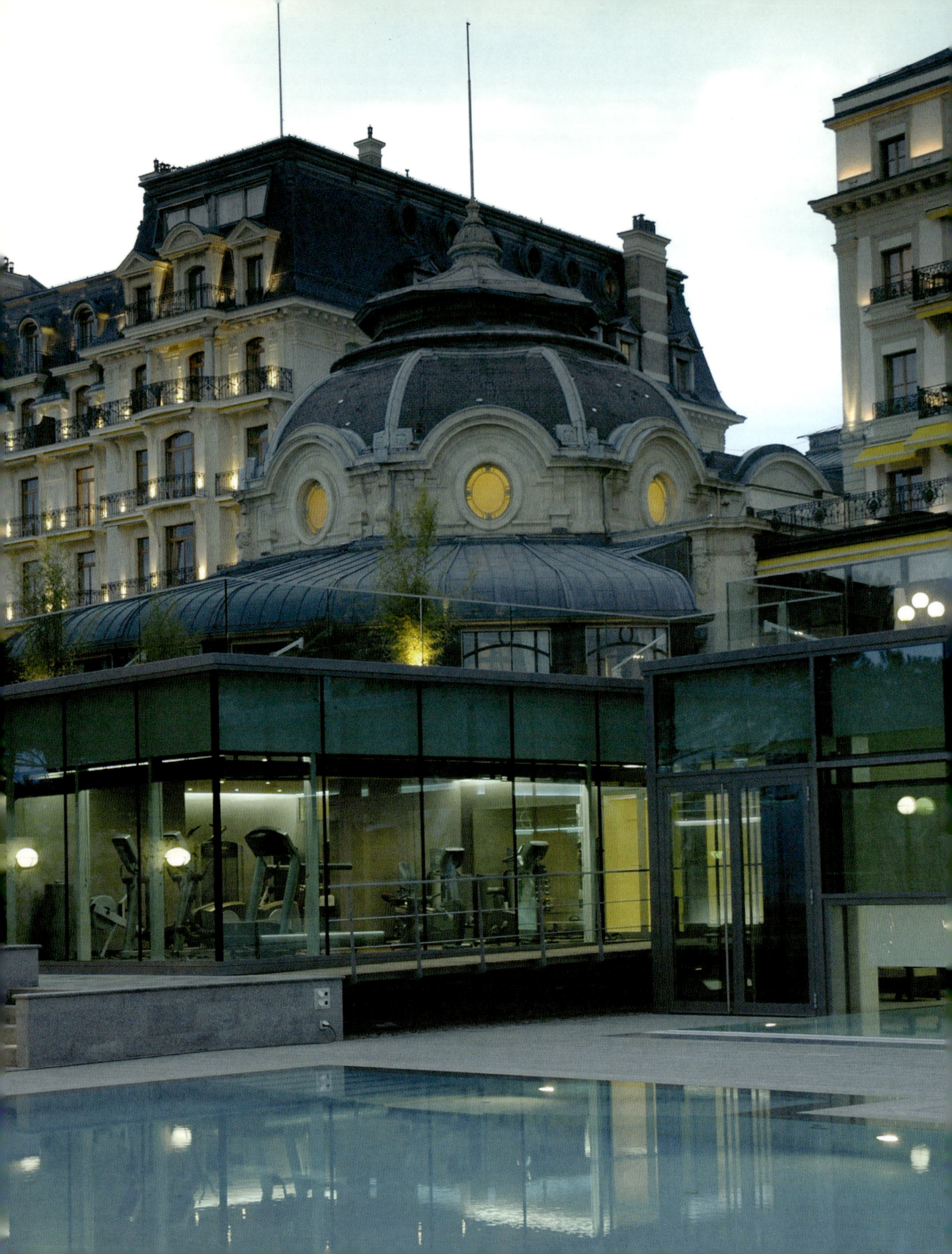

Beau-Rivage Palace Hotel Spa

Dieses 1.400 qm große Spa zählt zu den exklusivsten der Schweiz. Sein Konzept fußt auf einer Philosophie, die sich uralte Gesundheits- und Schönheitsrituale zueigen macht. Kulturelle Einflüsse aus Japan, Indien, Nordafrika, China und Bali offenbaren sich nicht nur im Design der acht Behandlungsräume, der beiden Pools und des Fitnessraums, sondern auch in den Gesundheits- und Schönheitstherapien, die die Weisheiten jahrtausendealter Kulturen auf die heutige Zeit übertragen.

This exclusive wellness area of 15,000 square feet is first among its type in Switzerland. It was designed with a philosophy that incorporates ancient rituals of health and beauty. Cultural influences from Japan, India, Northern Africa, China and Bali are evident not only in specific items of the design of the eight treatment rooms, the two pools and the fitness room, but also in the health and beauty therapies that apply the wisdom of millenary cultures to the present.

Cette adresse à part, dédiant ses 1.500 m² au bien-être, est la première du genre en Suisse. Le concept présidant à sa rénovation repose sur des rituels ancestraux de santé et de beauté. Les influences culturelles japonaise, indienne, nord-africaine, chinoise et balinaise sont perceptibles non seulement dans la décoration des 8 cabines de soins, des deux piscines et de la salle de remise en forme, mais aussi et surtout dans les soins de santé et de beauté, issus de la sagesse de ces cultures millénaires.

Dit 1500 m² omvattende kuurcomplex was het eerste in zijn soort in Zwitserland. Het is ontworpen volgens een filosofie die oeroude rituelen rond gezondheid en schoonheid in zich verenigt. Culturele invloeden uit Japan, India, Noord-Afrika, China en Bali komen niet alleen terug in designelementen in de acht behandelkamers, twee zwembaden en de fitnessruimte, maar ook in de gezondheids- en schoonheidsbehandelingen, die de wijsheid van oude culturen overbrengen naar het heden.

Lausanne, Switzerland

LES CINQ MONDES SPA

Photos © Beau-Rivage Palace

www.brp.ch

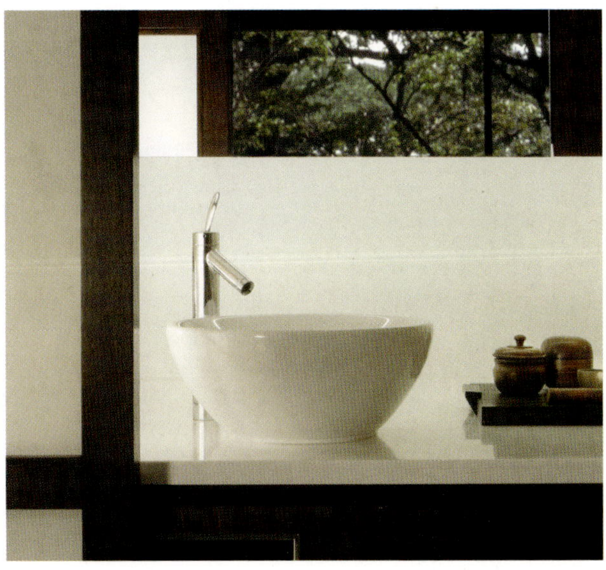

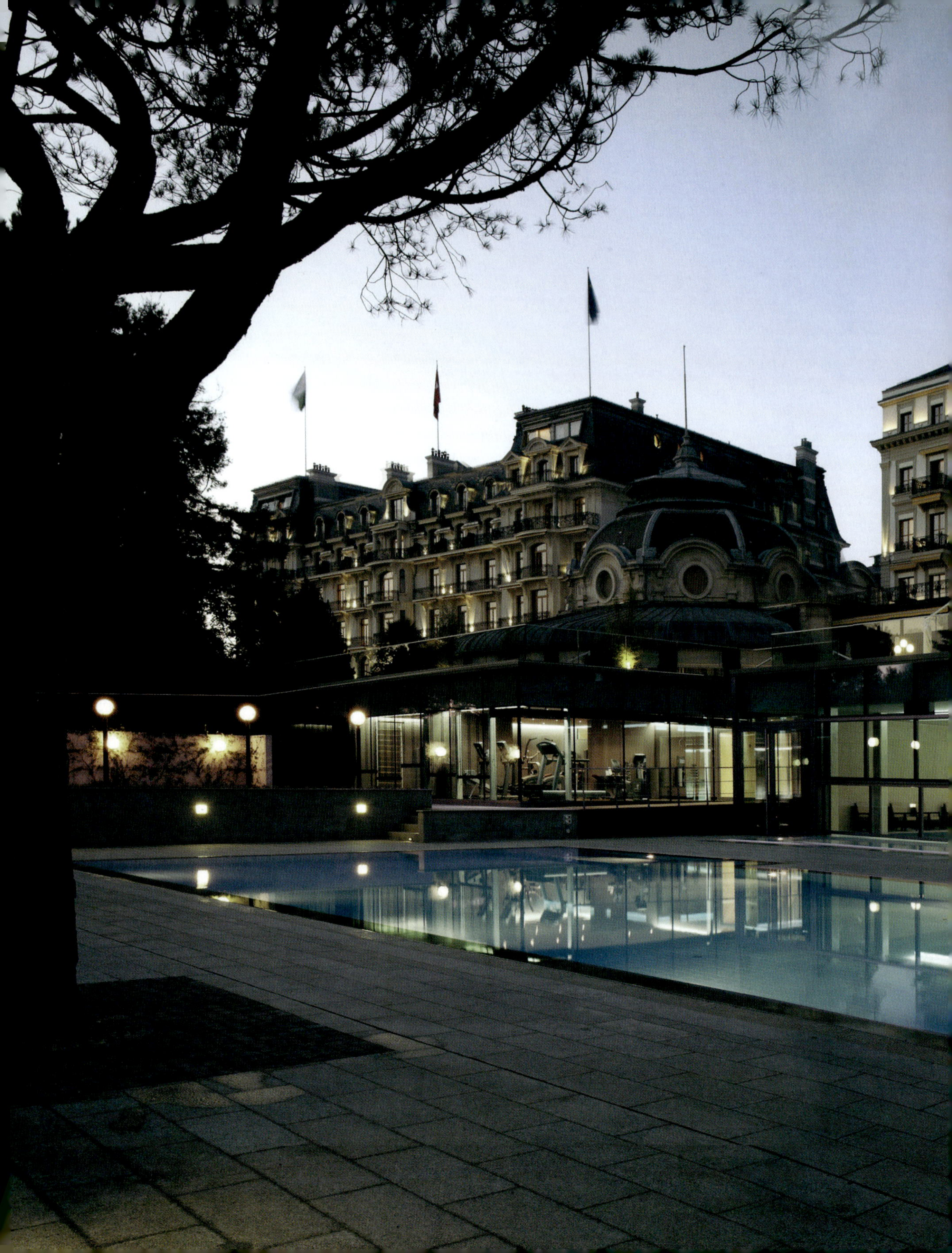

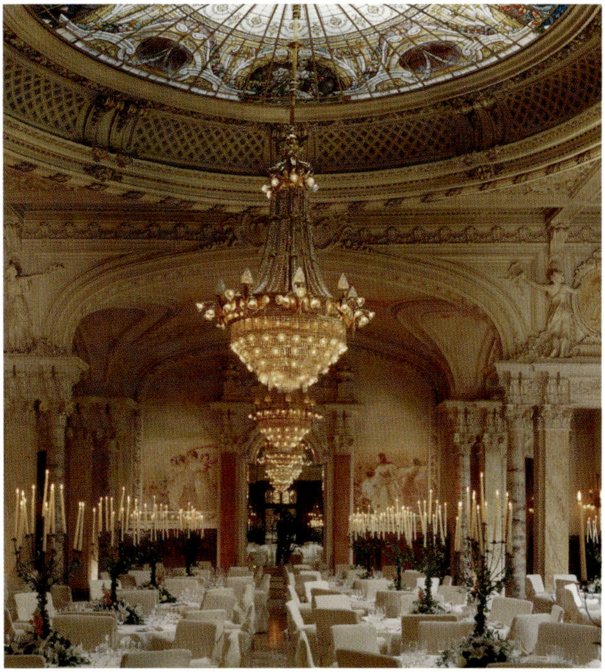

Zwischen der Entstehung beider Bauten liegen 70 Jahre. Das Spa entstand im Rahmen einer umfassenden Renovierung.

The two buildings were built seventy years apart, and the spa belongs to a recent renovation.

Soixante-dix années séparent la construction des deux bâtiments, et le spa est le fruit d'une rénovation récente.

De twee gebouwen zijn zeventig jaar na elkaar neergezet. Het kuurcomplex is het product van een recente renovatie.

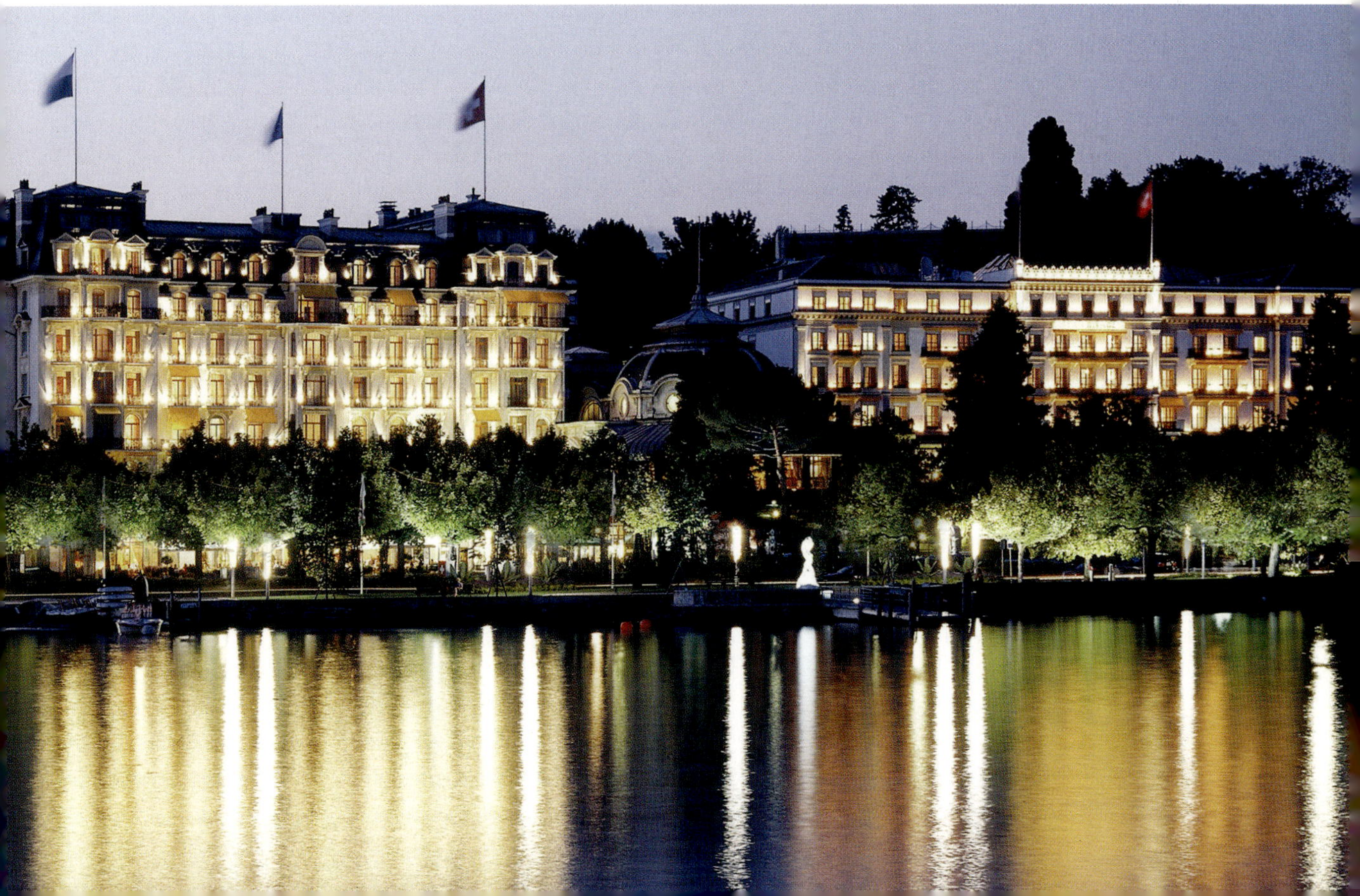

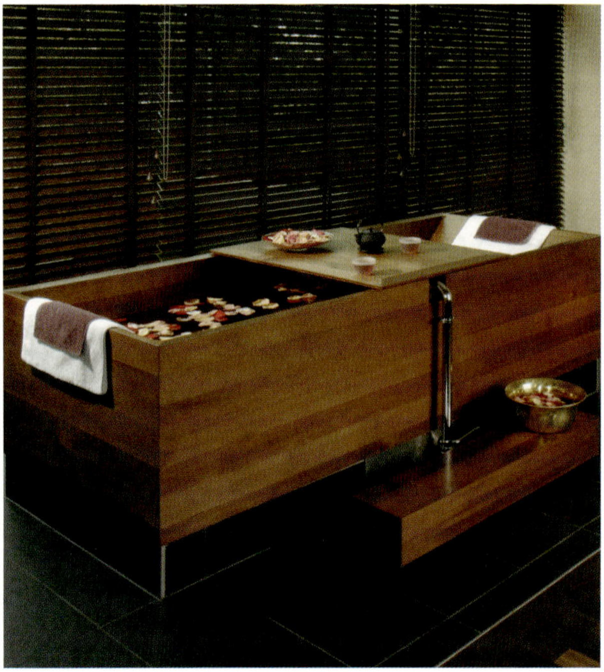

Indische Öle, japanische Massagen und ägyptisches Wasser: eine virtuelle Reise zu den schönsten Oasen.

Indian oils, tropical balms, Japanese massages and Egyptian waters: a virtual journey to the most serene sanctuaries.

Huiles indiennes, baumes tropicaux, massages japonais et eaux égyptiennes : tout invite ici à un voyage virtuel dans les temples de sérénité.

Indiase oliën, tropische balsems, Japanse massages en Egyptisch water: een virtuele reis naar serene toevluchtsoorden.

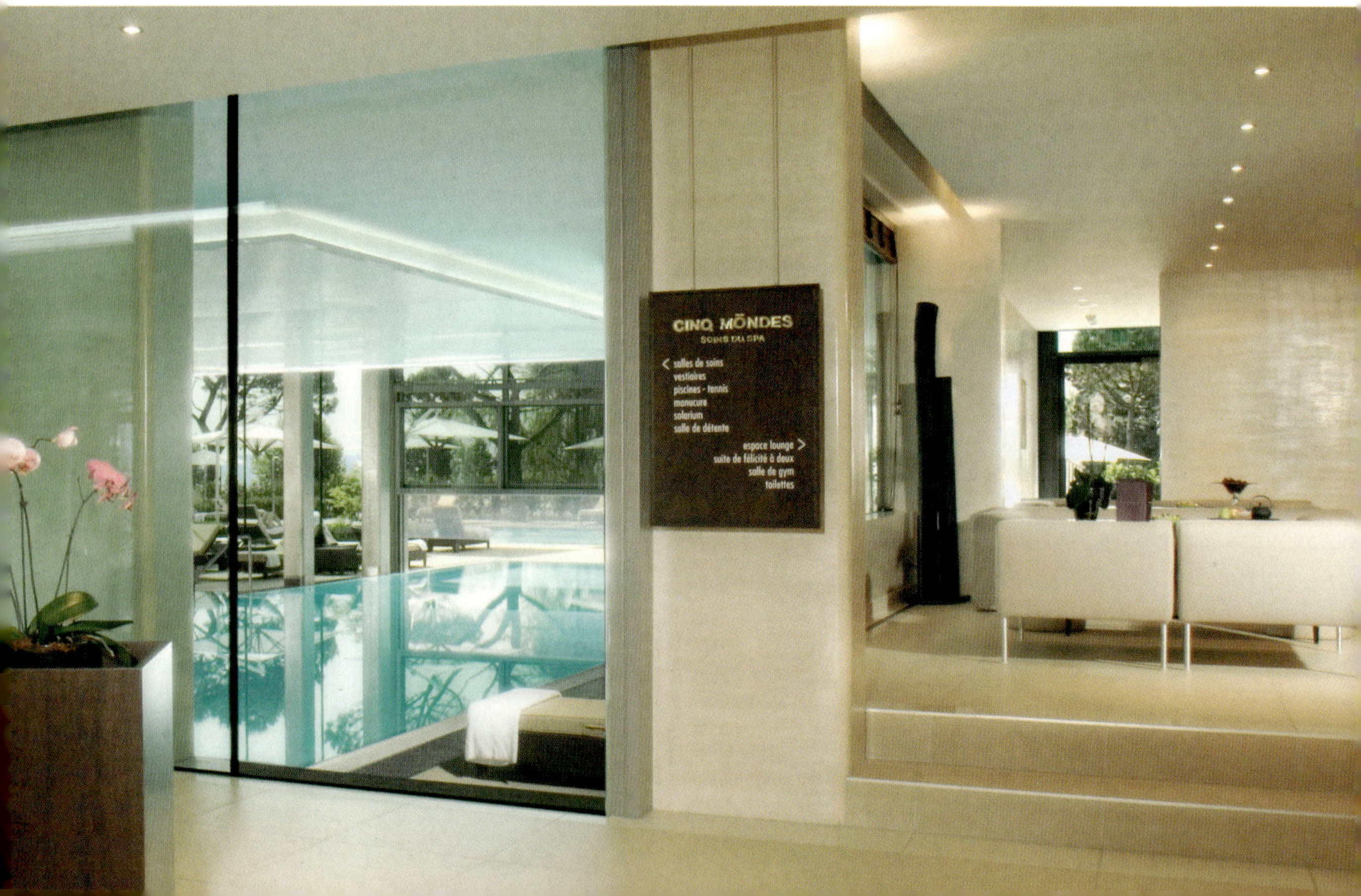

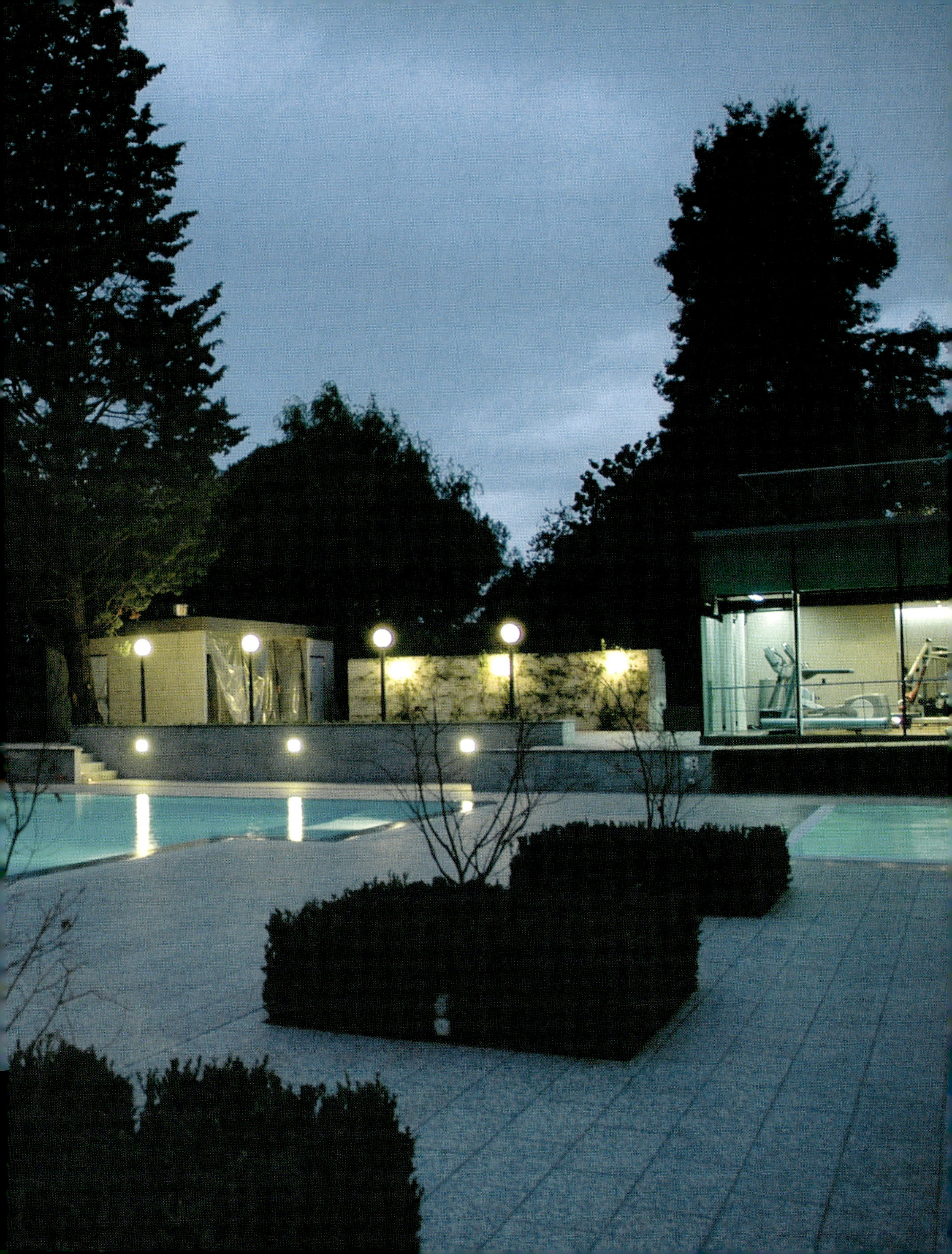

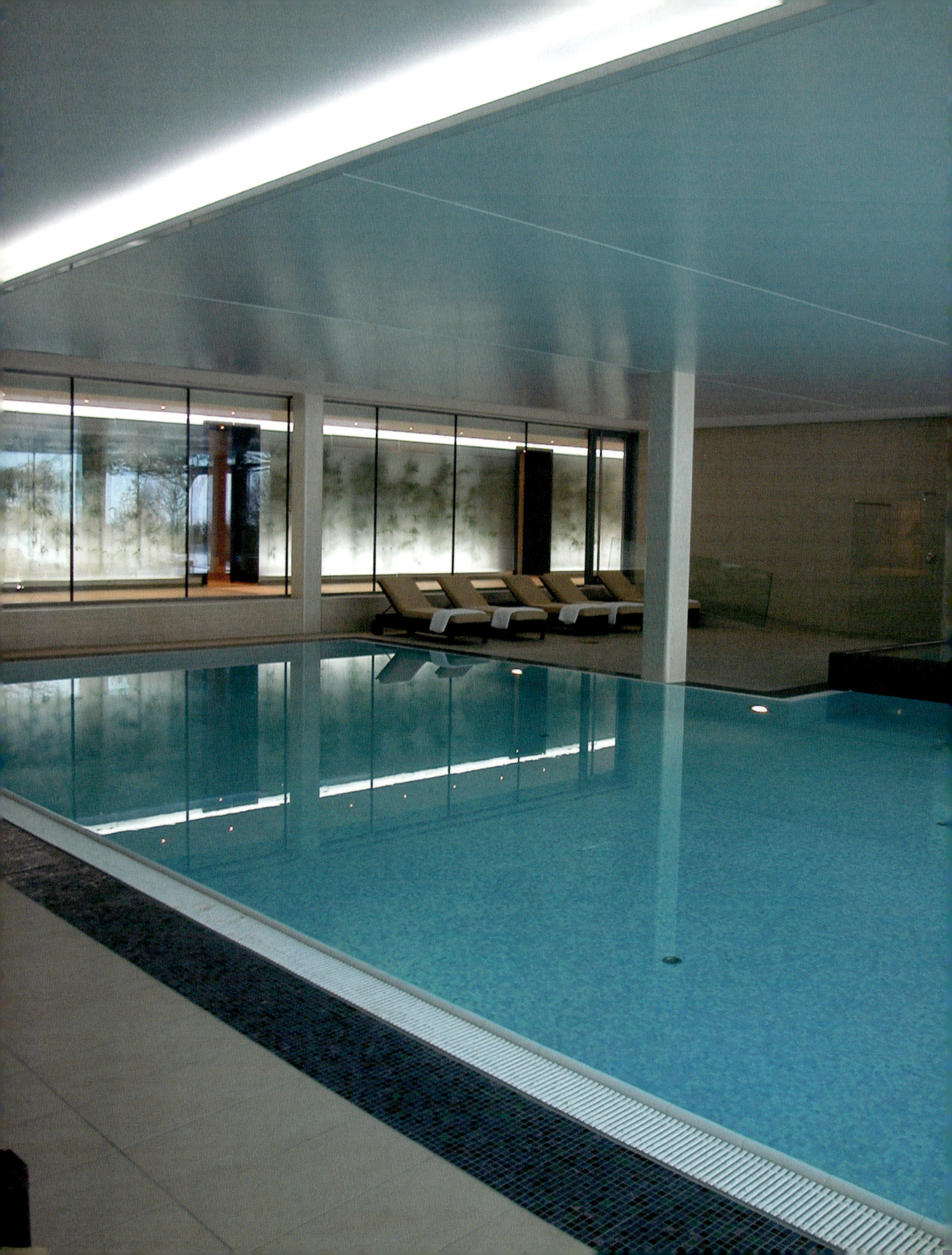

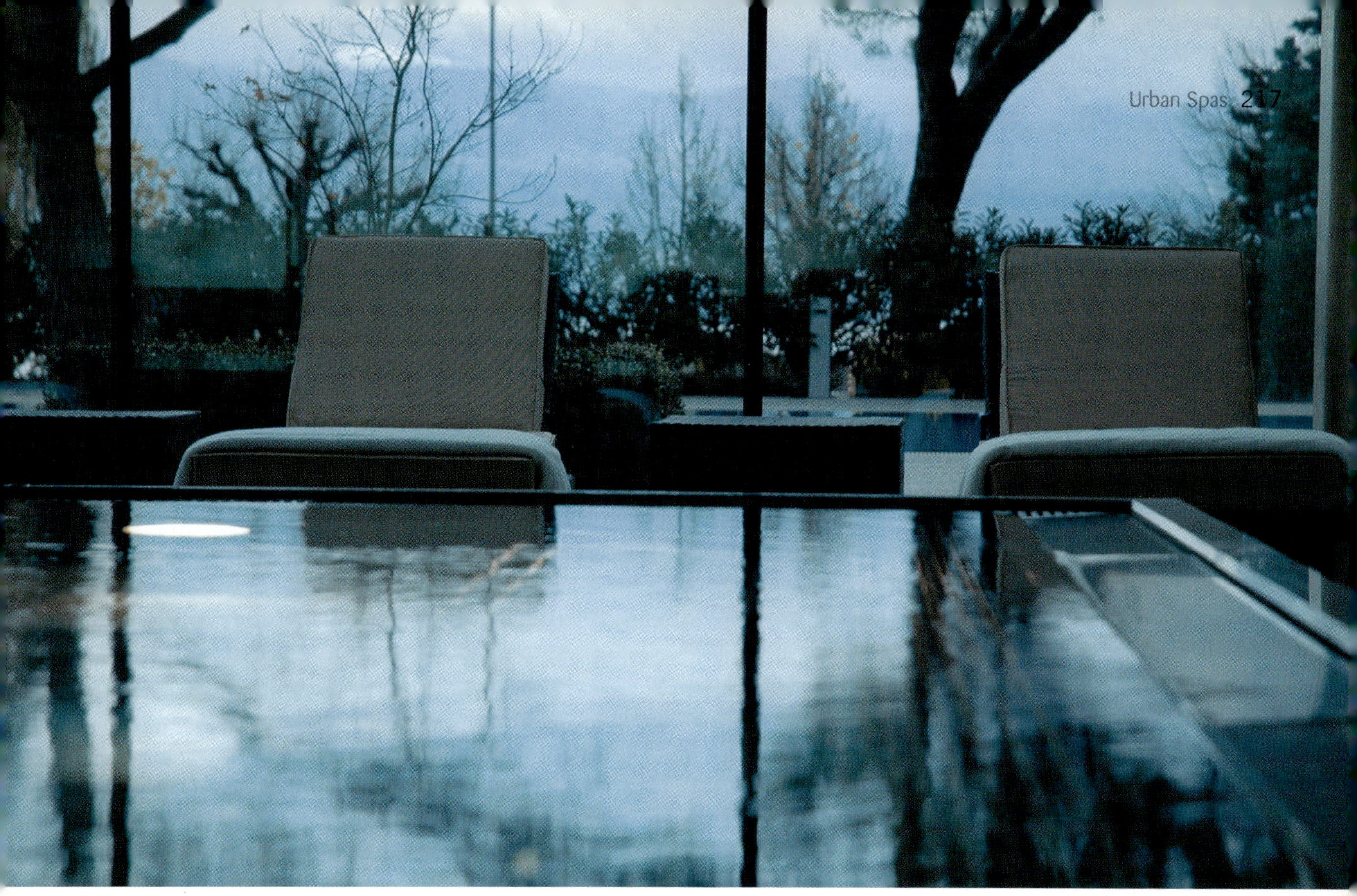

Das Spa verfügt über einen 15 m langen Innenpool mit Gartenblick und einen 20 m langen Außenpool.

The spa boasts an indoor pool of 49 feet overlooking the gardens, as well as an outdoor pool of 66 feet.

Le spa peut être se vanter de posséder une piscine intérieure de 15 m dominant les jardins, en même temps qu'une piscine extérieure de 20 m.

Het badcomplex bevat een vijftienmeterbad met uitzicht op de tuinen en een twintigmeterbad in de open lucht.

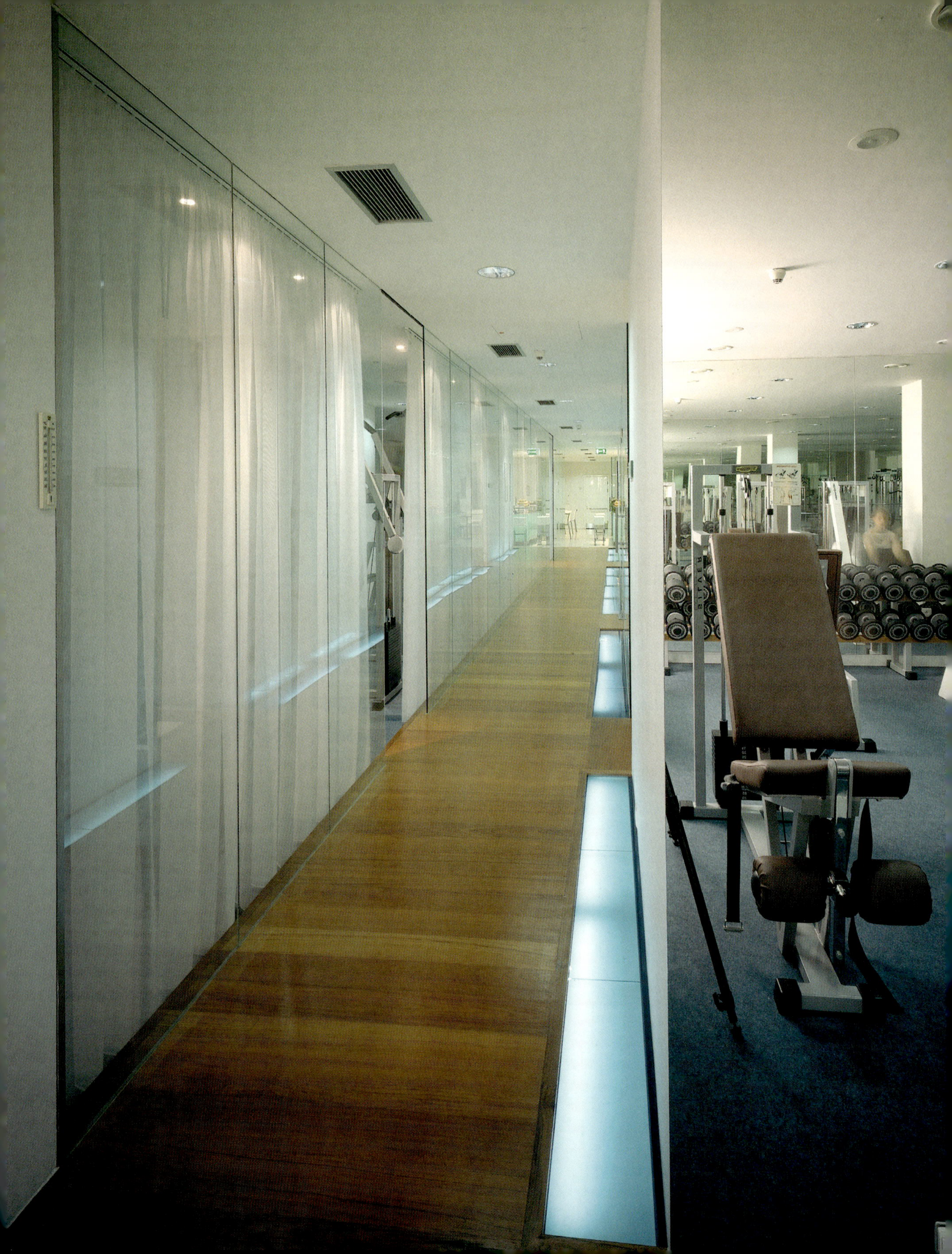

Health Club at Andel's Hotel

Die Räume dieses Spas sind durch eine „Brücke" miteinander verbunden, die an der Rezeption beginnt und beim Überqueren einen diskreten Blick auf die unterschiedlichen Bereiche gewährt. Der durch Glaswände und Voile-Stores abgegrenzte Durchgang verbindet Fitness- und Entspannungsräume auf der einen und Massagekabinen, Sauna und Dampfbäder auf der anderen Seite. Je mehr Privatsphäre die Aktivitäten erfordern, desto weiter liegen die Räume von der Brücke entfernt.

The spaces of this urban spa are connected by a "bridge" that starts at the luminous reception and that, as one crosses it, reveals the different activities without breaking into their intimacy. This wooden floored hallway with its glass and voile walls, connects the gym with the relaxation rooms on one side, and the massage cabins, sauna and steam baths on the other. The more privacy the activities require, the further the spaces are from the central bridge.

Partant d'une réception baignée de lumière, une passerelle relie les espaces de ce spa urbain. Lorsqu'on l'emprunte, cette passerelle révèle les différentes activités du spa, tout en préservant l'intimité des clients. Ce couloir au sol parqueté et aux murs de verres et de voilages, relie d'un côté la salle de gymnastique à celle de relaxation et, de l'autre côté, les cabines de massage, le sauna et le hammam. Plus les activités exigent un cadre intime, plus elles se trouvent éloignées de cette passerelle centrale.

De afdelingen van dit stedelijke kuuroord zijn met elkaar verbonden via een 'brug' die begint in de lichte entreehal en onder het lopen zicht biedt op de verschillende activiteiten, zonder die te verstoren. Dit houten voetpad met wanden van glas en gaas verbindt de sportzaal met de ontspanningsruimten aan de ene kant en de massagecabines, sauna en stoombaden aan de andere kant. Naarmate behandelingen meer privacy vereisen, liggen ze verder weg van de loopbrug.

Prague, Czech Republic

JESTICO & WHILES

Photos © Ales Jungmann

www.andelshotel.cz

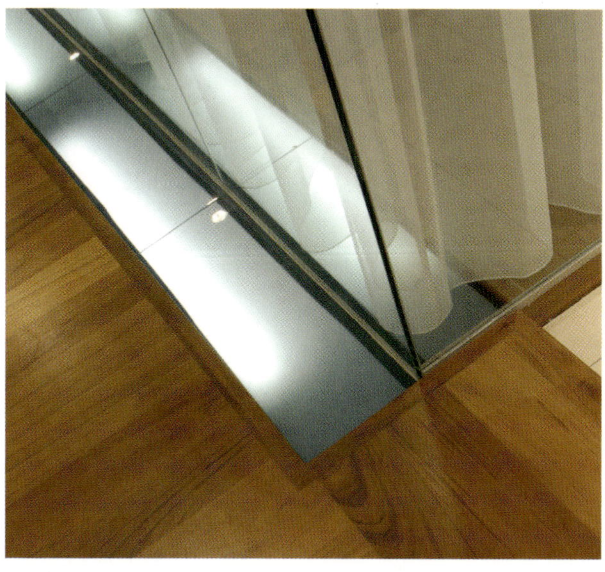

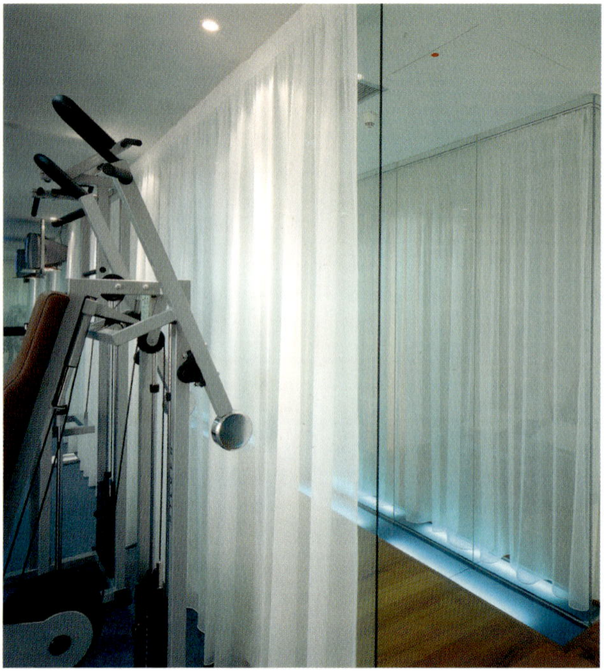

An der hell erleuchteten Rezeption befinden sich eine Saftbar und eine Boutique mit Therapieprodukten.

The luminous reception holds a fruit juice bar and a shop that sells therapeutic products.

La réception très lumineuse accueille à la fois un bar à jus de fruit et un espace de commercialisation de produits de santé.

De lichte entreehal bevat een sapbar en een winkel waar therapeutische producten worden verkocht.

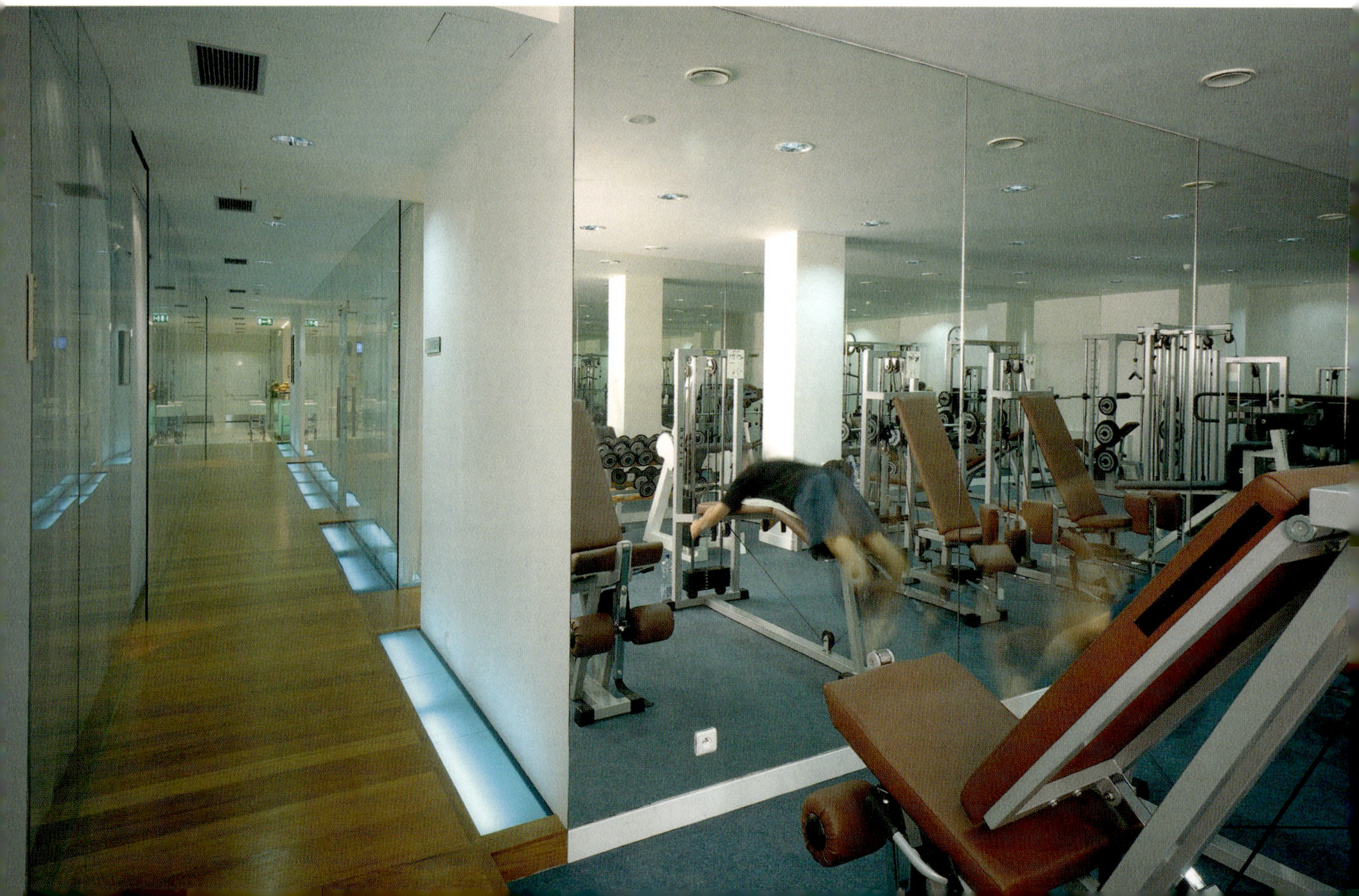

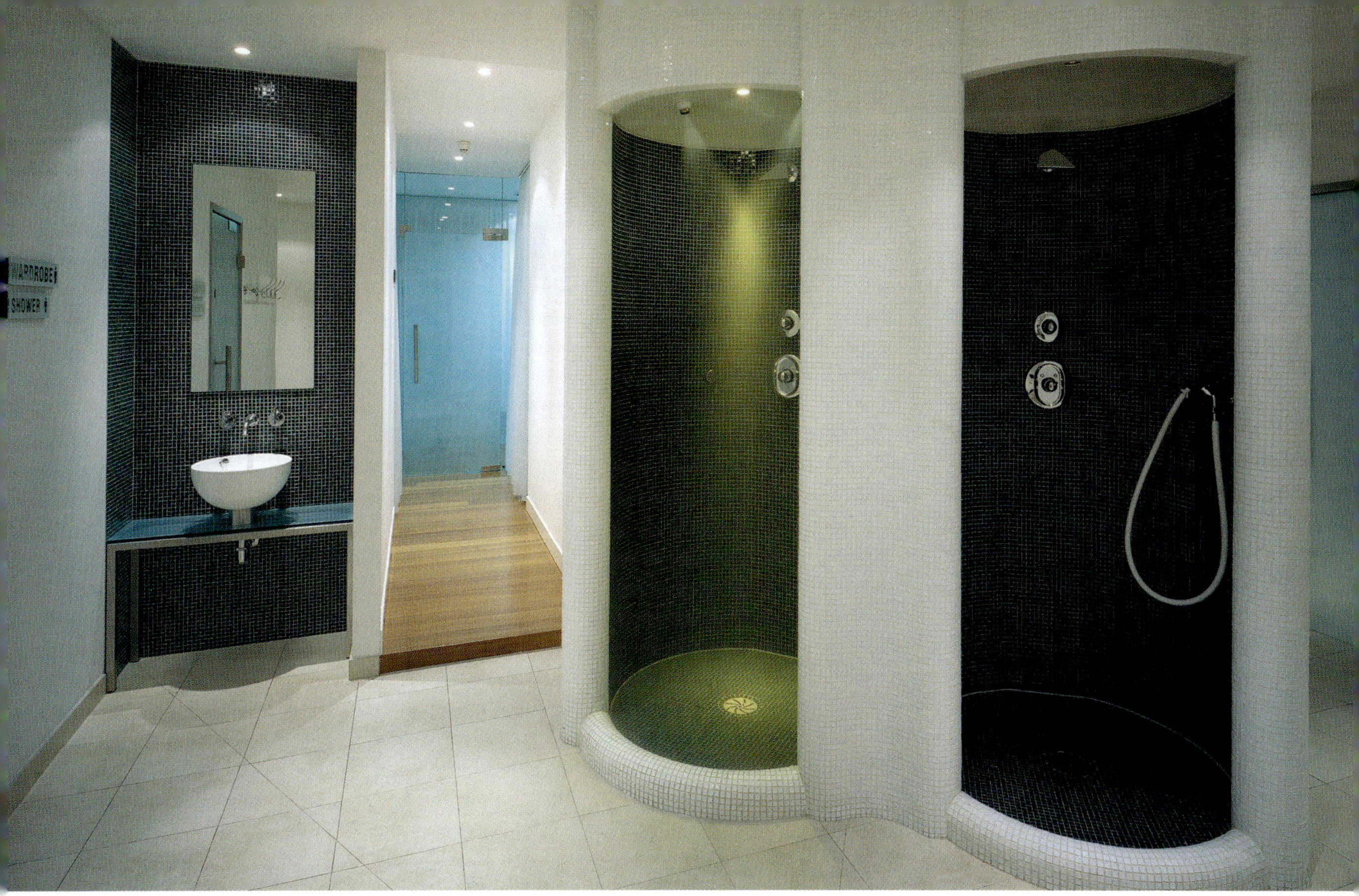
WARDROBE
SHOWER

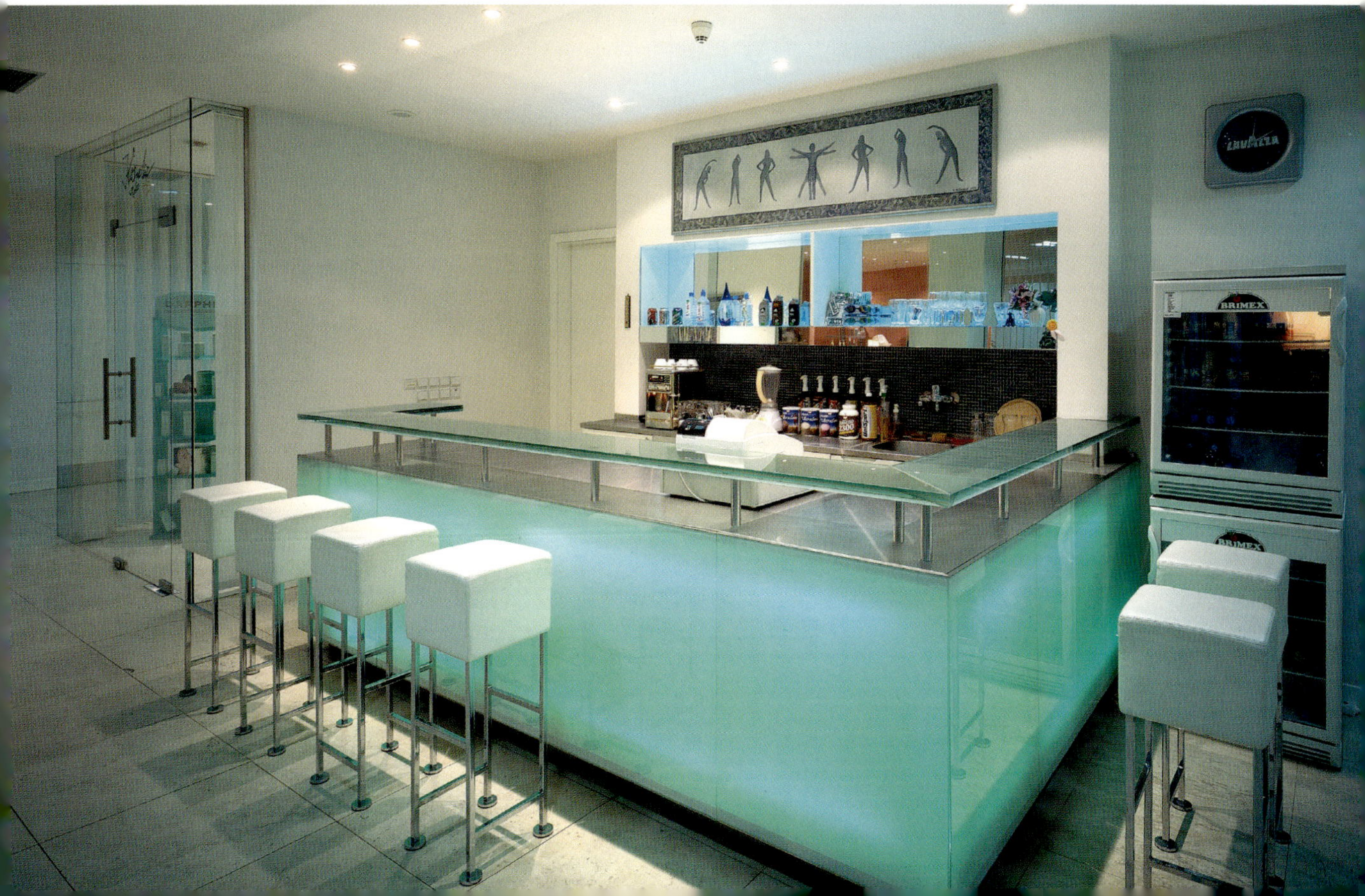
BRIMEX
BRIMEX

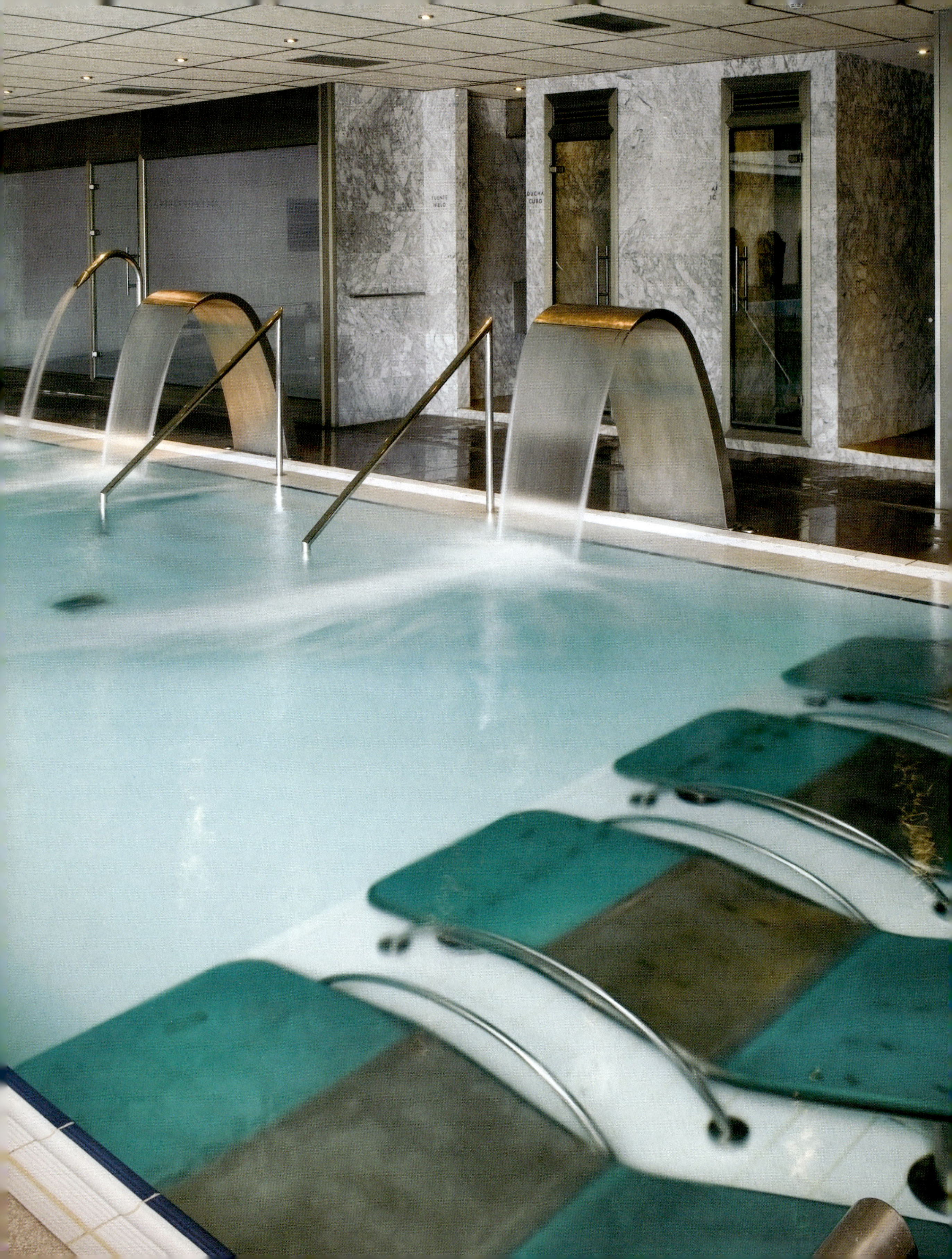
FUENTE HIELO
DUCHA CUBO

Health Club & Spa Metropolitan Gran Vía

Das 2006 eröffnete Hesperia Tower Hotel zählt zu den höchsten und beeindruckendsten Bauten Barcelonas. Saunen, türkische Bäder, Whirlpools, Wasserbetten, Zervikaldüsen und ein beheizter Pool bilden den Nassbereich des Spas, das durch Räume für Gesundheits- und Schönheitsbehandlungen ergänzt wird. Beide Bereiche sind durch ein 25-Meter-Becken und ein als Entspannungszone konzipiertes Holzdeck miteinander verbunden.

Inaugurated in 2006, Hesperia Tower hotel has become one of the tallest and most symbolic buildings in Barcelona. Saunas, Turkish baths, Jacuzzis, water beds, cervical jets and the heated pool constitute the spa's water circuit, which is complemented with its health and beauty treatments. An 82 feet swimming pool with a wooden deck equipped for relaxation, works as the space that integrates the two areas.

Inauguré en 2006, l'hôtel de la tour Hesperia est devenu l'une des constructions les plus hautes et les plus emblématiques de Barcelone. Saunas, bains turcs, jacuzzis, lits à eau, jets spéciaux pour les cervicales, et piscine chauffée constituent le circuit aquatique du spa, qui propose également des soins de santé et de beauté. Agrémentée d'une terrasse en bois dédiée à la relaxation, une piscine de 25 m constitue une zone de transition entre les deux espaces.

Het Hesperia Tower Hotel, geopend in 2006, was meteen al een van de hoogste, meest markante gebouwen van Barcelona. Sauna's, Turkse baden, jacuzzi's, waterbedden, hydromassagestralen en het verwarmde zwembad vormen samen het watercircuit, dat aan de andere kant wordt aangevuld met gezondheids- en schoonheidsbehandelingen. Een vijfentwintigmeterbad met een houten terras ter ontspanning smeedt deze twee afdelingen aaneen.

Barcelona, Spain

ALONSO BALAGUER Y ARQUITECTOS ASOCIADOS

Photos © David Cardelús, Pedro Pegenaute

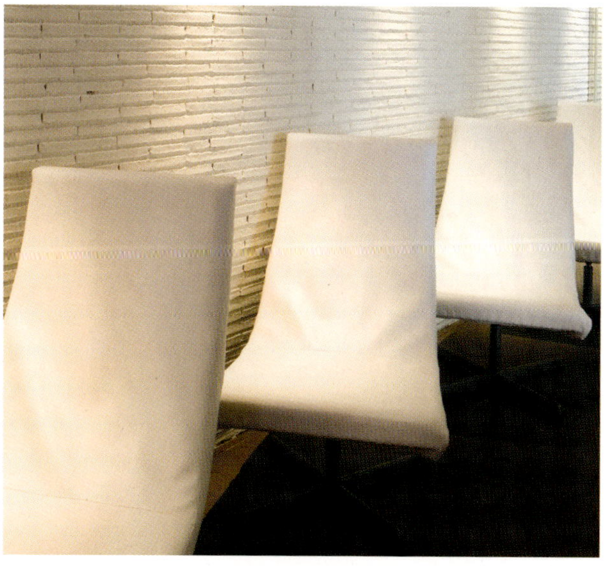

www.clubmetropolitan.net

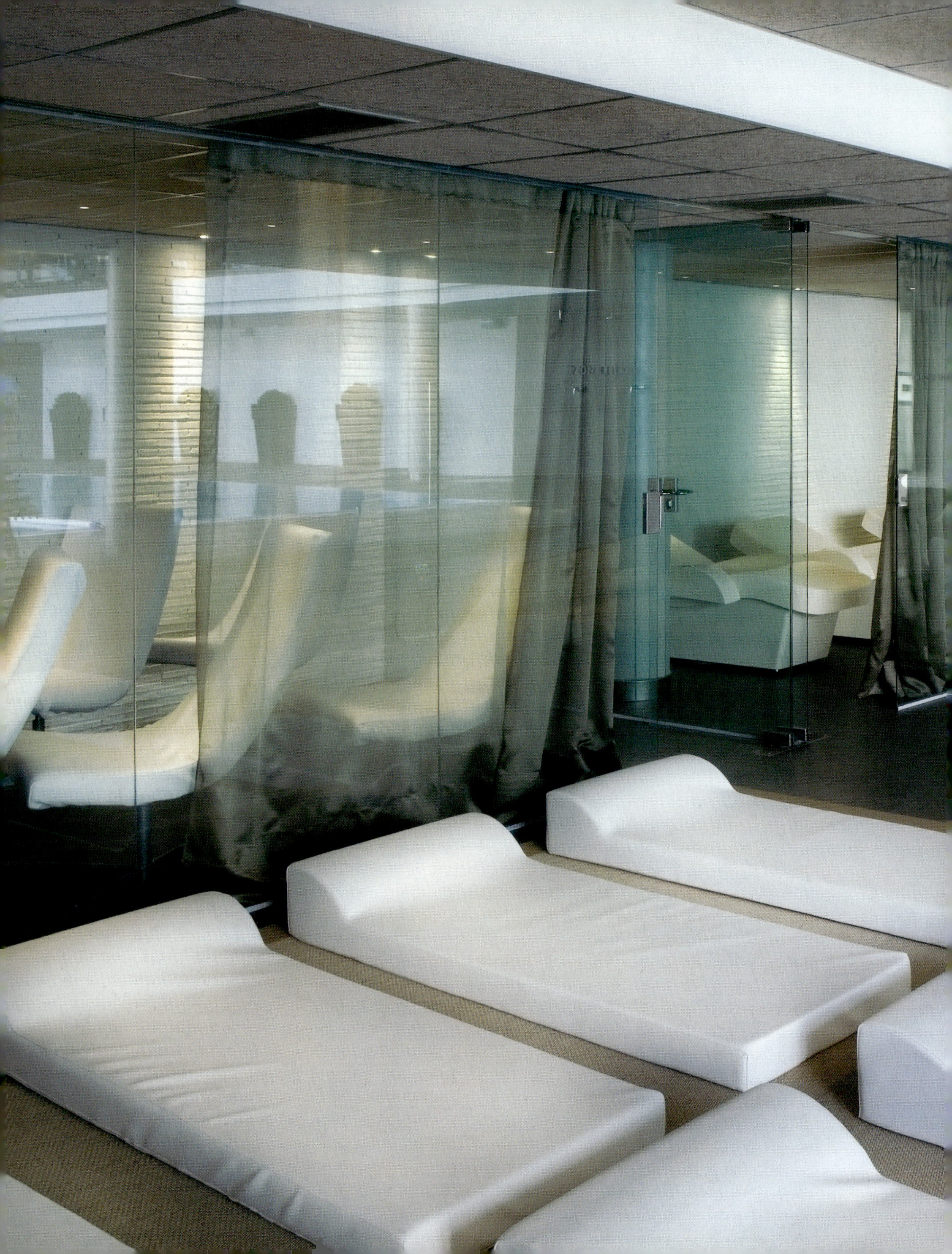

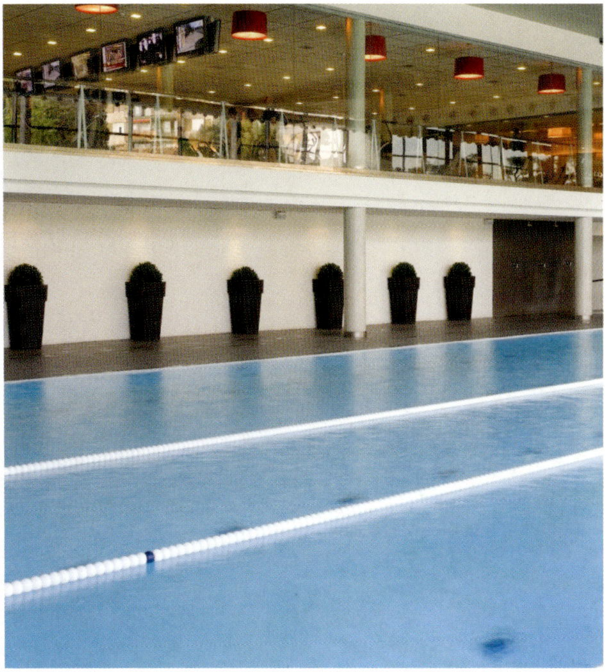

Sport, Gesundheit und Wellness sind die drei Grundpfeiler der Philosphie des Health Club & Spa Metropolitan Gran Vía.

Sport, health and wellbeing are the three fundamental activities that define Health Club & Spa Metropolitan Gran Vía.

Sport, santé et bien-être sont les trois éléments essentiels qui définissent le Health Club & Spa Gran Metropolitan Gran Via.

Sport, gezondheid en wellness zijn de drie uitgangspunten van de Health Club & Spa Metropolitan Gran Via.

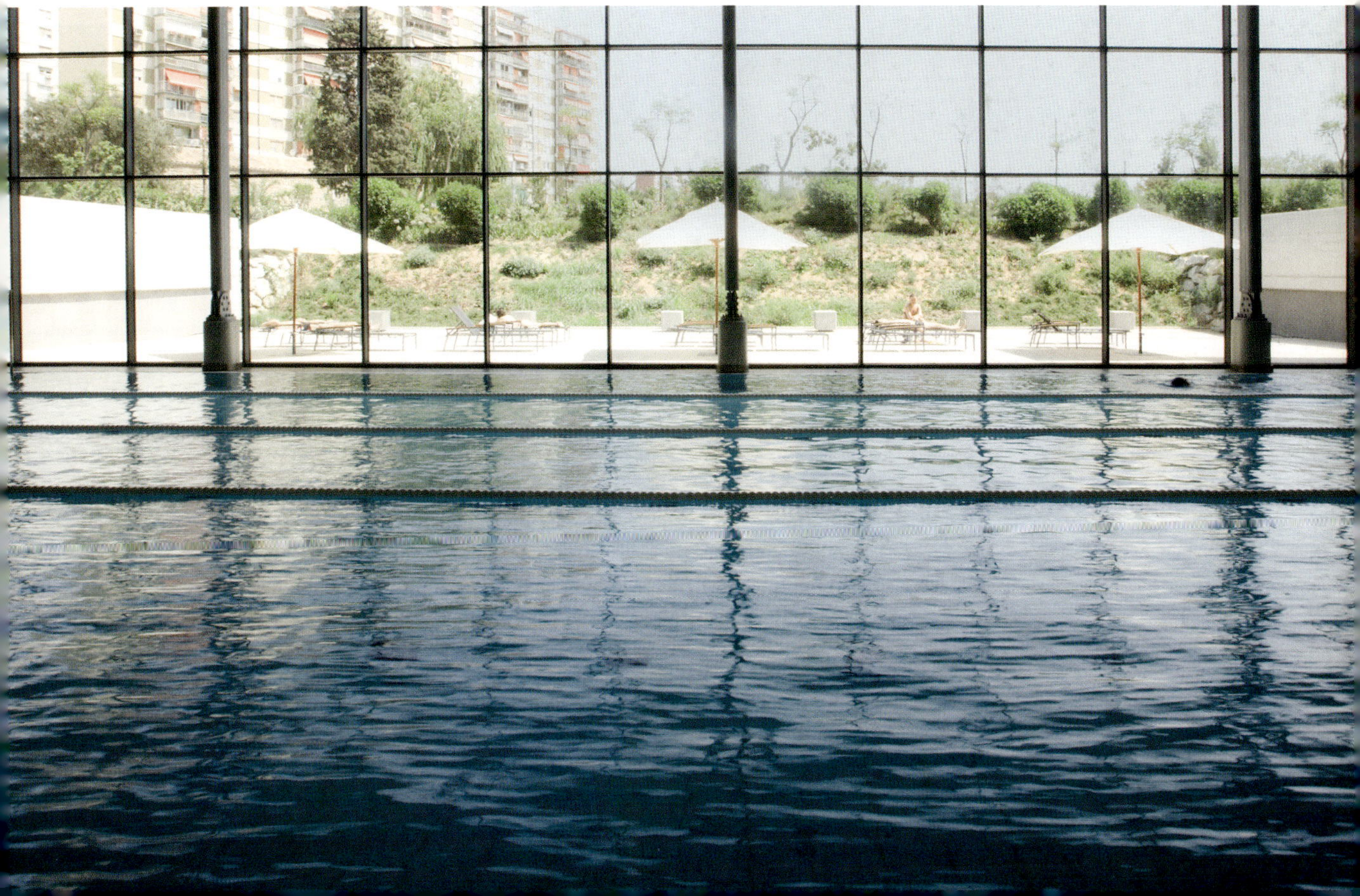

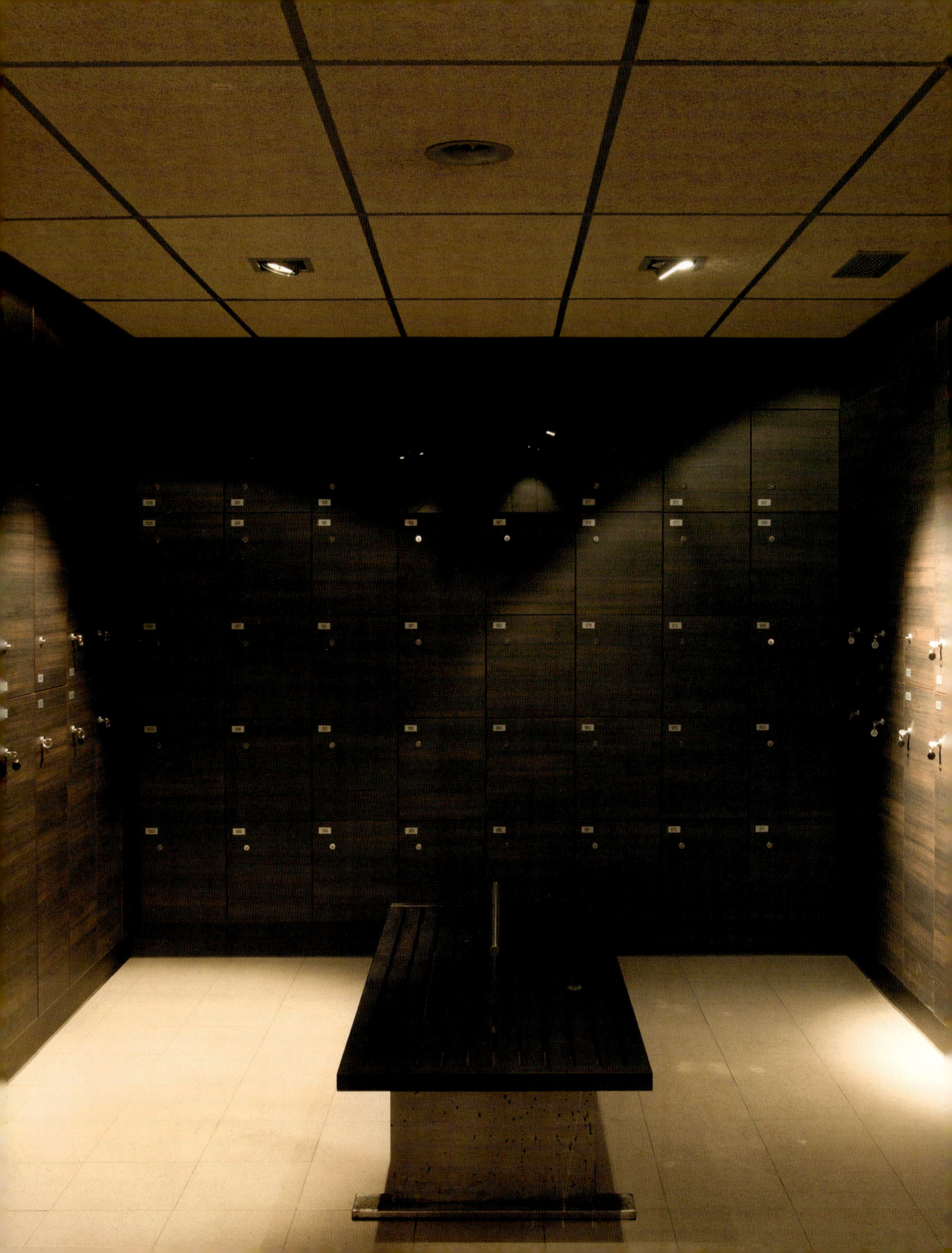

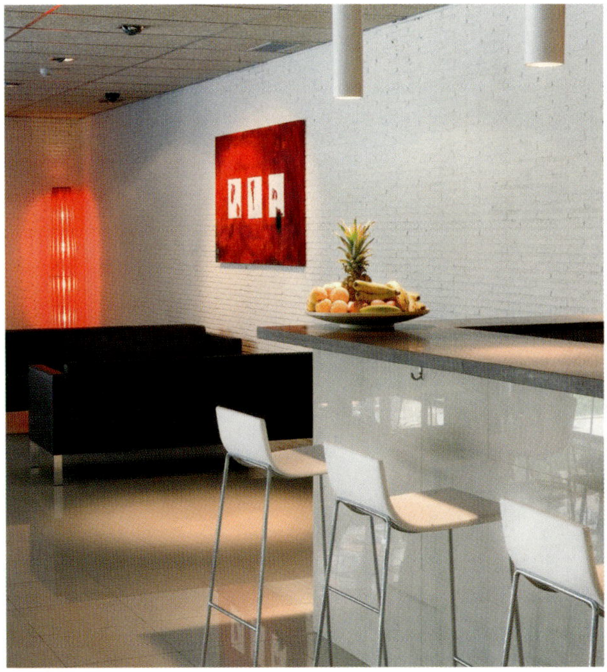

Dieses Spa bietet ein 25-Meter-Becken, Saunen, türkische Bäder, Whirlpools und Wasserbetten.

An 82 feet pool, saunas, Turkish baths, Jacuzzis and water beds are essential items in this spa.

La piscine de 25 m de long, les saunas, les hammams, les jacuzzis et les lits à eau sont les atouts majeurs de ce spa.

Een vijfentwintigmeterbad, sauna's, Turkse baden, jacuzzi's en waterbedden zijn wezenlijk voor deze kuurinrichting.

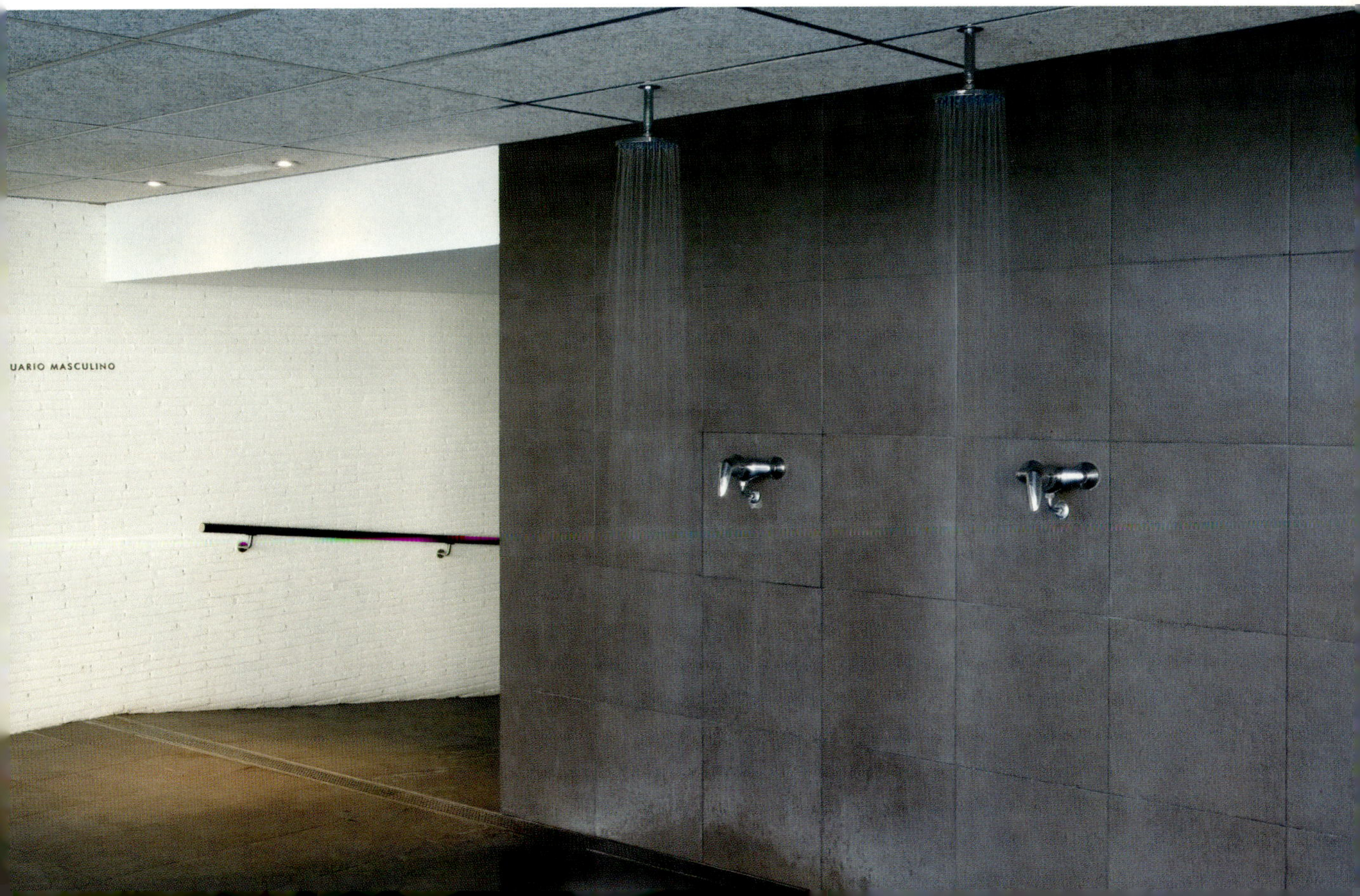

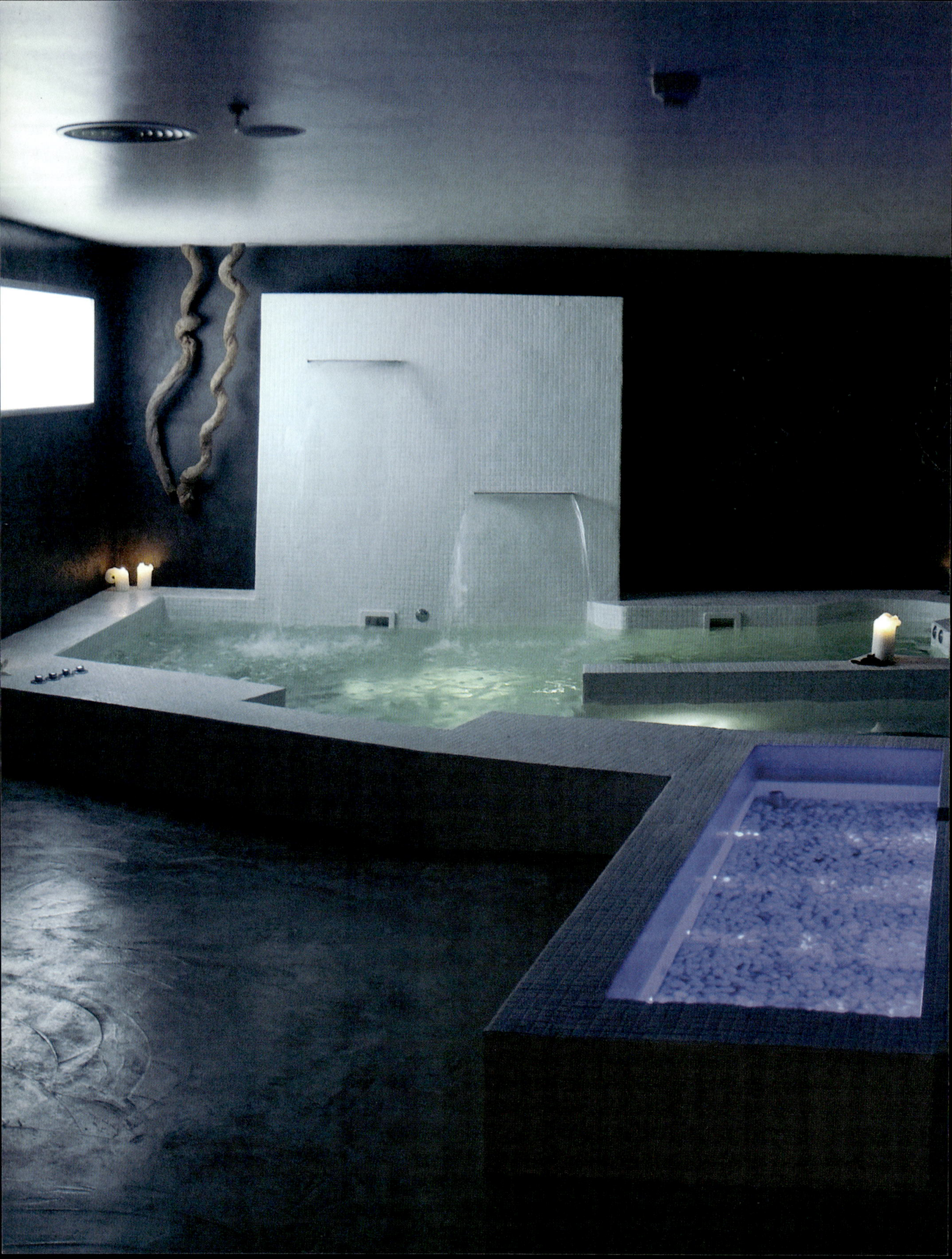

Caroli Health Club La Moraleja

Dieses Spa baut auf einem Konzept von verschiedenen Routen mit einander abwechselnden Erholungs- und Anregungszonen, bei dem Wasserspiele, Licht, Aromatherapie und Wärmekontraste zur Entspannung beitragen. Ein Beauty Center befindet sich hier ebenfalls. Zum Angebot gehören stressslösende Hydromassagen, revitalisierende Wasserbetten, finnische Sauna, Hammam und Aromatherapieduschen. Jede Route endet im Entspannungsbereich, wo Körper und Geist zur verdienten Ruhe kommen.

Conceived to liberate tensions through water games, light, aromatherapy and thermal contrasts, the spa is organized in circuits of relaxation and stimulation. The aesthetics center is on the same floor. Programs include hydromassage treatments to release stress, revitalizing water-beds, Finnish sauna to eliminate toxins, hammam, contrast therapies and aromatherapy showers. All routes end in the relaxation area, where body and mind are deservedly dedicated to serenity.

Conçu pour libérer des tensions corporelles par des jeux aquatiques, la lumière, l'aromathérapie et des contrastes thermiques, le spa s'organise autour de circuits de relaxation et de stimulation. L'institut de beauté est au même étage. Les programmes proposent des traitements anti-stress par hydromassage, des lits à eau revitalisants, du sauna finlandais pour éliminer les toxines, un hammam, des soins basés sur un jeu de contrastes et des douches d'aromathérapie. Tous les itinéraires aboutissent à l'espace relaxation, où le corps et l'esprit peuvent à juste titre s'adonner à la sérénité.

Dit kuuroord heeft circuits voor ontspanning en stimulatie, om stress te verlichten met wateractiviteiten, licht, aromatherapie en thermale contrasten. Het schoonheidscentrum ligt op dezelfde verdieping. Er zijn hydromassagebehandelingen tegen stress, revitaliserende baden, Finse sauna's om te ontgiften, hammams, contrasttherapieën en aromatherapiedouches. Alle trajecten eindigen in de ontspanningsruimte, waar lichaam en geest zich kunnen overgeven aan een welverdiende rust.

Madrid, Spain

COLOMBO & ASSOCIATES SRL

Photos © Pablo Alemán

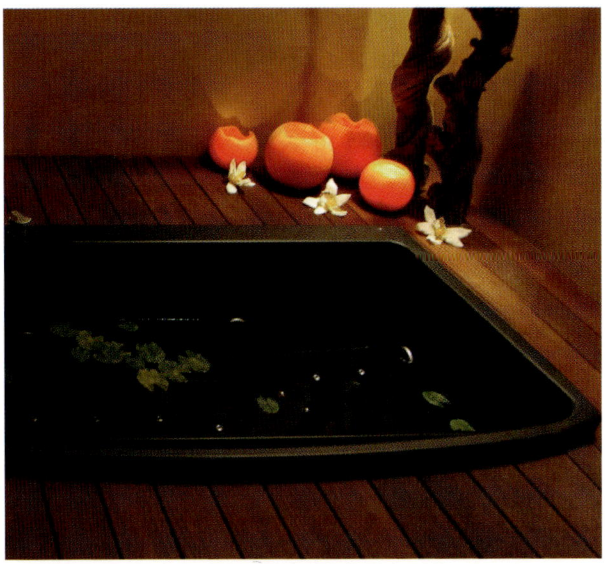

www.carolihealthclub.com

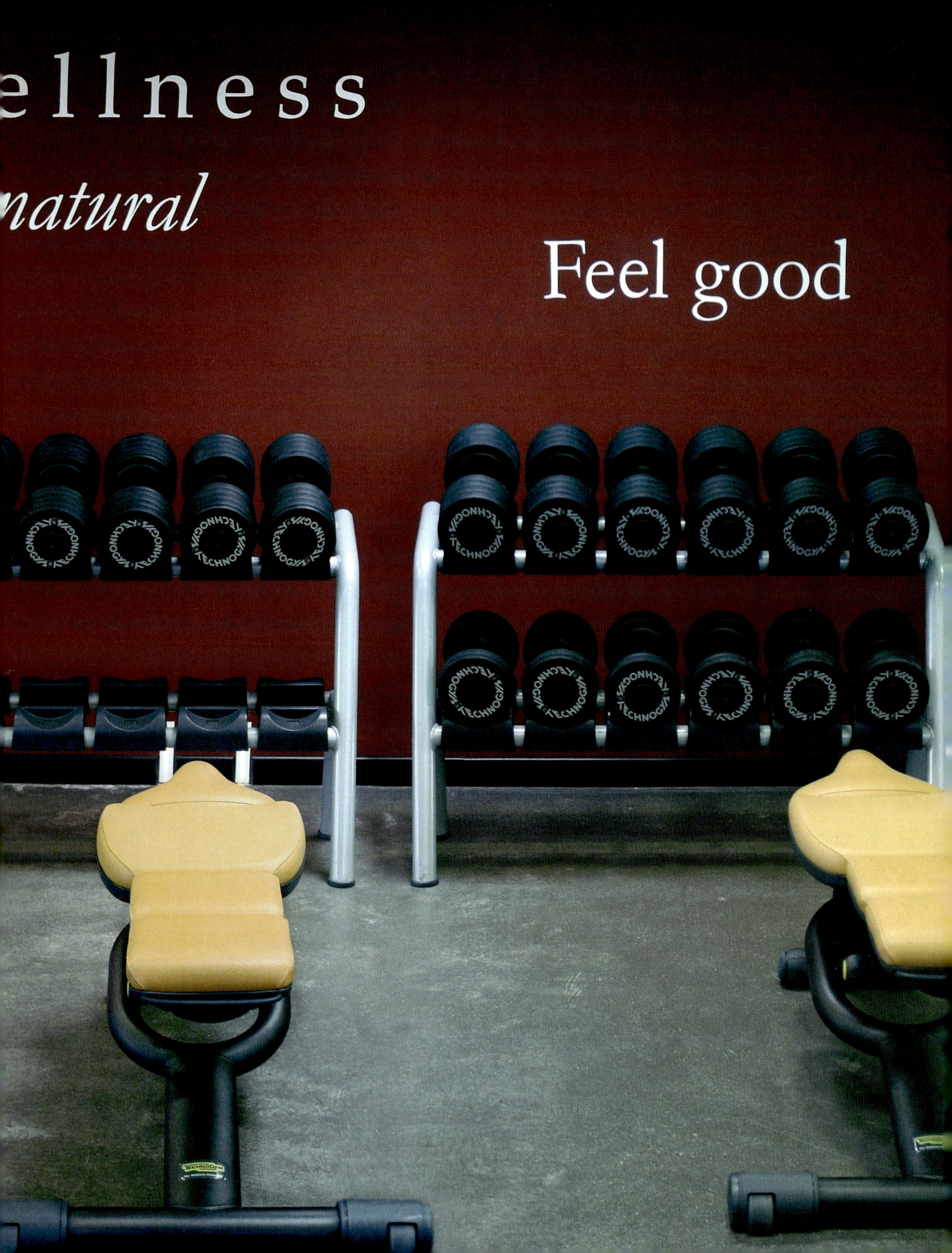
ellness
natural
Feel good
TECHNOGYM

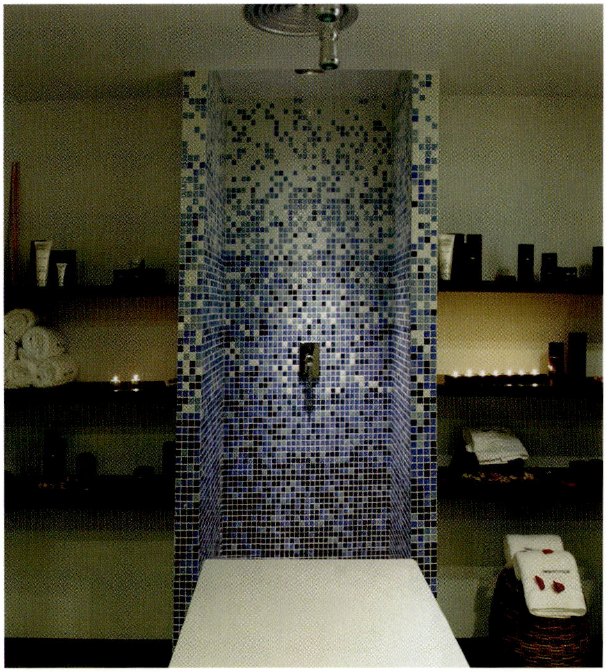

Zu den drei Spa-Routen zählt auch die Kneippkur, deren Heiß- und Kaltwasseranwendungen die Abwehrkräfte stärken.

The three spa circuits include the Kneipp route: an interplay of contrasts between cold and hot water at different pressures.

Les trois circuits du spa incluent un parcours Kneipp, basé sur un jeu de différentes pressions et de contrastes entre eau froide et eau chaude.

In de Kneipp-route, een van drie trajecten, gaat het om contrasten tussen koud en warm water en harde en zachte stralen.

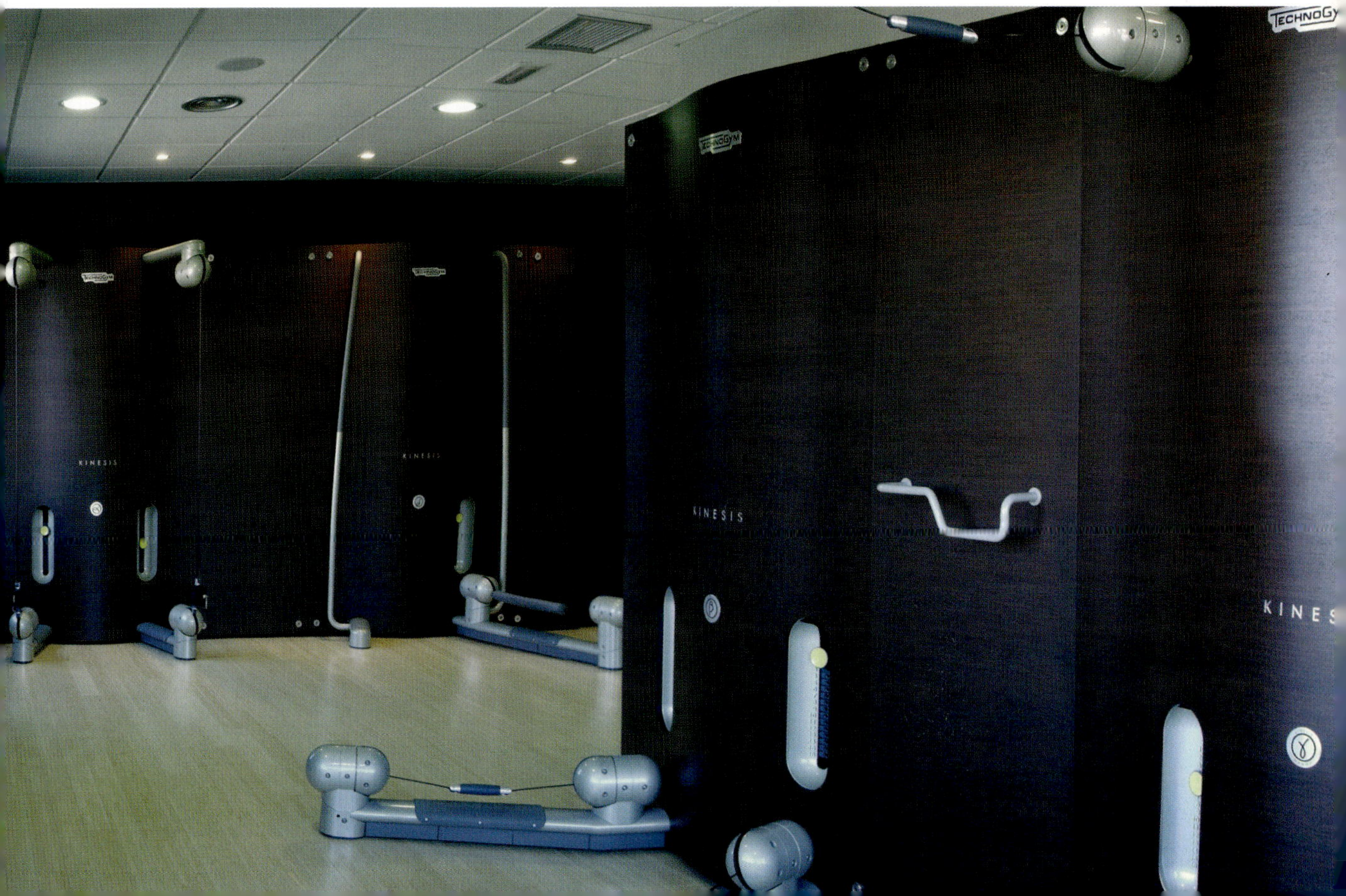

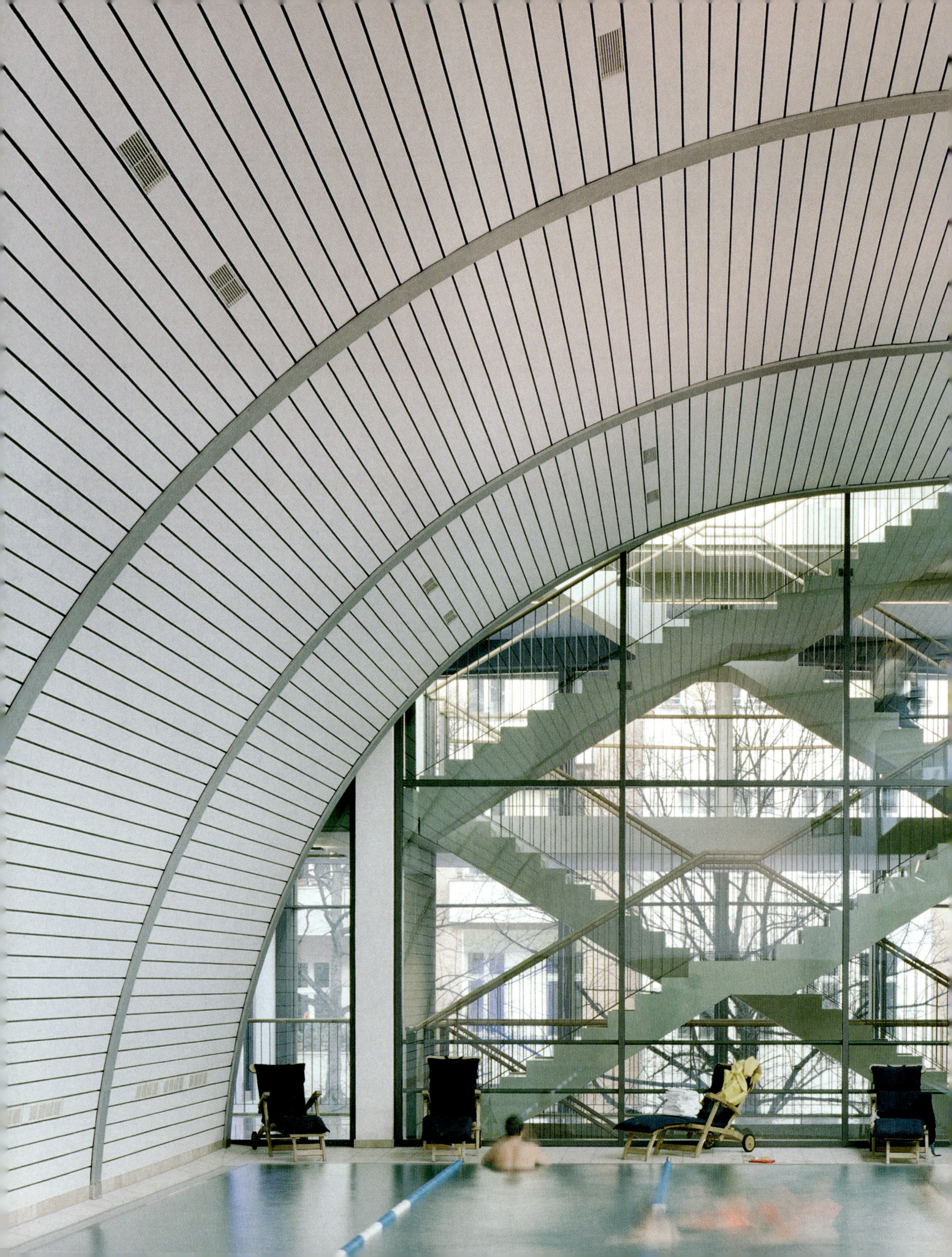

Aspria Spa & Sports

Nach umfassender Renovierung präsentiert sich dieses Spa mitten in Berlin als Wellnessoase mit moderner Ästhetik. Der 2.000 qm große Behandlungsbereich verfügt über einen Whirlpool, zwei Saunen, Sanarium mit Farb- und Aromatherapie, Dampfbäder, Eisraum, eine traumhafte Terrasse mit einem 600 qm großen Garten sowie ein Wellness-Bistro mit einem erfrischenden Angebot an gesunden Drinks und leichten Speisen.

After a complete structural reformation, Aspria Berlin has acquired a new dimension. The spa is defined by the warmth of its spaces, covered in wood and with oriental aesthetics. The 21,500 square feet treatment area includes a whirlpool bath, two saunas, a sanarium with chromotherapy and aromatherapy, steam baths, an ice room, a fantastic terrace with a 6,450 square feet garden and a wellness bistro specialized in dishes that are conceived for balanced nutrition.

Après une rénovation complète, l'Aspria de Berlin a acquis une nouvelle dimension. Couvert de bois, évoquant une esthétique orientale, le spa se caractérise par la chaleur de ses espaces. La zone de traitement de 2.000 m² comprend un bain bouillonnant, deux saunas, un sanarium avec chromothérapie et aromathérapie, un hammam, une cabine glacée, ainsi qu'une superbe terrasse arborée de 600 m², et un restaurant dont la carte ne propose que des plats diététiques.

Na een grondige renovatie heeft Aspria in Berlijn een nieuwe dimensie gekregen. Het badcomplex wordt getypeerd door een warme sfeer, veelvuldig gebruik van hout en een oosters aandoende inrichting. Op een oppervlak van 2000 m² liggen whirlpoolbaden, twee sauna's, een sanarium met chromotherapie en aromatherapie, stoombaden, een ijskamer, een fantastisch terras met een 600 m² grote tuin en een restaurant waar uitgebalanceerde gerechten worden geserveerd.

Berlin, Germany

FLETCHER PRIEST BÖESL ARCHITEKTEN (RENOVATION)

Photos © Jan Bitter Fotografie

www.aspria.com

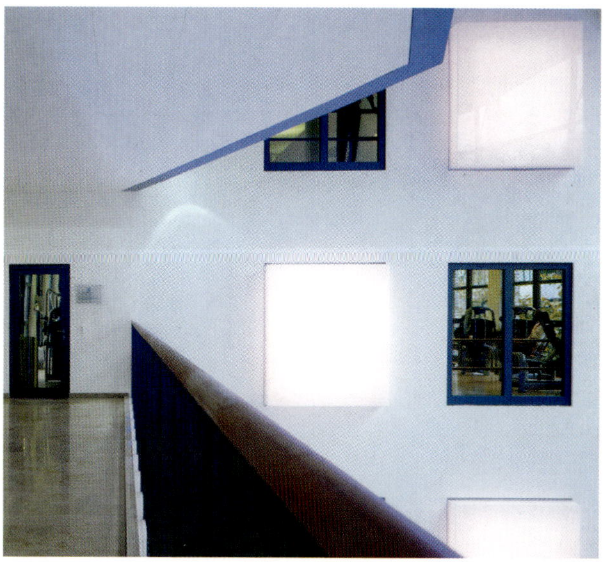

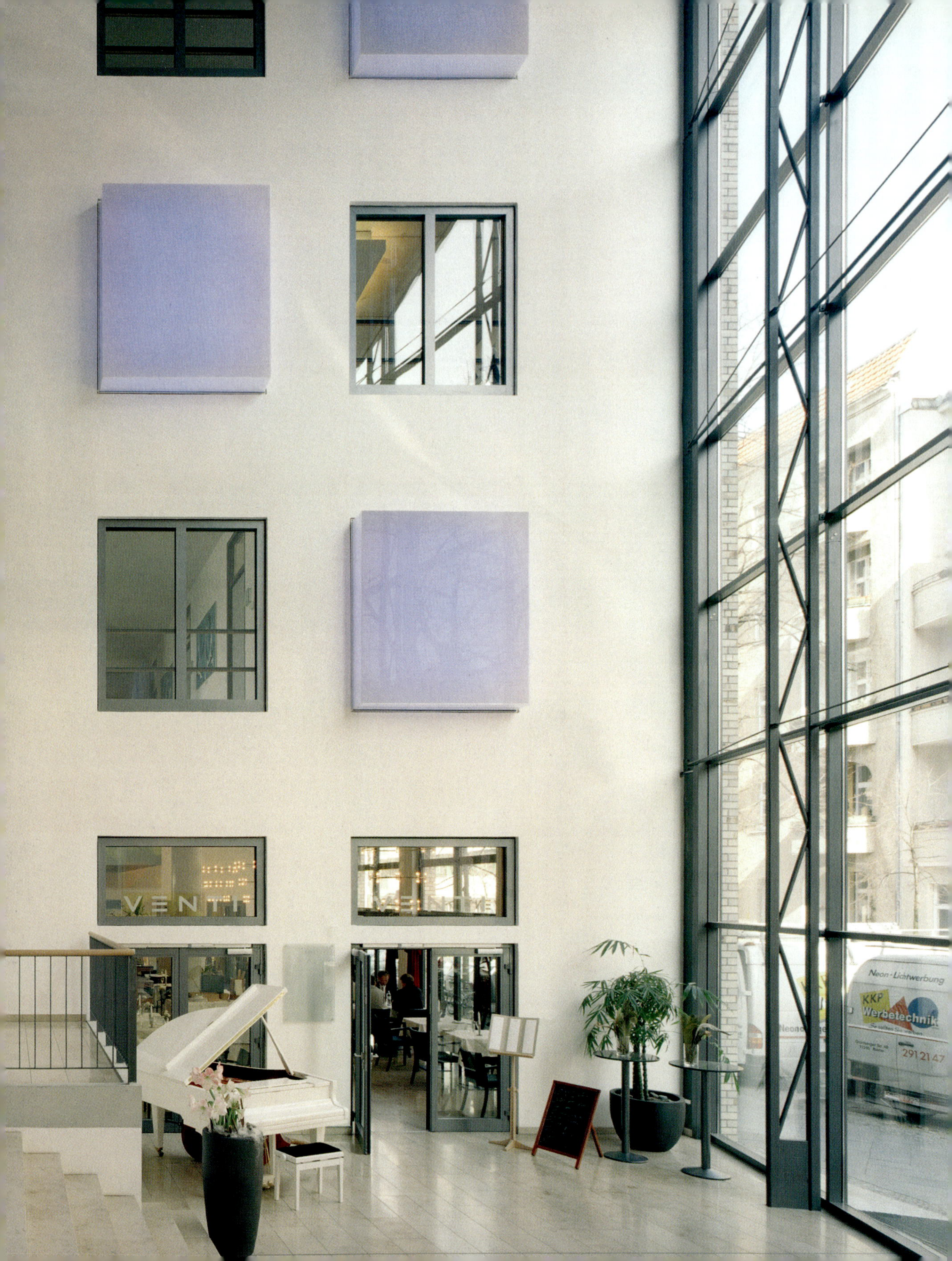
VENTI
Neon · Lichtwerbung
KKP
Werbetechnik
291 21 47

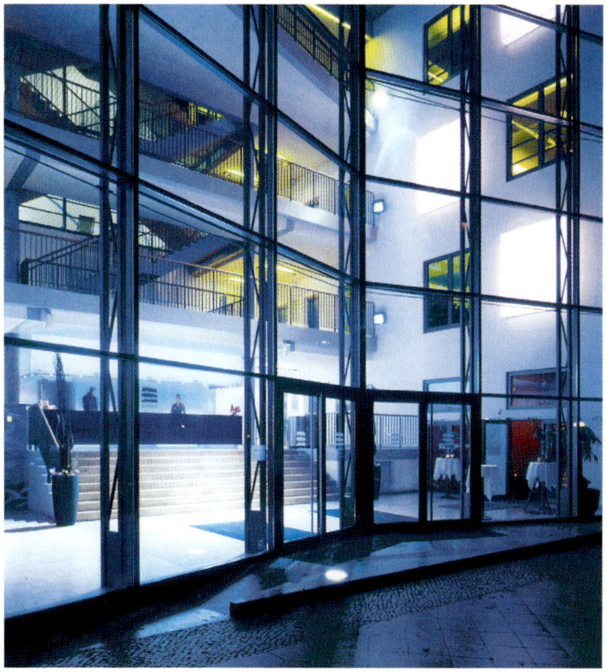

Schwedische Massagen, Thai-Massagen und Hot-Stone-Therapie gehören zum Behandlungsangebot des Oasis Day Spa.

Swedish and Thai massages, and warm stone therapies are some of the treatments offered at the Oasis Day Spa.

Des massages suédois, thaïs ou avec pierres chaudes sont quelques-uns des soins offerts à l'Oasis Day Spa.

Diverse massages en therapieën met warme stenen vormen een greep uit de behandelingen die de Oasis Day Spa aanbiedt.

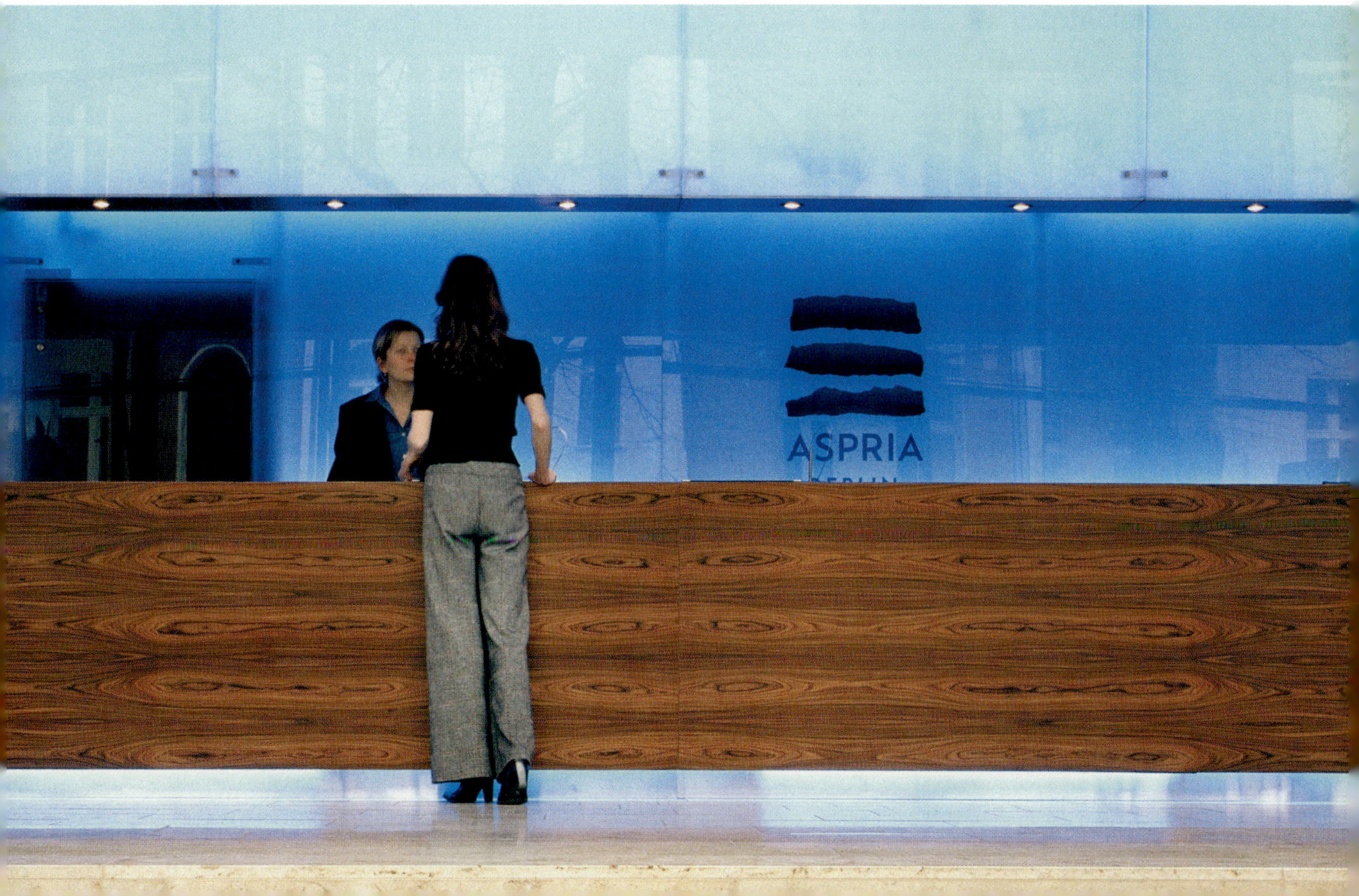

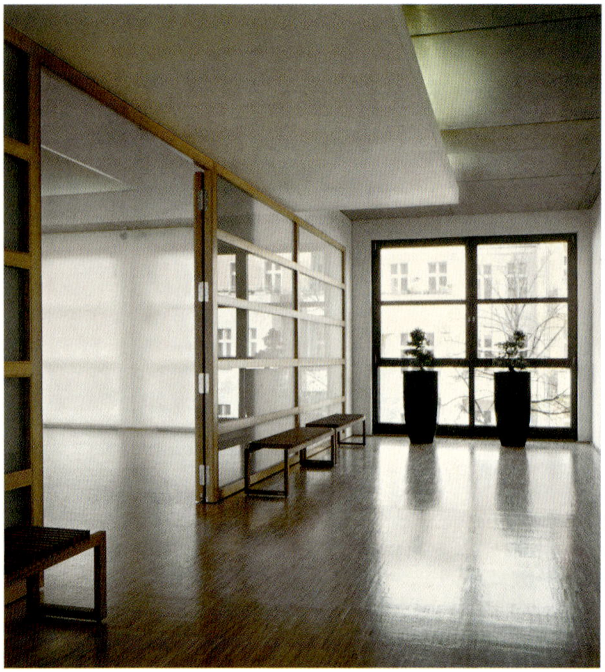

Industrielles Ambiente im Poolbereich, Zen-Atmosphäre im Spa und Farbenfreude im Fitnessbereich prägen den Design-Mix.

Each space has its own identity: industrial airs in the swimming pool, Zen in the spa and colorful at the fitness area.

Chaque espace possède son propre style : industriel pour la piscine, zen pour le spa et coloré pour la zone de remise en forme.

Elke ruimte heeft zijn eigen sfeer: het zwembad oogt industrieel, het spa-gedeelte is zen en de fitnessruimte kleurig.

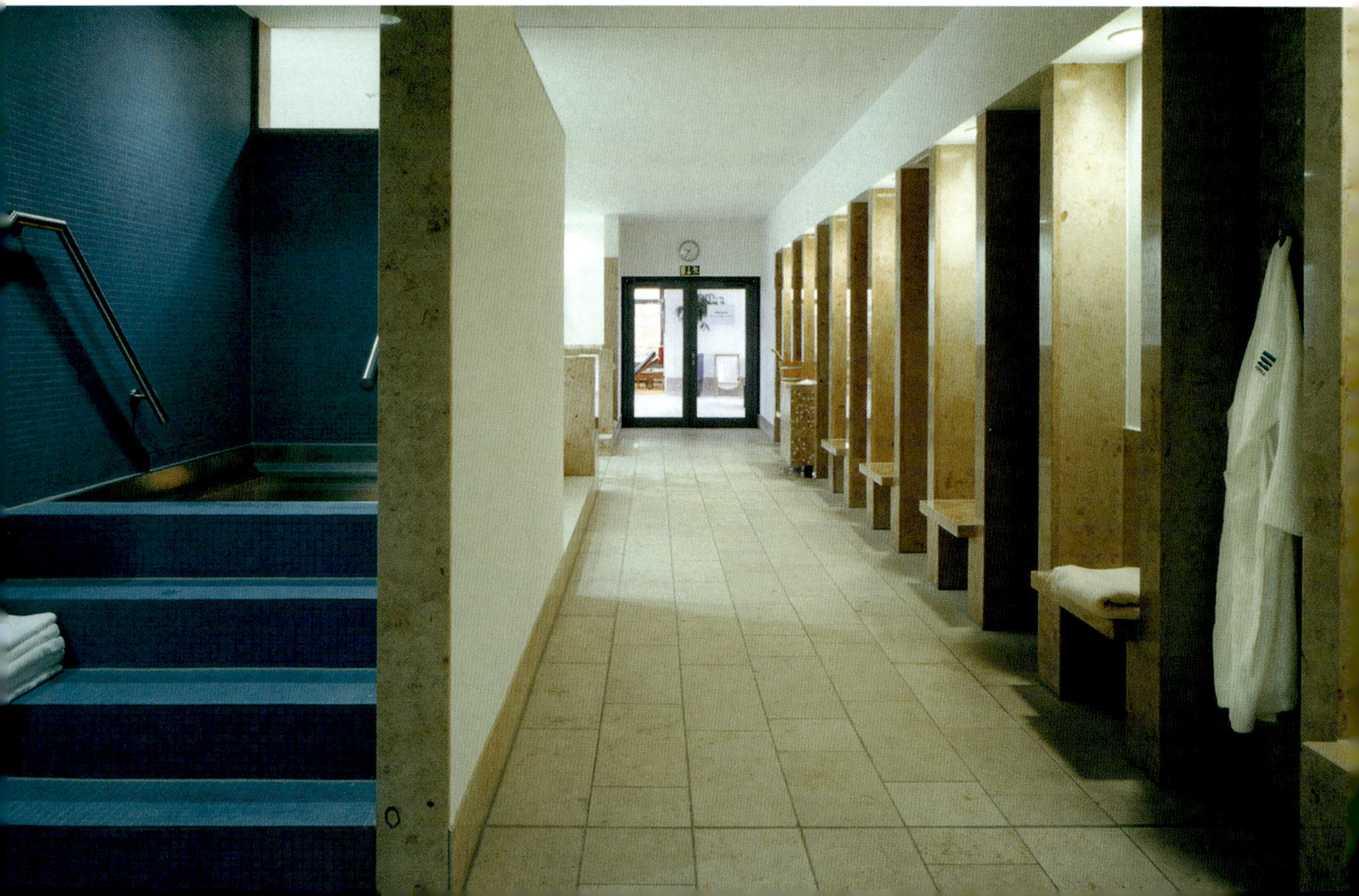

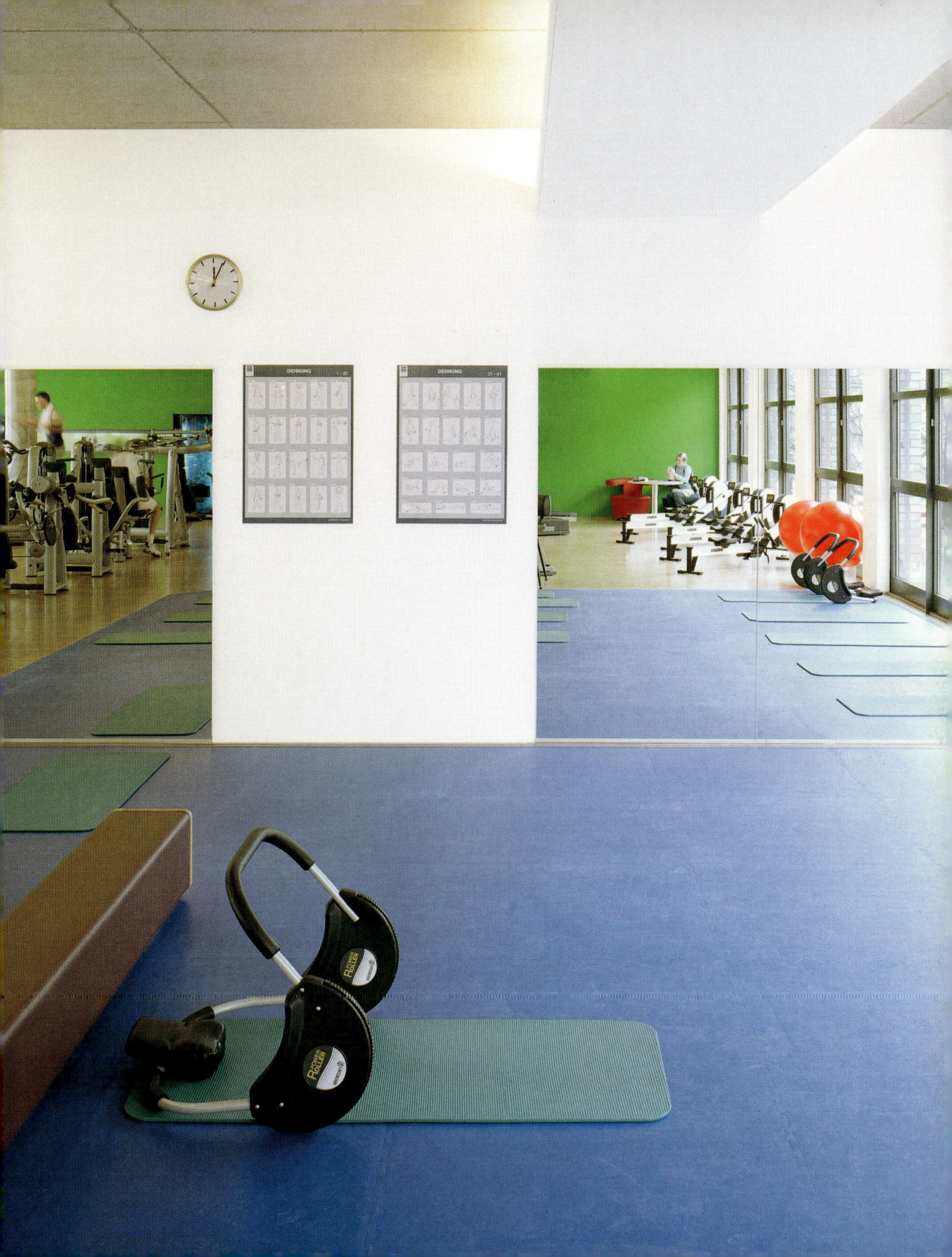
DEHNUNG 1 - 22
DEHNUNG 21 - 41

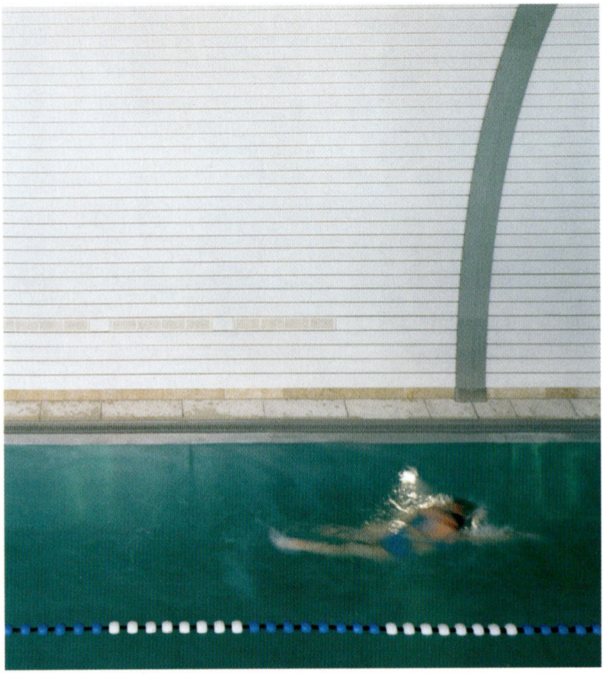

Der klimatisierte Fitnessbereich bietet unter anderem 4 Studios, ein Body & Mind Studio und ein 25-Meter-Becken.

The fitness area includes 4 studios, Mind & Body Studio, air conditioned fitness area and an 82 feet swimming pool.

La zone de remise en forme comprend quatre salles, un Mind & Body Studio, un espace de remise en forme climatisé et une piscine de 25 m.

Het fitnessdeel heeft 4 studio's, een Mind & Body-studio, een fitnessruimte met airco en een vijfentwintigmeterbad.

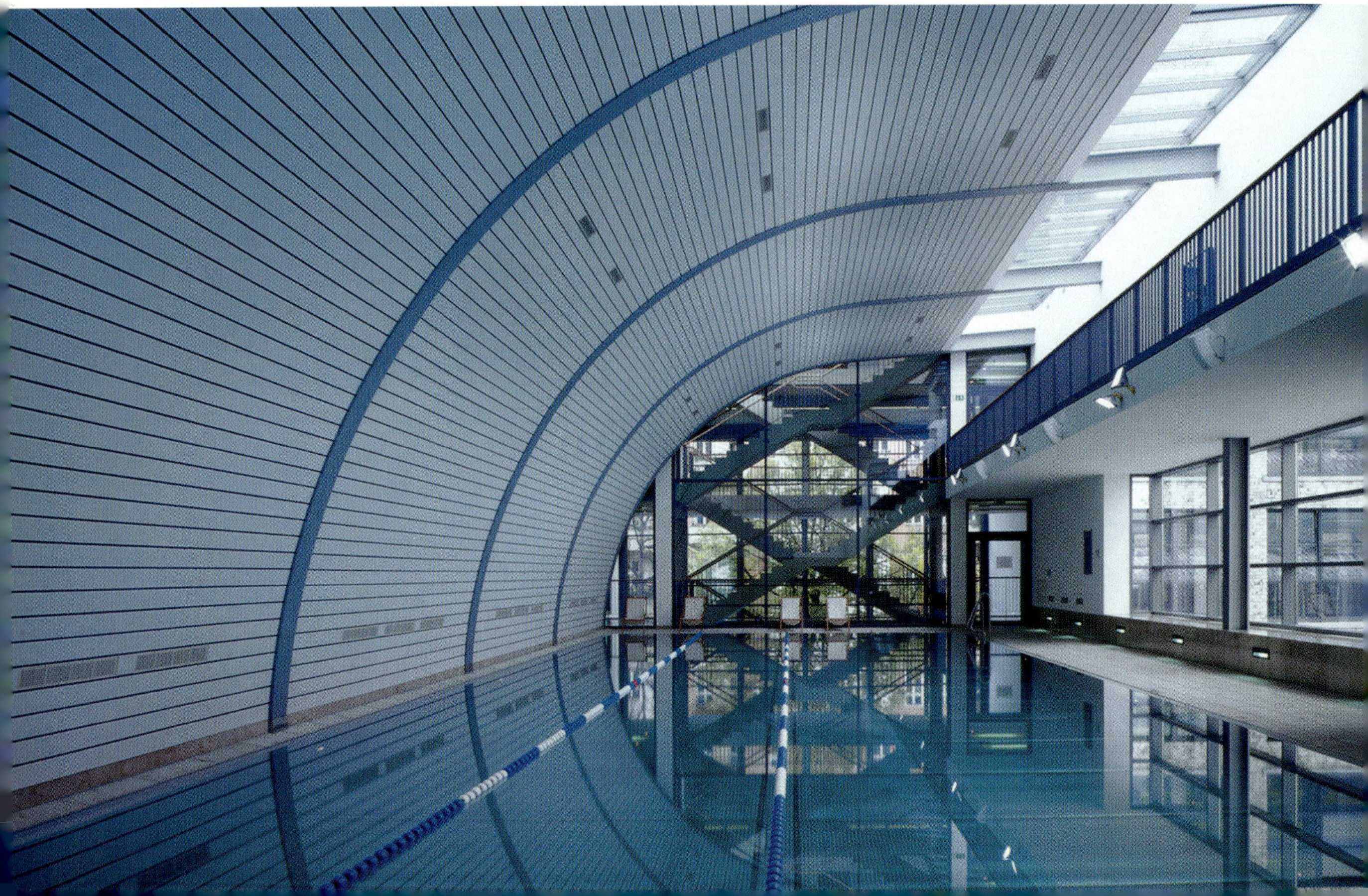

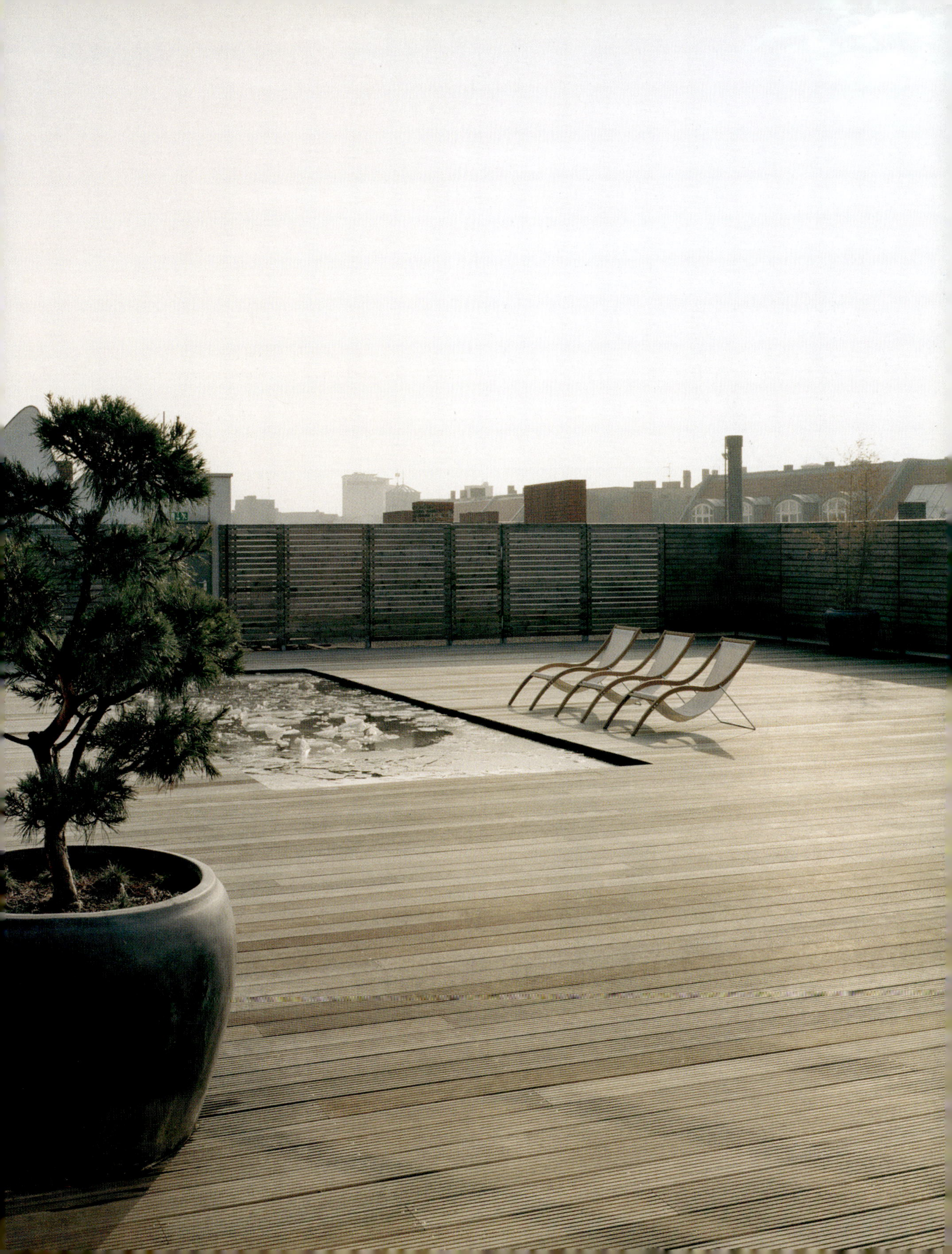

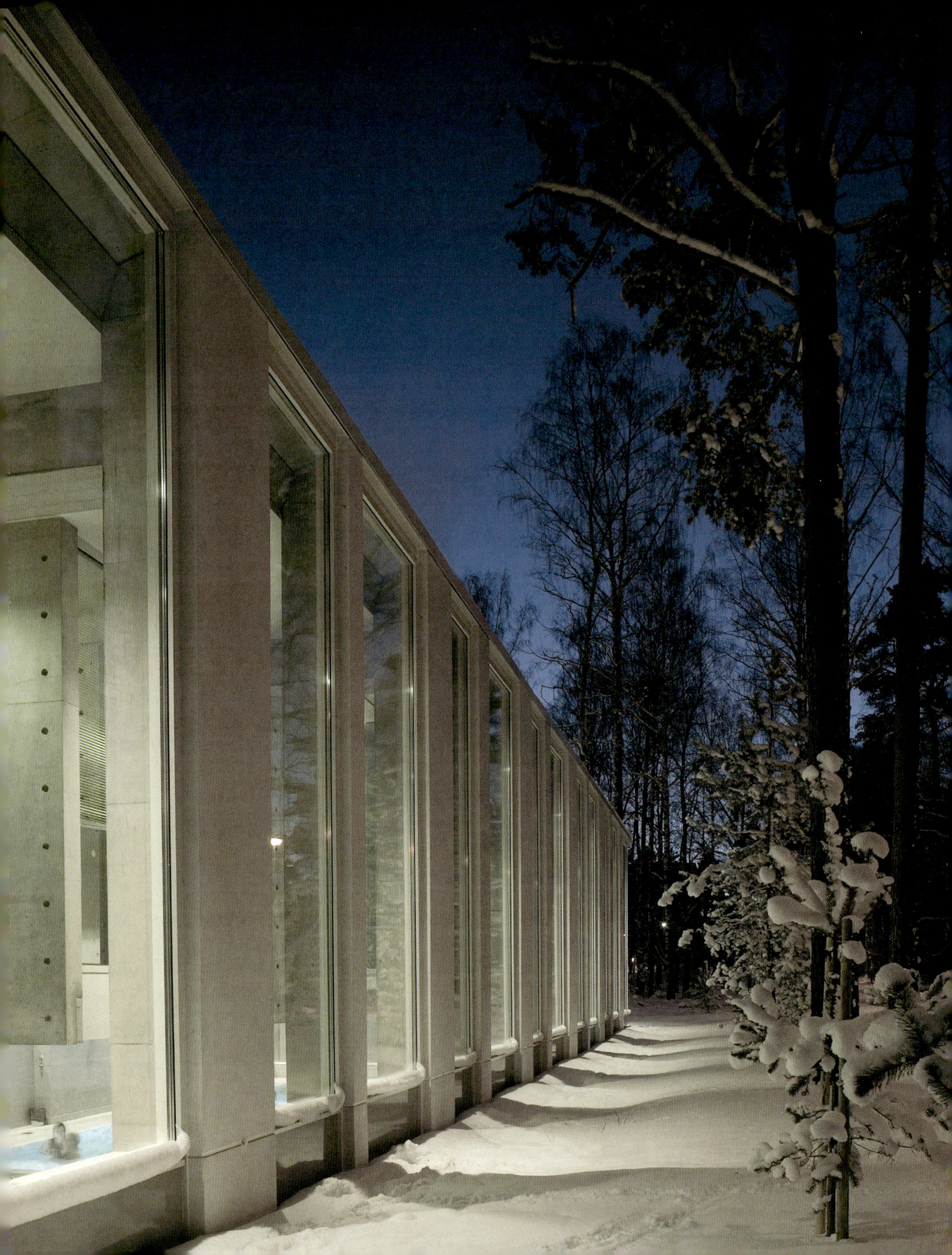

Tapiola

Die Wohnsiedlung Tapiola wurde in den 1960ern als Gartenstadt mit zentralem Schwimmbad konzipiert. Die finnische Regierung erklärte sie zu einem historisch bedeutsamen Ort. Der neue Poolbereich gehört zu einem Trakt jüngeren Baudatums, der mit dem alten Gebäude durch eine Glasrampe verbunden ist. Hier wurde ein Fitnessstudio als Deckenkonstruktion angelegt. Der Raum unter der Tribüne, wo sich früher die Wasseraufbereitungsanlage befand, behergt nun Saunen und Whirlpools.

Tapiola was designed during the 60s as a garden city with a central pool and a number of public buildings around it and has been declared of historical interest by the Finnish government. The new sector of the pool extends over one wing of recent construction that is connected with the old building by a glass ramp. The gym is suspended from the ceiling and underneath the stand, the room that used to house the water treatment plant now holds the saunas and Jacuzzis.

Déclaré patrimoine historique par le gouvernement finlandais, Tapiola a été conçu dans les années 1960 comme une « ville-jardin » , avec une piscine centrale entourée de nombreux bâtiments. Le nouvel espace de la piscine s'étend sur une aile récemment construite, reliée à l'ancien bâtiment par une passerelle vitrée. Suspendue au plafond, la salle de fitness a trouvé place au-dessus de la piscine, tandis que l'ancienne salle de traitement des eaux héberge maintenant les saunas et les jacuzzis.

Tapiola is in de jaren zestig ontworpen als een tuinstad met een zwembad en enkele openbare voorzieningen. De Finse regering heeft het zwembad inmiddels aangemerkt als historisch interessant. Het nieuwe gedeelte van het zwembad beslaat een vleugel van een recente aanbouw, die via een glazen helling is verbonden met het oude gebouw, dat een hangende fitnessruimte bevat. Onder de tribune is de ruimte waar vroeger de waterzuivering was. Nu zijn er sauna's en jacuzzi's.

Espoo, Finland

ARKKITEHTITOIMISTO NURMELA, RAIMORANTA, TASA OY

Photos © Antti Luutonen

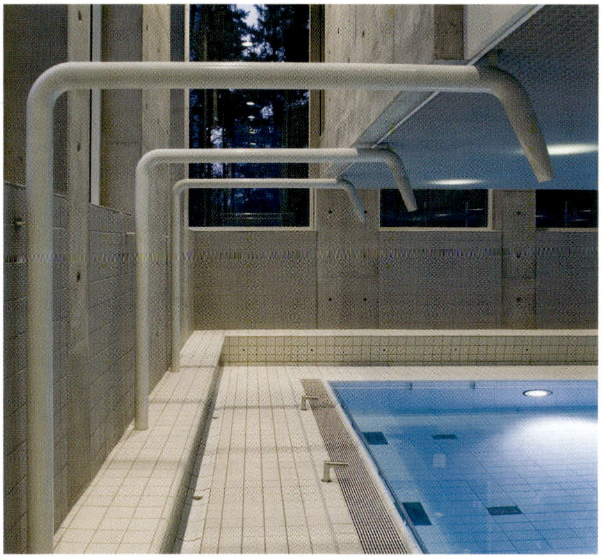

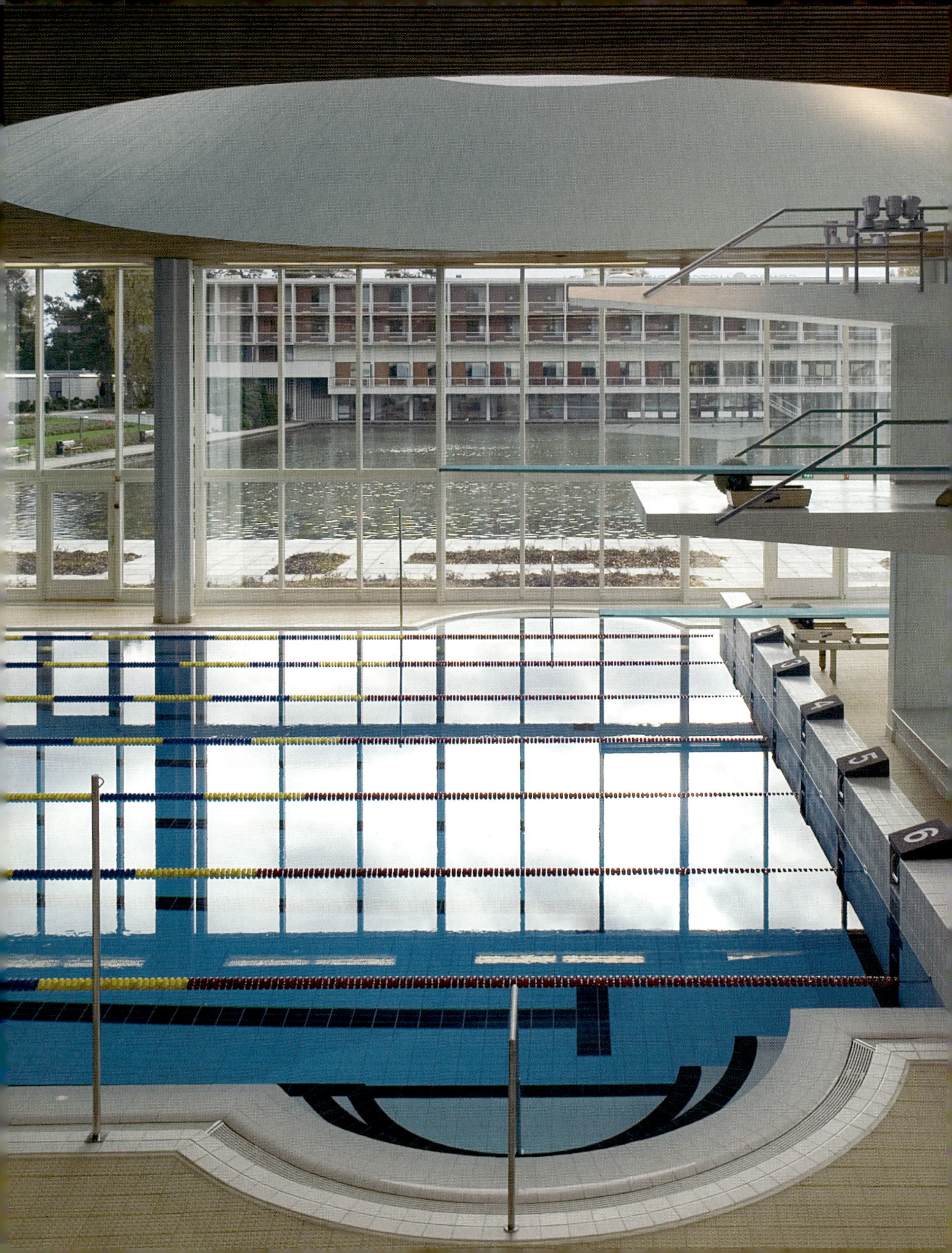
2
3
4
5
6

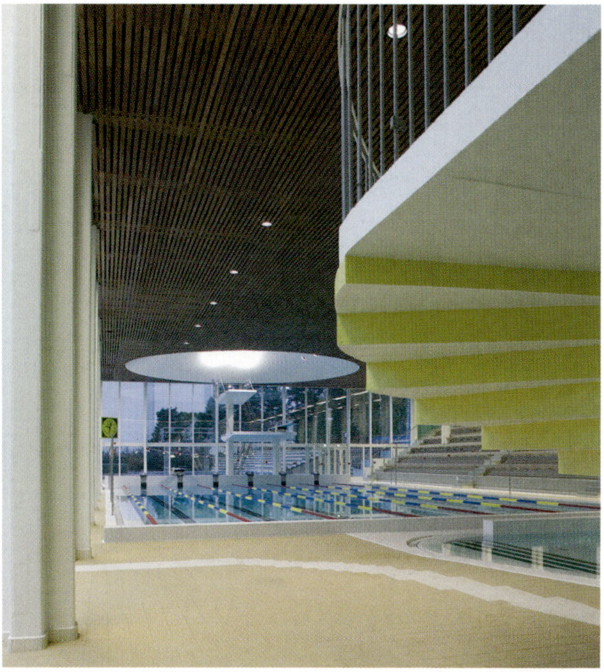

Das Außenschwimmbecken ist mit dem Gebäudeinneren durch eine hermetisch verschließbare Rampe verbunden.

The outside swimming pool is connected with the inside of the building through a hermetically sealed ramp.

La piscine en plein air est reliée au bâtiment principal par une passerelle étanche.

Het buitenbad is met de binnenkant van het gebouw verbonden via een hermetisch afgesloten helling.

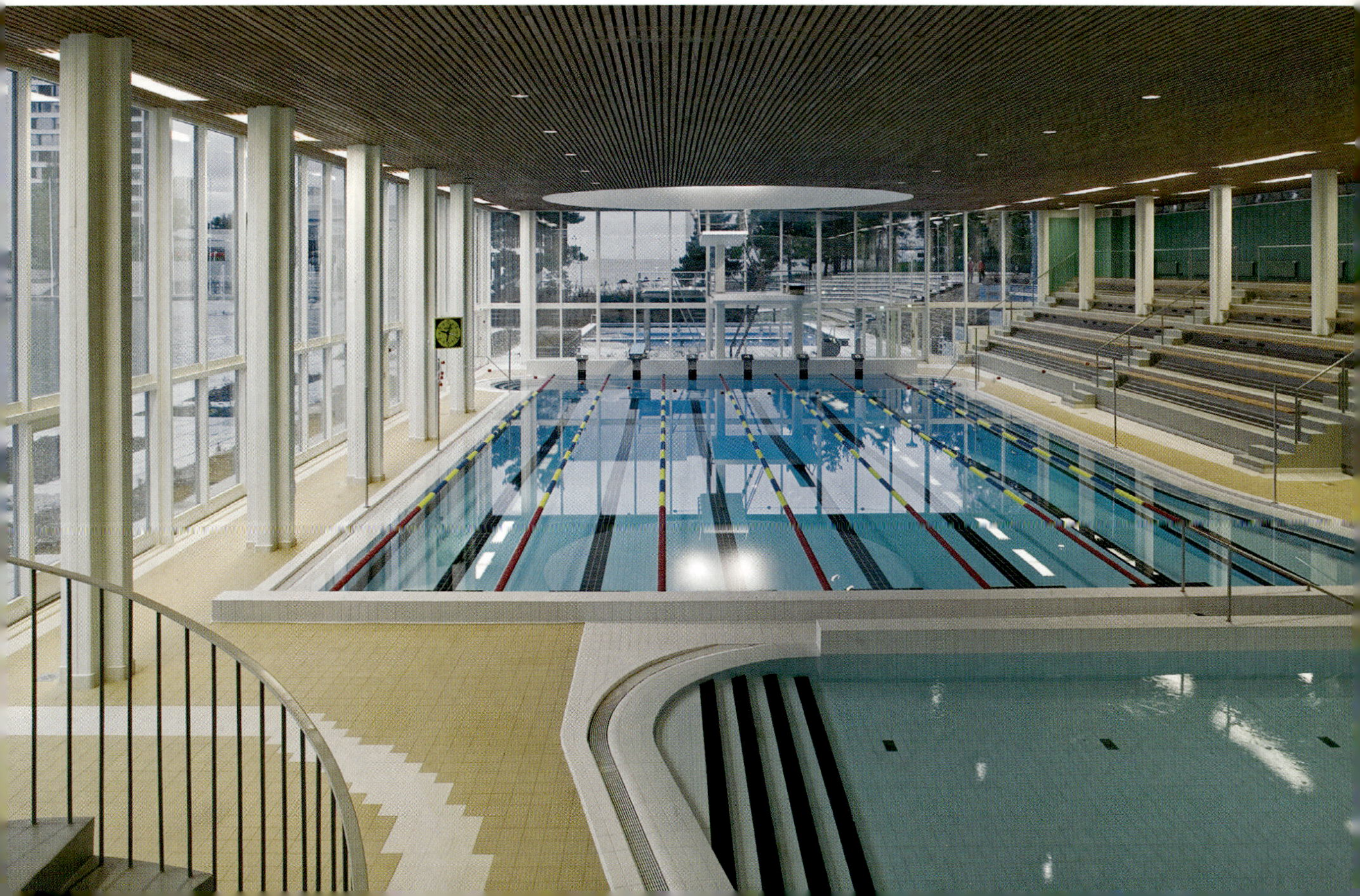

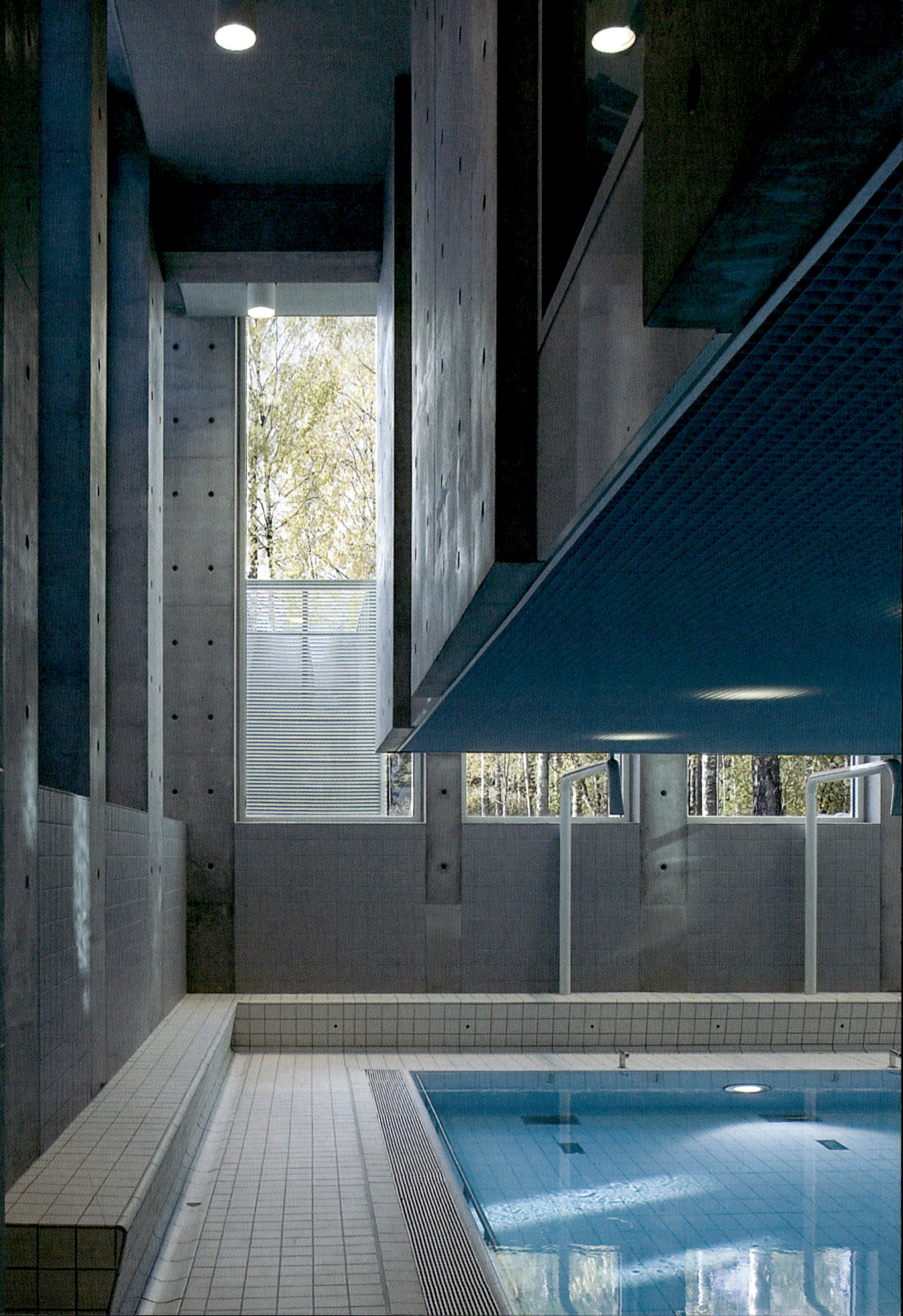

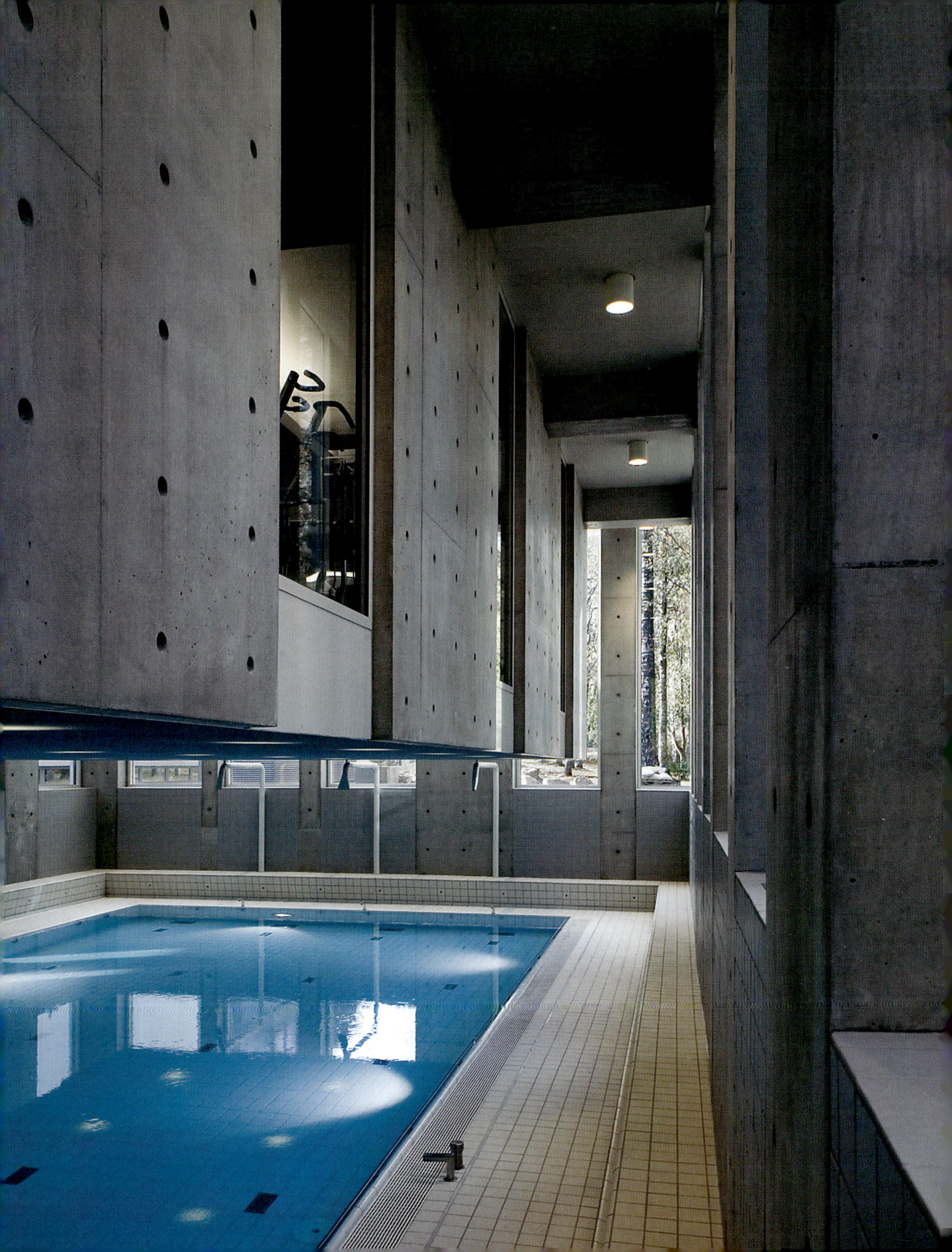

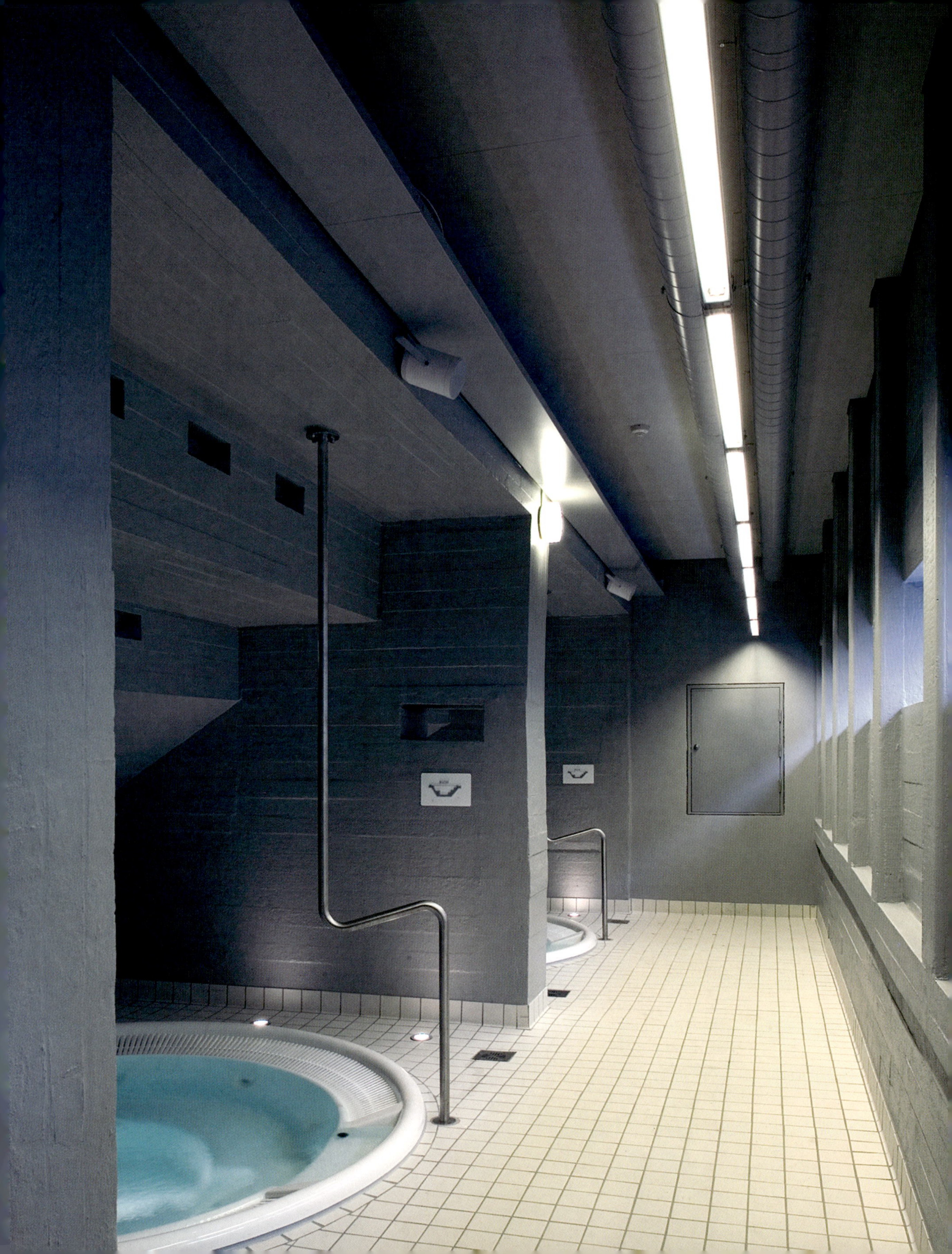

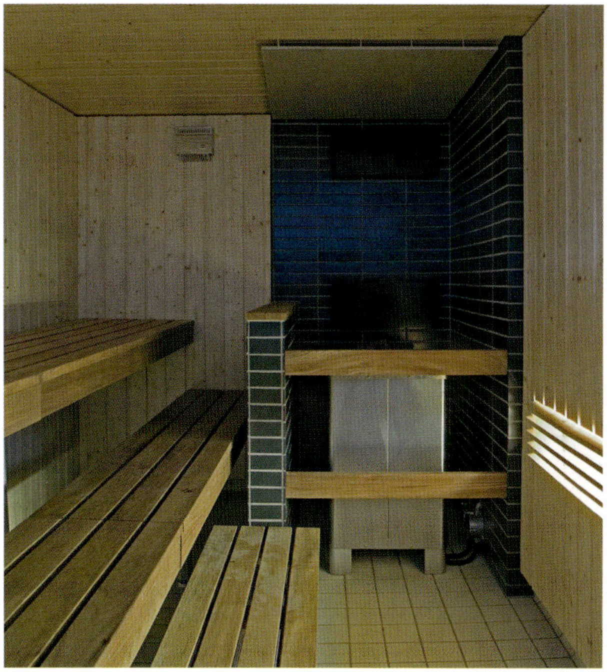

Das Fitnessstudio wurde als Deckenkonstruktion über dem neuen Pool- und Whirlpoolbereich angelegt.

The gym is suspended from the ceiling and towers over a new pool and the Jacuzzi area.

La salle de remise en forme, suspendue au plafond, domine largement la nouvelle piscine et l'espace jacuzzis.

De fitnessruimte hangt aan het plafond, hoog verheven boven een nieuw zwembad en het gedeelte met jacuzzi.

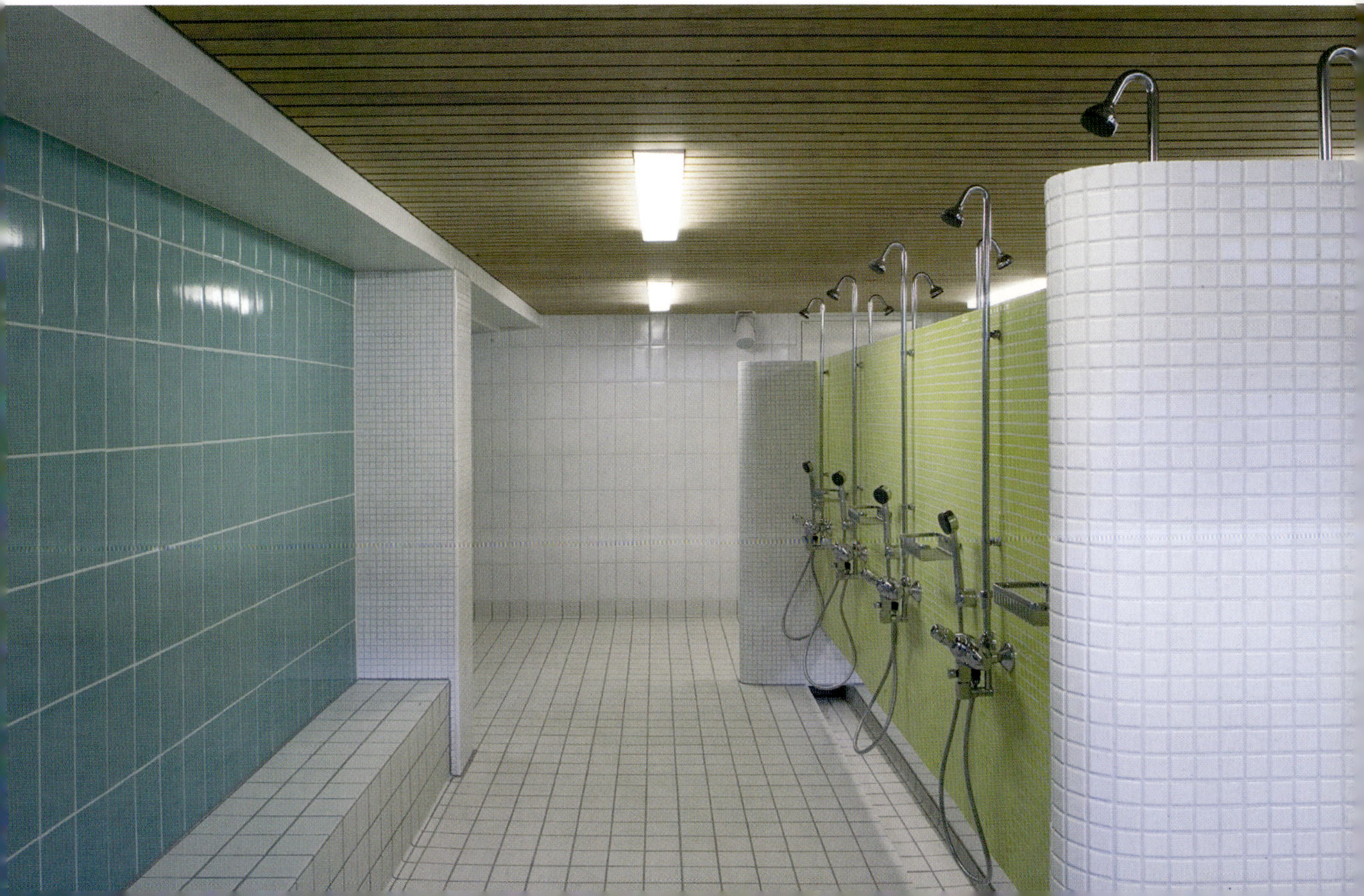

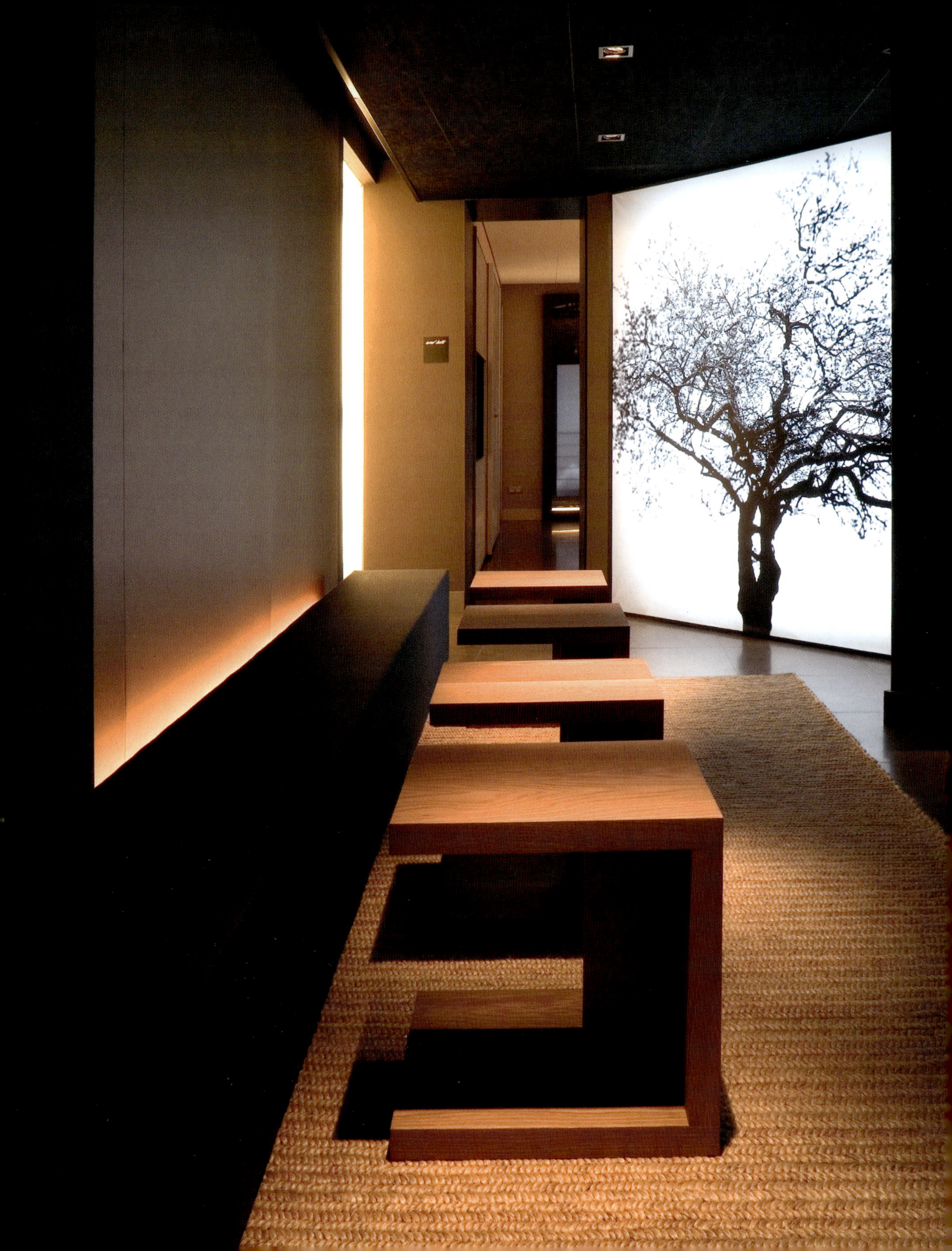

SpaciOmm

Das exklusive Spa des Designhotels Omm in Barcelona ist vom gleichen minimalistischen Stil geprägt wie das gesamte Gebäude.
Zum Thermalparcours des Spa gehören ein Aktivbecken mit Entspannungsmatten, ein Wasserfall, Behandlungsdüsen, ein Hammam, ein Eisbrunnen und ein Fußbad mit Regenzonen. Ein Fitnessstudio, ein Schönheitssalon und eine Bar vervollständigen den Service dieses 400 qm großen Spas, das seinen Gästen Entspannung in luxuriöser und intimer Atmosphäre bietet.

Hotel Omm, Barcelona is a reference of quality and design and its recently inaugurated spa enjoys the same minimalist spirit that predominates in the building. The spa's thermal circuit consists of an active pool with relaxation beds inside the water, a waterfall, treatment jets, a hammam bath, an ice fountain and a foot-bath with rain routes. A gym and a beauty parlor, as well as a bar, complement the services of this 4,300 square feet spa with an intimate personality.

Garant d'une qualité irréprochable à Barcelone, l'hôtel Omm a récemment inauguré un spa qui répond à l'esprit minimaliste caractérisant déjà la construction. Il propose un parcours composé d'une piscine équipée de lits relaxants immergés, d'une cascade d'eau, de jets thérapeutiques, d'un hammam, d'une fontaine glacée et de bains de pieds. Une salle de remise en forme, un salon de beauté et un bar complètent les services de ce spa de 400 m² au charme discret.

Hotel Omm in Barcelona staat symbool voor kwaliteit en design en de recent geopende spa heeft dezelfde minimalistische sfeer als de rest van het gebouw. Het thermale circuit bestaat uit een 'active pool' met ligstoelen in het water, een waterval, therapeutische waterstralen, een hammam, een ijsreservoir en een voetbad met regenwater.
Een fitnessruimte, een schoonheidssalon en een bar maken de faciliteiten van dit 400 m² grote complex met zijn intieme sfeer compleet.

Barcelona, Spain

SANDRA TARRUELLA & ISABEL LÓPEZ

Photos © Lourdes Jansana, Eva Balart, Anne Soderberg, Olga Planas

www.hotelomm.es

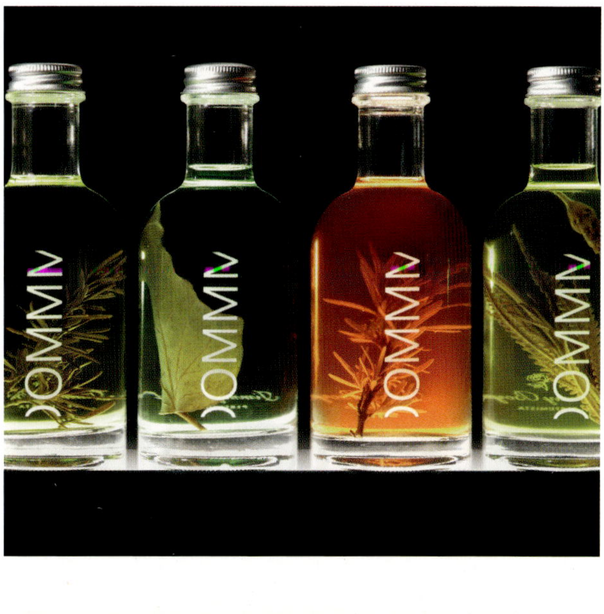

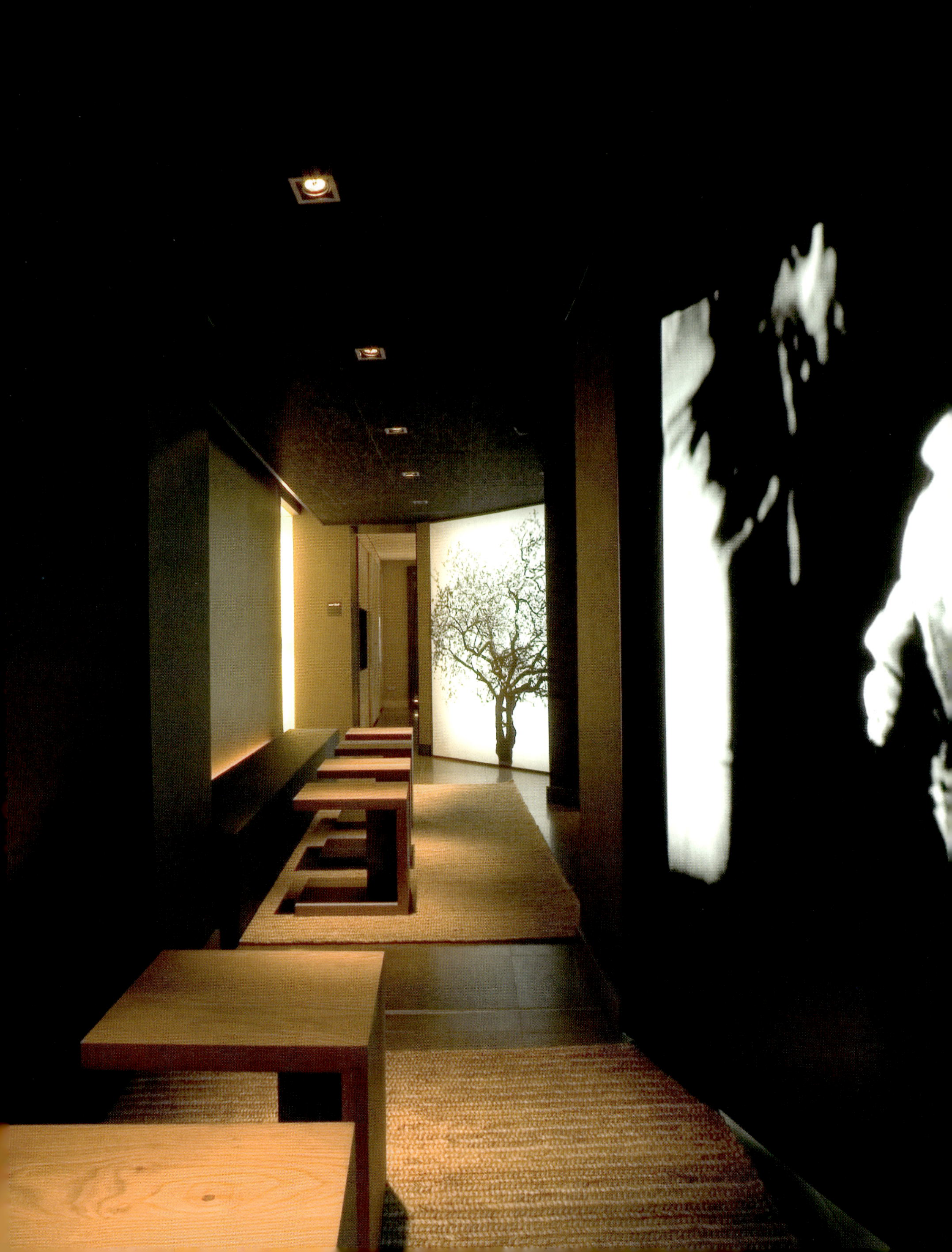

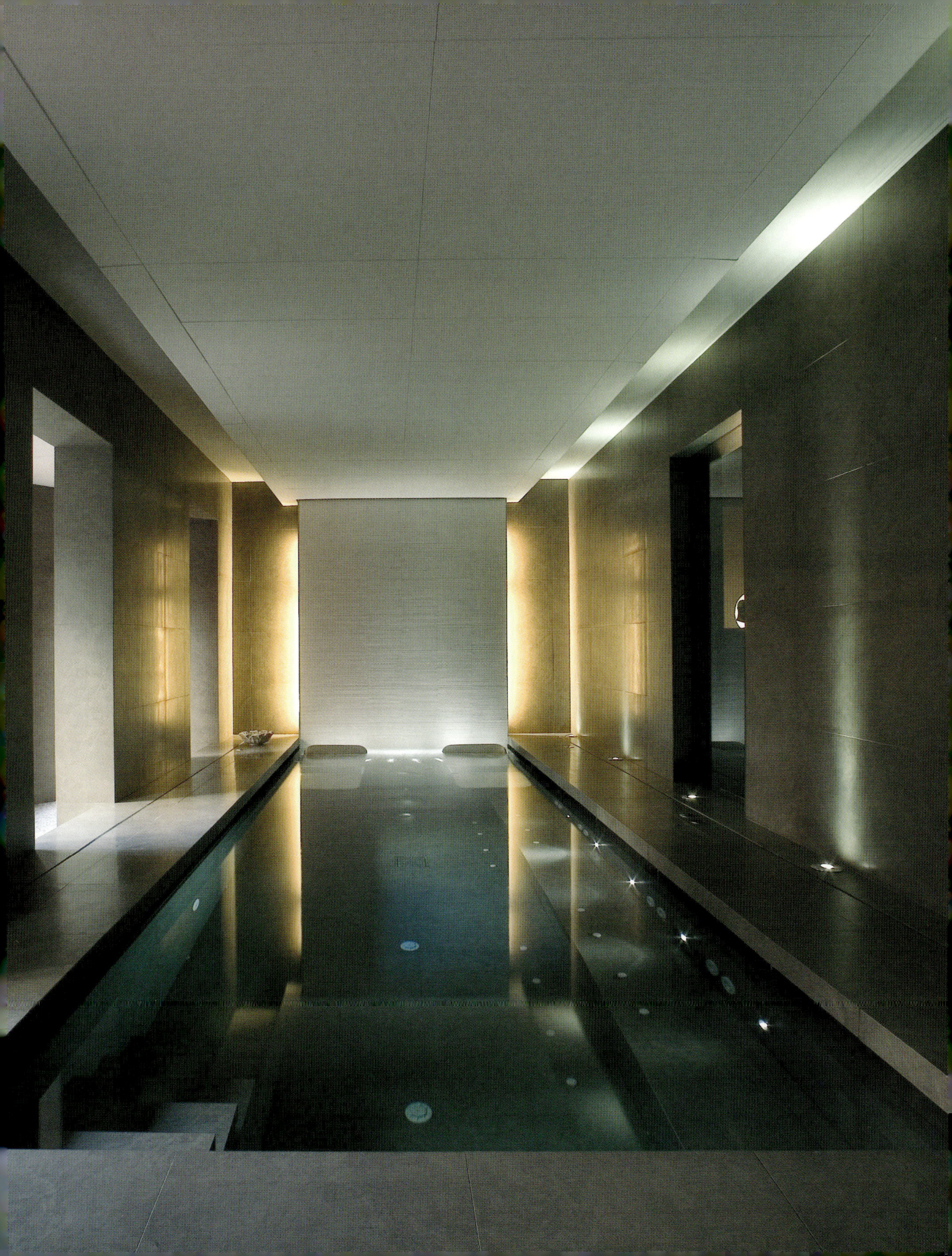

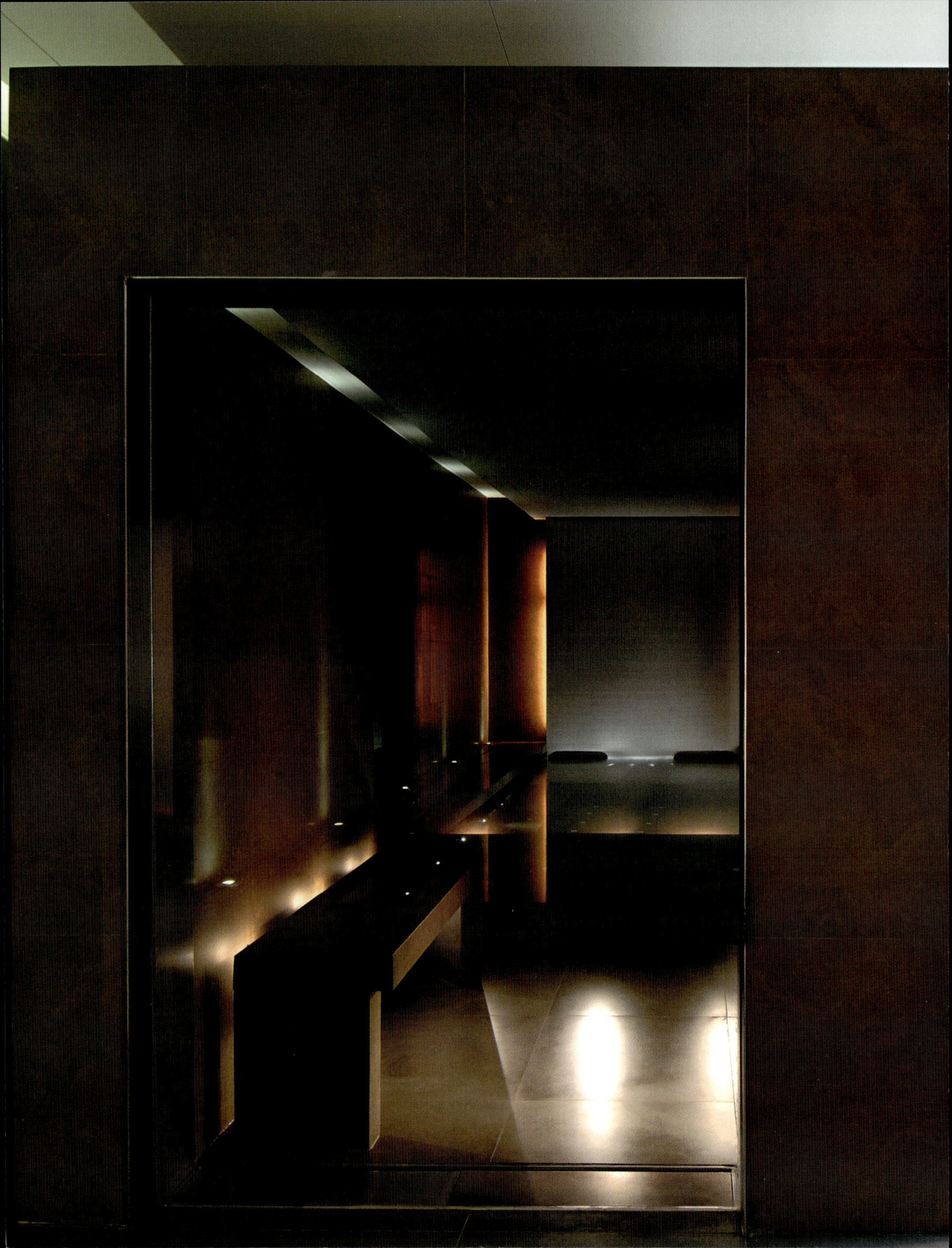

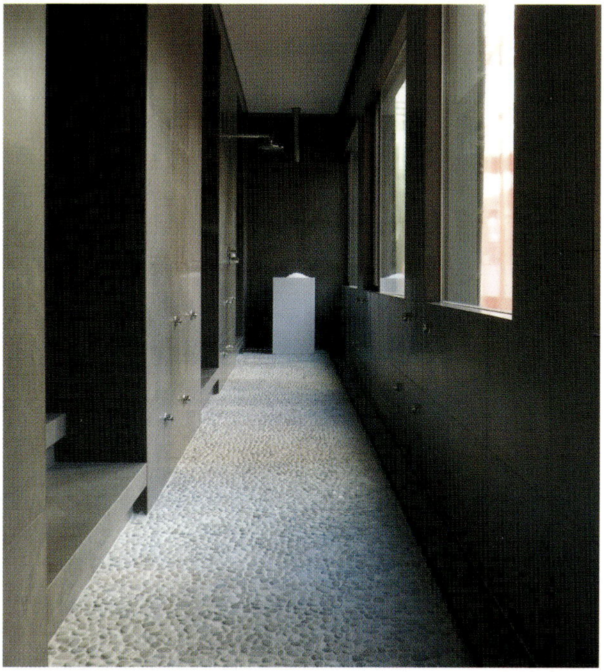

Für seine wohltuenden Behandlungen verwendet das SpaciOmm exklusive Produkte aus aller Welt.

Products coming from various countries are used to mitigate low moods as part of the treatments offered at SpaciOmm.

Des produits, venant de différents pays, et utilisés pour chasser les coups de déprime, font partie des traitements offerts à SpaciOmm.

Producten uit verschillende landen worden in SpaciOmm gebruikt tegen lichte klachten van depressiviteit.

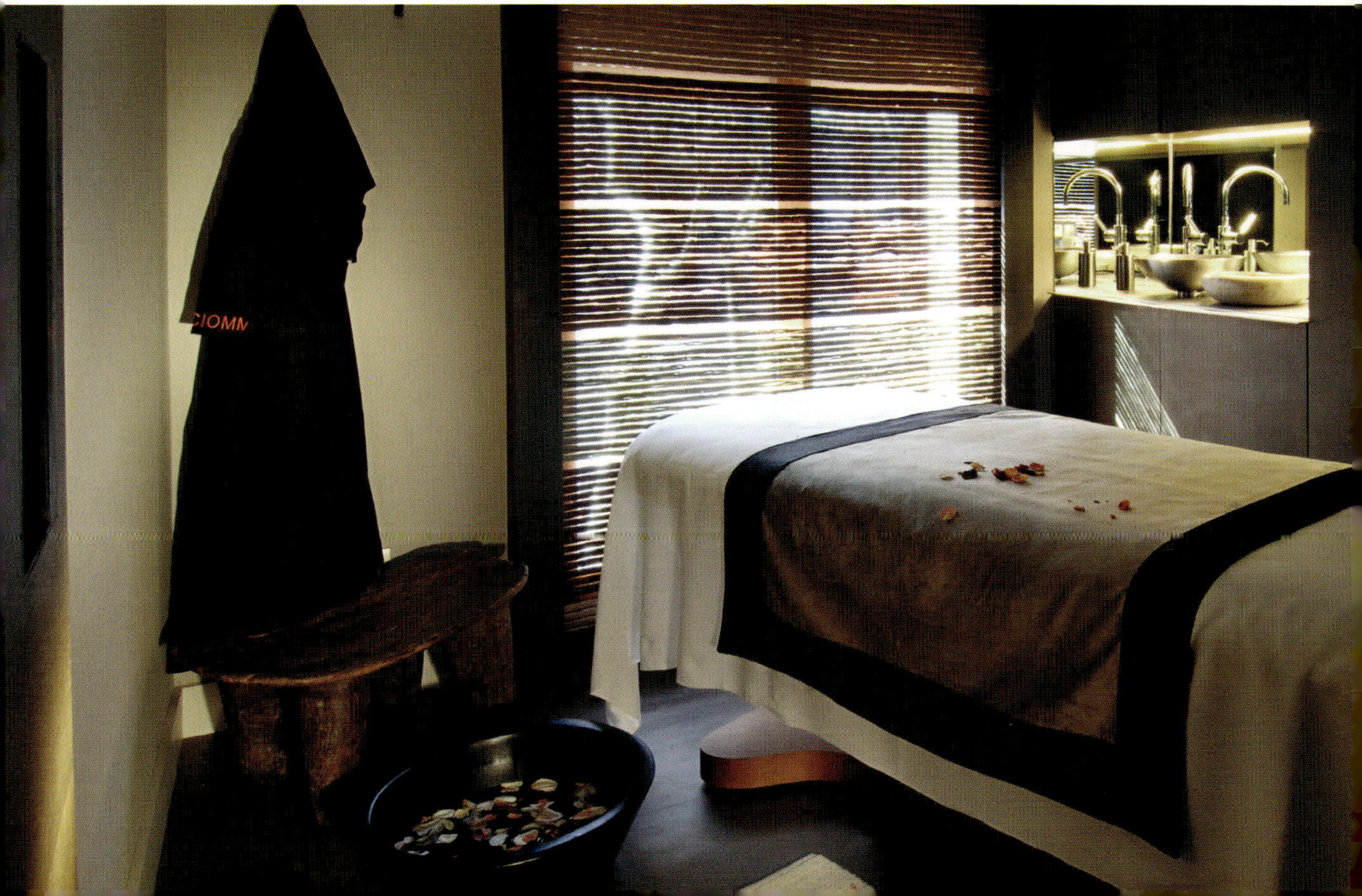

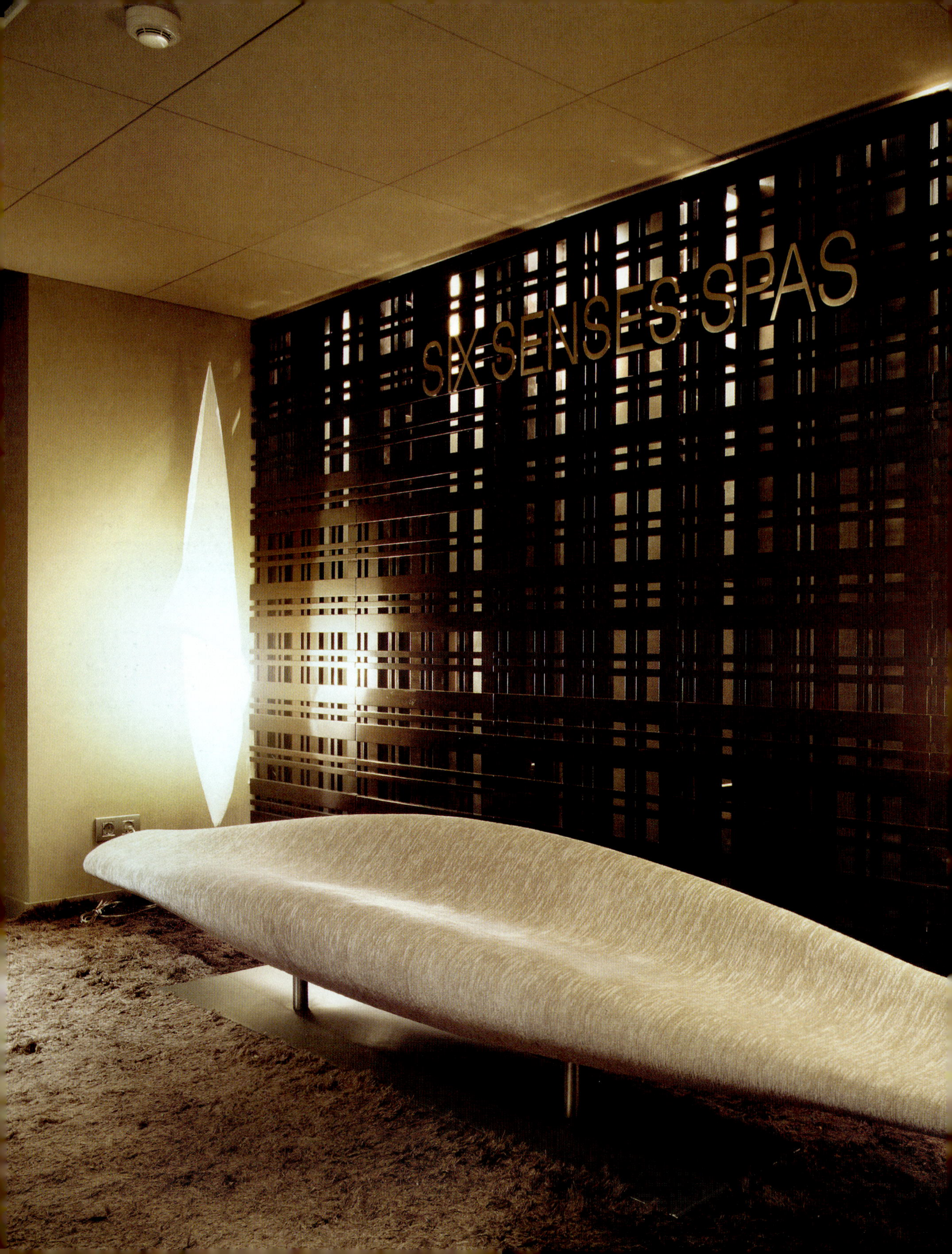
SIX SENSES SPAS

Hotel Arts Spa

Auf den Etagen 42 und 43 des Hotel Arts präsentiert sich dieses 900 qm große Spa als exklusive Wellnessoase mit fantastischem Blick auf Barcelona und das Meer. Die von der Rezeption aus zu erreichenden Räumlichkeiten umfassen Umkleideräume, Nassbereiche, Behandlungskabinen und Entspannungsräume für Damen und Herren. Schwarzer Granit und warme Farben prägen das avantgardistische Ambiente, das den Gästen pure Entspannung in eleganter Atmosphäre verspricht.

Located on floors 42 and 43 of the Hotel Arts, the Spa occupies 9,690 square feet, a space of pure wellbeing offering privileged views of Barcelona and the coast. From the reception one can access the dressing rooms, the wet areas, the treatment cabins and the relaxation rooms for men and women. The predominant materials, such as the black stone, the relief coating of the pool and the lace curtains that cover the windows create a fantastic ambiance that helps the mind to escape.

Occupant sur 900 m² les 42e et 43e étages de l'hôtel Arts, le spa éponyme est un espace de pur bien-être, offrant une vue privilégiée sur Barcelone et sa côte. Depuis la réception, on peut accéder aux vestiaires, aux zones aquatiques, aux cabines de soins et aux salons de relaxation pour hommes et femmes. La pierre noire, la fresque en relief de la piscine, et les rideaux tout en volutes des fenêtres, sont les éléments prédominants, créant une ambiance fantastique propice au dépaysement.

De spa op de 42e en 43e verdiepingen van het Arts Hotel biedt 800 m² aan pure wellness met schitterende uitzichten op Barcelona en de kust. De receptieruimte biedt toegang tot de kleedkamers, baden, therapieruimten en rustruimten voor mannen en vrouwen. De gebruikte materialen, zoals zwarte steen, de reliëflaag op het zwembad en de halftransparante gordijnen voor de ramen creëren een fantastische sfeer die de geest helpt om spanningen los te laten.

Barcelona, Spain

GCA ARQUITECTES ASSOCIATS

Photos © Jordi Miralles, Imanol Sistiaga

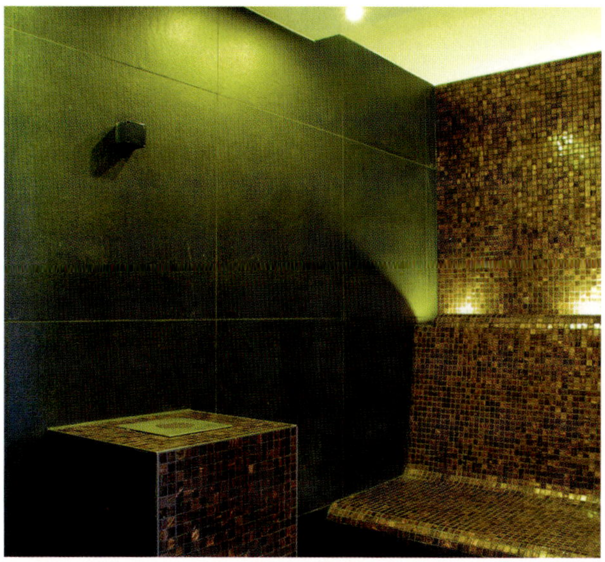

www.hotelartsbarcelona.com

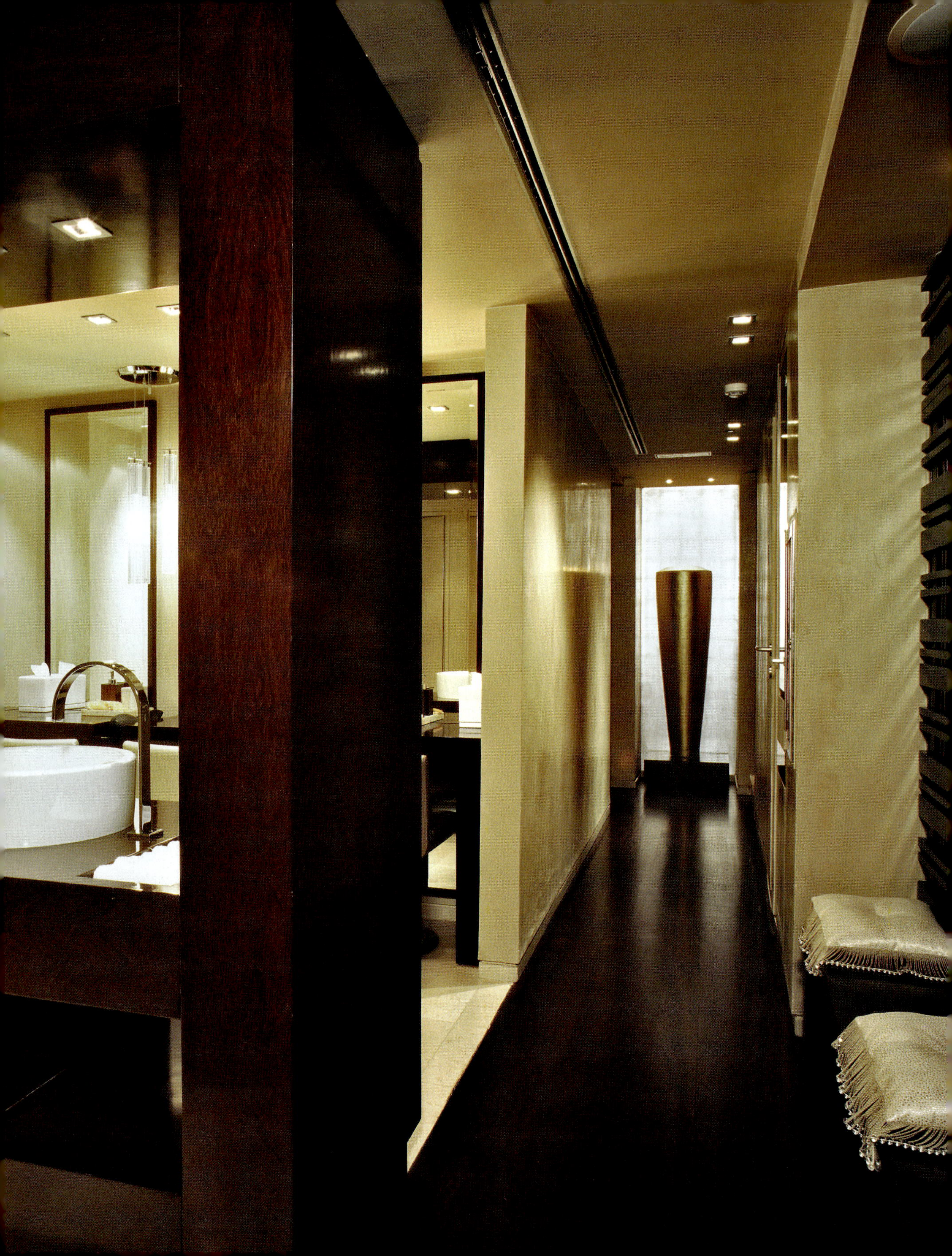

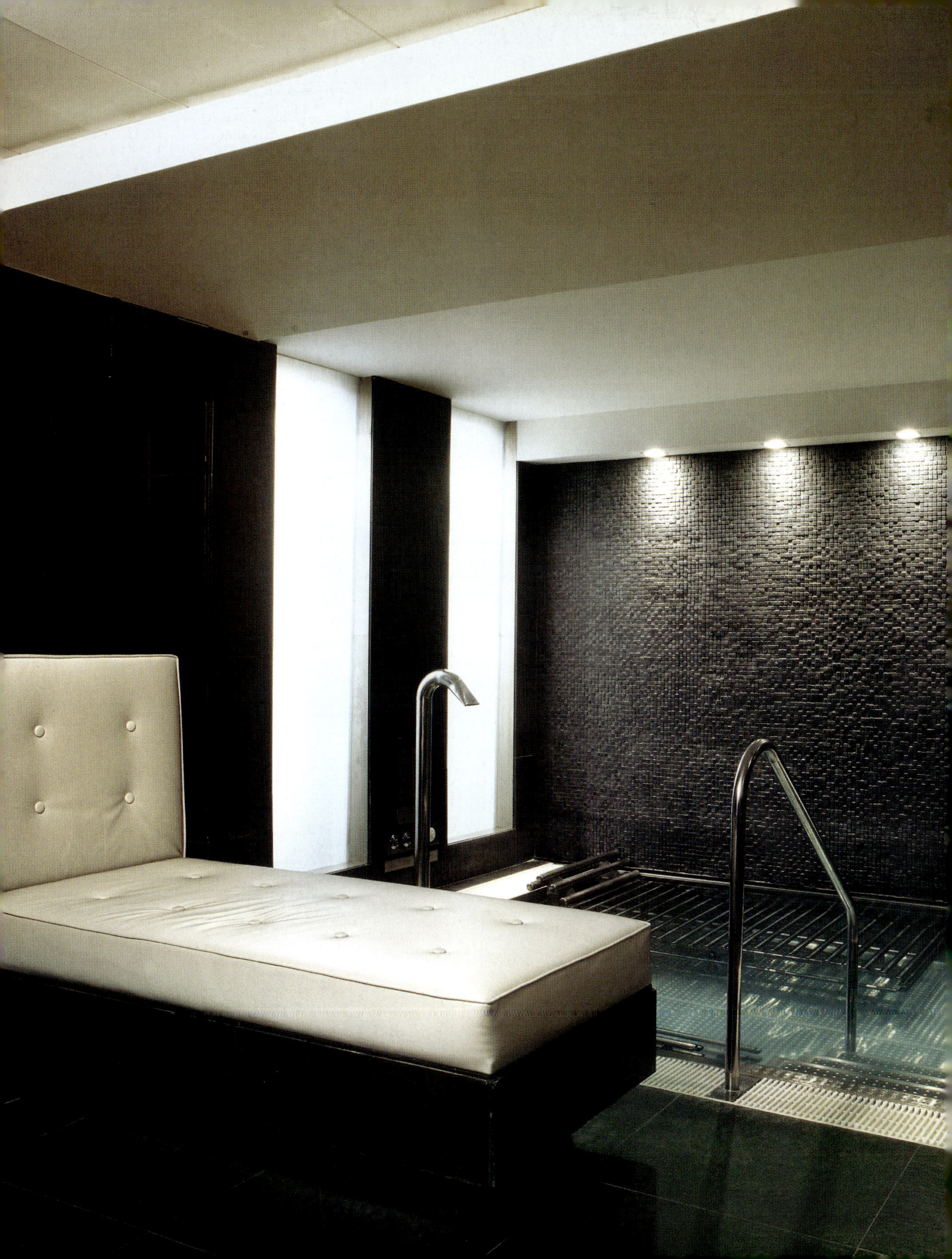

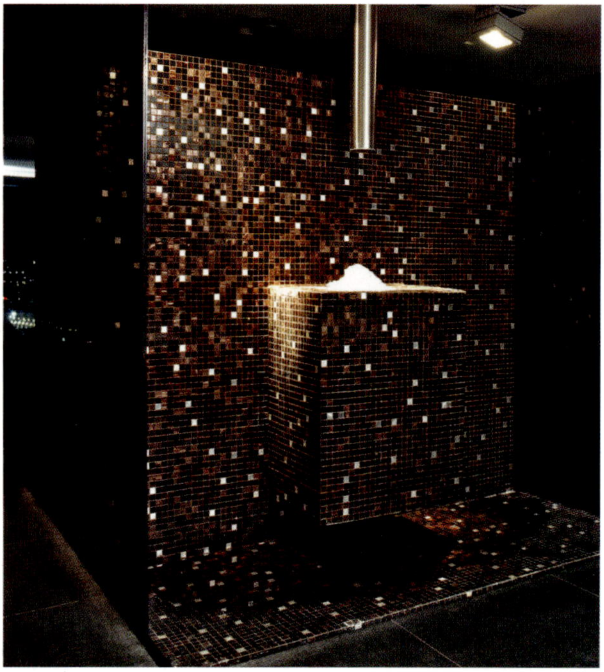

Farben und Einrichtung verleihen dem Spa eine sehr elegante und entspannte Atmosphäre.

The range of colors and the furniture used throughout the spa give the place a warm vanguard feeling.

Le choix des couleurs et des meubles confère au spa un caractère avant-gardiste et chaleureux à la fois.

Het gebruikte kleurenpalet en het meubilair zorgen voor een warme, avant-gardistische sfeer.

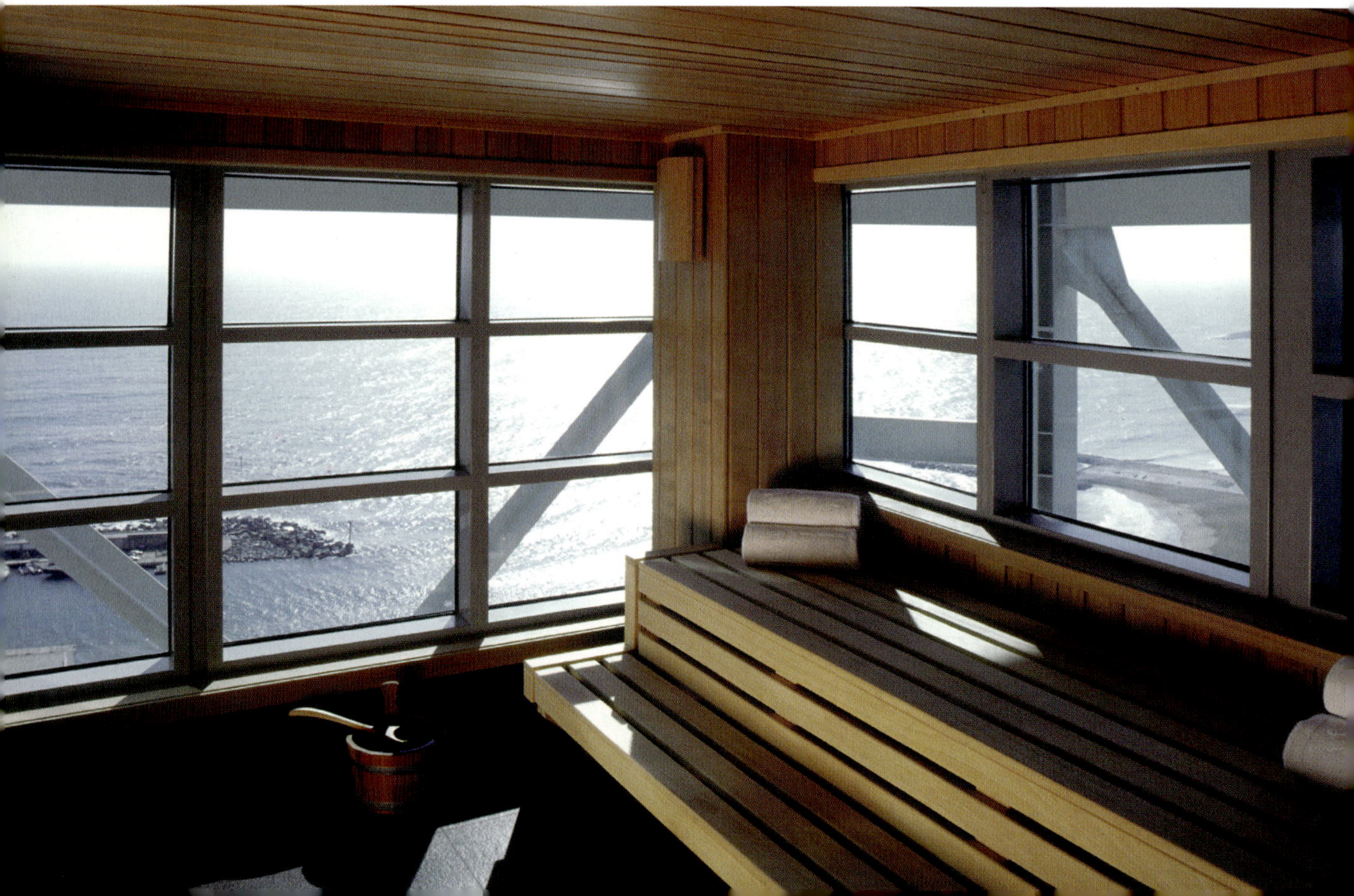

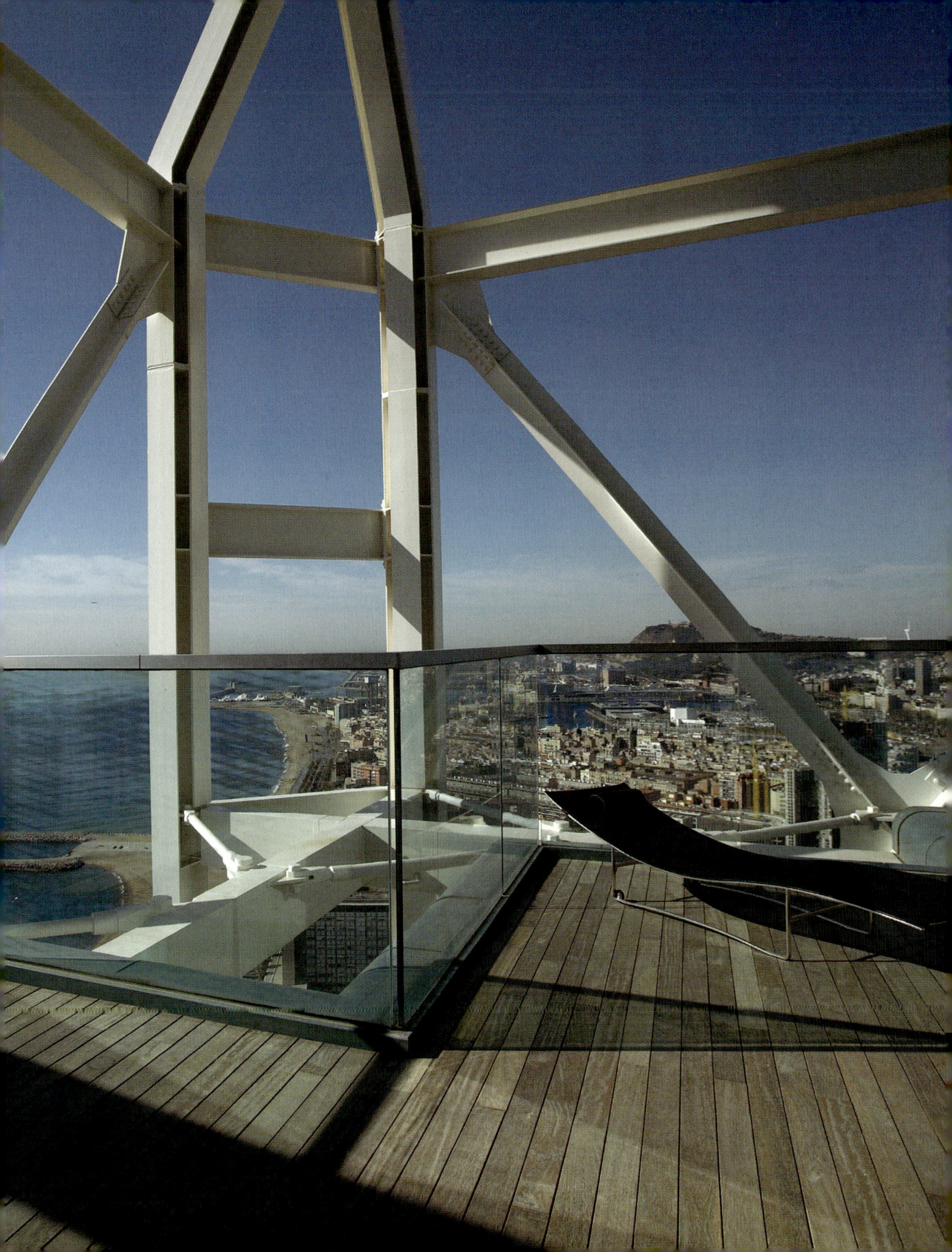

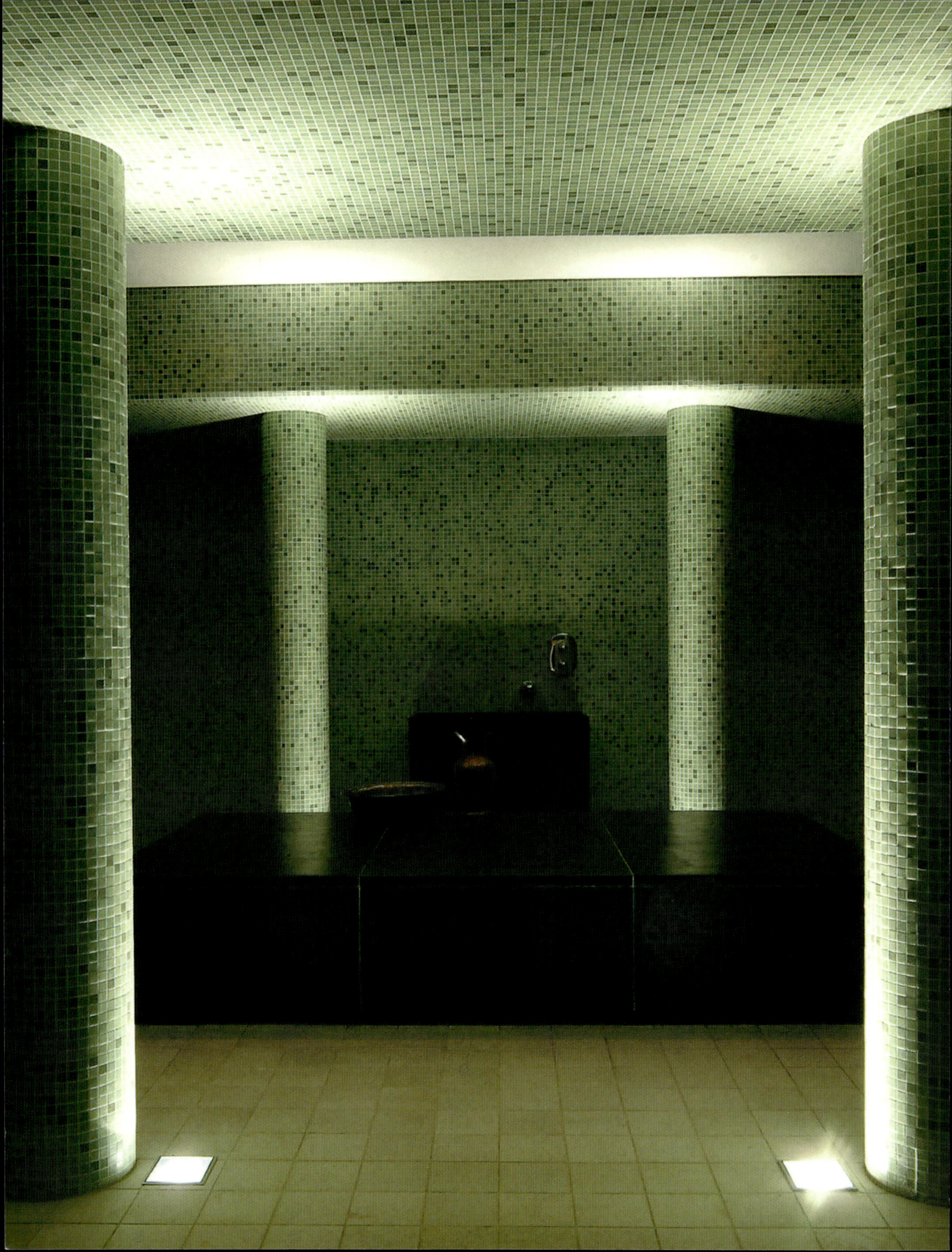

Wave Urbanspa

Diese Spa im Zentrum von Verona bietet ein umfangreiches Wellnesskonzept. Im Erdgeschoss weist der schmale Empfangskorridor den Weg zum Hauptpool und zum Japanischen Garten. Auf der ersten Etage befindet sich die Behandlungszone mit Massageräumen und Nassbereich, dessen Mittelpunkt ein Hammam bildet. Travertinmarmor und grüne Mosaikkacheln erinnern an römische Bäder.

Wave Urbanspa is located in the middle of the city, especially built to offer all the activities comprised in the concept of wellness. On the ground floor, the small welcome hallway leads the way to the area where the main pool and the Japanese garden lie. On the first floor one finds the treatment area that includes the massage rooms and the wet area, presided by a hammam, coated in green because of the travertine marble and the mosaics that remind one of the Roman baths.

Situé en plein cœur de la ville, Wave Urbanspa a été conçu pour offrir toutes les prestations dédiées au bien-être. Au rez-de-chaussée, un vestibule de taille modeste mène à la piscine principale ainsi qu'à un jardin japonais. Le premier étage héberge la zone des soins qui comprend les cabines de massage, et l'espace fraîcheur, dominé par un hammam, dont les mosaïques vertes qui évoquent les bains romains répondent au vert du marbre travertine.

Wave Urbanspa ligt midden in de stad en is speciaal gebouwd voor allerlei activiteiten die met wellness te maken hebben. Op de begane grond bevindt zich een kleine ontvangsthal, die toegang biedt tot het zwembad en de Japanse tuin. Op de eerste verdieping ligt het behandelcentrum met massagekamers en badencomplex, waaronder een hammam uitgevoerd in groen travertijn en mozaïeken die doen denken aan Romeinse baden.

Verona, Italy

PAGANI & DI MAURO ARCHITETTI

Photos © Dario Lasagni

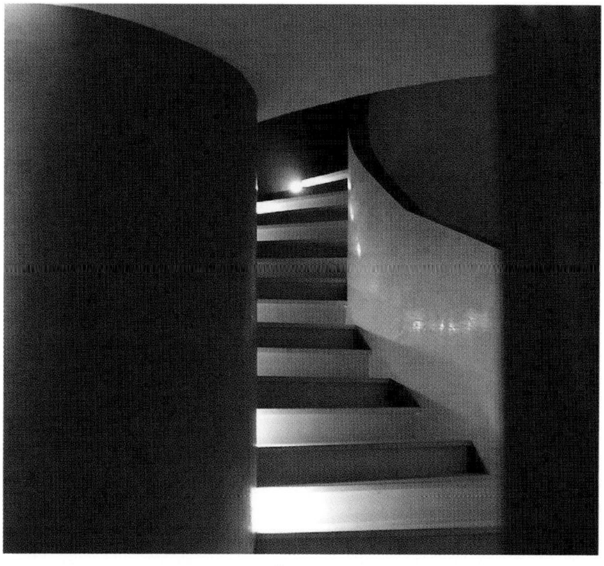

www.waveurbanspa.it

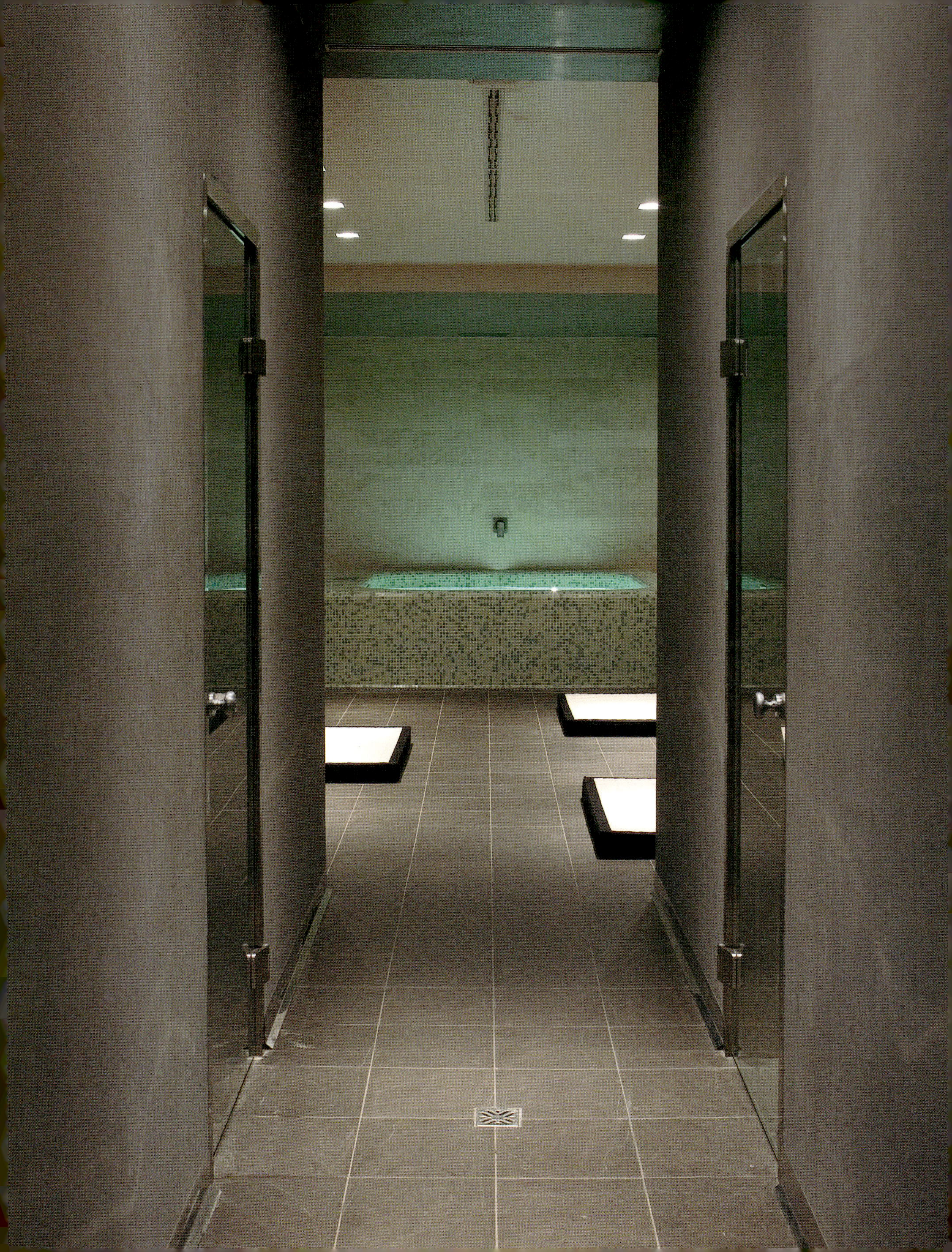

Der Hauptpool und ein Japanischer Garten nehmen das Erdgeschoss ein.

The main pool and a Japanese garden occupy the ground floor.

Une piscine principale et un jardin japonais occupent le rez-de-chaussée.

Het zwembad en een Japanse tuin liggen op de eerste verdieping.

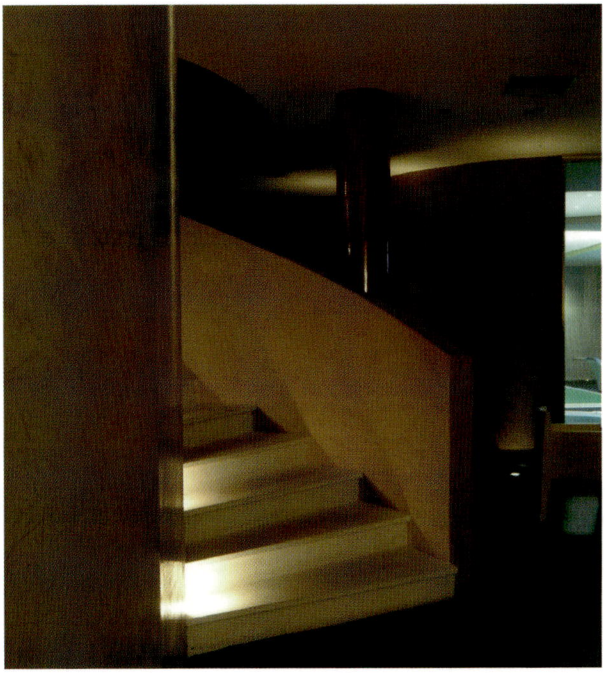

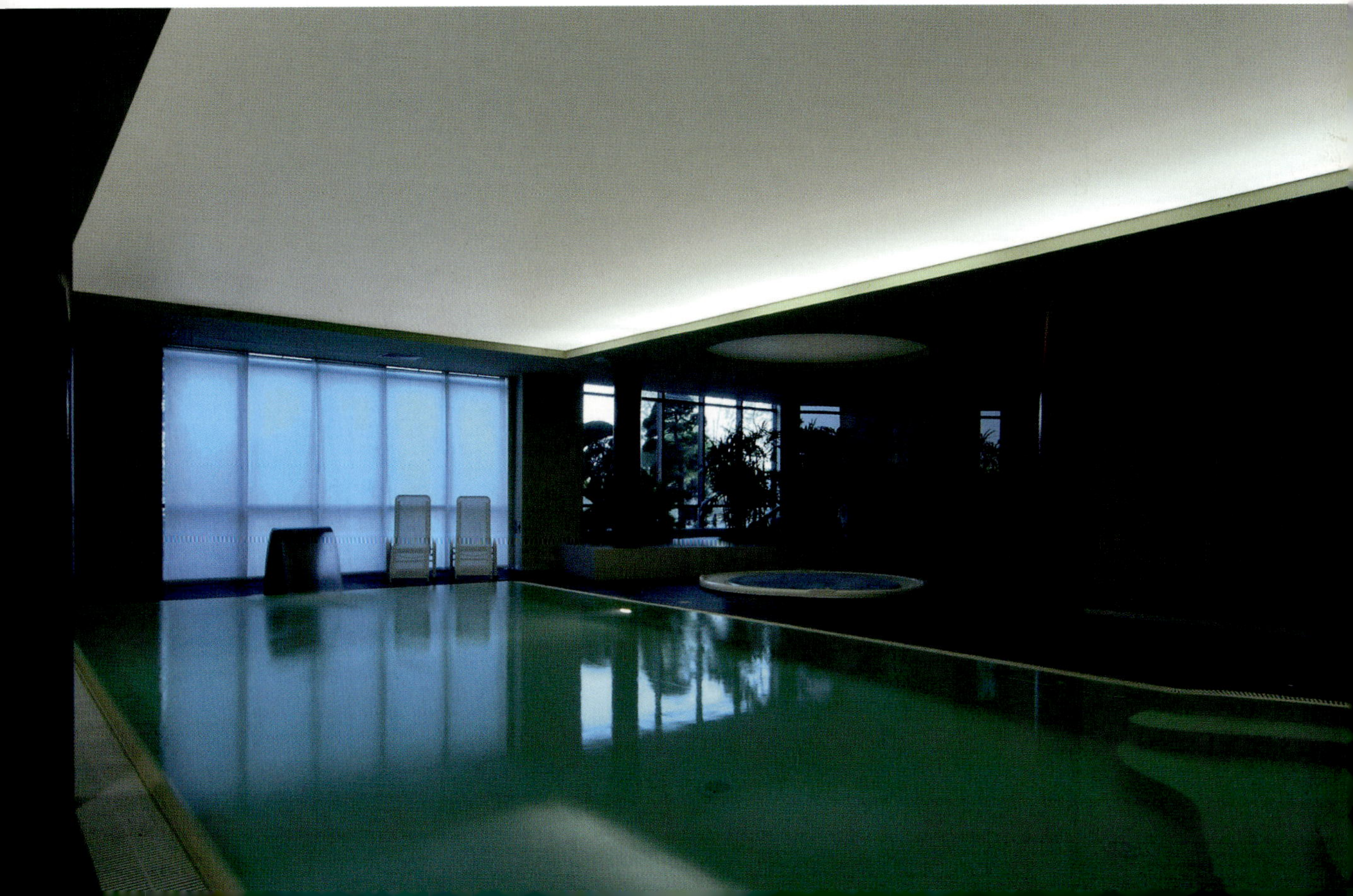

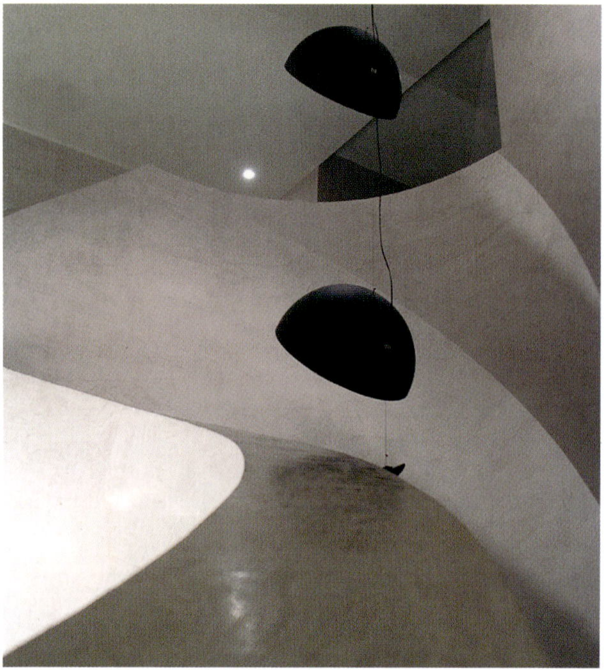

Die Einrichtung wird von Travertinmarmor und Mosaikkacheln dominiert.

The predominant materials are travertine marble and mosaics.

Les matériaux prédominants sont le marbre travertine et les mosaïques.

Travertijn en mozaïeken domineren de inrichting.

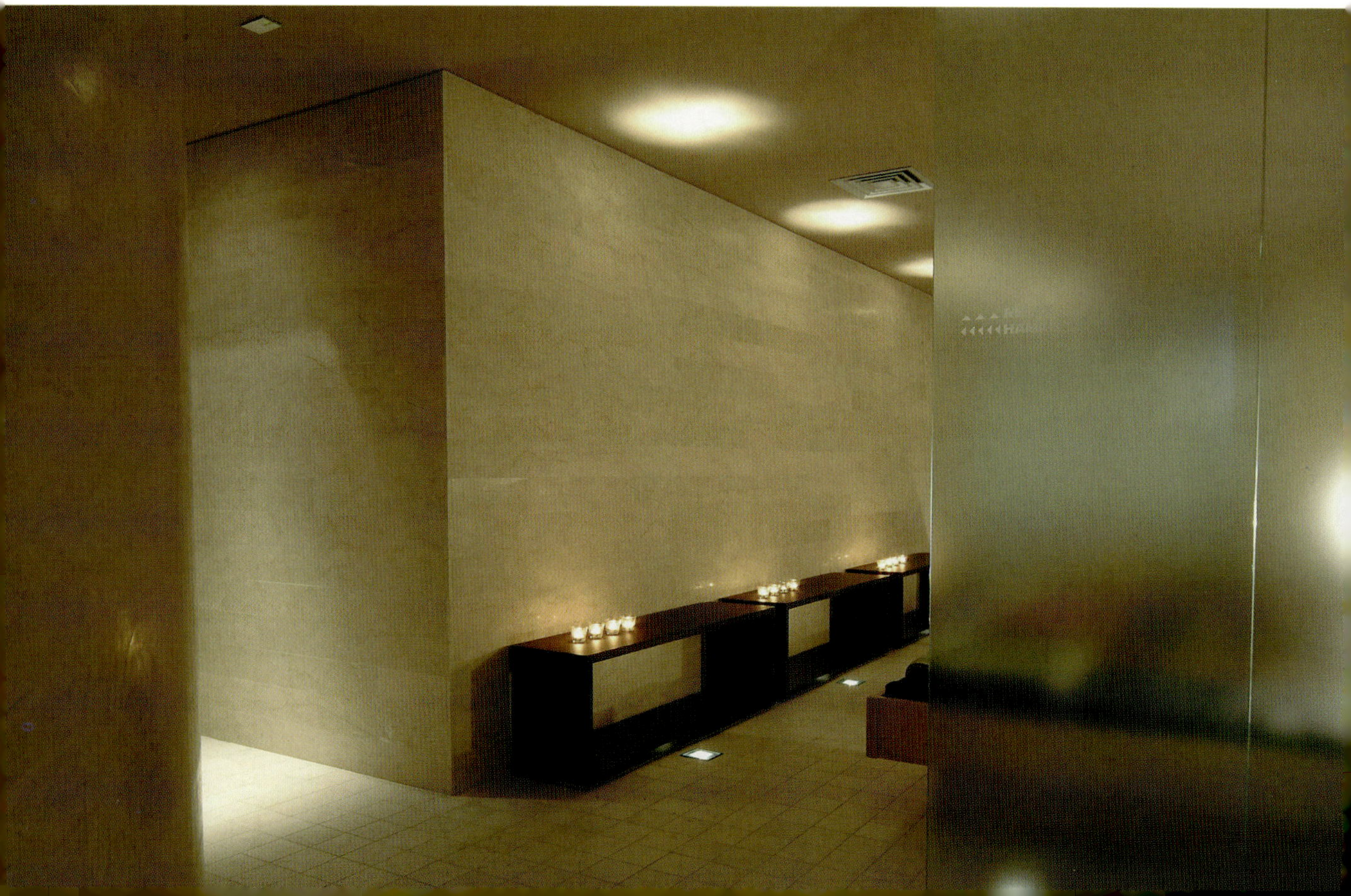

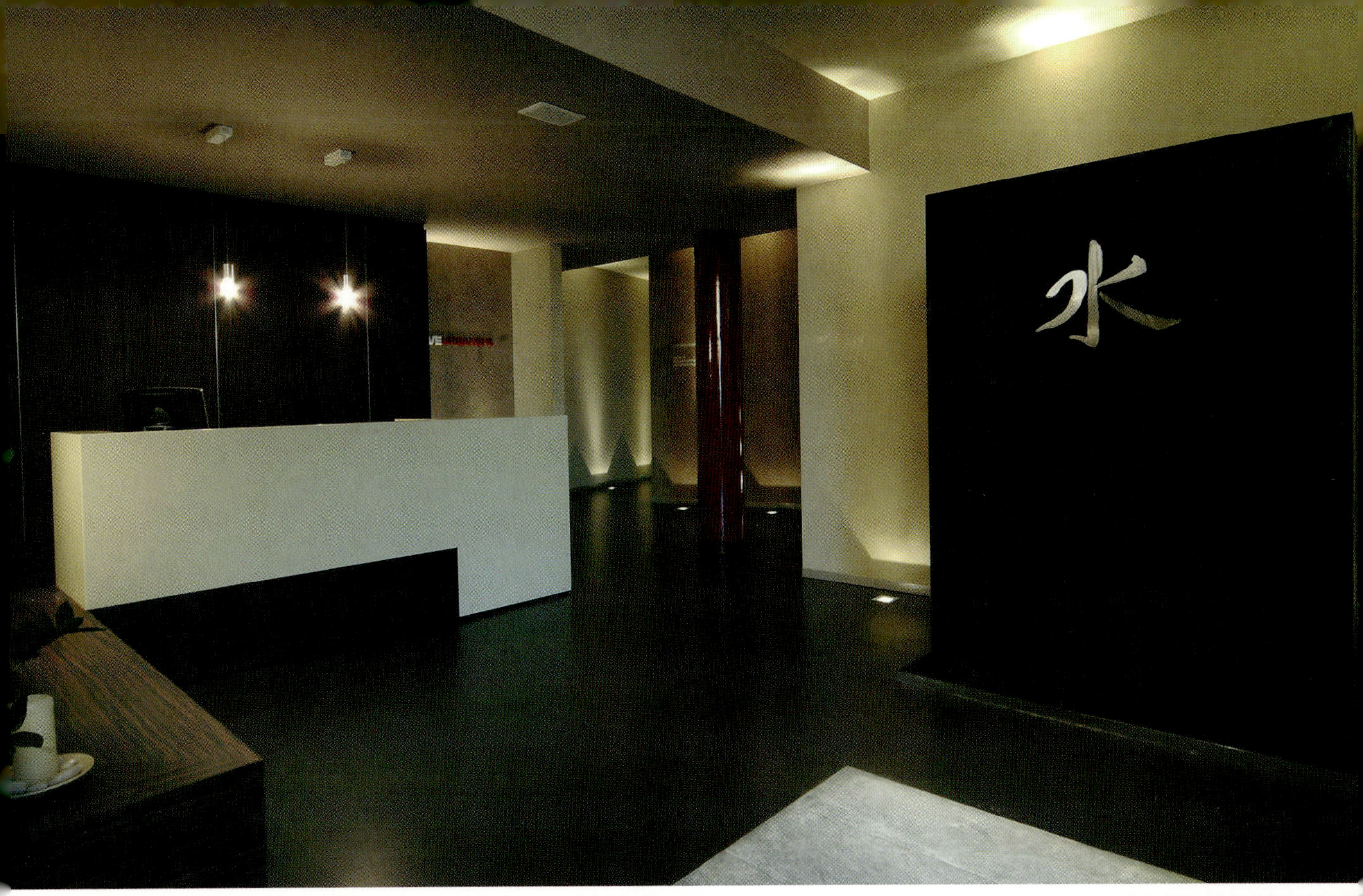
水
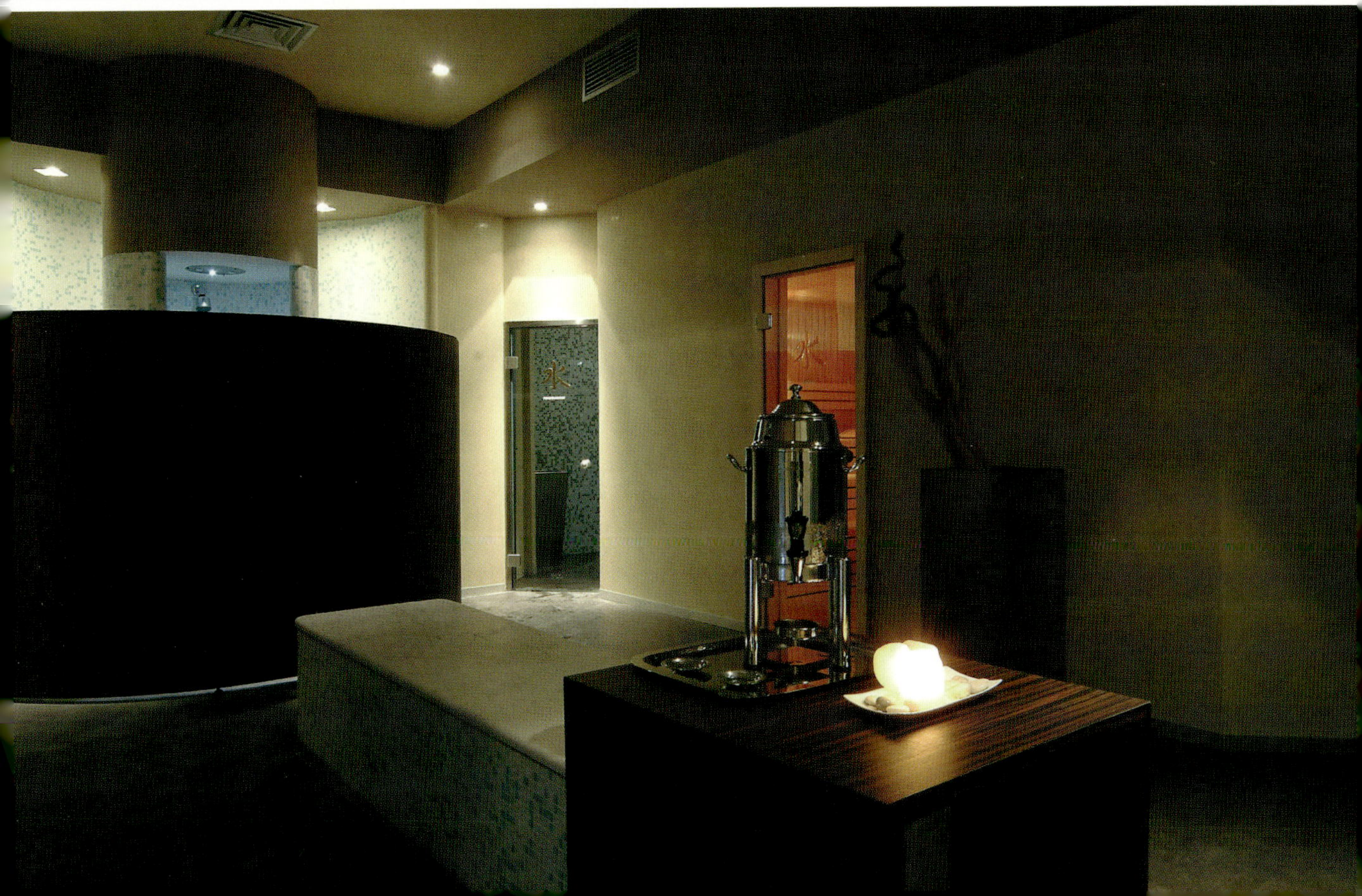

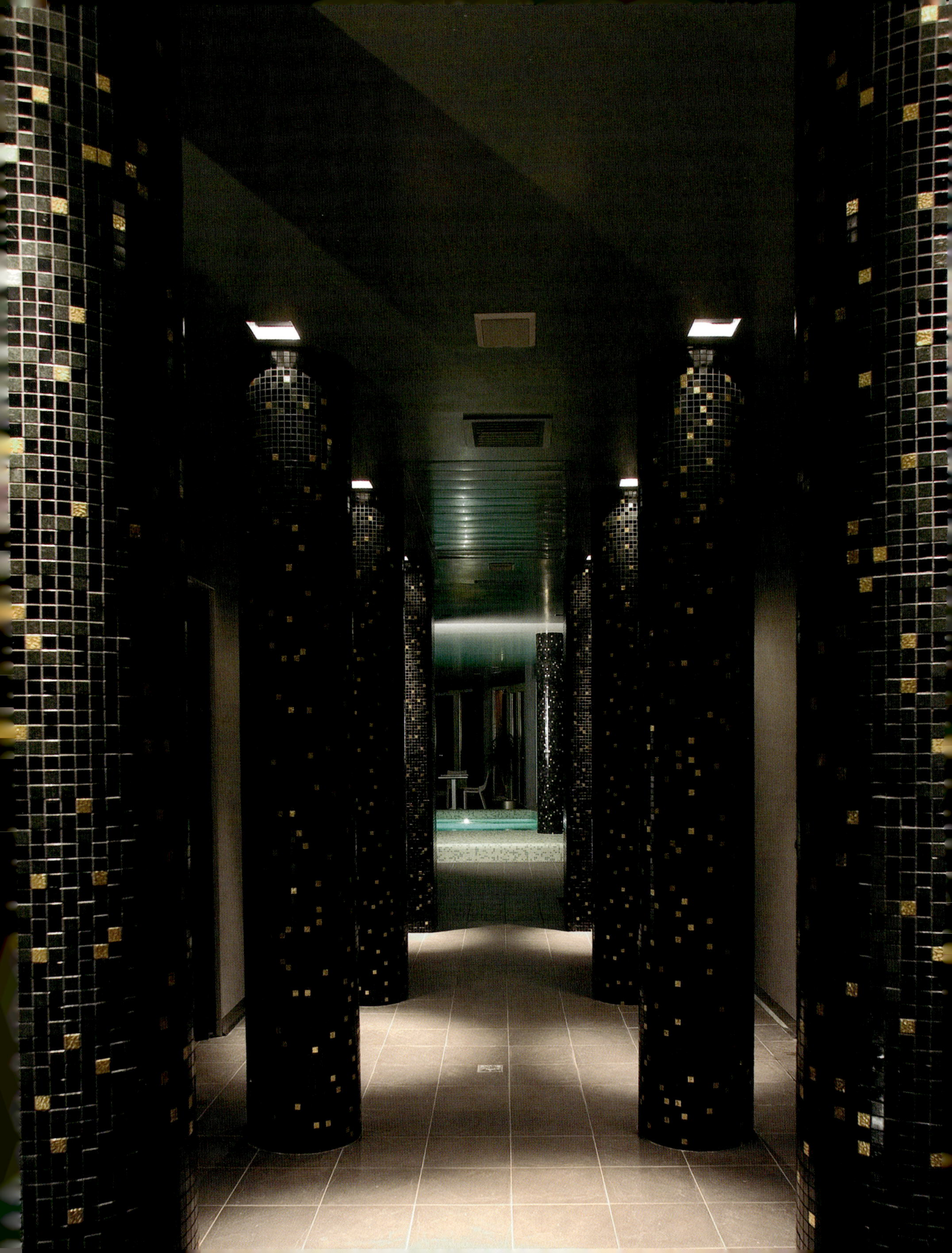

Notos Spa

Das Altafiumara ist ein altes Schloss, das modernen Hotelstandards angepasst wurde. Es beherbergt das Notos Spa, eine über 1.000 qm große Anlage, die einer modernen Ästhetik mit klaren Linien und ruhigen Farben folgt. Der mit Whirlpooldüsen ausgestattete Hauptpool ist durch eine Glaswand geteilt: Eine Hälfte ist überdacht und liegt neben der Entspannungszone; die andere Hälfte befindet sich im Freien und lockt mit einem herrlichen Blick auf die offene Landschaft.

The Altafiumara is an ancient castle that has been adapted to the standards of the modern hotel industry and, as such, it holds the Notos Spa, with over 10,800 square feet, provided with contemporary aesthetics of pure lines and serene colors. The main pool, equipped with Jacuzzi jets, is divided by a glass wall: half of it is under a roof, near the relaxation zone, and the other half looks outside thus becoming a water balcony with views over the open country.

Ancien château par la suite adapté aux normes de l'hôtellerie moderne, l'Altafiumara comprend le spa Notos, de plus de 1.000 m², où se déclinent dans une esthétique contemporaine lignes pures et couleurs sobres. La piscine principale, équipée de jets jacuzzis, est divisée en deux parties par un mur de verre. La première moitié, proche de la zone de relaxation, est couverte ; l'autre, partiellement tournée vers l'extérieur, devient ainsi un balcon aquatique et offre un panorama dégagé sur la campagne.

Het Altafiumara is een oeroud kasteel dat is aangepast aan de eisen van de moderne hotelindustrie en o.a. de Notos Spa bevat, een ruim 1000 m² groot, modern, in heldere lijnen en serene kleuren vormgegeven complex. Het grote zwembad bezit massagestralen en wordt in tweeën gedeeld door een glazen muur: de ene helft is binnen, vlak bij de rustruimte, en de andere helft steekt uit naar buiten, als een soort waterbalkon met uitzicht op het omringende landschap.

Calabria, Italy

PAGANI & DI MAURO ARCHITETTI

Photos © Dario Lasagni

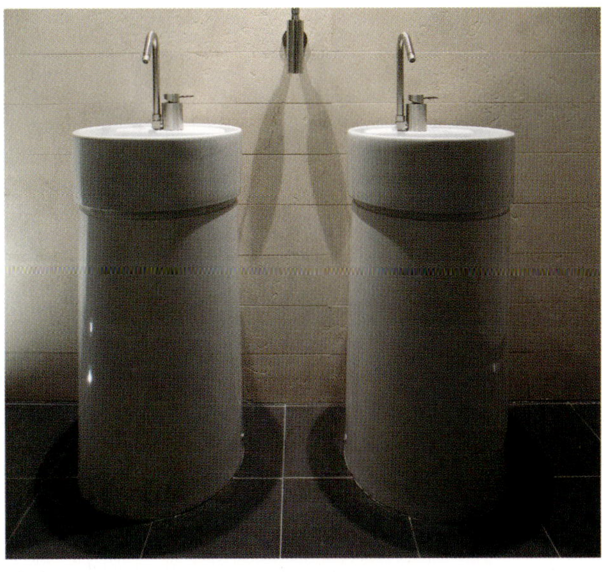

www.altafiumara.it

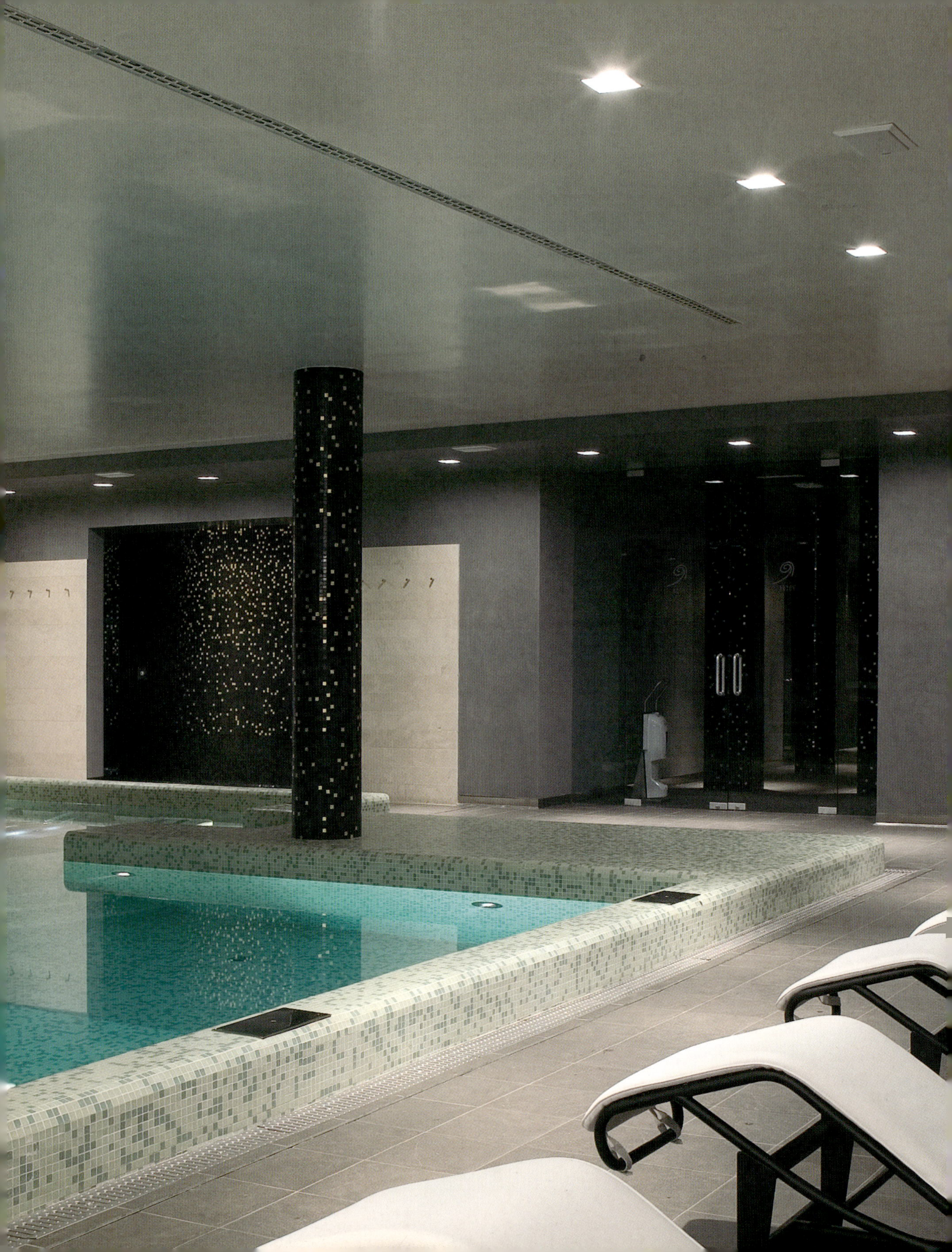

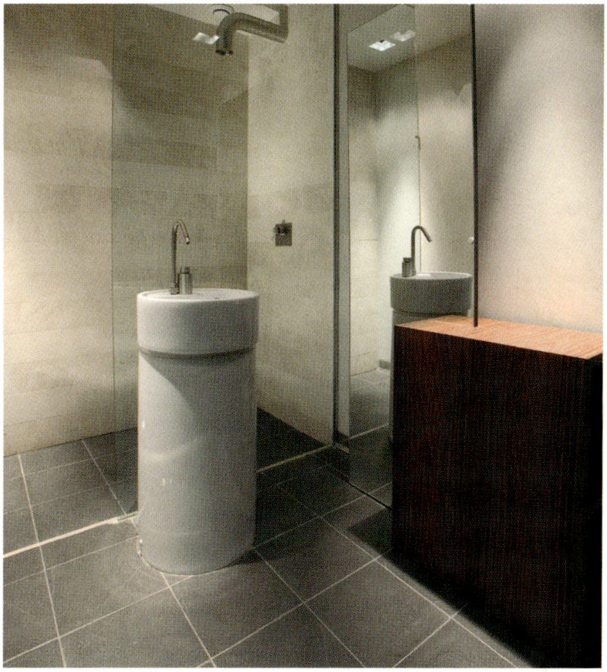

In der ersten Etage des Spa werden ausschließlich Massagen und Anwendungen zur Körperpflege angeboten.

The spa's first floor is completely dedicated to massages and other treatments for body care.

Le premier étage du spa est entièrement réservé aux massages et autres soins pour le corps.

De eerste verdieping is volledig gewijd aan massages en andere lichaamsbehandelingen.

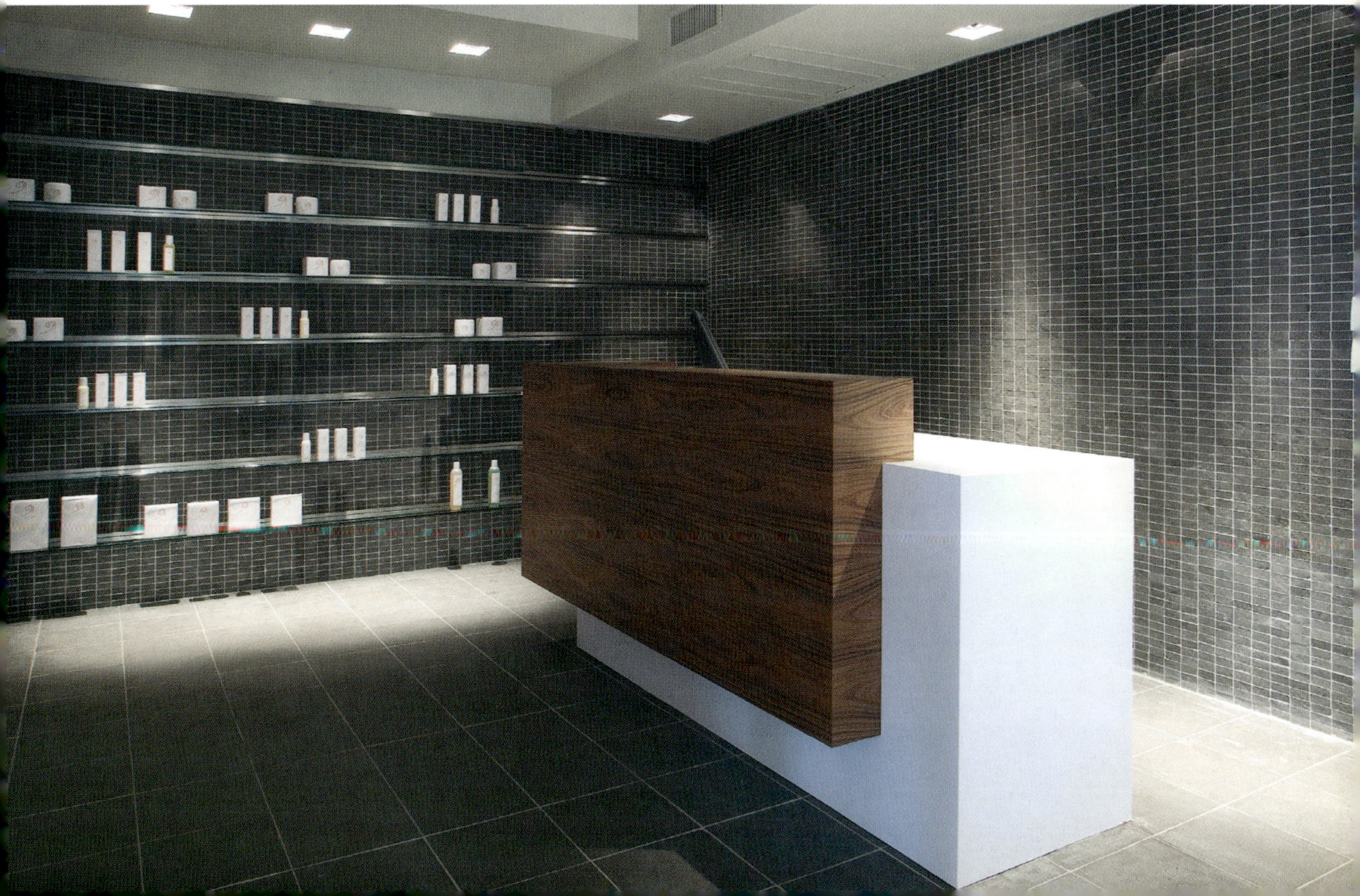

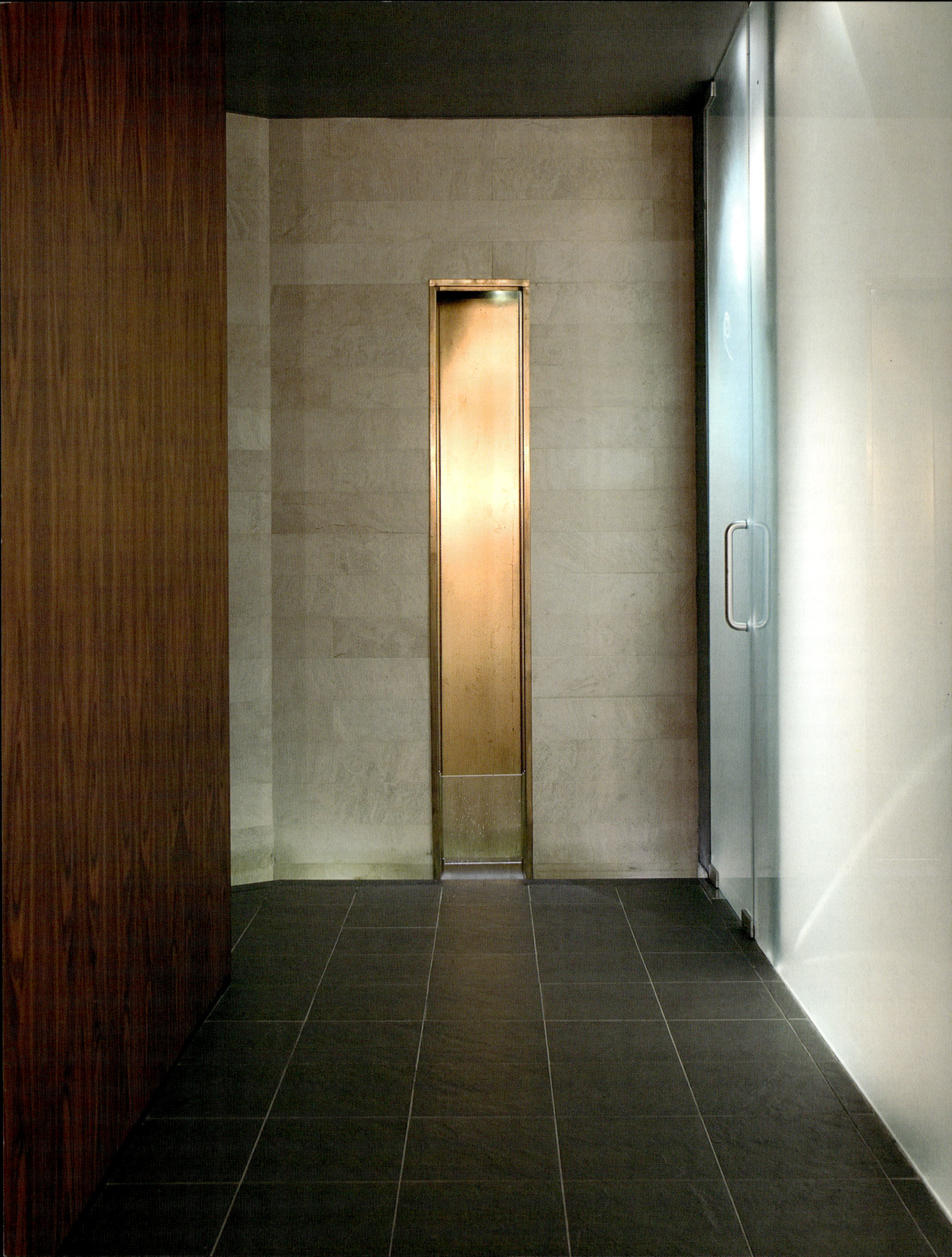

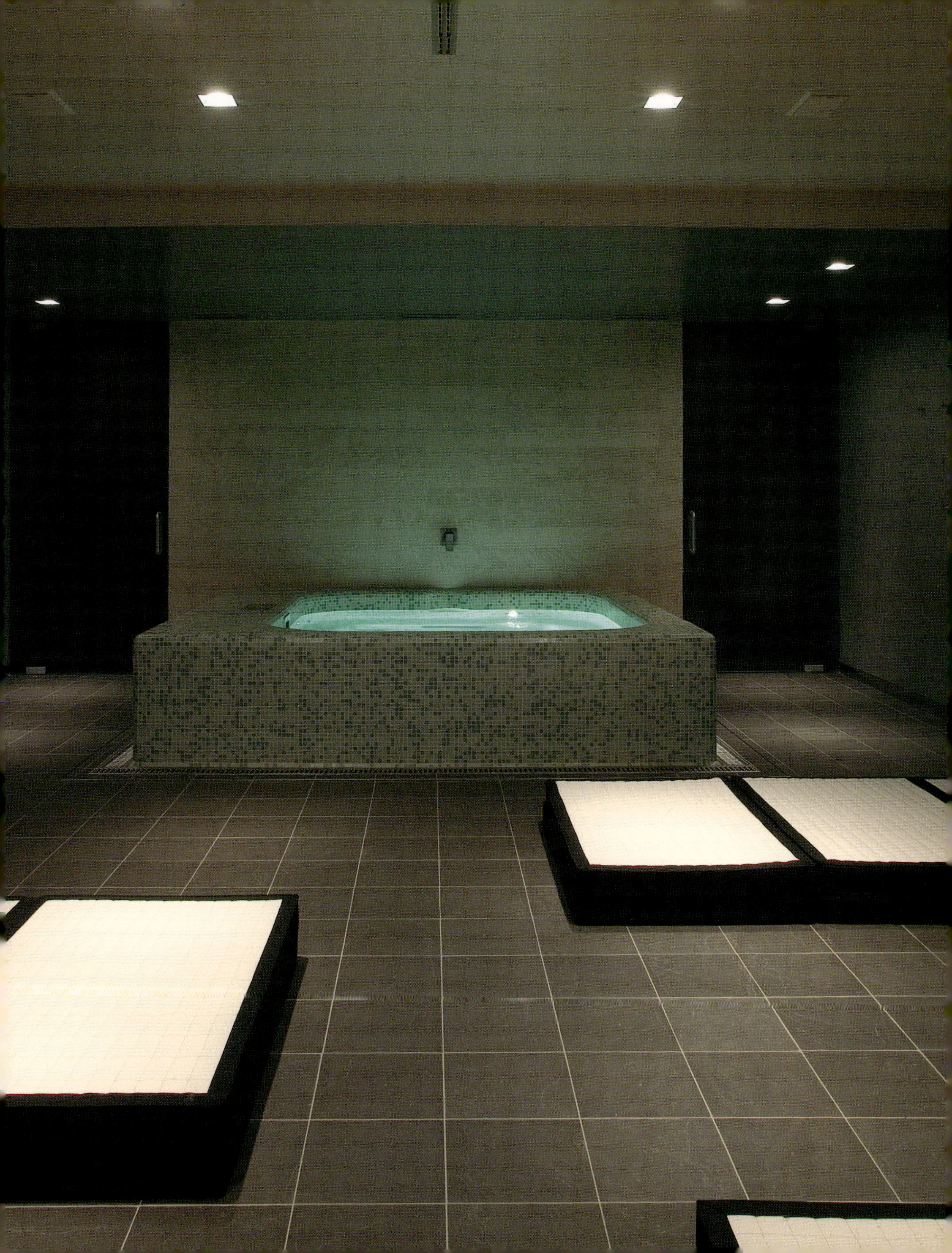

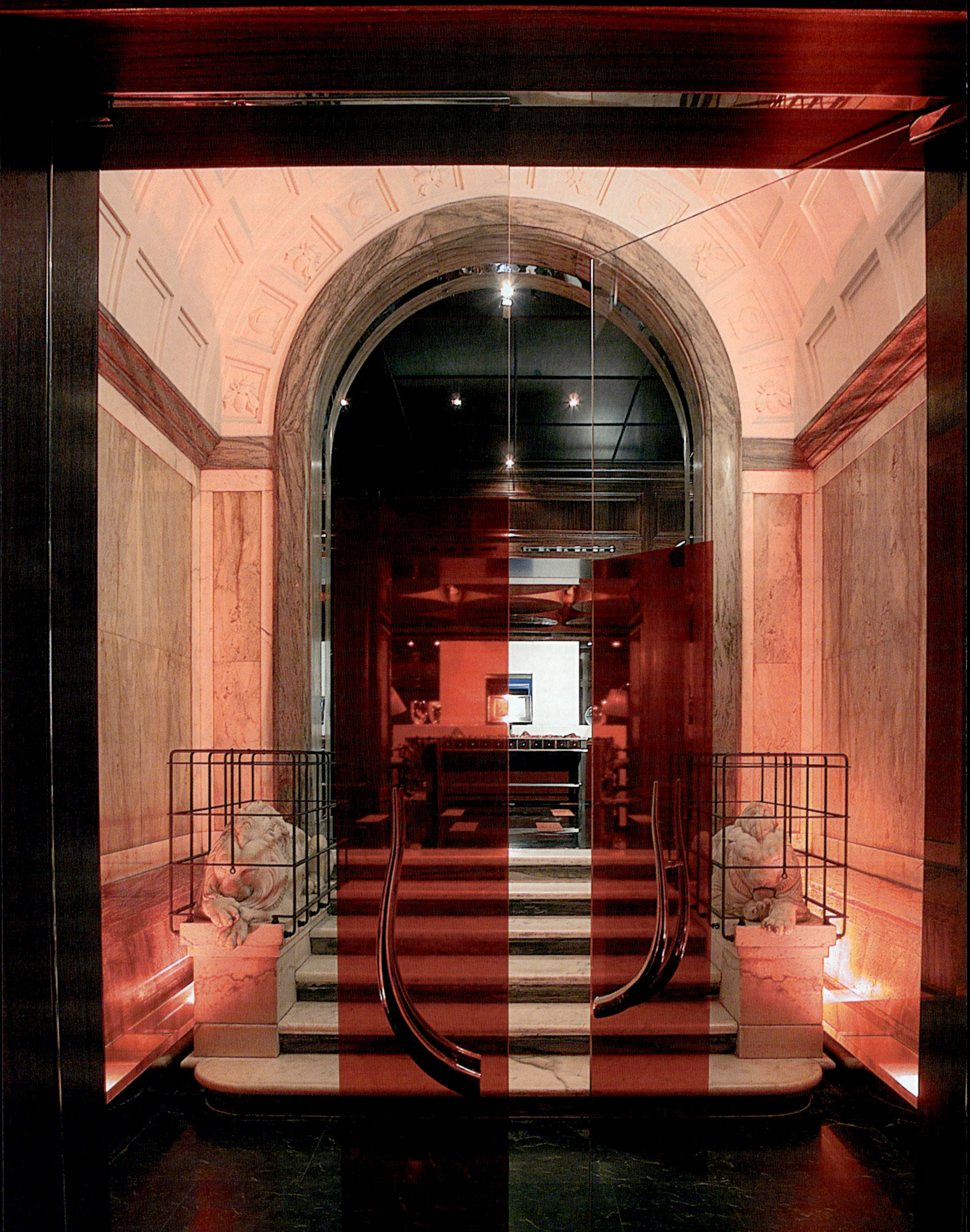

Spa Paraiso at the Aleph

Dieses Spa bietet Hotelgästen und externen Besucher zahlreiche Wohlfühlanwendungen, darunter Schokoladen-Treatments, Honig-Maismehl-Hautkuren, Shiatsu, Ayurveda-Massagen und chinesische Reflexzonenmassage. Neben Saunen, türkischen Bädern und einem Thermal-Whirlpool gibt es auch ein kleines, aber gut ausgestattetes Fitnessstudio. Der Pool besteht aus zwei miteinander verbundenen Becken; eines ist lang und schmal, das andere sehr breit mit Stufen, die als Ruhezone dienen.

Open to guests and to external visitors of the hotel, the spa's offer includes treatments with melted chocolate, skin cleansing with honey and corn flour, shiatsu, Ayurvedic massages and Chinese reflexology. Saunas, Turkish baths and a thermal whirlpool are complemented by a small but well equipped gym. Two communicating pools, one long and narrow, the other one very wide with steps that serve as a rest area, form the swimming pool.

Ouvert aux clients de l'hôtel, mais pas seulement, l'offre de ce spa propose des enveloppements au chocolat, des nettoyages de peau à base de miel et de farine de blé, du shiatsu, des massages ayurvédiques, et de la réflexologie chinoise. Saunas, hammams et jacuzzis sont complétés par une petite salle de fitness très bien équipée. Deux bassins communicants, l'un long et étroit, l'autre très large, et dont les marches servent de zone de repos, forment la piscine.

Dit complex is ook toegankelijk voor gasten die niet in het hotel logeren. Het biedt behandelingen aan met gesmolten chocolade, huidreiniging met honing en maïsmeel, shiatsu, ayurvedische massages en Chinese reflexzonetherapie. De sauna's, Turkse baden en thermale whirlpool worden aangevuld met een kleine, maar volledig ingerichte fitnessruimte. Het zwembad bestaat uit twee communicerende vaten, het ene lang en dun, het andere met brede traptreden om op uit te rusten.

Rome, Italy

ADAM D. TIHANY/TIHANY DESIGN

Photos © Alberto Ferrero, Boscolo Hotels

www.aleph.boscolohotels.com

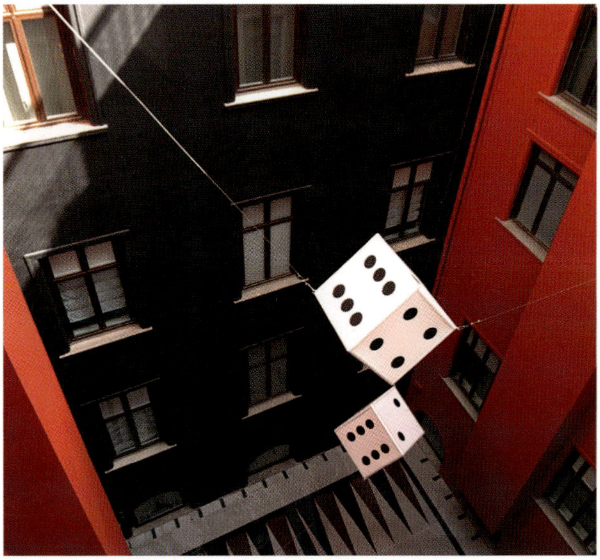

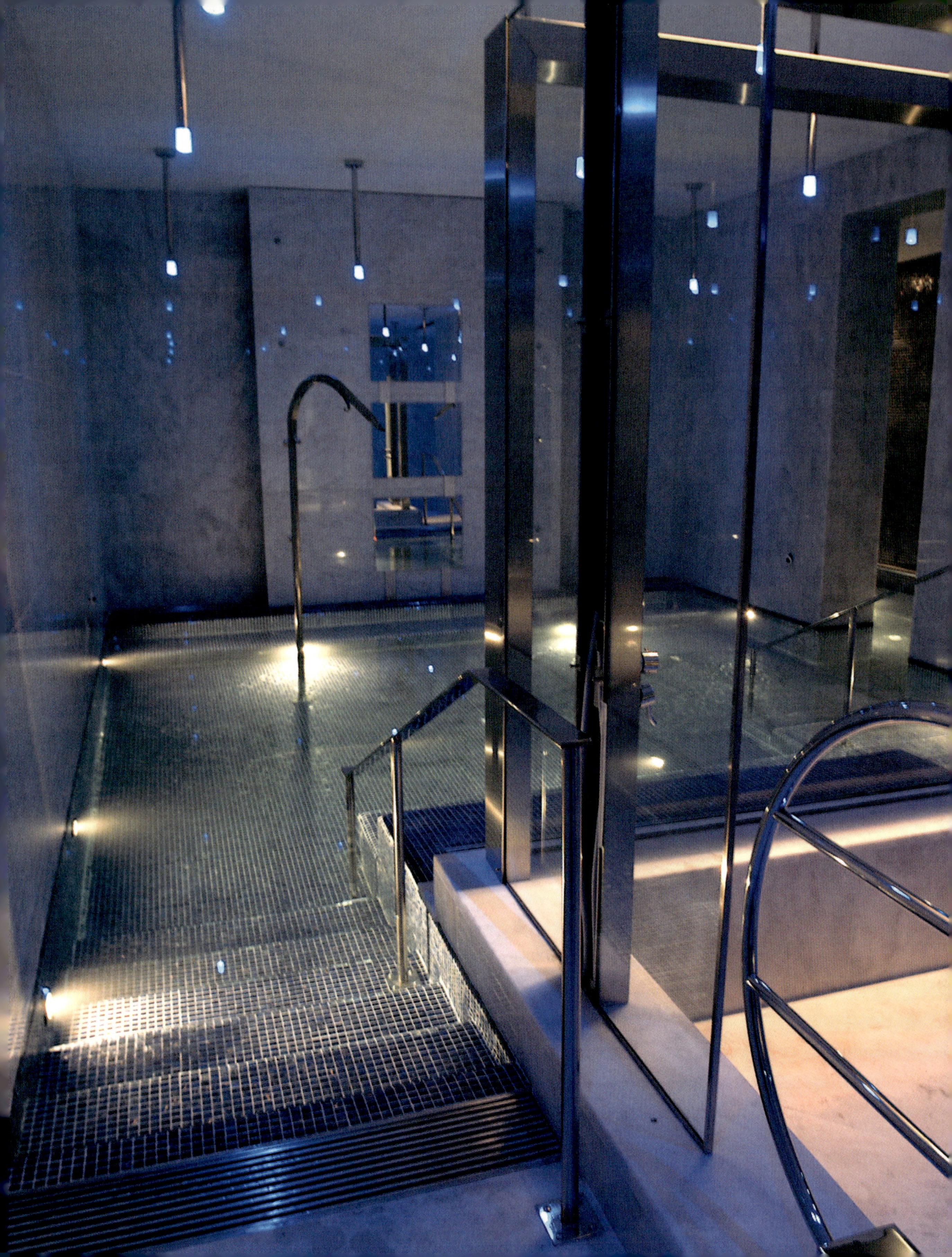

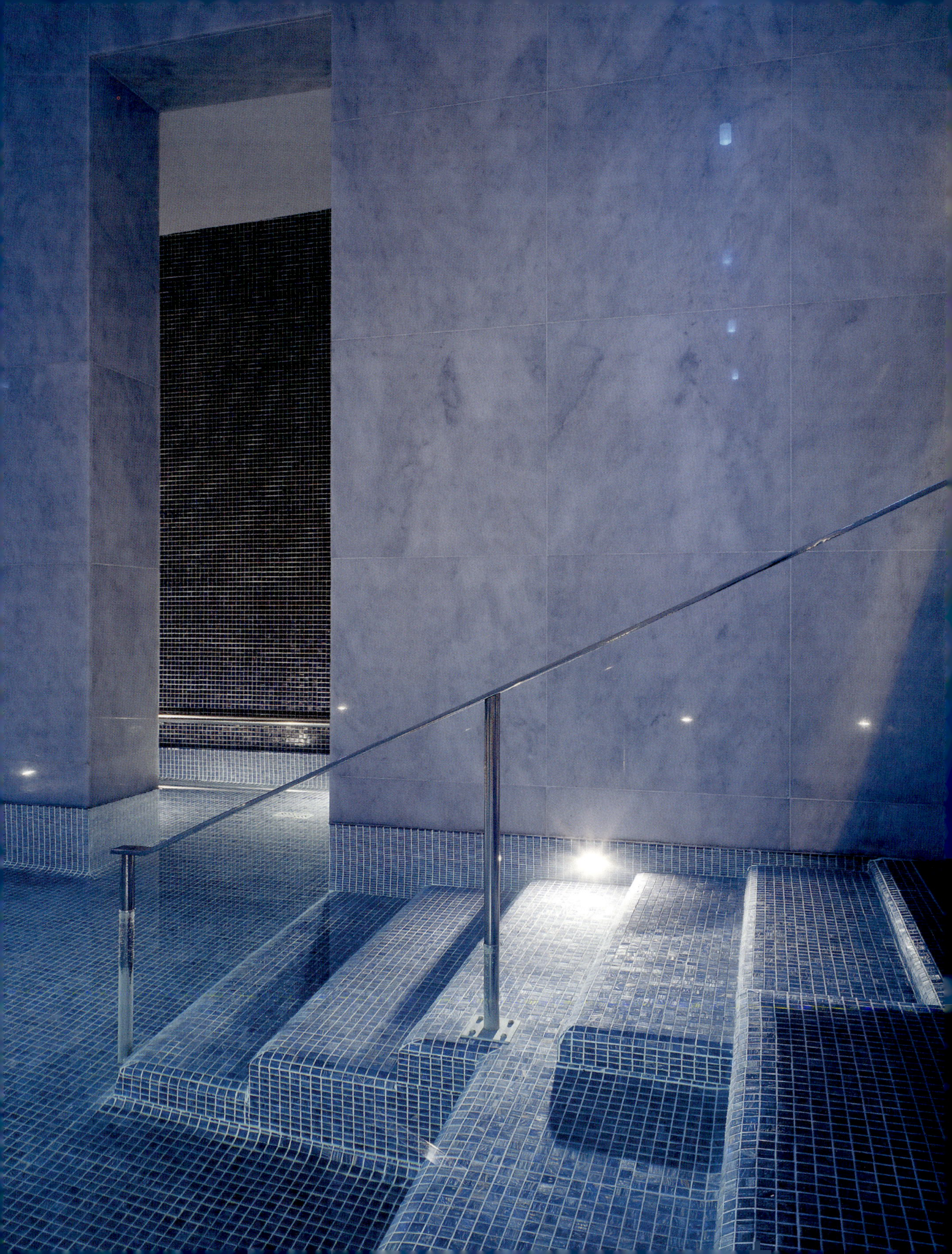

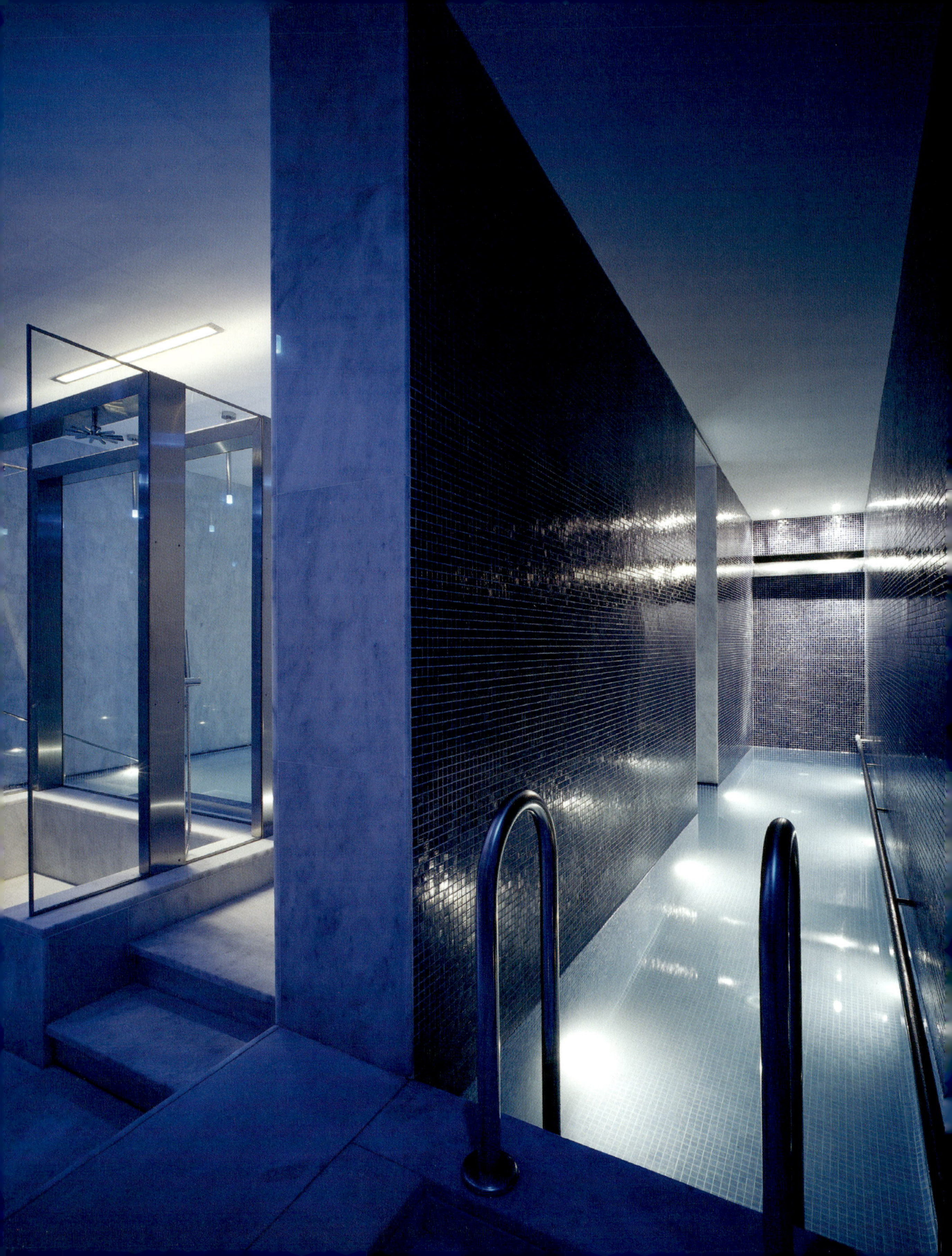

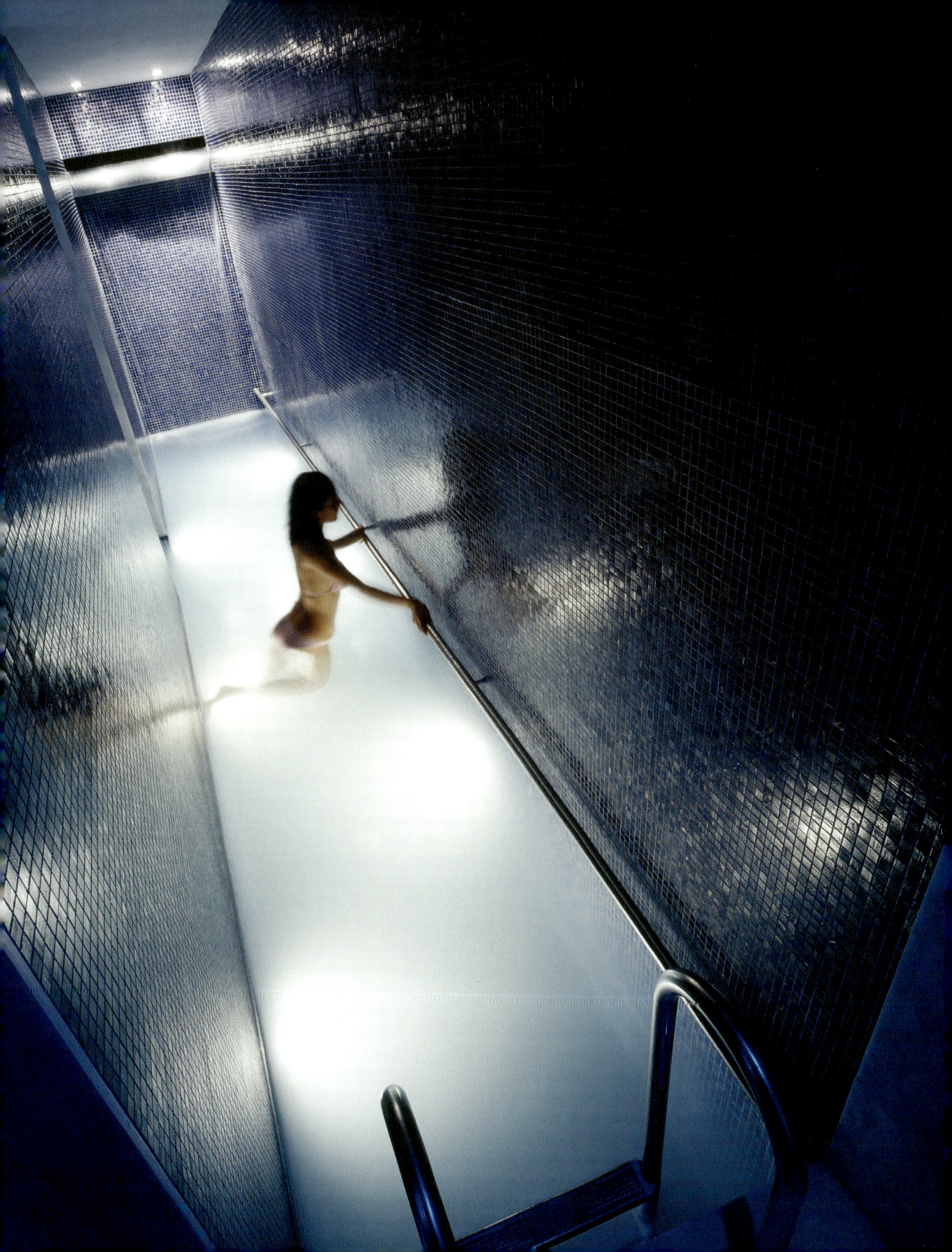

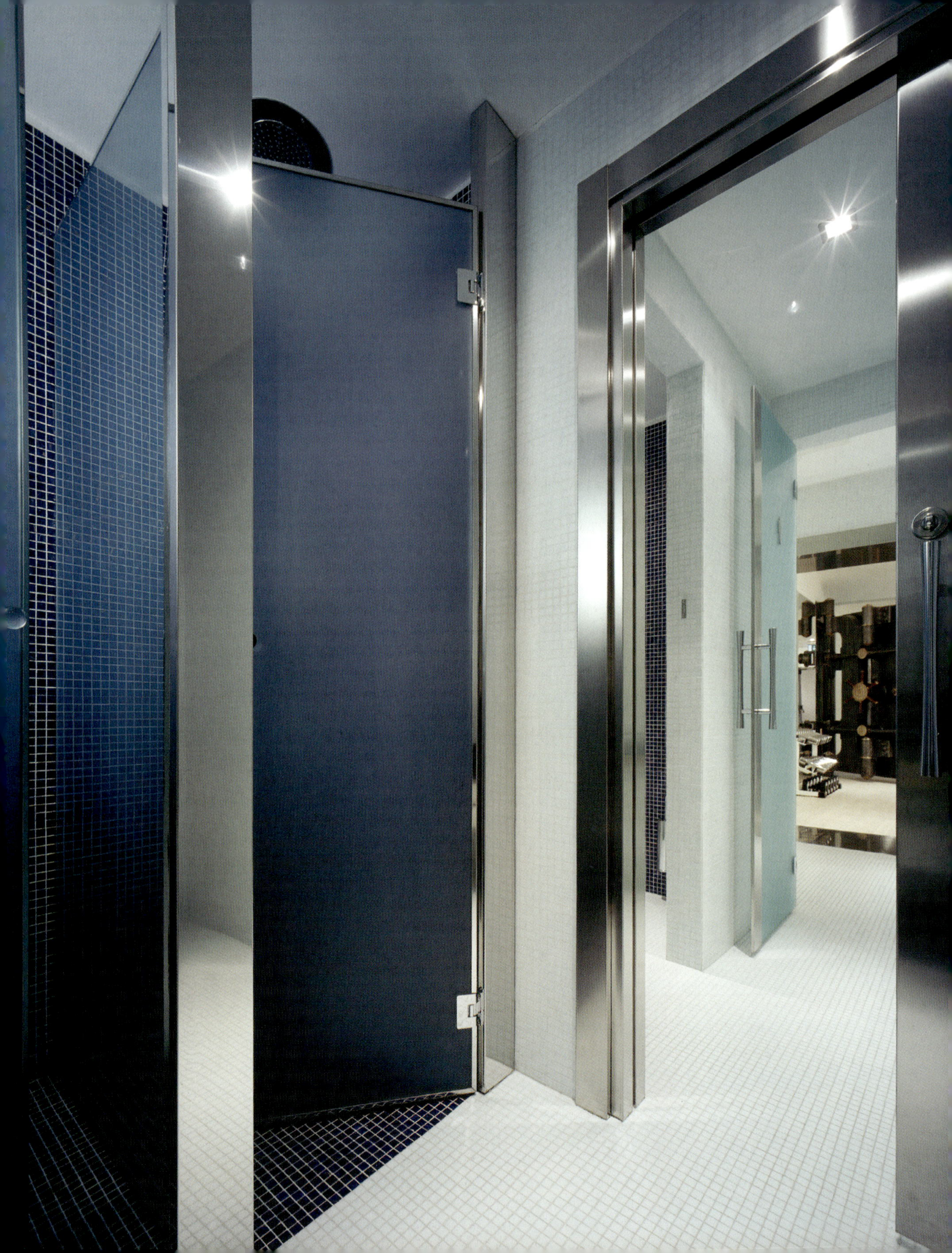

Blaue Mosaikkacheln und harmonisches Licht schaffen eine wahrhaft paradiesische Atmosphäre.

The blue mosaic tiling and precise lighting create an almost celestial atmosphere, honoring the spa's name.

Comme un hommage au nom du spa, le carrelage en mosaïque bleu et l'éclairage directionnel créent une atmosphère presque céleste.

De blauwe mozaïektegeltjes en slimme belichting creëren een hemelse sfeer, die de naam van dit complex eer aandoet.

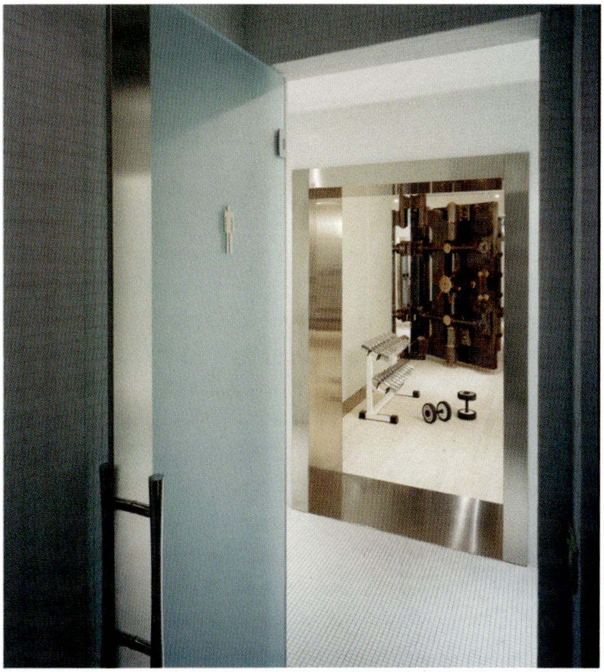

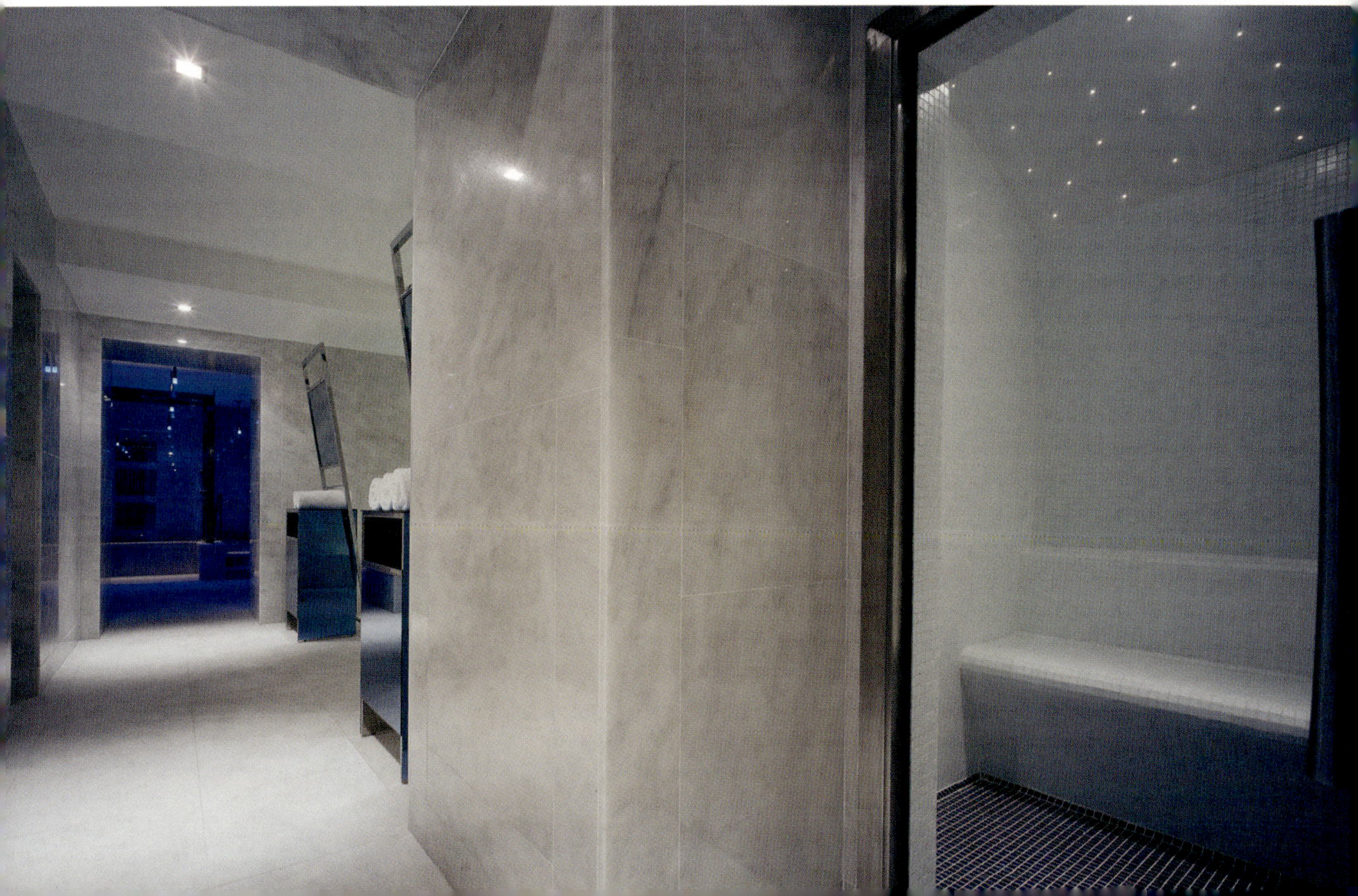

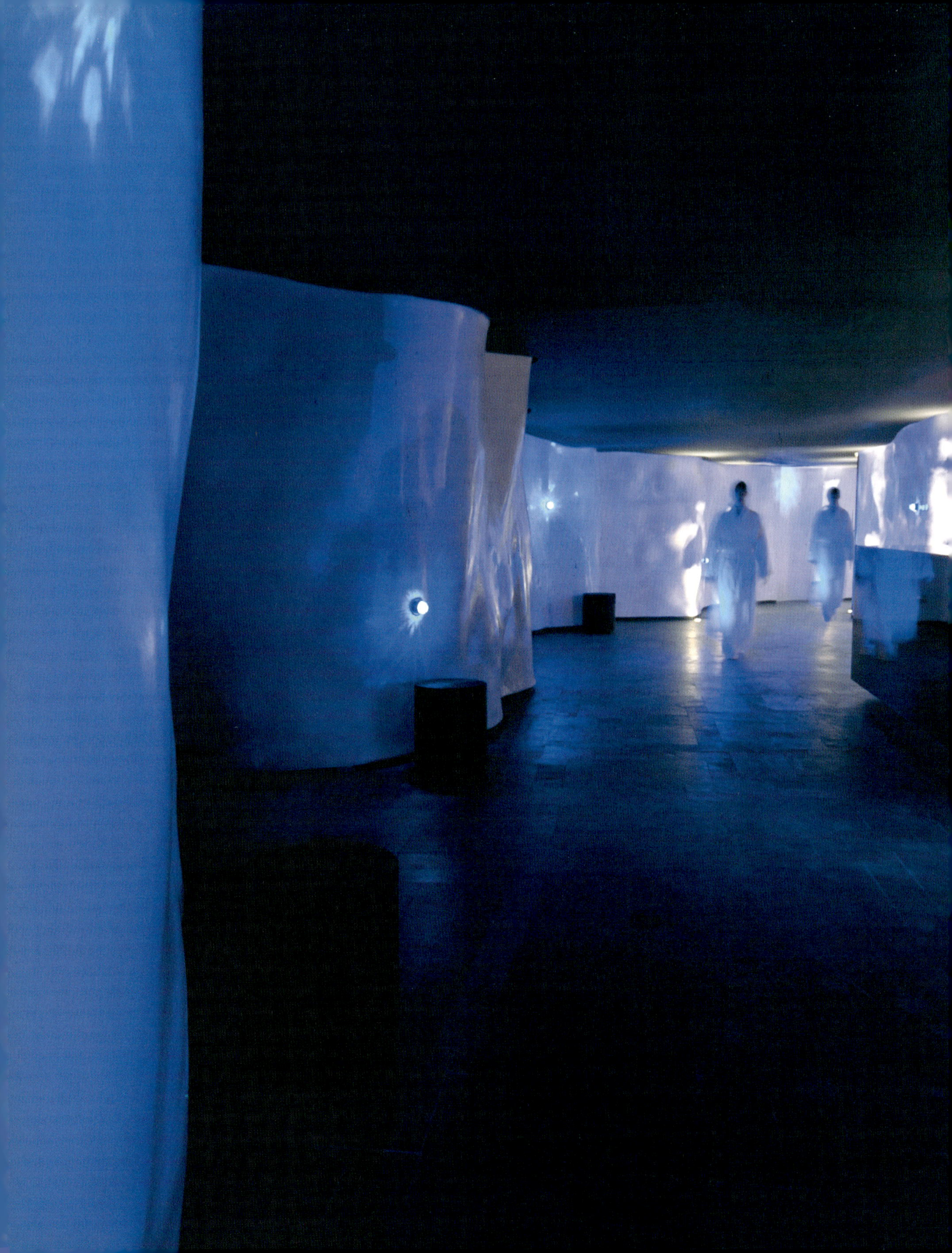

New York Palace Hotel Spa

Dieses Spa offenbart sich als außergewöhnliche Sinneserfahrung, bei der Wirklichkeit und Traum miteinander verschmelzen.
Die gipsmodellierten Wände entfalten eine eigene Dynamik: Durch die Verkleidung mit leuchtend weißem Kunstharz nehmen sie organische Formen an und erzeugen ein einzigartiges Licht- und Schattenspiel.
Die Fläche teilt sich auf in Saunen, Behandlungskabinen, ein Fitnessstudio, Dampfbäder und eine Nasszone.

This spa is a scenario of seductive drama, conceived as a sensory experience in which the reality is mixed with a dream world. The walls, covered in plastic, become dynamic surfaces built with plaster. Thanks to the finishes in bright, white resin, they adopt organic shapes and provoke a play of lights and shadows that makes them visually lighter. The space is divided into saunas, treatment cabins, a gym, steam baths and a wet zone.

Ce spa, digne d'un décor de film, est conçu comme une expérience multi-sensorielle dans laquelle la réalité se transforme en univers onirique. Les murs de plâtre, aux formes dynamiques, ont été recouverts de plastique ; grâce à une finition en résine brillante, ils adoptent des formes organiques et provoquent un jeu d'ombres et de lumières qui les rendent visuellement aériens. L'espace est composé de saunas, de cabines de soins, d'une salle de remise en forme, de hammams, et d'une zone fraîcheur.

Deze spa is ontworpen als een zintuiglijke ervaring waarin dromen en werkelijkheid worden vermengd. De met kunststof overtrokken muren vormen dynamische vlakken. Dankzij de afwerking met helderwitte hars nemen ze organische vormen aan en zorgen ze voor een spel van licht en schaduw dat ze visueel lichter maakt. De ruimte is verdeeld in sauna's, behandelcabines, een fitnessruimte, stoombaden en een badencomplex.

Budapest, Hungary

SIMONE MICHELI

Photos © S.M.A.H.

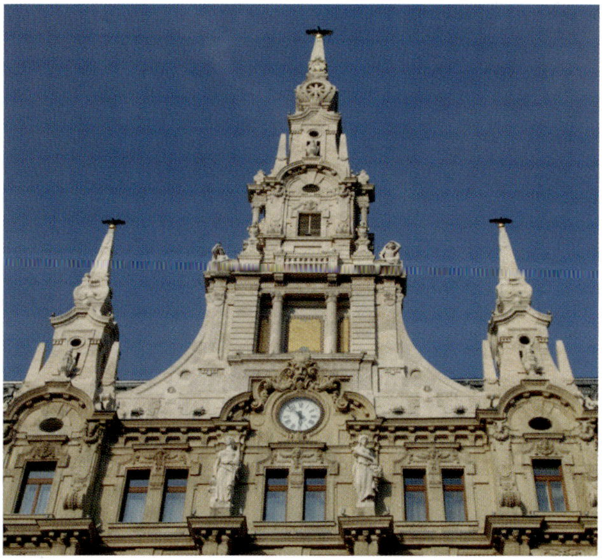

www.boscolohotels.com

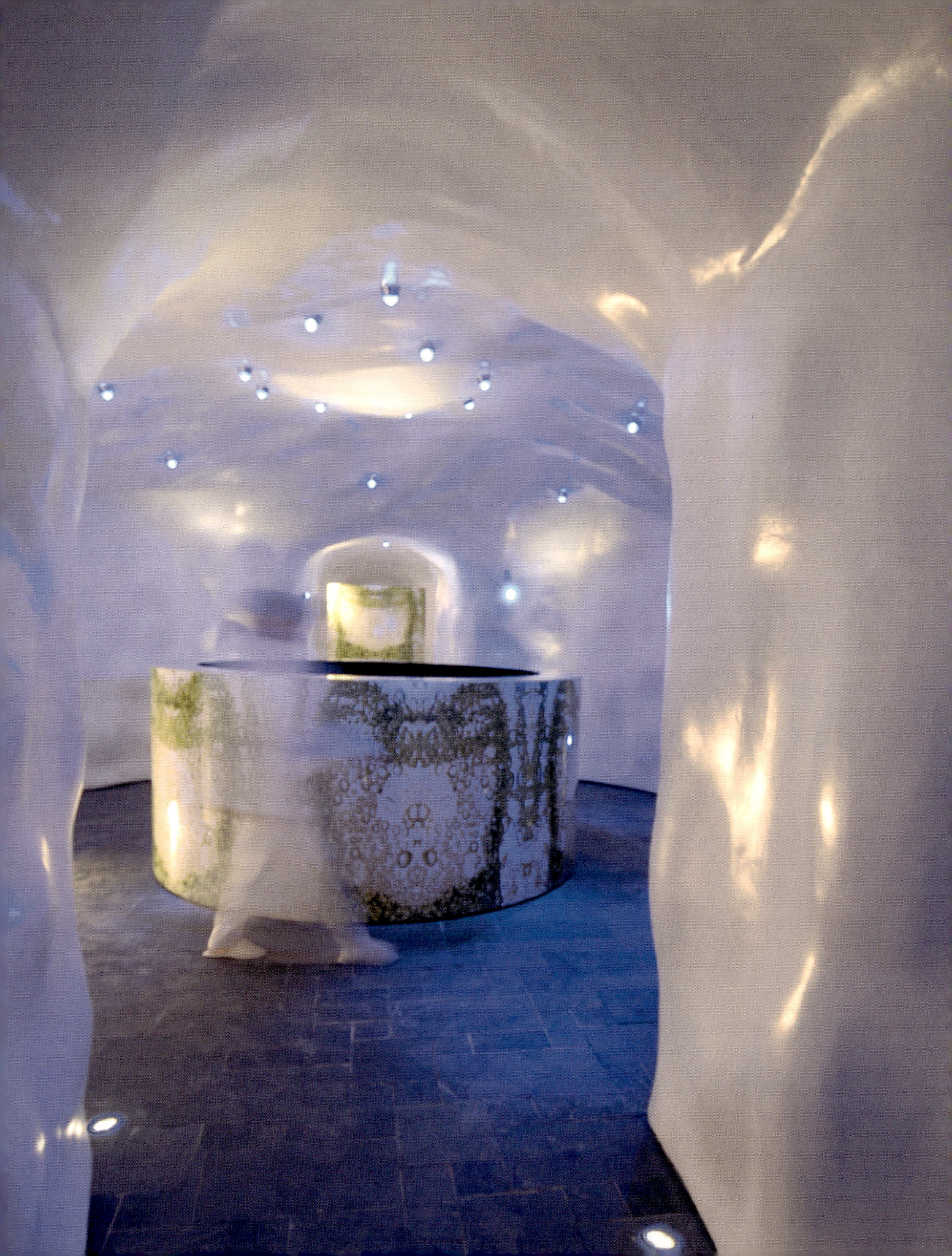

Mit fließenden Formen und beruhigenden Farben verbreitet das Spa eine wohltuende Wirkung.

Thanks to its design of fluid shapes and relaxing colors, the spa at the New York Palace Hotel is a therapy in itself.

Le design aux formes fluides et aux couleurs relaxantes du spa du New York Palace Hotel constitue déjà en soi une forme de thérapie.

De vloeibare vormen en ontspannende kleuren van het ontwerp maken de New Hork Palace Hotel Spa al een therapie op zich.

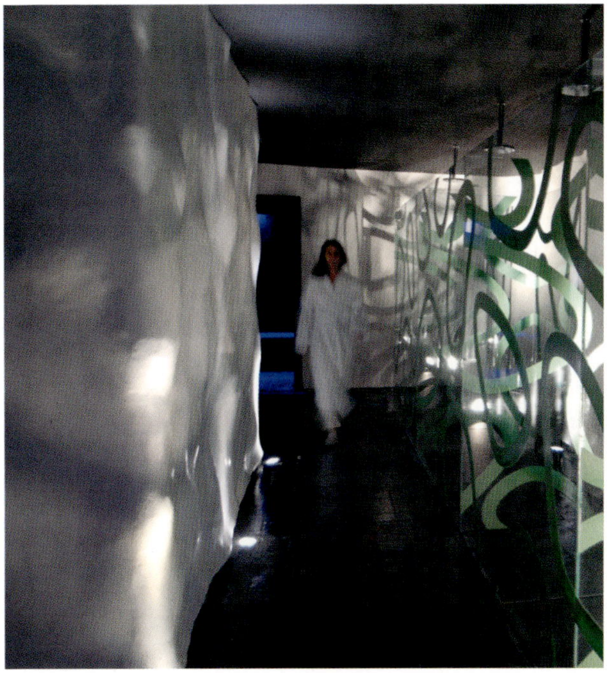

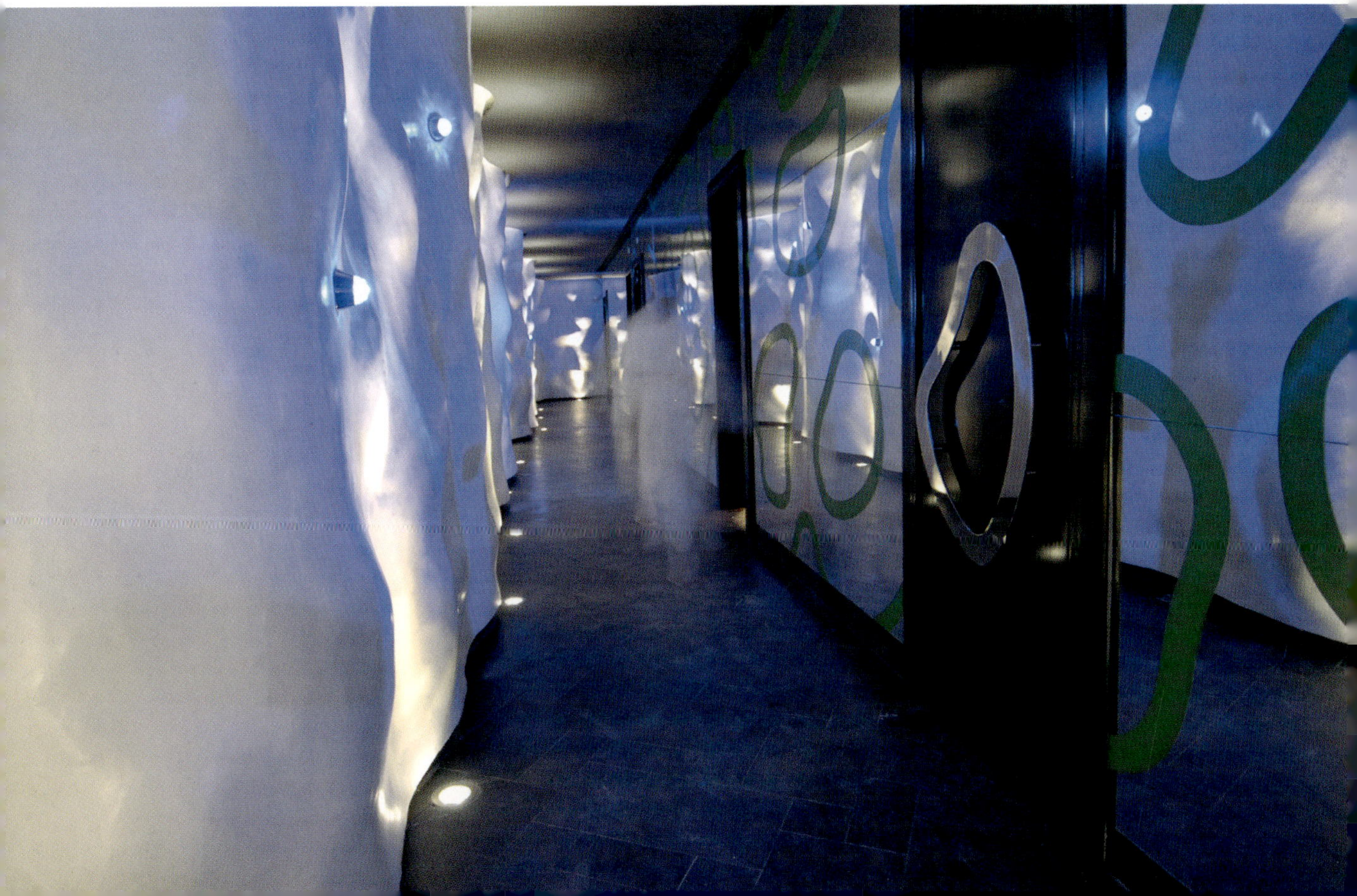

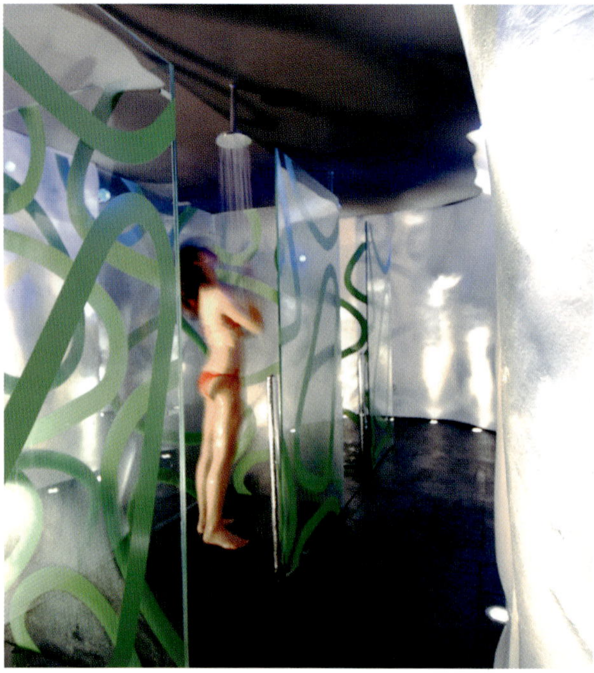

Die Hydromassageduschen sind durch transparente Wände mit fluoreszierenden Motiven separiert.

The showers with hydro-massage to release shoulder tension are divided by transparent walls with fluorescent imprints.

Les douches à hydro-massage, idéales pour chasser la tension au niveau des épaules, sont séparées par des murs transparents à empreintes fluorescentes.

De hydromassagedouches zijn afgescheiden door middel van transparante muren met fluorescerende sjablonen.

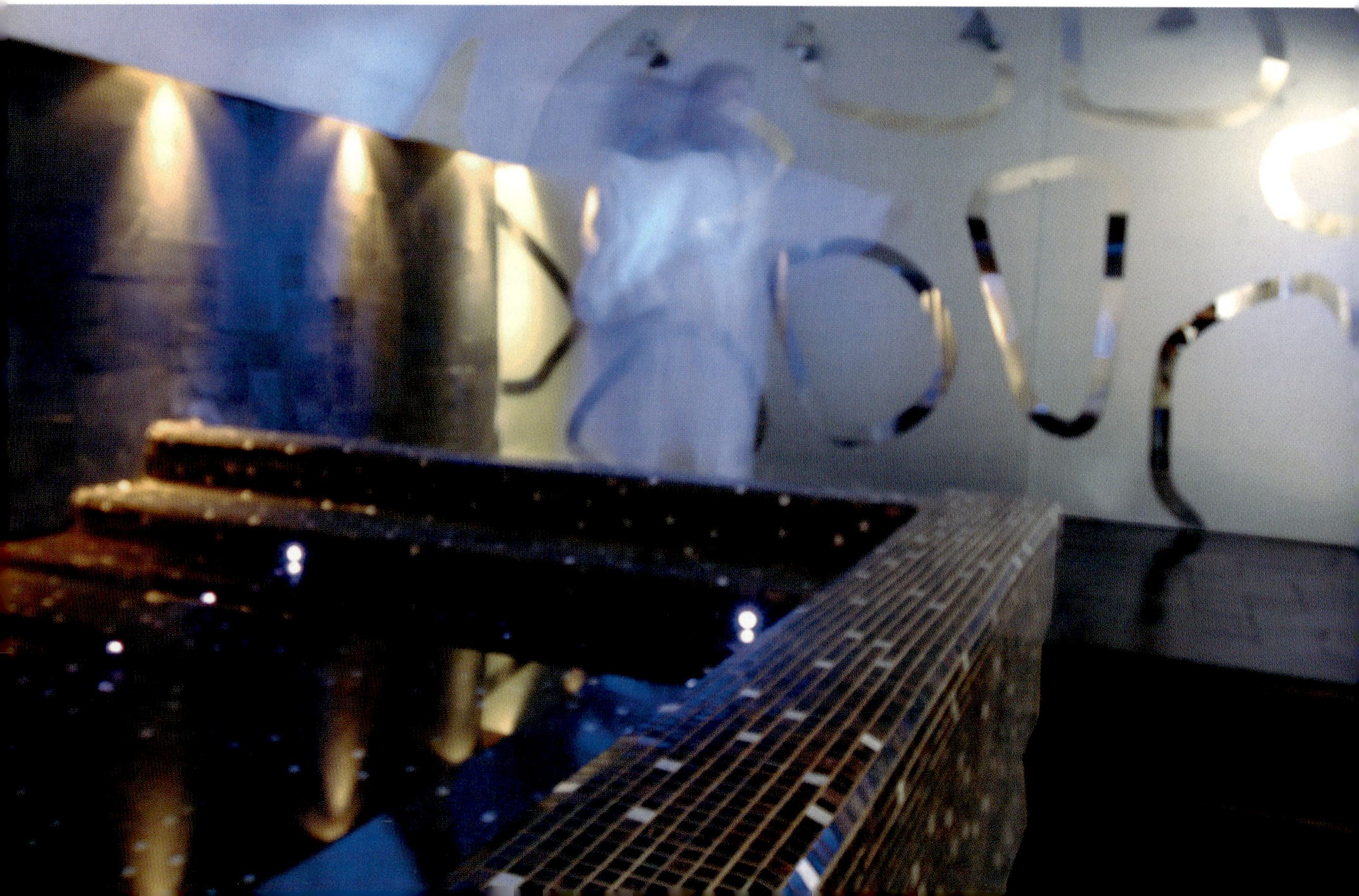

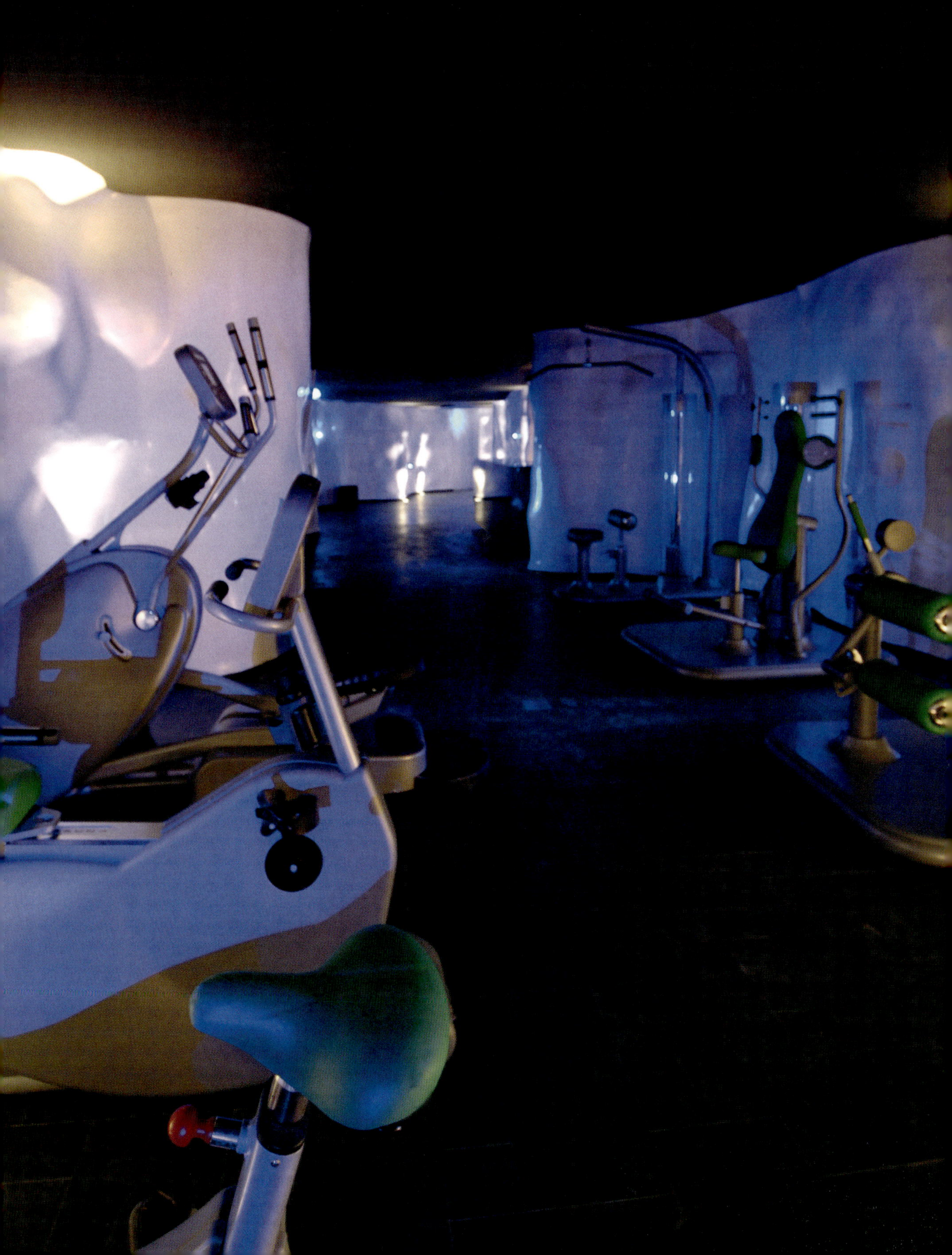

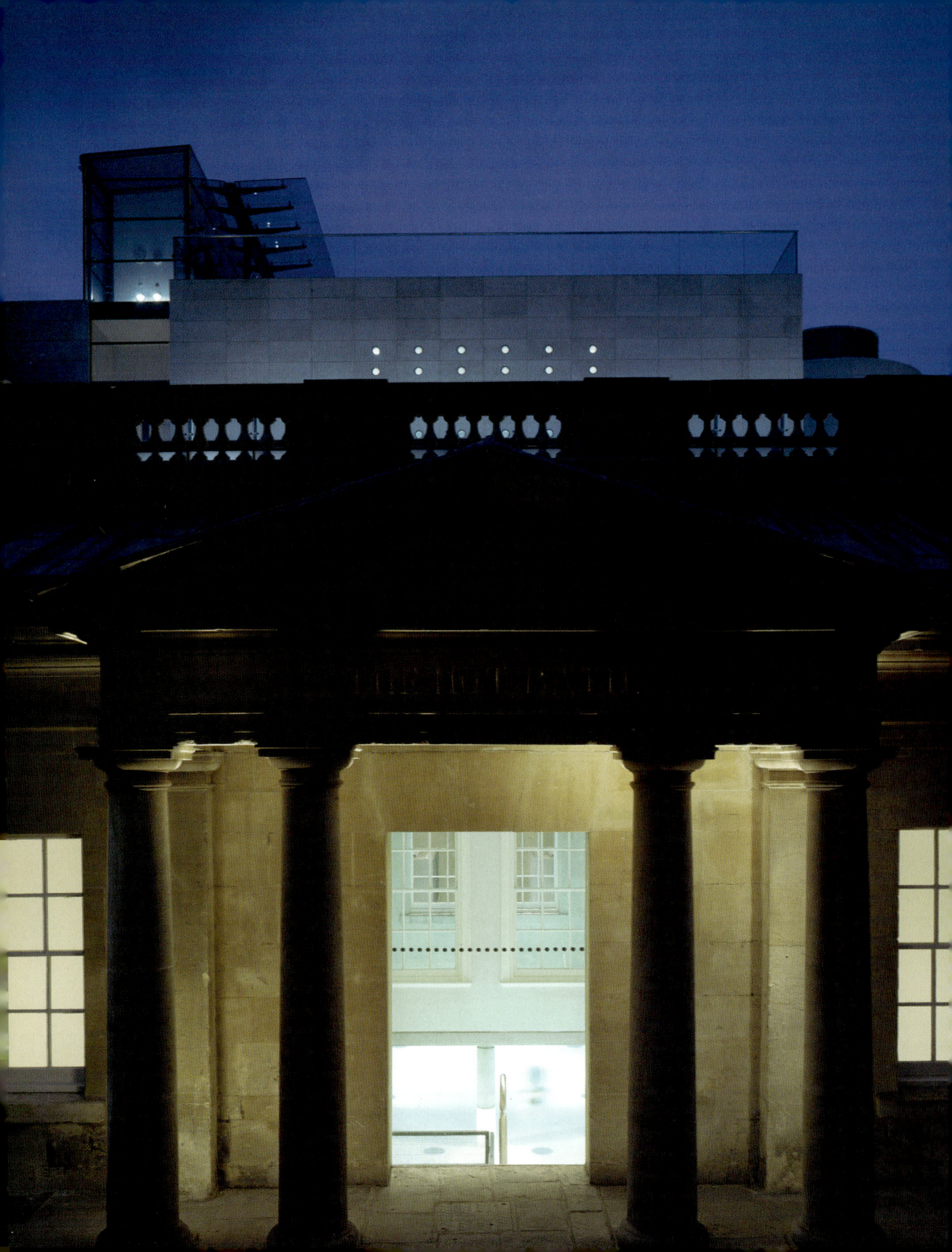

Thermae Bath Spa

Nach jahrelanger aufwändiger Renovierung öffnete die einzige Mineraltherme Großbritanniens im Jahr 2006 erneut ihre Pforten. Die fünf bestehenden Gebäude wurden komplett umgestaltet und durch einen Neubau bereichert. Das New Royal Bath lockt mit zwei Schwimmbecken: einem Hallenbad mit Whirlpool und einem Dachpool mit herrlicher Aussicht. Moderne Glaselemente bilden einen reizvollen architektonischen Kontrast zu jahrhundertetaltem Stein, Granit und Holz.

After having remained closed for 28 years, Thermae Bath reopened in 2006, totally renovated. Architects reformed five existing buildings and built a completely new one. The New Royal Bath holds two pools, one inside that features a whirlpool and another one, on the roof, that has breathtaking views. The result is an interplay of architectural contrasts: the semi transparencies of modern glass stand out over the stone, granite and wood, which have remained there for centuries.

Après être resté fermé pendant vingt-huit ans, le spa Thermae Bath, totalement rénové, a réouvert en 2006. Les architectes ont reconverti les cinq bâtiments existants, et ajouté une extension. Le New Royal Bath compte deux piscines : une couverte, à remous ; une autre, sur le toit, qui offre une vue à couper le souffle. Le résultat donne à voir un jeu de contrastes architecturaux où les vitres semi-opaques se détachent de la pierre, du granit et du bois, plusieurs fois centenaires.

Na 28 jaar gesloten te zijn geweest, ging Thermae Bath in 2006 weer open, compleet gerenoveerd. De vijf bestaande gebouwen werden omgewerkt door architecten en er werd een heel nieuw gebouw bij gebouwd. New Royal Bath heeft twee zwembaden, een binnenbad met een whirlpool en een buitenbad op het dak met adembenemend uitzicht. Het resultaat is een samenspel van architectonische contrasten, van de transparantie van modern glas tegenover eeuwenoude steen, graniet en hout.

Bath, United Kingdom

GRIMSHAW ARCHITECTS

Photos © Matt Cardy, Nick Smith, Edmund Sumner

www.thermaebathspa.com

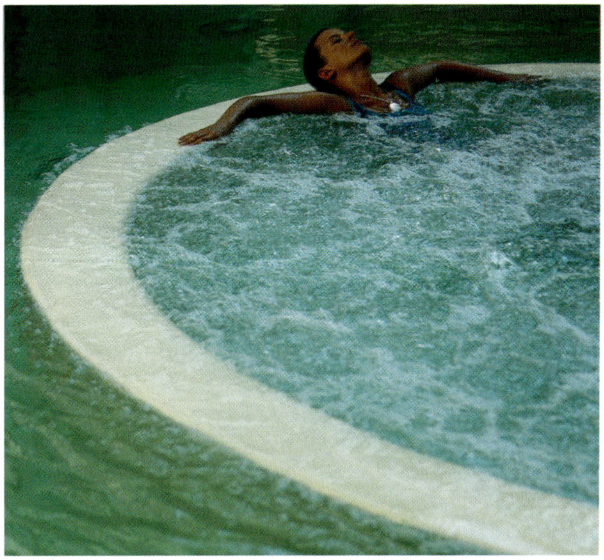

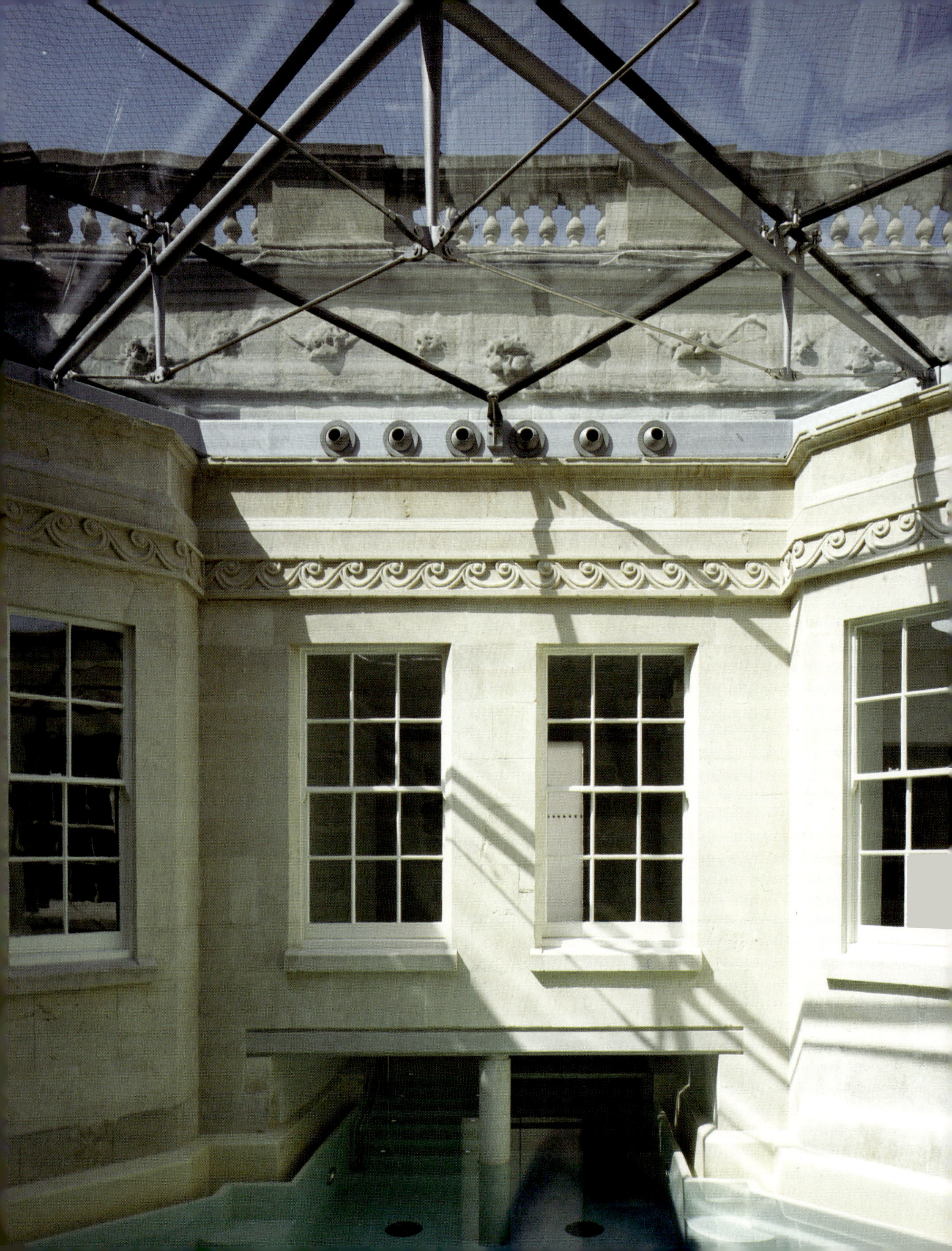

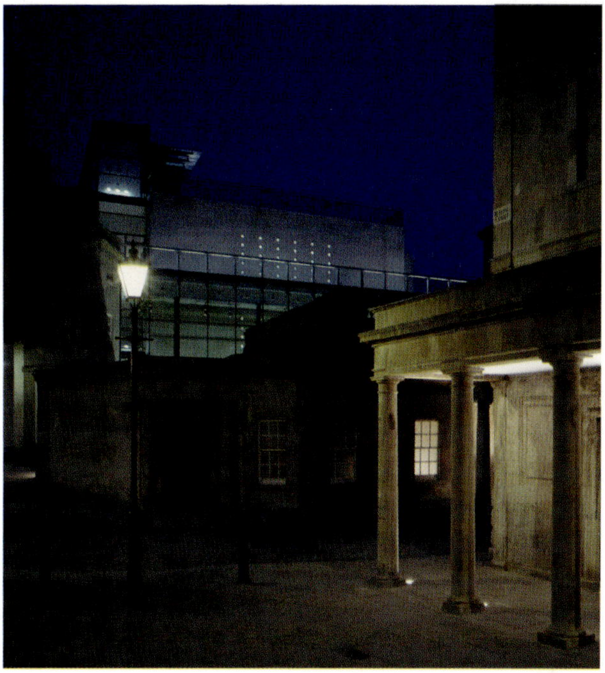

Der Pool auf dem Dach bietet einen herrlichen Blick auf die malerische Innenstadt von Bath.

From the pool located on the rooftop one can enjoy breathtaking views of the beautiful city of Bath.

La piscine, située sur le toit, offre une vue à couper le souffle sur la charmante ville de Bath.

Vanaf het zwembad op het dak heb je een adembenemend uitzicht over de mooie stad Bath.

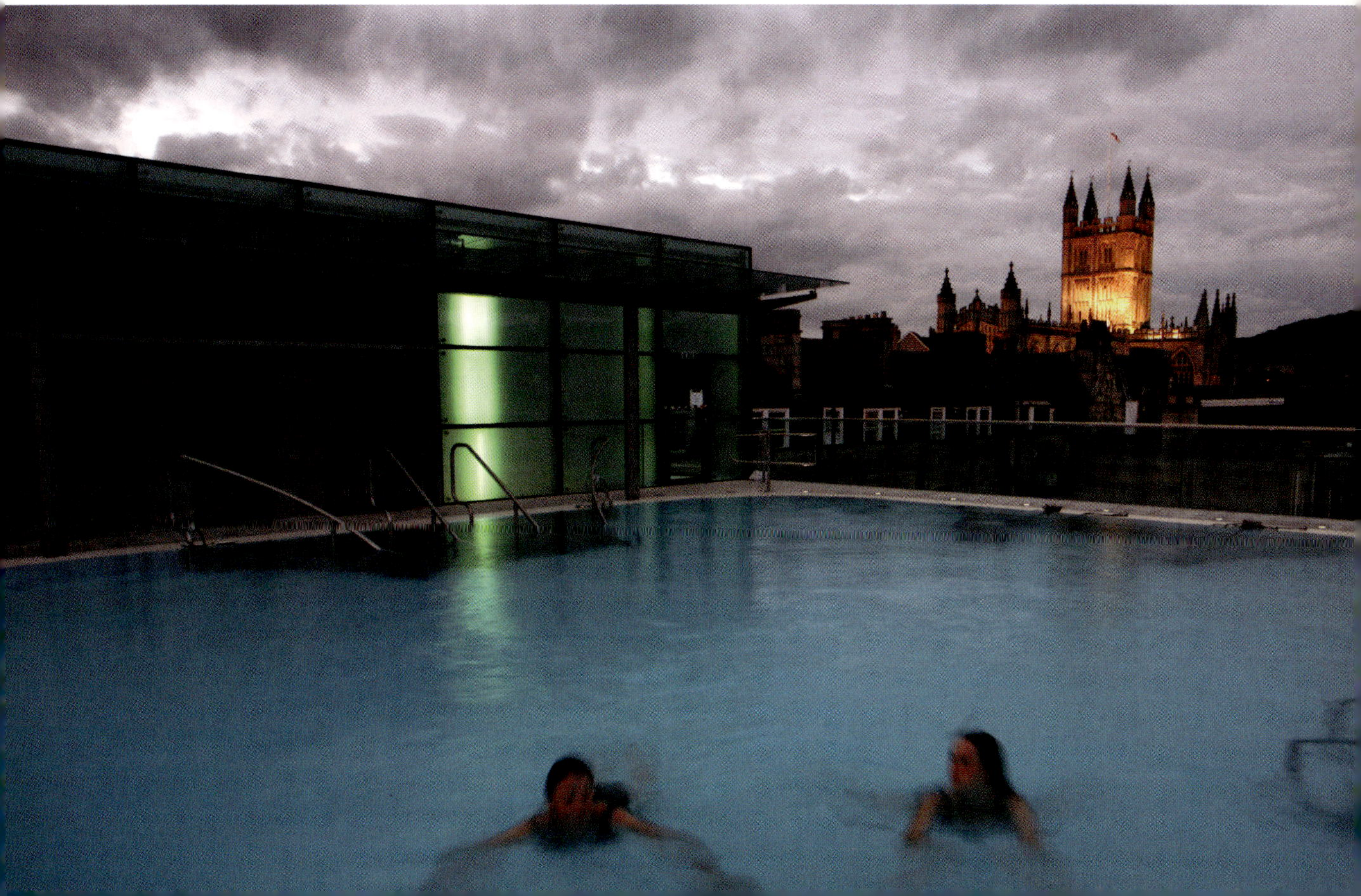

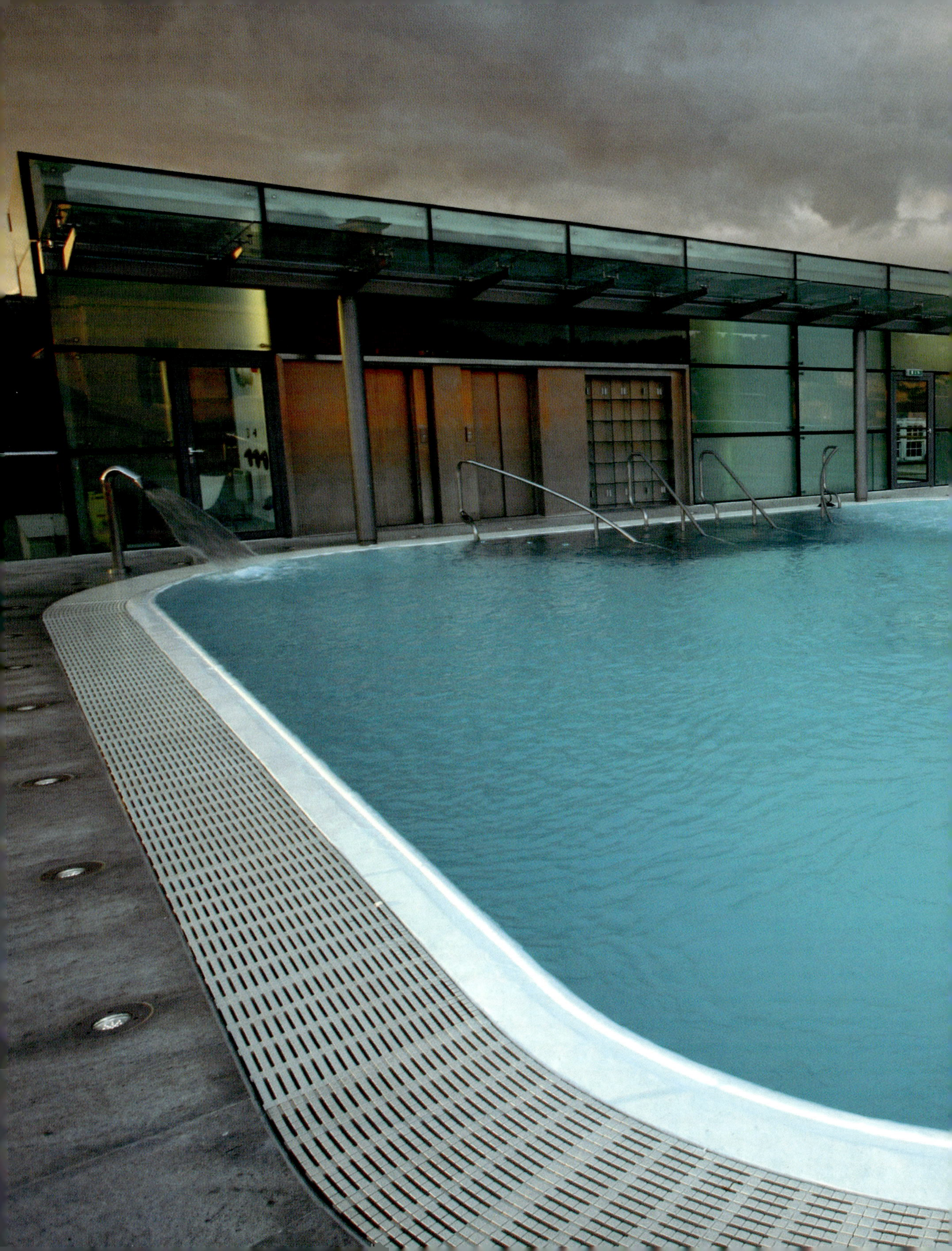

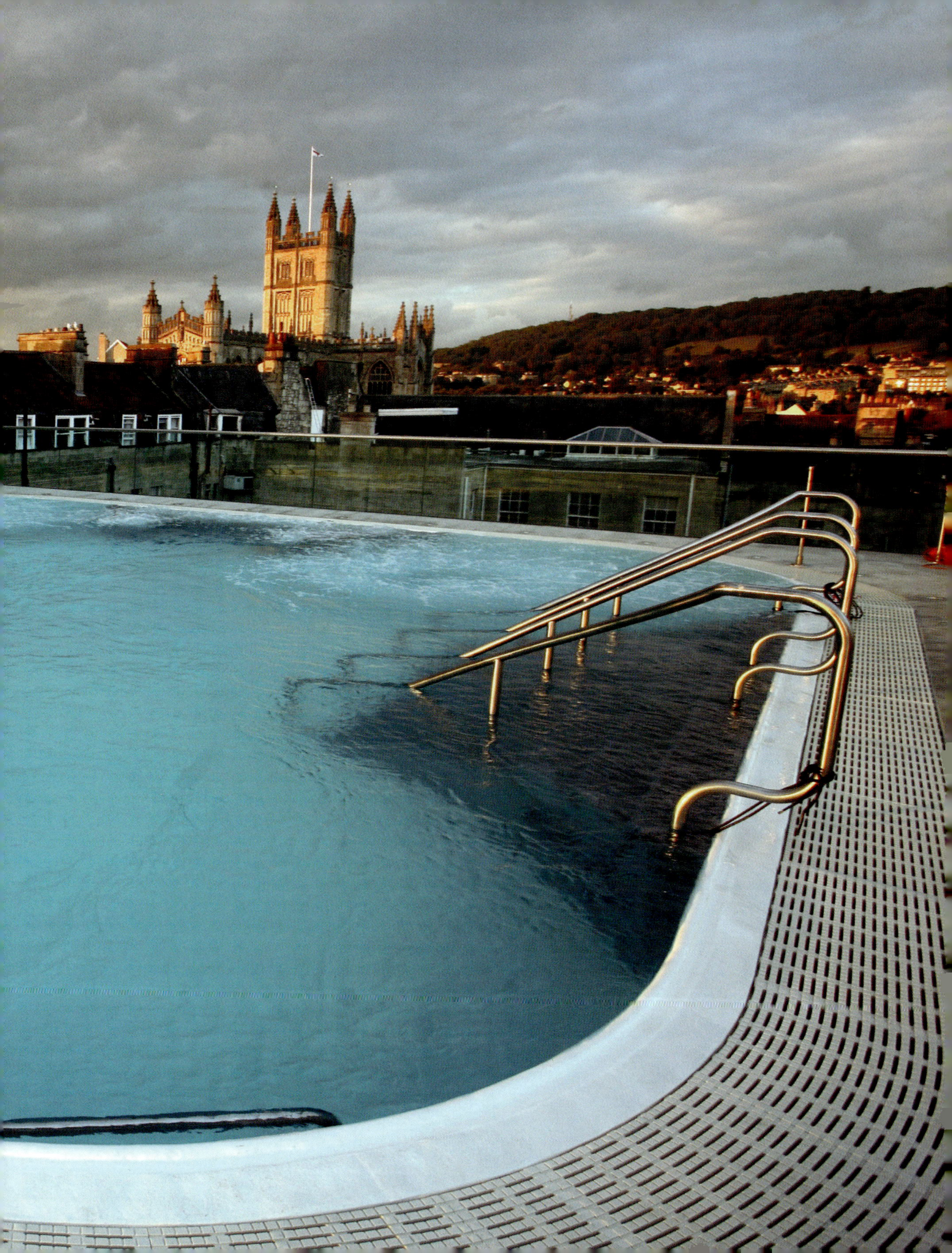

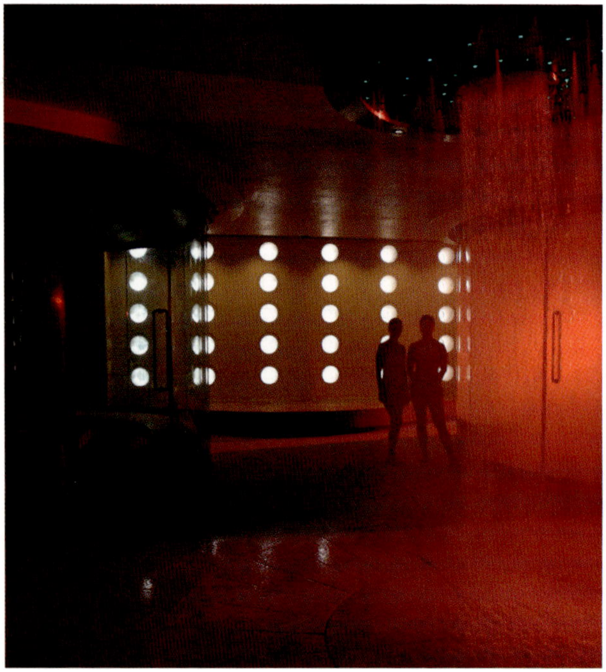

Das Wasser dieser heißen Quellen soll vor 10.000 Jahren durch Regenfälle entstanden sein.

It is believed that the water from these hot springs fell as rain 10,000 years ago.

L'eau de ces sources chaudes semble provenir des cieux, comme une pluie millénaire.

Er wordt aangenomen dat het water uit deze warmwaterbronnen 10.000 jaar geleden is neergevallen als regen.

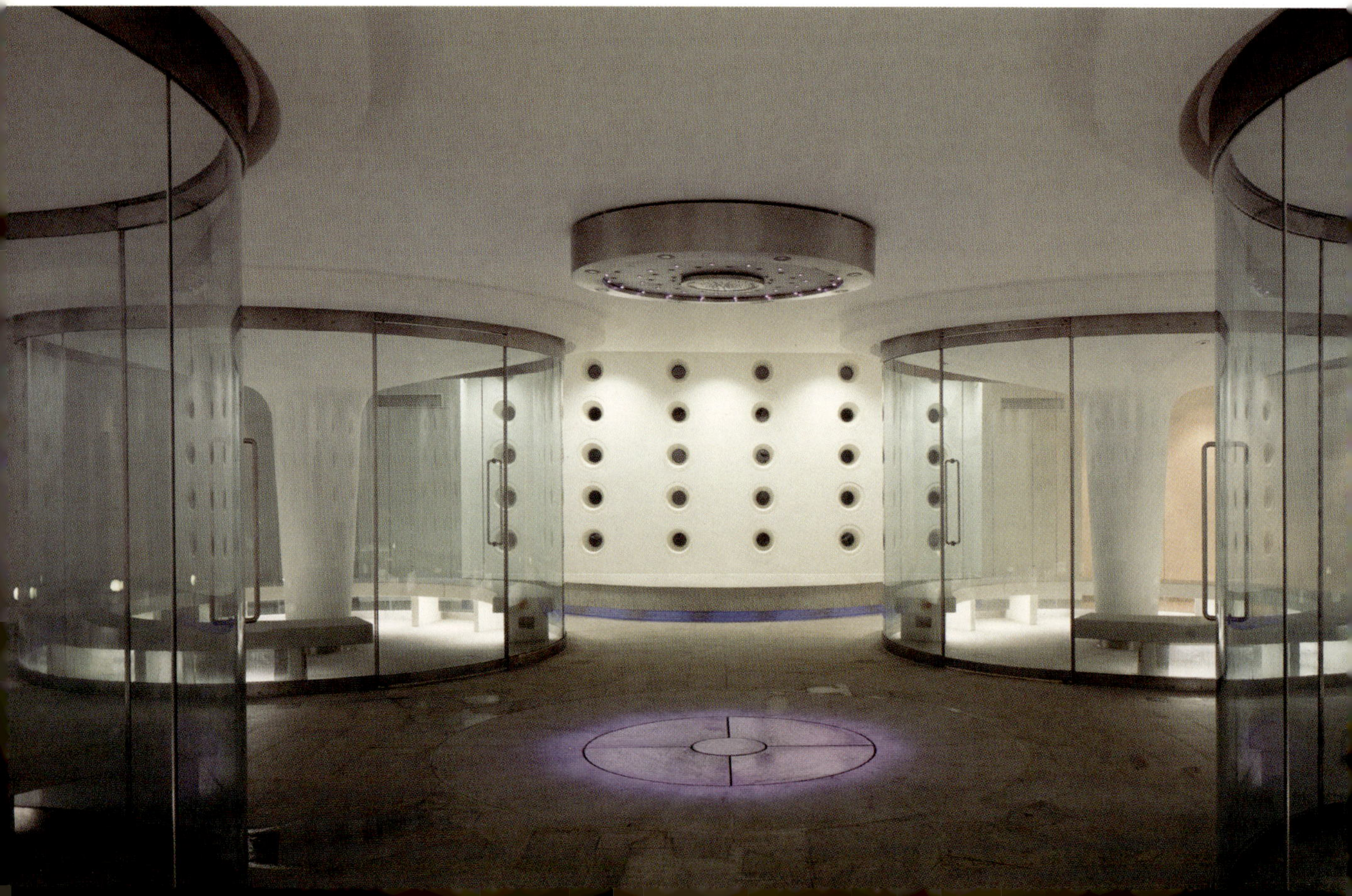

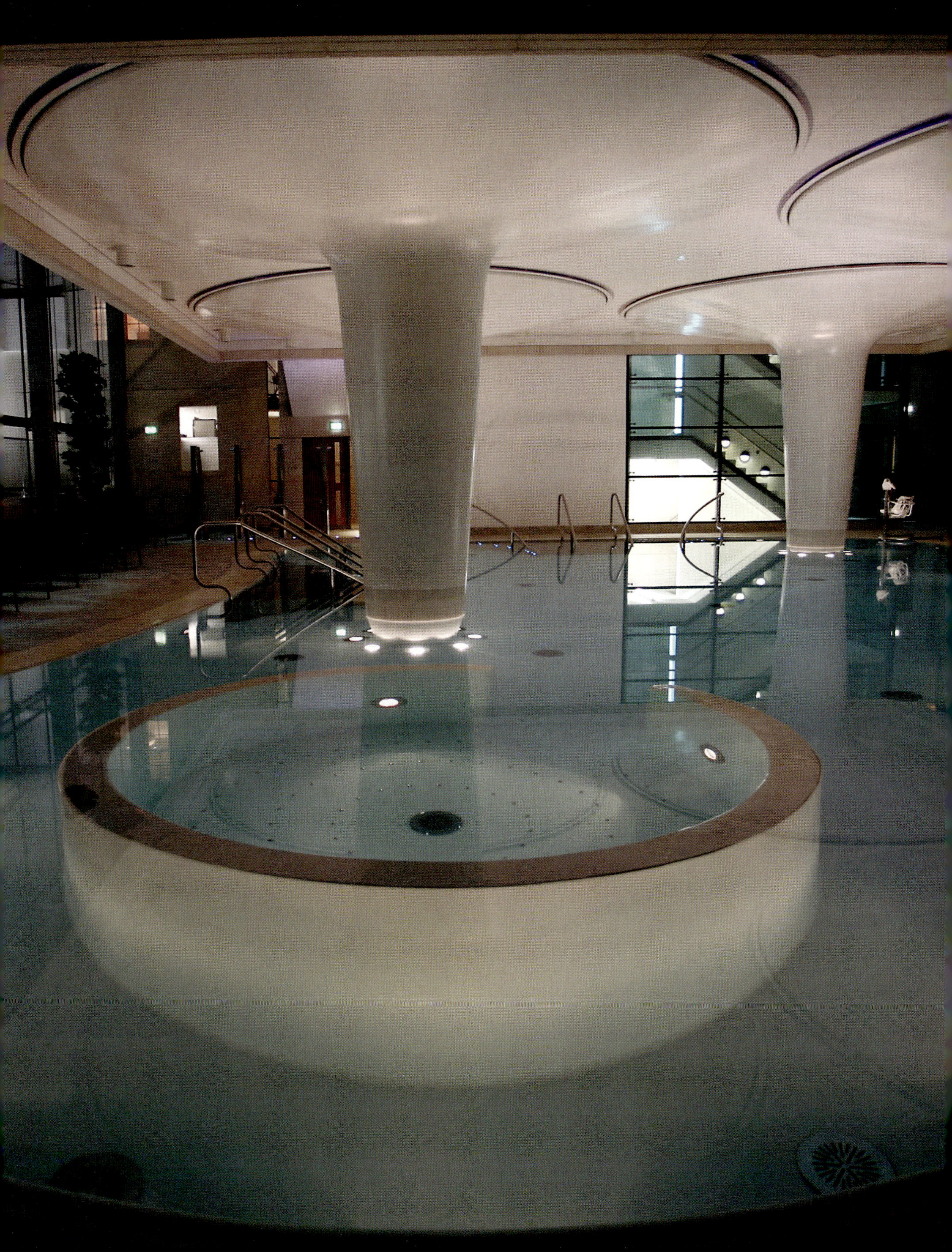

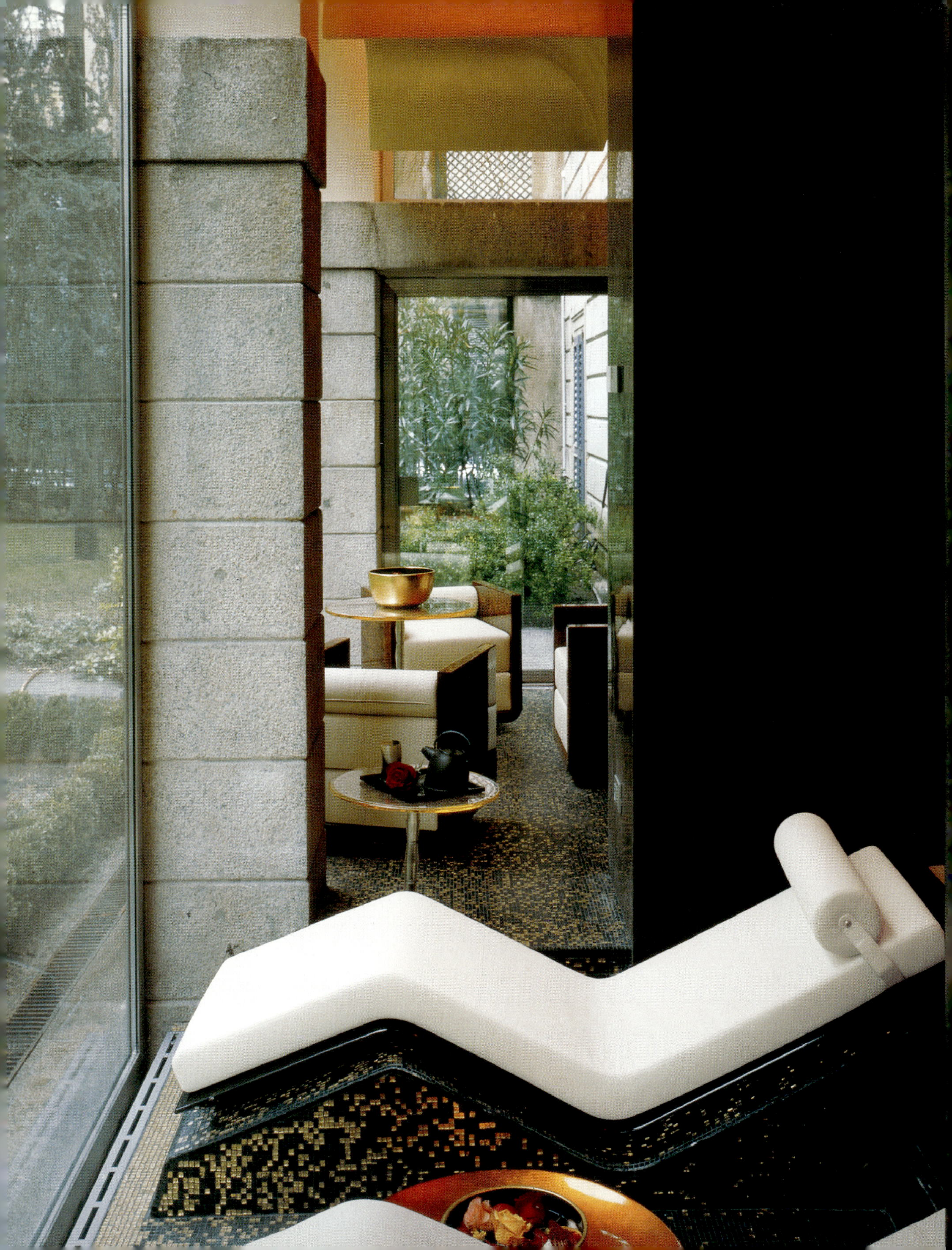

ESPA by Gianfranco Ferré

Die Ästhetik dieses Spas im hinteren Bereich der Mailänder Gianfranco Ferré Boutique trägt die unverwechselbare Handschrift des Modeschöpfers: Luxus mit klaren Linien. Zwischen Wänden aus poliertem Zement und hellem Holz tritt immer wieder das ursprüngliche Gestein hervor. Die Treatments umfassen traditionelle Methoden verschiedener Kulturen in modernem Gewand. Jeden der sechs Gäste, die gleichzeitig Zutritt erhalten, erwartet ein exklusives maßgeschneidertes Programm.

The spa, located in the back of the shop at Via Sant'Andrea, has aesthetics that continue with the characteristic identity of Ferré: luxury and sobriety. The walls are covered in polished cement and bright wood and they alternate with the original stone of the location. The treatments are a fusion between techniques from ancient cultures and philosophies from the whole world. This spa, that admits only six people at a time, offers exclusive treatments for each customer.

Situé derrière la boutique de la Via Sant'Andrea, le spa possède une esthétique en parfaite harmonie avec le style caractéristique de Ferré, qui allie luxe et sobriété. Les murs offrent une alternance de ciment ciré et de bois brillant qui contrastent avec la pierre d'origine du lieu. Les soins sont la parfaite fusion entre des techniques à la fois ancestrales et internationales. Ce spa, qui ne peut recevoir que six personnes à la fois, propose des soins exclusifs pour chaque client.

Deze kuurinrichting achter in de winkel aan de Via Sant' Andrea heeft een stijl die perfect samengaat met de sobere luxe van zijn opzet. De muren zijn uitgevoerd in gepolijst cement en licht hout, afgewisseld met de originele steen van het gebouw. De behandelingen behelzen een fusie van technieken uit oude culturen en filosofieën van over de hele wereld. Deze spa, waar maar zes mensen tegelijk in mogen, biedt exclusieve behandelingen voor iedere gast.

Milan, Italy

ESPA

Photos © Paola Di Pietri, Bisazza

www.gianfrancoferre.com

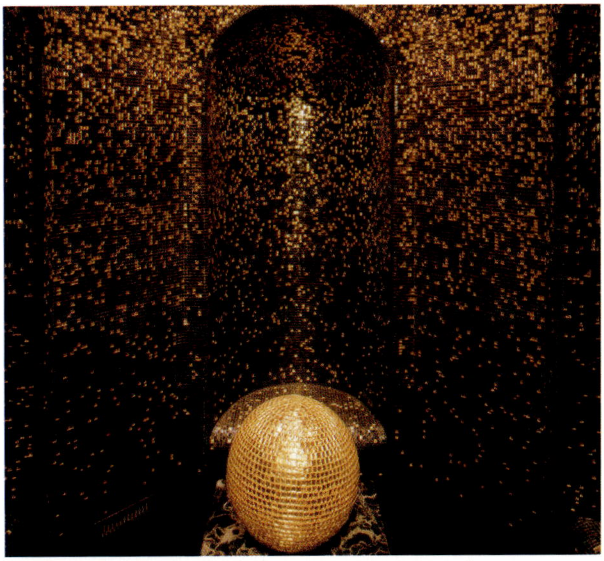

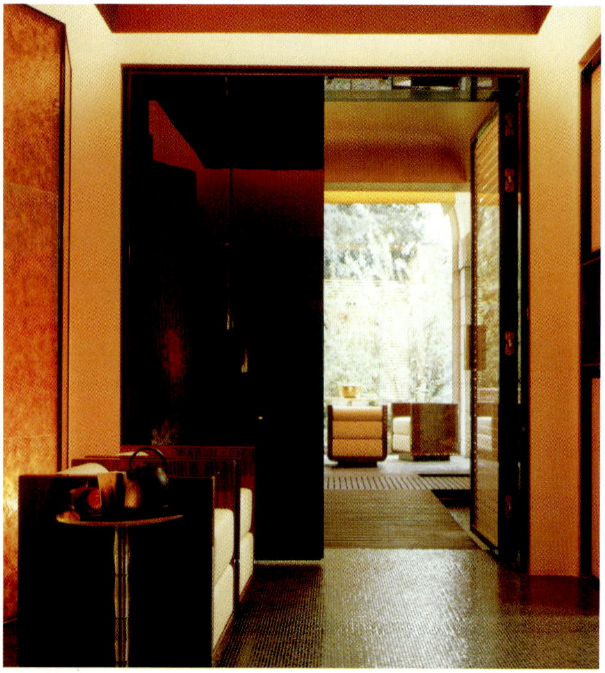

Möbel aus beigefarbenem Leder und Walnussholz prägen den Entspannungsraum mit Blick auf den Innengarten.

The beige leather and walnut wood furniture characterize the relaxation room which has views over the inner garden.

Le cuir beige et les meubles en noyer caractérisent le salon de relaxation, qui offre une vue sur le jardin intérieur.

Het walnotenhouten meubilair met beige leer zet de toon in de rustruimte met uitzicht op de binnentuin.

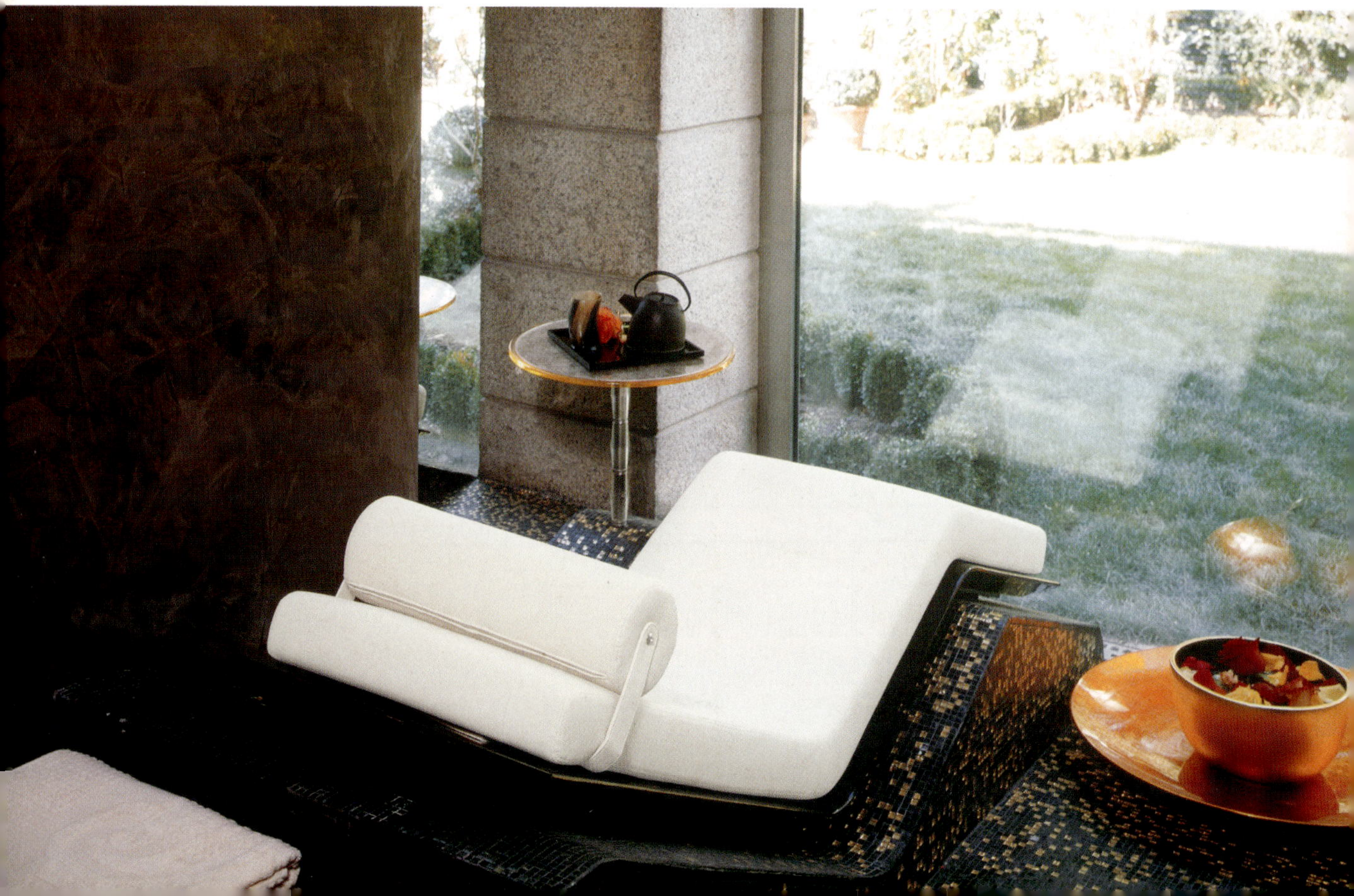

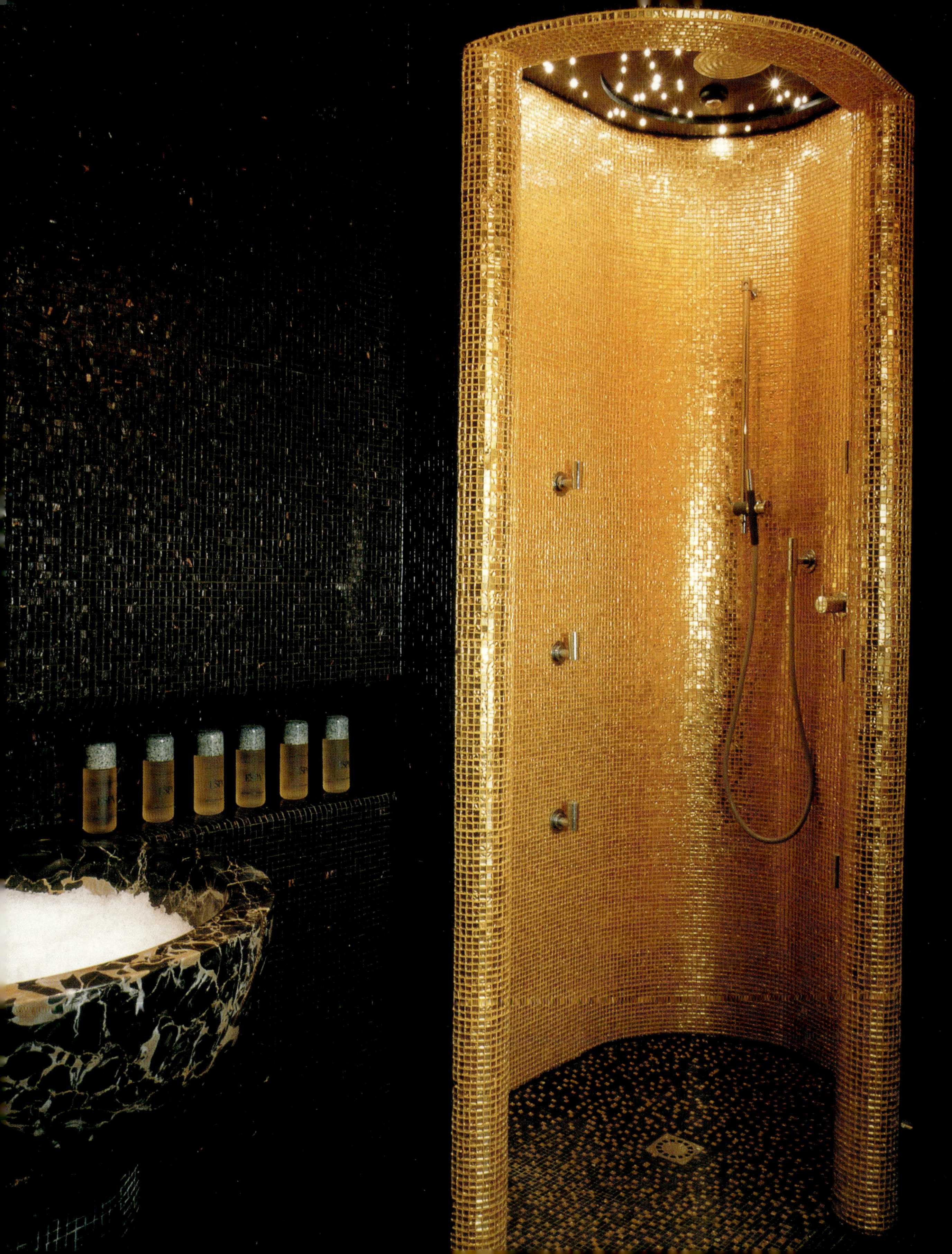

Directory of Architects and Designers

Alonso Balaguer y Arquitectos Asociados
Bac de Roda, 40
Barcelona 08019, Spain
T +34 93 303 41 60
estudi@alonsobalaguer.com
www.alonsobalaguer.com

Archisphere Architects and Designers
Neubaugasse, 44/2/13
Vienna 1070, Austria
T +43 1573 327 10
office@archisphere.at
www.archisphere.at

Atelier Mendini
Via Sannio, 24
Milan 20137, Italy
T +39 02 5518 5185
mendini@ateliermendini.it
www.ateliermendini.it

Colombo & Associates SRL
Viale Biancamaria, 13
Milan 20122, Italy
T +39 02 780 414
paolo.colombo@colombo-online.com
www.colombo-online.com

Corporate Edge
149 Hammersmith Road
London W14 0QL, United Kingdom
T +44 20 7855 5888
www.corporateedge.com

Daniel Jouvance
41 rue Camilla Desmoulins
3 allée de Grenelle
Issy-les-Moulineaux Cedex 92444, France
T +33 1410 85 500
www.danieljouvance.com

De Matos Storey Ryan Ltd
99-100 Turnmill Street
London EC1M 5QP, United Kingdom
T +44 20 7336 0100
mail@dmsr.co.uk
www.dmsr.co.uk

Dietrich Untertrifaller Architekten
Flachgasse 35-37
Vienna A-1150, Austria
T +43 5574 78888-0
arch@dietrich.untertrifaller.com
www.dietrich.untertrifaller.com

Douglas Wallace Architects
St Kevins Female School
1 Grantham Street
Dublin 8, Ireland
T +353 1 478 7500
dublindesign@douglaswallace.com
www.douglaswallace.com

Fadesa
Av. Alfonso Molina, s/n
Edificio Fadesa
A Coruña 15008, Spain
T +34 98 117 92 00
www.fadesa.es

Fletcher Priest Böesl Architekten
United Kingdom:
Middlesex House
34/42 Cleveland Street
London W1T 4JE, United Kingdom
T +44 20 7034 2200
enquiries@fletcherpriest.com
Germany:
Marsiliusstrasse 20
Cologne 50937, Germany
T +49 221 941 050
enquiries@fpb-europe.com
www.fletcherpriest.com

Frank Gehry & Partners
12541 Beatrice Street
Los Angeles, CA 90066, USA
T +1 310 482 3000
info@foga.com
www.foga.com

GCA Arquitectes Associats
Valencia 289
Barcelona 08009, Spain
T +34 93 476 18 00
info@gcaarq.com
www.gcaarq.com

Grimshaw Architects
57 Clerkenwell Road
London EC1M 5NG, United Kingdom
T +44 20 7291 4141
info@grimshaw-architects.com
www.grimshaw-architects.com

Halter Architekten AG
Rathausstrasse 2
Postfach 1439
Rapperswil SG 8640, Switzerland
T +41 055 220 62 62
www.halter-architekten.ch

Jestico & Whiles
1 Cobourg Street
London NW1 2HP, United Kingdom
T +44 207 380 0382
jk@jesticowhiles.com
www.jesticowhiles.co.uk

Les Cinq Mondes
51, rue de la Chaussée d'Antin
75009 Paris, France
T +33 1 42 66 00 60
www.cinqmondes.com

Mario Botta
Via Ciani 16
Lugano CH-6904, Switzerland
T +41 91 972 86 25
info@botta.ch
www.botta.ch

Martin Kohlbauer ZT
Nestroyplatz 1/27
Vienna 1020, Austria
T +43 1 218 55 88
www.martinkohlbauer.com

Matteo Thun
Via Appiani 9, I
Milan 20121, Italy
T +39 02 655691
info@matteothun.com
www.matteothun.com

Michele Sweeney/Oppermann Associates
Unit D1, The Millhouse, The Steelworks
Foley Street
Dublin 1, Ireland
T +353 1 889 9800
architecture@oppermann.ie
www.oppermann.ie

Mireia Vila Merino
Rubí 16, 3º 3ª
Palma de Mallorca 07002, Spain
T +34 97 171 80 84
mireia@mireiavila.com
www.mireiavila.com

Niki Szilagyi
Viktualienmarkt 8
Kustermannhaus, 6 floor
Munich D-80331, Germany
T +49 89 26949280
info@niki-szilagyi.de
www.niki-szilagyi.de

Arkkitehtitoimisto Nurmela, Raimoranta, Tasa Oy
Kalevankatu 31
Helsinki 00100, Finland
T +358 9 6866 780
ark.tsto@n-r-t.fi
www.n-r-t.fi

Pagani & Di Mauro Architetti
Via Emilia, 14
Ponte Enza - Reggio Emilia, Italy
T +39 0522 902145
studio@paganidimauro.com
www.paganidimauro.com

Patrice Reynaud
Route de Frontenex 78
Genève 1208, Switzerland
T +41 22 786 90 40
bureau@reynaud.ch
www.reynaud.ch

Plajer & Franz Studio
Erkelenzdamm 59/61
Berlin 10999, Germany
T +49 30 616 55 80
studio@plajer-franz.de
www.plajer-franz.de

Richter & Dahl Rocha Architects
Avenue Dapples 54
Lausanne CH-1001, Switzerland
T +41 021 612 01 01
architectes@rdr.ch
www.rdr.ch

Sandra Tarruella & Isabel López
Putget 6, local 8
Barcelona 08006, Spain
T/F +34 93 253 11 69
isabel@tarruellalopez.com
sandra@tarruellalopez.com
www.tarruellalopez.com

Schletterer Wellness & Spa Design GmbH
Bundesstrasse 190
Strass 6261, Austria
T +43 5244 62005
office@schletterer.com
www.schletterer.com

Schnögass & Partner Ziviltechniker
Hietzinger Hauptstraße 122b
Vienna 1130, Austria
T +43 1 877 77 78
office@splusn.at
www.splusn.at

Simone Micheli
Via Aretina 197r/199r/201r
Florence 50136, Italy
T +39 05569 12 16
simone@simonemicheli.com
www.simonemicheli.com

Studio Tecnico di Architettura Lorenzo Bellini Associates di L. Bellini
Via Umberto Moricca, 90
Rome 00167, Italy
info@lorenzobellini.com
www.lorenzobellini.com

The Syntax Group
The Old Boathouse
Mill Lane, Taplow
Maidenhead, Berkshire SL6 0AA
United Kingdom
T +44 1628 789646
info@syntaxuk.com
www.syntaxuk.com

Tihany Design
New York:
135 West 27th Street, 9th Floor
New York, NY 10001, USA
T +1 212 366 5544
Rome:
Via di Villa Emiliani, 21, int. 3
Rome 00197, Italy
T +39 06 4542 3490
mail@tihanydesign.com
www.tihanydesign.com

VA Arkitektar
Skólavör_ustígur 12,
Reykjavík 101, Iceland
T +354 530 6990
vaarkitektar@vaarkitektar.is
www.vaarkitektar.is